T0134595

METHODS IN PHARMACOLOGY AND TOXICOLOGY

Series Editor
Y. James Kang
Department of Pharmacology & Toxicology
University of Louisville
Louisville, Kentucky, USA

For further volumes:
http://www.springer.com/series/7653

Drug-Induced Liver Toxicity

Edited by

Minjun Chen

Division of Bioinformatics and Biostatistics, National Center for Toxicological Research,
U.S. Food and Drug Administration, Jefferson, AR, USA

Yvonne Will

Drug Safety Research and Development, Pfizer Inc., Groton, CT, USA

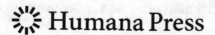

Editors
Minjun Chen
Division of Bioinformatics and Biostatistics
National Center for Toxicological Research
U.S. Food and Drug Administration
Jefferson, AR, USA

Yvonne Will
Drug Safety Research and Development
Pfizer Inc.
Groton, CT, USA

ISSN 1557-2153   ISSN 1940-6053   (electronic)
Methods in Pharmacology and Toxicology
ISBN 978-1-4939-9256-0   ISBN 978-1-4939-7677-5   (eBook)
https://doi.org/10.1007/978-1-4939-7677-5

Printed on acid-free paper

This Humana Press imprint is published by the registered company Springer Science+Business Media, LLC part
of Springer Nature.
The registered company address is: 233 Spring Street, New York, NY 10013, U.S.A.

Foreword

I am honored to have been asked to help introduce this unique monograph on a subject that has inspired and piqued my clinical and research interest for more than 35 years. Having been mentored in drug-induced liver injury (DILI) by the late Hyman J Zimmerman for more than 20 years, I know he would appreciate how far the field has come in expanding the mechanisms of hepatotoxicity and the clinical signatures of old and new agents causing liver injury, and would welcome the new regulatory approaches and perspectives of drug developers that he helped to define before his passing in 1999. While DILI is still infrequently encountered in clinical practice, its impact on the drug development process and regulatory actions taken for adverse hepatic effects remains significant. Despite advances in the ability to define the various forms of hepatotoxicity from hundreds of drugs, weight loss and dietary supplements, and herbal products, the diagnosis of DILI continues to remain one of exclusion. No specific liver enzyme pattern or histological finding is considered pathognomonic, as DILI can mimic all forms of acute and chronic liver diseases. As a result, the diagnosis has come to depend on a constellation of clinically, genetically, and pharmacologically based elements for which no other cause seems more likely.

Efforts devoted to assigning causality to specific agents suspected to have led to liver injury have grown considerably over the past 25 years since pioneers in drug hepatotoxicity established the Roussel-Uclaf Causality Assessment Method (RUCAM), and whose diagnostic elements remain the basis upon which most assessments are determined. In the past 10–15 years, numerous global drug registries have been chronicling the clinical and biochemical signatures, outcomes, and prognosis of DILI, and several international consortia have been convened to help determine potential DILI mechanisms and identify diagnostic biomarkers. However, without a specific, confirmatory, validated tool to diagnose DILI, much of our causality assessment process remains circumstantial and dependent on expert opinion. Even RUCAM, which was developed by expert consensus opinion, remains imperfect as a methodology. The US DILI Network method that incorporates an expert opinion process into the RUCAM elements is considered by many to be the most rigorous causality method, but can be time consuming, and may still lack complete agreement among its knowledgeable assessors. Similarly, attempts to identify a "one size fits all" biomarker to diagnose the innumerable faces of DILI remain incomplete. Moreover, since there are no specific antidotes to treat acute idiopathic DILI from non-acetaminophen-based drugs, discontinuation of the suspected agent is generally required. Having to withdraw a drug that turns out not to be the actual cause of the injury results in several adverse outcomes, including depriving a patient of a useful treatment for which no good alternatives might exist, adding erroneous safety information to a drug's profile, and leading to costly regulatory and even medical-legal consequences.

The risks and expenses associated with bringing a new chemical entity to market can be extremely high, especially since hepatotoxicity is one of the two most common preclinical toxicities identified and has been responsible for prematurely ending the further development of various agents. Although the FDA has not approved any drug since the late 1990s that has been withdrawn specifically for hepatotoxicity, some agents approved elsewhere have been shown to be the cause of severe liver injury and numerous compounds have been abandoned in early phase development in the past two decades due to the risk of DILI. As a result, DILI stakeholders from all corners of the development globe are turning to various forms of in silico or in vitro modeling and pharmacoinformatics to help identify which new chemical entities have a propensity to cause liver injury prior to their expensive entry into later phase studies.

To help educate drug developers, toxicologists, biochemists, clinicians, and regulators alike on the diverse aspects and processes involved with identifying DILI, Drs. Minjun Chen from the FDA's National Center for Toxicological Research and Yvonne Will from Pfizer Inc. have brought together the leading scientific and clinical experts in the field of drug-induced hepatotoxicity to create a timely handbook where all of the latest preclinical and clinical disciplines converge. Seminal textbooks authored by the late Hyman Zimmerman and newer compendiums and websites on DILI (such as LiverTox) have provided much of the clinical information that often aids in identifying the clinical signatures of DILI, and in understanding its mechanisms of injury, but this current effort emphasizes the newly discovered pharmacologic as well as the most up-to-date clinical and genetic risk factors associated with DILI while the search for a diagnostic DILI biomarker continues. Erudite discussions on the latest mechanisms of DILI, modeling of hepatotoxins, and the structural alerts that are currently employed to help predict and/or prevent potentially hepatotoxic compounds from entering further clinical development are among the 30 authoritative chapters that cover nearly the entire field of hepatotoxicity. The readership of this volume will benefit from the in-depth reviews on the recent observations derived from the emerging fields of pharmacogenetics, pharmacoinformatics, proteomics, transcriptomics, among others applied specifically to DILI, along with discussions on several clinical and preclinical in vitro and in vivo aspects of liver injury that enhance our understanding of hepatotoxicity. Chapters devoted to the regulatory science of evaluation and approval of new drugs and challenges that remain in drug discovery and post-marketing surveillance specifically related to DILI provide the information that is most helpful to ensure drug safety. In particular, the chapter by John Senior and Ted Guo of the FDA is one of the most useful summaries on the history of DILI dating back to the 1950s—providing the necessary clinical and regulatory context for many of the current efforts in the field of hepatotoxicity.

Specific topics that readers will find most helpful include the latest reviews of the physico-chemical properties of drugs that form the basis for structural alerts regarding hepatotoxicity. The usefulness of combining the dose of a drug, the degree of its hepatic metabolism, lipophilicity, and formation of reactive metabolites into the novel "Rule of Two" and other predictors has offered significant insight into these pharmacologic risk factors. At the preclinical level, the use of various hepatocyte cell lines, the ability to simulate populations at risk of hepatotoxicity using DILI-sym™, and other novel technologies are proving to be quite useful in identifying agents that may be hepatotoxic well before the need to expose such agents to animals or humans. Delving into the development of potentially toxic metabolites, assessing the role of BSEP and hepatic transporters, and examining the role of drugs on mitochondrial toxicity are among other in vitro technologies that are bringing us closer to a fuller understanding of DILI mechanisms. On the clinical side, the current state of micro-RNAs and other mechanistic biomarkers to help foretell the severity of acute DILI, defining the various genetic and other host risk modifiers that help predict who is most likely to develop DILI, and a review of the regulatory and diagnostic tools at our disposal to best establish the causality of DILI round out the additional chapters that are included.

I very much look forward to having this text on my bookshelf as the authoritative resource on the diverse preclinical, clinical, and regulatory topics that comprise what we have all come to recognize as a challenging disorder. Drs. Chen and Will are to be congratulated for assembling such an all-star team of hepatotoxicity experts. Their timely and informative reviews and discussions will no doubt serve the field of drug-induced liver injury extremely well now and into the foreseeable future.

James H. Lewis
Georgetown University Hospital
Washington, DC, USA

Preface

Drug-induced liver toxicity remains a leading cause of acute liver failure and a major contributor to black box warnings and market withdrawal. Despite tremendous efforts towards developing new methodologies to better understand, evaluate, and manage liver toxicity, progress is still limited, and liver toxicity remains a challenging issue for drug developers, regulators, and clinicians.

Twenty years ago, Dr. Hyman Zimmerman published his monograph, *Hepatotoxicity: The Adverse Effects of Drugs and Other Chemicals on the Liver*. In the book, Dr. Zimmerman postulated the need to develop a database that contained the assessment of hepatotoxic potential and characteristics of medications. In addition, he suggested that maintaining an up-to-date list of hepatotoxins would permit the prediction of untested medications by correlating structural features of compounds with hepatotoxic potential.

The strategy Dr. Zimmerman suggested 20 years ago is still valid today. Databases, such as the LiverTox by the U.S. National Institutes of Health and the Liver Toxicity Knowledge Base (LTKB) by the U.S. Food and Drug Administration, serve as valuable resources in the development of new methodologies that aim to assess hepatotoxic risk in humans. New tools and models have been developed, including "rule-of-two" (Chap. 3), DILI-Sym (Chap. 6), risk matrix (Chap. 17), and e-DISH (Chap. 20). New technologies are rapidly advancing, which would help improve assessment and understanding of hepatotoxic potentials of new medications and marketed drugs.

This book provides a comprehensive view of the methodologies for the study of liver toxicity encountered throughout the whole life cycle of a drug, from drug discovery, to clinical trial, post-marketing, and even clinical practice. It is organized into six parts. The first part begins with an introduction to the mechanisms contributing to drug-induced liver toxicity. The second and third parts introduce in silico and in vitro approaches used to help mitigate hepatotoxicity liability at the early stages of drug development. The fourth part describes methodologies applied in regulatory processes, including preclinical studies, clinical trials, and post-marketing surveillance. The fifth part discusses clinical hepatotoxicity. Emerging technologies are introduced in the final part of the book.

All chapters are written by internationally recognized experts from Big Pharma, regulatory agencies, universities, or clinical centers. The in-depth hepatotoxic knowledge provided in this multiauthor volume will benefit toxicologists, pharmacologists, biochemists, bioinformaticians, drug discovery and development researchers, clinicians with interest in liver diseases, and government regulators. Finally, the editors would like to acknowledge all the authors for their enthusiasm and contributions to this book and the publisher, Springer, for their ongoing support in this project.

Jefferson, AR, USA
Groton, CT, USA

Minjun Chen
Yvonne Will

Disclaimer

The opinions expressed by the authors do not reflect the opinions or policies of their respective institutions. Any statements in this article should not be considered present or future policy of any regulatory agency.

Contents

Contributors

MICHAEL D. ALEO • *Drug Safety Research and Development, Investigative Toxicology, Pfizer Inc., Groton, CT, USA*

EILEEN NAVARRO ALMARIO • *Office of Computational Science, Center for Drug Evaluation and Research, U.S. Food and Drug Administration, Silver Spring, MD, USA*

RAÚL J. ANDRADE • *Unidad de Gestión de Aparato Digestivo, Servicio de Farmacología Clínica, Instituto de Investigación Biomédica de Málaga (IBIMA), Hospital Universitario Virgen de la Victoria, Universidad de Málaga, Málaga, Spain*

DANIEL J. ANTOINE • *MRC Centre for Inflammation Research, The Queen's Medical Research Institute, The University of Edinburgh, Edinburgh, UK*

FRANCK A. ATIENZAR • *Non-Clinical Development, Investigative Toxicology Group, UCB BioPharma SPRL, Braine-l'Alleud, Belgium*

MARK I. AVIGAN • *Office of Surveillance and Epidemiology, Center for Drug Evaluation and Research, U.S. Food and Drug Administration, Silver Spring, MD, USA*

CHRISTINA BATTISTA • *Institute for Drug Safety Sciences, Eshelman School of Pharmacy, The University of North Carolina at Chapel Hill, Chapel Hill, NC, USA; DILIsym Services, Inc., Research Triangle Park, NC, USA*

ANDREAS BAUDY • *Merck & Co., West Point, PA, USA*

ANNIE BORGNE-SANCHEZ • *MITOLOGICS Research Lab, Hôpital Robert Debré, Paris, France; MITOLOGICS SAS, Parc Biocitech, Romainville, France*

BAS TER BRAAK • *Division of Toxicology, Leiden Academic Centre for Drug Research, Leiden University, Leiden, The Netherlands*

ALLEN D. BRINKER • *Division of Pharmacovigilance, Office of Surveillance and Epidemiology, Center for Drug Evaluation and Research, U.S. Food and Drug Administration, Silver Spring, MD, USA*

NELLY BURON • *MITOLOGICS Research Lab, Hôpital Robert Debré, Paris, France; MITOLOGICS SAS, Parc Biocitech, Romainville, France*

MINJUN CHEN • *Division of Bioinformatics and Biostatistics, National Center for Toxicological Research, U.S. Food and Drug Administration, Jefferson, AR, USA*

SI CHEN • *Division of Biochemical Toxicology, National Center for Toxicological Research, U.S. Food and Drug Administration, Jefferson, AR, USA*

GYORGY CSAKO • *National Heart, Lung, and Blood Institute, National Institutes of Health, Bethesda, MD, USA*

ANN K. DALY • *Institute of Cellular Medicine, Newcastle University, Newcastle upon Tyne, UK*

GABY DANAN • *Pharmacovigilance Consultancy, Paris, France*

RUITANG DENG • *Department of Biomedical and Pharmaceutical Sciences, College of Pharmacy, University of Rhode Island, Kingston, RI, USA*

HONG FANG • *Office of Scientific Coordination, National Center for Toxicological Research, U.S. Food and Drug Administration, Jefferson, AR, USA*

LILIA FISK • *Lhasa Limited, Leeds, UK*

BERNARD FROMENTY • *INSERM, INRA, Univ Rennes 1, Univ Bretagne Loire, Nutrition, Metabolism and Cancer (NuMeCan), Rennes, France*

ALEKSANDRA GALETIN • *University of Manchester, Manchester, UK*

JINPING GAN • *Metabolism and Pharmacokinetics, Bristol-Myers Squibb, Princeton, NJ, USA*

CHRISTOPHER E.P. GOLDRING • *Department of Molecular and Clinical Pharmacology, MRC Centre for Drug Safety Science, University of Liverpool, Liverpool, UK*

PING GONG • *Environmental Laboratory, U.S. Army Engineer Research and Development Center, Vicksburg, MS, USA*

NIGEL GREENE • *Astra Zeneca, Waltham, MA, USA*

LEI GUO • *Division of Biochemical Toxicology, National Center for Toxicological, Research, U.S. Food and Drug Administration, Jefferson, AR, USA*

TED GUO • *Office of Biostatistics, Office of Translational Sciences, Center for Drug Evaluation and Research, U.S. Food and Drug Administration, Silver Spring, MD, USA*

ELIZABETH HAUSNER • *Division of Cardiovascular and Renal Products, Center for Drug Evaluation and Research, U.S. Food and Drug Administration, Silver Spring, MD, USA*

STEVEN HIEMSTRA • *Division of Toxicology, Leiden Academic Centre for Drug Research, Leiden University, Leiden, The Netherlands*

CATHERINE D.G. HINES • *Merck & Co., West Point, PA, USA*

PAUL HOCKINGS • *Antaros Medical, BioVenture Hub, Mölndal, Sweden; MedTech West, Chalmers University of Technology, Gothenburg, Sweden*

WOUTER DEN HOLLANDER • *Division of Toxicology, Leiden Academic Centre for Drug Research, Leiden University, Leiden, The Netherlands*

HUIXIAO HONG • *Division of Bioinformatics and Biostatistics, National Center for Toxicological Research, U.S. Food and Drug Administration, Jefferson, AR, USA*

BRETT A. HOWELL • *DILIsym Services, Inc., Research Triangle Park, NC, USA*

HARTMUT JAESCHKE • *Department of Pharmacology, Toxicology and Therapeutics, University of Kansas Medical Center, Kansas City, KS, USA*

S. CHRISTOPHER JONES • *Division of Pharmacovigilance, Office of Surveillance and Epidemiology, Center for Drug Evaluation and Research, U.S. Food and Drug Administration, Silver Spring, MD, USA*

NEIL KAPLOWITZ • *USC Research Center for Liver Disease, Keck School of Medicine, University of Southern California, Los Angeles, CA, USA*

J. GERRY KENNA • *Bioxydyn, Manchester Science Park, Manchester, UK; Safer Medicines Trust, Kingsbridge, UK*

IMRAN KHAN • *Division of Anesthesia, Analgesia and Addiction Products, Center for Drug Evaluation and Research, U.S. Food and Drug Administration, Silver Spring, MD, USA*

SALMAN R. KHETANI • *Department of Bioengineering, University of Illinois at Chicago, Chicago, IL, USA*

JOS C. KLEINJANS • *Department of Toxicogenomics, Maastricht University, Maastricht, The Netherlands*

THEO M. DE KOK • *Department of Toxicogenomics, Maastricht University, Maastricht, The Netherlands*

CINDY KORTEPETER • *Division of Pharmacovigilance, Office of Surveillance and Epidemiology, Center for Drug Evaluation and Research, U.S. Food and Drug Administration, Silver Spring, MD, USA*

JULIAN KRAUSKOPF • *Department of Toxicogenomics, Maastricht University, Maastricht, The Netherlands; Department of Toxicogenomics, GROW School for Oncology and Developmental Biology, Maastricht University, Maastricht, The Netherlands*

ALBERT P. LI • *In Vitro ADMET Laboratories Inc., Columbia, MD, USA*

DEBORAH S. LIGHT • *Drug Safety Research and Development, Investigative Toxicology, Pfizer Inc., Groton, CT, USA*

ZHICHAO LIU • *Division of Bioinformatics and Biostatistics, National Center for Toxicological Research, U.S. Food and Drug Administration, Jefferson, AR, USA*

M. ISABEL LUCENA • *Unidad de Gestión de Aparato Digestivo, Servicio de Farmacología Clínica, Instituto de Investigación Biomédica de Málaga (IBIMA), Hospital Universitario Virgen de la Victoria, Universidad de Málaga, Málaga, Spain*

CHASE P. MONCKTON • *Department of Bioengineering, University of Illinois at Chicago, Chicago, IL, USA*

MONICA A. MUÑOZ • *Office of Surveillance and Epidemiology, Center for Drug Evaluation and Research, U.S. Food and Drug Administration, Silver Spring, MD, USA*

DEAN J. NAISBITT • *Department of Molecular and Clinical Pharmacology, MRC Centre for Drug Safety Science, University of Liverpool, Liverpool, UK*

RUSS NAVEN • *Takeda International, Cambridge, MA, USA*

JEAN-MARIE NICOLAS • *Non-Clinical Development, Development DMPK/PKPD, UCB BioPharma SPRL, Braine-l'Alleud, Belgium*

MARIJE NIEMEIJER • *Division of Toxicology, Leiden Academic Centre for Drug Research, Leiden University, Leiden, The Netherlands*

BAITANG NING • *Division of Systems Biology, National Center for Toxicological, Research, U.S. Food and Drug Administration, Jefferson, AR, USA*

NABIL NOUREDDIN • *USC Research Center for Liver Disease, Keck School of Medicine, University of Southern California, Los Angeles, CA, USA*

MONICAH A. OTIENO • *Preclinical Development & Safety, Janssen Pharmaceuticals, Spring House, PA, USA*

AXEL PÄHLER • *Pharmaceutical Sciences, Roche Pharmaceutical Research and Early Development, pRED, Roche Innovation Center Basel, F. Hoffmann-La Roche Ltd, Basel, Switzerland*

B. KEVIN PARK • *Department of Molecular and Clinical Pharmacology, MRC Centre for Drug Safety Science, University of Liverpool, Liverpool, UK*

MANISHKUMAR PATEL • *Merck & Co., West Point, PA, USA*

TEJAS PATEL • *Office of Computational Science, Center for Drug Evaluation and Research, U.S. Food and Drug Administration, Silver Spring, MD, USA*

MIKAEL PERSSON • *Drug Safety and Metabolism, Innovative Medicines and Early Development, AstraZeneca R&D Gothenburg, Mölndal, Sweden*

FRANCOIS POGNAN • *Discovery Investigative Safety, PreClinical Safety, Novartis Pharmaceutical AG, Basel, Switzerland*

MATHIEU PORCEDDU • *MITOLOGICS Research Lab, Hôpital Robert Debré, Paris, France; MITOLOGICS SAS, Parc Biocitech, Romainville, France*

CHRIS S. PRIDGEON • *Department of Molecular and Clinical Pharmacology, MRC Centre for Drug Safety Science, University of Liverpool, Liverpool, UK*

WILLIAM PROCTOR • *Department of Safety Assessment, Genentech Inc., South San Francisco, CA, USA*

ZHEN REN • *Division of Biochemical Toxicology, National Center for Toxicological, Research, U.S. Food and Drug Administration, Jefferson, AR, USA*

PIERRE RUSTIN • *INSERM, UMR1141-PROTECT, Hôpital Robert Debré, Paris, France*

CONSTANZE SCHLOTT • *Department of Molecular and Clinical Pharmacology, MRC Centre for Drug Safety Science, University of Liverpool, Liverpool, UK*

GUNNAR SCHUETZ • *Bayer Pharma AG, Berlin, Germany*

DANIEL SCOTCHER • *University of Manchester, Manchester, UK*

JOHN SENIOR • *Office of Surveillance and Epidemiology, Center for Drug Evaluation and Research, U.S. Food and Drug Administration, Silver Spring, MD, USA*

MD SHAMSUZZAMAN • *Office of Computational Science, Center for Drug Evaluation and Research, U.S. Food and Drug Administration, Silver Spring, MD, USA*

SCOTT Q. SILER • *DILIsym Services, Inc., Research Triangle Park, NC, USA*

STEVEN SOURBRON • *University of Leeds, Leeds, UK*

CAMILLA STEPHENS • *Unidad de Gestión de Aparato Digestivo, Servicio de Farmacología Clínica, Instituto de Investigación Biomédica de Málaga (IBIMA), Hospital Universitario Virgen de la Victoria, Universidad de Málaga, Málaga, Spain*

ROLF TESCHKE • *Division of Gastroenterology and Hepatology, Department of Internal Medicine II, Klinikum Hanau, Hanau, Germany; Academic Teaching Hospital of the Medical Faculty, Goethe University Frankfurt/Main, Frankfurt am Main, Germany*

BEREKET TESFALDET • *Office of Computational Science, Center for Drug Evaluation and Research, U.S. Food and Drug Administration, Silver Spring, MD, USA*

SHRADDHA THAKKAR • *Division of Bioinformatics and Biostatistics, National Center for Toxicological Research, U.S. Food and Drug Administration, Jefferson, AR, USA*

WEIDA TONG • *Division of Bioinformatics and Biostatistics, National Center for Toxicological Research, U.S. Food and Drug Administration, Jefferson, AR, USA*

BOB VAN DE WATER • *Division of Toxicology, Leiden Academic Centre for Drug Research, Leiden University, Leiden, The Netherlands*

JOHN C. WATERTON • *Bioxydyn, Manchester Science Park, Manchester, UK; University of Manchester, Manchester, UK; Alderley Imaging, Macclesfield, UK*

PAUL B. WATKINS • *Institute for Drug Safety Sciences, Eshelman School of Pharmacy, The University of North Carolina at Chapel Hill, Chapel Hill, NC, USA; DILIsym Services, Inc., Research Triangle Park, NC, USA*

STEVEN WINK • *Division of Toxicology, Leiden Academic Centre for Drug Research, Leiden University, Leiden, The Netherlands*

MIN WEI WONG • *Department of Molecular and Clinical Pharmacology, MRC Centre for Drug Safety Science, University of Liverpool, Liverpool, UK*

CHAOYANG ZHANG • *School of Computer Science, University of Southern Mississippi, Hattiesburg, MS, USA*

JIEQIANG ZHU • *Division of Bioinformatics and Biostatistics, National Center for Toxicological Research, U.S. Food and Drug Administration, Jefferson, AR, USA*

SABINA ZIEMIAN • *Bayer Pharma AG, Berlin, Germany*

Part I

Introduction

Part I

Introduction

Chapter 1

Overview of Mechanisms of Drug-Induced Liver Injury (DILI) and Key Challenges in DILI Research

Nabil Noureddin and Neil Kaplowitz

Abstract

The liver is an important target for foreign chemicals, such as drugs, which are metabolized and excreted by the liver. Reactive metabolites, or in some cases parent drug, elicit a variety of biochemical consequences such as covalent binding and oxidative stress which trigger signal transduction, transcription factors, mitochondrial and endoplasmic reticulum (ER) stress which can lead directly to cell death or activate adaptive responses which mitigate these hazards. Alternatively, these stress responses may predict the development of idiosyncratic drug-induced liver injury (IDILI). Current evidence supports the hypothesis that IDILI is often mediated by adaptive immunity in genetically susceptible individuals which is modulated by the robustness of immune tolerance.

Key words Hepatotoxicity, Liver injury, Adaptive immunity, Stress responses, Adaptation, Tolerance

1 Introduction

Drug-induced liver injury (DILI) is a diagnosis of exclusion which manifests as a spectrum of clinical presentations such as acute hepatocellular liver injury presenting as acute hepatitis, cholestatic jaundice, nodular regenerative hyperplasia, sinusoidal obstruction syndrome, steatohepatitis, or subclinical injury which is detected during routine testing of serum chemistries [1, 2]. DILI is infrequently observed in clinical practice with an incidence ranging from 0.014% in a French population-based cohort study, 0.019% in the Iceland population, to 1.4% in an in-patient study from Switzerland [3–5]. Despite its rarity, because of the wide use of medications, DILI remains an important clinical problem. Although most of the DILI seen postmarketing is due to drugs approved before 1990 (Hoofnagle, personal communication), DILI remains an ongoing problem for the pharmaceutical industry during preclinical and clinical drug development. New drugs with DILI potential are usually identified in preclinical and premarketing

Minjun Chen and Yvonne Will (eds.), *Drug-Induced Liver Toxicity*, Methods in Pharmacology and Toxicology,
https://doi.org/10.1007/978-1-4939-7677-5_1, © Springer Science+Business Media, LLC, part of Springer Nature 2018

clinical development due to the vigilance of regulatory bodies and Industry.

DILI imposes major clinical, economic, regulatory, and scientific challenges. DILI is the leading cause of acute liver failure (ALF) in the United States. In fact, more than half of all ALF cases in the USA are a result of DILI, most of which are due to acetaminophen [6], but idiosyncratic DILI represents an important contributor [7]. According to Liver Tox analysis which excluded drugs marketed in the past 5 years, of 673 marketed drugs evaluated, 53% had published convincing cases of DILI [8]. It is one of the most frequently cited reasons for drug nonapproval, withdrawal, abandonment, and postmarketing regulatory actions [9]. Mainly because of the dreaded risk of ALF and its reliable predictor, Hy's law, much effort is made to identify or predict the risk during preclinical drug development by the pharmaceutical industry.

DILI can be broadly divided into predictable, dose dependent, direct (intrinsic) toxicity, such as acetaminophen (APAP) toxicity, and unpredictable or idiosyncratic DILI (IDILI), such as isoniazid and amoxicillin-clavulanic acid. This chapter will provide a broad overview of the mechanisms of DILI, and the key challenges in the field.

2   Mechanisms and Pathogenesis

The central role of the liver in removal of lipophilic drugs and their hepatic metabolism places the liver as a prime target for reactive metabolites of drugs. After the exposure to reactive metabolites, or in some cases the parent drug, the ensuing fundamental processes in DILI are biochemical and organelle stress and/or the death of hepatocytes accompanied by inflammation (innate immunity) and, in many cases, the participation of the adaptive immune system. All these processes are potentially mitigated by biochemical and immunological adaptive responses. The cascade of events that lead to direct hepatotoxicity or IDILI have many similarities in the upstream processes but fundamental differences which are determined by the individual drug and host factors, especially genetic [10–12].

3   Direct Hepatocyte Toxicity

Drugs or reactive metabolites can cause intrinsic predictable toxicity by covalent binding to intracellular proteins, generating reactive oxygen species (ROS), and inducing organelle stress (such as endoplasmic reticulum (ER) and mitochondrial stress). If the stress is minor, organelle adaptive responses (such as the unfolded protein responses in the ER or mitochondria) will compensate and the development of the injury will be dampened. If these responses are overwhelmed, organelle stress can activate the intrinsic pathway of apoptosis via mitochondrial outer membrane permeabilization (MOMP) or lead to necrosis by mitochondrial permeability transition (MPT) and cell death will occur [12]. The roles of other forms of cell death in DILI, such as necroptosis, ferroptosis, or pyroptosis are not well understood. Understanding the mode of cell death and mechanisms leading to cell death is critical for developing therapeutic strategies to treat DILI before it becomes severe (Hy's law or ALF).

3.1 Acetaminophen (APAP) Toxicity

The most prominent example of direct hepatotoxin is acetaminophen (APAP). A brief summary of the cascade of events in acetaminophen metabolism and toxicity follows, which illustrates some of the critical events in direct intrinsic toxicity.

The major metabolites of APAP are the glucuronide and sulfate conjugates, while a minor fraction is converted in the liver by the cytochrome P450 system (mainly CYP2E1) to a highly reactive toxic electrophilic arylating metabolite, NAPQI. NAPQI is normally quickly inactivated by being preferentially conjugated with reduced glutathione in the liver. When large doses of APAP are ingested, NAPQI production increases and glutathione becomes depleted [13]. The dose of APAP sufficient to induce toxicity in humans is very variable and depends on the many known and unknown factors that influence APAP metabolism and the downstream events that induce injury and repair. NAPQI can covalently bind to cell protein thiols and also can oxidize them leading to the formation of inter-protein crosslinking, disulfide bridges or mixed disulfides [14]. This causes ER stress [15] but the contribution of ER stress in APAP toxicity has not been clearly elucidated. NAPQI is sufficiently stable so as to enter the mitochondria, where it leads to impairment in electron transport, resulting in the generation of ROS [16]. NAPQI and consequent mitochondrial-derived ROS damage mitochondrial DNA, and the release of mitochondrial ROS activates upstream kinases such as GSK3β [19], RIPK1 [21], PKC [20], MLK3 [23], ASK1 [24] and MKK4 [25] leading to c-Jun N terminal Kinase (JNK) activation in the cytoplasm [16–18]. Activated JNK (p-JNK) then binds to its target Sab [22] and phosphorylates it on the outer mitochondrial membrane, leading to the intermembrane release of protein tyrosine phosphatase type 6 (PTPN6) from Sab. PTPN6 dephosphorylates and inactivates Src in the intermembrane space [22]. Active Src is required to maintain electron transport in the inner membrane. When Src is inactivated, the ETC chain is blocked and ROS production is amplified, ultimately leading to MPT. This results in the collapse of mitochondrial membrane potential, and thus the cessation of ATP synthesis, as well as to the release of mitochondrial proteins which damage nuclear DNA. Necrotic cell death ensues, characterized by cell swelling and lysis, referred to as oncosis.

3.2 Cellular Stress Responses and Adaptive Responses in DILI

When exposure is sufficient, many possible biochemical and organelle stress responses are triggered by reactive metabolites which are generated in hepatocytes. These mechanisms can induce cell dysfunction, potentially generate danger signals such as danger-associated molecular patterns (DAMPS), sensitize hepatocytes to death receptor-induced cell death, or induce sufficient stress to mediate hepatocyte death through intrinsic death mechanisms. Alternatively, hepatocytes have a variety of adaptive mechanisms which can arrest the progression of cell dysfunction or lethality. The major stressors and adaptive mechanisms are listed in Table 1. Reactive metabolites can undergo covalent interaction with proteins or induce redox perturbations leading to oxidative stress. These upstream biochemical events play a role in causing or worsening organelle dysfunction in the ER and mitochondria. Hepatotoxic drugs commonly induce oxidative stress, ER stress, and mitochondrial stress (any or all). Aside from a pivotal role for ROS generated in mitochondria, accumulation of bile acids due to drug or metabolite inhibition of BSEP may play an important role, not only in inhibiting bile secretion (cholestasis), but in affecting ER and mitochondrial function [26]. Although less is known about the stress-inducing effects of fatty acids in the context of DILI, saturated fatty acids also impair ER and mitochondrial function [27]. A key feature of all these biochemical and stress responses is the involvement of signaling kinases, such as MAPK, in causing or responding to organelle and oxidative stress to perpetuate and amplify cellular dysfunction [28].

Table 1
Intracellular stress responses and adaptive responses

Stress initiator	Adaptive responses
CYP-mediated reactive metabolite formation	CYP inactivation Enhanced detoxification
Reactive oxygen species (redox perturbations and signal transduction)	Antioxidant defense [Nrf2, etc.]
Mitochondrial impairment	Mitophagy, fission/fusion, biogenesis and UPR^{Mito}
ER stress	UPR^{ER}
BSEP inhibition (bile acid toxicity)	FXR mediated enhancement of bile acid export
Innate immunity, cytokines, chemokines, inflammation	Anti-inflammatory responses

Intracellular adaptive responses, when not successful in restoring homeostasis, might sensitize "stressed hepatocytes" to greater immune-mediated toxicity and T cell or cytokine induced apoptosis. Similar hypotheses can be generated for adaptation to ER stress, commonly seen in response to covalent binding, as well as adaptive responses to mitochondrial stress. In both instances the cell responds to organelle specific stress through unfolded protein responses (ER or mitochondria), which upregulate the transcription of chaperones and improve protein folding. In addition, damaged mitochondria elicit other adaptive responses such as mitophagy (a form of autophagy selectively involving damaged, ROS producing mitochondria) to remove them, or biogenesis to replace them. Retrograde signaling from stressed mitochondria or ER leads to transcriptional programs for both protective UPR and organelle biogenesis to replace the damaged organelles removed by nonselective or selective (mitophagy) autophagy.

UPR^{ER} retrograde signaling mainly occurs through activation of transcription factors such as sXBP1 and ATF6 which induce chaperones which mitigate impaired folding. At the same time translational arrest occurs through the activation of ER PERK which reduces client load. When these adaptive mechanisms fail, the ER signals apoptosis through the activation of JNK, which along with Ca^{2+} released from the ER targets mitochondria leading to ROS production and intrinsic cell death (apoptosis) mediated by Bcl family mediated permeabilization of the outer membrane of mitochondria [29, 30].

UPR^{mito} has been more recently elucidated and involves a novel regulatory mechanism of mitochondrial protease mediated degradation of cytoplasmic proteins taken up by normal mitochondria. For example, ATFS-1 is a transcription factor with both mitochondrial and nuclear localization peptide sequences. Mitochondrial uptake and degradation dominates under basal conditions. However, when its mitochondrial uptake is impaired (depolarized or damaged mitochondria), this transcription factor is stabilized and translocates from the cytoplasm to the nucleus to activate expression of mitochondrial chaperones and import machinery [31]. Interestingly, this type of novel protein regulatory turnover mechanism also plays a role in mitophagy. PINK1 is a kinase which continuously enters mitochondria and is degraded. When mitochondria depolarize, PINK1 stabilizes on the outer membrane and recruits and phosphorylates PARKIN, an E3 ligase which ubiquitinates outer membrane proteins which target mitochondria for mitophagy after p62 binding to the ubiquitinated proteins. PINK1 also inactivates mitochondrial fusion allowing fission to occur so that mitochondrial fragments are able to undergo mitophagy [32]. The regulation and importance of fission/fusion in DILI is largely unexplored.

The role of autophagy/mitophagy has been studied in APAP induced hepatotoxicity. APAP resulted in formation of autophagosomes that engulfed mitochondria and pharmacological inhibition of autophagy by 3-methyladenine or chloroquine exacerbated APAP toxicity while this was attenuated by rapamycin-induced enhanced autophagy, even if administered two hours after APAP [33].

Direct toxicity is generally identified readily in preclinical and/or the early phase of clinical testing and only is acceptable in the extension of drug development when the benefit far outweighs the risk. The latter scenario mainly applies to cancer chemotherapy drugs. An overview of the principles of direct hepatotoxicity is illustrated in Fig. 1. These concepts of cellular stress and death also seem to be relevant to IDILI. There are many approaches to preclinical screening of drugs which have been validated using panels of drugs known to cause IDILI compared to drugs which have no or minimal risk. The study models include isolated mitochondria or microsomes, hepatocytes, liver cancer cell lines, collaborative cross of inbred mouse strains, humanized mice, organoids, liver on a chip, micropatterned culture, iPS derived liver-like cells, and other emerging technologies. Assessment for various hazards include transcriptomics, cellular respiration, ATP, ROS, covalent binding, apoptosis or necrosis, and BSEP inhibition with the aim of identifying hazards such as oxidative stress, lipid peroxidation, transcriptomic changes, ER or mitochondrial stress, or the footprint

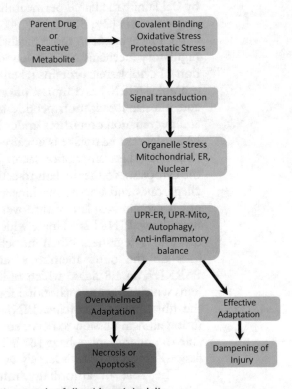

Fig. 1 Pathogenesis of direct hepatotoxicity

of these hazards as reflected in robust adaptive responses. The challenging aspect of the findings relates to the reason for good predictive performance of most of these model systems in identifying IDILI risk in the face of the fact that these approaches are largely identifying direct toxicity and may not necessarily reflect the idiosyncratic mechanism. Are these predictable hazards a surrogate for drugs which are potentially immunogenic without informing on specific mechanism or are these hazards important contributing factors to the development of adaptive immunity through the generation of danger signals and/or are these hazards contributing to the unmasking of IDILI by sensitizing to adaptive immune-mediated killing? Further complicating these possibilities is the question of whether variations in the adaptive responses to cellular hazards contribute to susceptibility to direct or idiosyncratic DILI.

4   IDILI

The pathophysiology of IDILI is multifactorial, involving drug/pharmacological factors, host factors, and factors affecting the adaptive immune system. Current evidence strongly favors the concept that IDILI is usually mediated by the adaptive immune system. Recent work has shown that many examples of IDILI are associated with genetic susceptibility in the MHC genes [34]. However, in most examples only a small proportion of individuals carrying the risk allele develop liver injury.

4.1 Factors Contributing to Development of IDILI

- *Pharmacological*: Certain drug properties such as dosage and lipophilicity have been associated with IDILI. In fact, drugs that are both taken at a high dose (greater than 50–100 mg/day) and have a calculated octanol-water partition coefficient (log $P > 3$) rendering them lipophilic have a higher positive predictive value for inducing toxicity than a dose alone, indicating the need for a threshold level of hepatic exposure [35]. Thus, although IDILI is not strictly dose-related, a dose threshold to meet some level of exposure to the drug, its metabolites, and or its hazards appears to be needed for the development of adaptive immune response.

- *Host factors*: Age and sex are well-known risk factors for toxicity of specific drugs. It is possible that age influences the adaptive immune response. Of course, medication use increases with age and polypharmacy is more prevalent [36]. Women tend to be at higher risk for IDILI in many studies. However, in the Spanish DILI registry, Lucena et al. did not find an association between female sex and overall increased incidence of DILI [37].

- *Hepatic metabolism and transport*: Most often, the first step for an IDILI event is for the parent drug to form a reactive metabolite capable of covalently binding intracellular proteins and generating cellular stress. There is considerable individual variation in the activity of the cytochromes P-450 (CYP) determined by environmental and genetic effects. Similarly, exposure may be greatly influenced by the status of phase 2 conjugation and phase 3 transporters which are also subject to environmental and genetic influences. Surprisingly, GWAS and exome sequencing studies have only infrequently found genetic polymorphisms in IDILI related to hepatic metabolism or transport [38, 39]. However, nongenetic variations in hepatic metabolism and transport likely play a role in susceptibility to direct toxicity and by extension to hazards elicited by IDILI drugs. The fact that hazards in preclinical testing are usually studied at high drug concentrations could obscure the contribution of variations in drug metabolism and transport to risk. Certainly, potency of BSEP inhibition in predicting IDILI suggests that effects of transporters maybe be of importance.

- *Genetic variations and polymorphisms in human leukocyte antigens*: The idiosyncratic nature of most drug reactions has long been viewed as evidence of a genetic predisposition to hepatotoxicity. Polymorphisms in HLA genes have been clearly demonstrated to be associated with many recent IDILI drugs [34]. The implication of these studies is that IDILI is the result of the activation of an adaptive immune response. These HLA haplotype associations suggest that DILI occurs due to a genetic predisposition to an adaptive immune response due to the presentation and recognition of a drug-related antigen.

  Although HLA restriction has been evident for years, the underlying mechanisms of the immune response have not been fully elucidated. Several hypotheses of the immune system activation in IDILI have been proposed [34]. These are supported by earlier studies identifying the occurrence of anti-drug hapten antibodies and autoantibodies in some cases as well as by the occurrence of systemic hypersensitivity as evidenced by fever, rash, eosinophilia with a latency of days to a few weeks in some cases. However, it is important to recognize that many examples of IDILI are not accompanied by such systemic manifestations of hypersensitivity and exhibit longer latency of months. It is remarkable that these IDILI scenarios selectively involving the liver were formerly considered to be due metabolic idiosyncrasy. This is not to say that metabolic idiosyncrasy does not occur due to cumulative direct effects of certain drugs, for example nucleosides and amiodarone toxicity.

**4.2   Hypotheses
of Immune System
Activation
and Involvement
in IDILI**

- *Hapten hypothesis.* This postulates that certain drugs are metabolized to reactive compounds which can bind to endogenous proteins and form neoantigenic or "hapten" peptides that are presented to and recognized as foreign antigens by the immune system of certain individuals with HLA polymorphisms [34, 40]. This is probably the most common mechanism. In certain cases, the parent drug (e.g., flucloxacillin [41]) may form covalent interactions with a peptide directly in the MHC groove. However, covalent binding probably occurs in nearly all exposed individuals including those with HLA risk, whereas even mild DILI occurs in only a small minority.

- *Pharmacological interaction (p-i) hypothesis.* This proposes that certain drugs can directly form noncovalent interactions with MHC molecules leading to the activation of the immune system [42, 43]. It is likely that the initial binding of the drug to the MHC molecule is labile, and serves as a scaffold for a T cell receptor (TCR) interaction of much higher relative affinity. This TCR interaction is capable of generating an immunological response, as it involves T cell activation. However, the specific sites of drug binding on the MHC-peptide complex remain unresolved for many drugs.

- *The altered peptide repertoire hypothesis.* This model suggests that certain drugs can cause mistargeting of endogenous peptides to the wrong HLA leading to autoimmunity. The mistargeting is drug dependent and may involve covalent or noncovalent binding of the parent drug to the MHC peptide binding groove. The mechanism of abacavir skin toxicity is the best example [44, 45].

- *Multiple determinant hypothesis.* An alternative hypothesis for IDILI is that multiple risk factors (such as polymorphisms, age, gender, preexisting conditions) could overlap together to induce DILI [46–48]. The mouse model of halothane-induced liver toxicity can be used as example. Among the known human risk factors for halothane hepatitis are female gender, middle age, genetic predisposition, and multiple exposures. Therefore, unless all conditions are met and the multiple determinants are fulfilled IDILI will not occur which may partly explain why the disease is so rare [49]. Nevertheless, this hypothesis is most likely a precursor for the development of adaptive immunity in susceptible individuals.

- *Inflammatory stress hypothesis.* The unpredictable nature of idiosyncratic DILI may also suggest that there could be another event occurring concomitantly with drug therapy. This raises the possibility that IDILI reactions could be unmasked by inflammation concomitantly occurring during drug therapy, which could interact with the action of the drug and escalate into liver injury. Such a response is often characterized by inflammatory cell infiltrates within liver lesions of patients suffering from IDILI. These inflammagens bind to "pattern recognition receptors" such as Toll-like receptors (TLRs) on immune system cells, which initiate the activation of transcription factors and the expression of inflammatory mediators such as TNFα and IFNγ [46–50]. This seems most plausible in the in the context of danger signals to promote adaptive immunity in genetically predisposed individuals. However, the adaptive immune response may not only be costimulated by cytokines, but may also lead to production of cytokines which are effectors of hepatocellular stress and death (e.g., TNF and IFNγ mediated necrosis). Thus, immune mediated cell death, the key manifestation of serious IDILI may be mediated by a repertoire of effector mechanisms including TCR engagement, granzyme/porin, FasL, cytokines, and antibody/complement.

4.3 Immune-Tolerance and Adaptation

Only a small proportion of individuals with susceptible HLA genotypes develop clinically significant liver injury when exposed to IDILI drugs. The adaptation hypothesis has been put forth as an explanation for why only a small percentage of susceptible individuals develop either no evidence of liver injury or overt IDILI and severe injury, while the majority with susceptible genotypes develop only mild abnormalities that usually resolve spontaneously despite continuation of the drug. This spontaneous resolution is referred to as clinical adaptation. This adaptation may be the result of liver's constant state of immune tolerance in order to avoid inflammatory reaction due to its routine exposure to foreign antigens [21] (Fig. 2).

The mechanisms of immune-tolerance can be broken down to the following key events: control of antigen presentation, clonal deletion (apoptosis of antigen-specific T cells) and immune deviation (switching fromTh2 to Th1 predominance).

The liver microenvironment plays a crucial role in the induction of immune tolerance toward dietary and foreign antigens. The liver contains various cell types, hepatocytes, along with the cholangiocytes, are the functional components of the liver. Other cell types referred to as nonparenchymal cells (NPC), essential to normal biologic and immunologic functions, include liver sinusoidal endothelial cells (LSECs, which constitute the wall of the liver sinusoids), Kupffer cells (KCs) which are resident liver macrophages, stellate cells (HSCs) which are pericytes found in perisinusoidal space, liver-associated lymphocytes and dendritic cells. LSECs function as a barrier between leukocytes or other macromolecules present in the sinusoidal lumen and hepatocytes, thus preventing direct contact between leukocytes and hepatocytes. LSECs take up antigens from the sinusoids for processing and

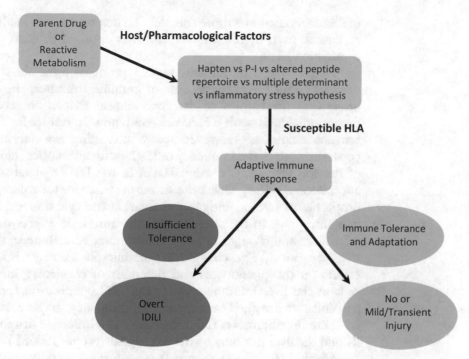

Fig. 2 Importance of status of immune tolerance in the pathogenesis of IDILI

antigen presentation. They can induce cytokine expression and proliferation and activation of CD4+ T cells. KCs, which are specialized macrophages, are located mainly in the periportal sinusoids so they can phagocytose and eliminate antigens and pathogens entering the liver parenchyma via portal venous blood from the intestines. KCs also play a pivotal role in regulating the liver's homeostasis in the face of constant exposure to ingested antigens. The liver's immune tolerance is dependent on the autocrine and paracrine effects of cytokines secreted by KCs as well as on LPS stimulation of immune cells and antigen presenting cells (KC and LSECs particularly). LPS from gut accompanies ingested food antigens and has been shown to have immune-tolerogenic properties. KCs and LSECs express cytokines such as IL-10, TGFβ, TNF, and prostaglandins either constitutively or in response to LPS, resulting in downregulation of leukocyte adhesion to LSECs, expansion of regulatory T cells (T-regs), and abrogation of T cell activation, all of which lead to an increased immune tolerance in the liver [21, 51].

Another proposed mechanism of peripheral immune-tolerance induction by the liver is the phenomenon of clonal deletion or induction of antigen-specific T cell apoptosis in the liver [52, 53]. While the elimination of T cell populations seems an attractive explanation, it does not seem to be the whole story since tolerance can be transferred from one animal to another. This can be achieved by adoptive transfer of γδ T cells, which suggests that the mechanism of this phenomenon is more complex and that tolerance is mediated, at least in part, by immune deviation as opposed to mass T cell elimination [21].

Despite these recent advances in proof of principle studies demonstrating the potential role of immune tolerance, the exact underlying mechanism of defective clinical adaptation, even in those individuals with HLA risk, and how it results in IDILI remains unknown. However, many interesting associations are apparent, such as the frequency of IDILI with antibiotics (nine out of the top ten agents causing IDILI in the DILIN database are antimicrobials) [54]. Given the strong evidence for the tolerogenic properties of LPS on antigen presentation and cytokine secretion, it is intriguing to hypothesize that the antibiotic effects on gut microflora and changes in LPS exposure may contribute to defective adaptation. The changes in gut microbiota may also have effects on the phenotypes and functions of regulatory immune cells in the liver immune system, e.g., KC polarization (pro- or anti-inflammatory), T-reg expansion/frequency, hepatic stellate cells, etc. Furthermore, the microbiome can influence drug toxicity and the liver not only by the tolerogenic properties of LPS, but by affecting drug metabolism. It is important to point out that these are only associations and intriguing as hypotheses but no evidence of causality exists [54]. Furthermore, complicating the role of the microbiome are its effects on drug metabolism and enterohepatic cycling of drugs which may influence exposure in the liver [55, 56]. In addition, since mitochondria, derived from ancestor protobacteria, retain similar machinery for protein synthesis, one could speculate that antibiotics have similar toxic effects on liver mitochondria, possibly inducing a costimulatory effect on adaptive immune response.

More recently several studies and animal models have shown that when the intrinsic liver autoimmunity checkpoints are experimentally bypassed, drugs that normally would not result in liver injury or only cause transient DILI, caused T cell activation with persistent and more severe DILI, which strengthens the immune tolerance and clinical adaptation theory [57–59].

It is tempting to speculate that clinical adaptation, during which liver tests reflecting mild injury resolve despite continued drug ingestion, is mainly driven by the development of immune tolerance which dampens the injury and conversely the inadequate development of tolerance may explain the progression to Hy's law and severe liver injury. Indeed, one could even entertain the hypothesis that hypertolerant individuals begin to dampen injury before it can be detected. Thus, despite the low incidence of clinical adaptors and even lower incidence of nonadaptors among those who have a genetic predisposition to an adaptive immune response to an IDILI drug, it is likely that far more of these individuals exhibit covalent binding. They may not progress to even mild DILI because of an

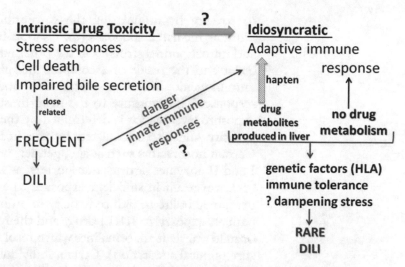

Fig. 3 Mechanistic relationship between intrinsic (direct) toxicity and DILI

effective early immune tolerance but also possibly because the hazardous biochemical stress responses may trigger robust cellular adaptive responses which dampen danger signals.

Elucidation of the relationship between the direct toxicity of IDILI drugs in preclinical studies and the development of adaptive immunity remains a major challenge: is there a mechanistically relevant relationship or is it fortuitous in the sense that the direct toxicity is a surrogate for something else? Much of this discussion is hypothetical but presents ideas which could be experimentally addressed. Ideally such studies would be best performed in humans and would involve noninvasive ways of expanding our limited repertoire to identify drug-induced hazards in the liver with unique biomarkers and imaging approaches. In addition, we need to better understand the mechanisms of immune tolerance, variations in how and when they are deployed, and how they can be enhanced to dampen early evidence of DILI (Fig. 3).

5   Conclusions

DILI is a very challenging diagnosis in clinical practice since it mimics a broad range of liver disease. Hepatocellular injury remains the most feared consequence as it can progress to acute liver failure. Concern for DILI greatly impacts drug development and regulatory bodies. DILI is divided into predictable (direct), dose dependent (such as APAP) or unpredictable, idiosyncratic. Exposure of hepatocytes to parent drug or reactive metabolites may induce a variety of stress responses and adaptive mechanisms, which can directly cause liver injury or illicit danger signals activating the innate and adaptive immune system. Drugs could also sensitize to toxicity by modulating the susceptibility of hepatocytes to immune mediated apoptosis (for example by causing oxidative ER and mitochondrial stress). On the other hand, IDILI is a rare disorder and the result of a complex interplay between potentially immunogenic drugs or metabolites and the host's immune response. The exposure to the drug must surpass a "threshold" exposure level, which is determined by the drug dosage and lipophilicity and also modulated by the host's metabolic capacity. Certain host factors such as age, gender, or variations in the phase I and II enzymes or drug transporters, as well as transcription factors, can result in sufficient exposure to a toxic and electrophilic drug metabolite to induce toxicity or an immune response. Most patients exposed to IDILI drugs and their metabolites develop no or mild transient abnormalities which resolve with continued exposure (clinical adaptation). Certain individuals with polymorphisms in HLA molecules when exposed to these IDILI drugs may develop overt clinical liver injury, although a multitude of conditions need to be met for IDILI to occur. There are several hypotheses for how drugs can lead to activation of the adaptive immune system leading to liver injury. All are probably relevant and depend on drug specific factors.

Our mechanistic understanding of direct DILI has greatly advanced through the identification of the role of stressors or hazards such as covalent binding, ROS, signal transduction and bile acids which elicit responses in organelles which promote injury at the functional and survival level. These responses lead to adaptive responses which dampen cellular and organelle dysfunction. These same mechanisms are commonly observed when IDILI drugs are examined in various preclinical models, suggesting but not proving that they represent relevant hazards mechanistically involved in the development of IDILI. However, IDILI is a rare disorder which impacts only a small minority of even genetically susceptible individuals. Adaptive immunity appears to be a dominant mechanism for IDILI and its modulation by immune tolerance may greatly impact the low frequency of its occurrence in genetically susceptible individuals. Overall the DILI field has benefited from enormous progress in our understanding of mechanisms and we now have more refined hypotheses to test as we look for better ways to predict risk, specifically identify DILI in humans, and clarify the specific hazards and their contribution to IDILI.

References

1. Chalasani N, Hayashi P, Bonkovsky H et al (2014) ACG clinical guideline: the diagnosis and management of idiosyncratic drug-induced liver injury. Am J Gastroenterol 109:950–966
2. Kaplowitz N (2005) Idiosyncratic drug hepatotoxicity. Nat Rev Drug Discov 4:489–499
3. Sgro C, Clinard F, Ouazir K et al (2002) Incidence of drug-induced hepatic injuries: a French population-based study. Hepatology 36:451–455
4. Björnsson E, Bergmann O, Björnsson H et al (2013) Incidence, presentation, and outcomes

in patients with drug-induced liver injury in the general population of Iceland. Gastroenterology 144:1419–1425

5. Meier Y, Cavallaro M, Roos M et al (2005) Incidence of drug-induced liver injury in medical inpatients. Eur J Clin Pharmacol 61:135–143

6. Larson A, Polson J, Fontana R et al (2005) Acetaminophen-induced acute liver failure: results of a United States multicenter, prospective study. Hepatology 42:1364–1372

7. Reuben A, Koch D, Lee W et al (2010) Drug-induced acute liver failure: results of a U.S. multicenter, prospective study. Hepatology 52:2065–2076

8. Björnsson E, Hoofnagle J (2016) Categorization of drugs implicated in causing liver injury: critical assessment based on published case reports. Hepatology 63:590–603

9. Senior J (2007) Drug hepatotoxicity from a regulatory perspective. Clin Liver Dis 11:507–524

10. Yuan L, Kaplowitz N (2013) Mechanisms of drug-induced liver injury. Clin Liver Dis 17:507–518

11. Kaplowitz N (2002) Biochemical and cellular mechanisms of toxic liver injury. Semin Liver Dis 22:137–144

12. Iorga A, Dara L, Kaplowitz N (2017) Drug-induced liver injury: cascade of events leading to cell death, apoptosis or necrosis. Int J Mol Sci 18:1018

13. Jaeschke H (2011) Reactive oxygen and mechanisms of inflammatory liver injury: present concepts. J Gastroenterol Hepatol 26:173–179

14. Gibson J, Pumford N, Samokyszyn V et al (1996) Mechanism of acetaminophen-induced hepatotoxicity: covalent binding versus oxidative stress. Chem Res Toxicol 9:580–585

15. Uzi D, Barda L, Scaiewicz V et al (2013) CHOP is a critical regulator of acetaminophen-induced hepatotoxicity. J Hepatol 59:495–503

16. Saito C, Lemasters J, Jaeschke H (2010) c-Jun N-terminal kinase modulates oxidant stress and peroxynitrite formation independent of inducible nitric oxide synthase in acetaminophen hepatotoxicity. Toxicol Appl Pharmacol 246:8–17

17. Gunawan B, Kaplowitz N (2004) Clinical perspectives on xenobiotic-induced hepatotoxicity. Drug Metab Rev 36:301–312

18. Hanawa N, Shinohara M, Saberi B et al (2008) Role of JNK translocation to mitochondria leading inhibition of mitochondria bioenergetics in acetaminophen-induced liver injury. J Biol Chem 283:13565–13577

19. Shinohara M, Ybanez M, Win S et al (2010) Silencing GSK-3β inhibits acetaminophen hepatotoxicity and attenuates JNK activation and loss of GCL and Mcl-1. J Biol Chem 285:8244–8255

20. Saberi B, Ybanez M, Johnson H et al (2014) Protein kinase C (PKC) participates in mediates acetaminophen hepatotoxicity through JNK dependent and independent signaling pathways. Hepatology 59:1543–1554

21. Dara L, Johnson H, Suda J et al (2015) Receptor interacting protein kinase-1 mediates murine acetaminophen toxicity independent of the necrosome and not through necroptosis. Hepatology 62:1847–1857

22. Win S, Than T, Min R et al (2016) c-Jun N-terminal kinase mediates mouse liver injury through a novel sab (SH3BP5)-dependent pathway leading to inactivation of intramitochondrial Src. Hepatology 63:1987–2003

23. Sharma M, Gadang V, Jaeschke A (2012) Critical role for mixed-lineage kinase 3 in acetaminophen-induced hepatotoxicity. Mol Pharmacol 82:1001–1007

24. Nakagawa H, Maeda S, Hikiba Y et al (2008) Deletion of apoptosis signal-regulating kinase 1 attenuates acetaminophen-induced liver injury by inhibiting c-Jun N-terminal kinase activation. Gastroenterology 135:1311–1321

25. Zhang J, Min R, Le N et al (2017) Role of MAPK2 and p38 kinase in acute liver injury. models. Cell Death Dis 8:e2903

26. Welch M, Köck K, Urban T et al (2015) Toward predicting drug-induced liver injury: parallel computational approaches to identify multidrug resistance protein 4 and bile salt export pump inhibitors. Drug Metab Dispos 43:725–734

27. Win S, Than T, Le B et al (2015) Sab (SH3BP5) dependence of JNK-mediated inhibition of mitochondrial respiration in palmitic acid induced hepatocyte lipotoxicity. J Hepatol 62:1367–1374

28. Han D, Dara L, Johnson H et al (2013) Regulation of drug-induced liver injury by signal transduction pathways: critical role of mitochondria. Trends Pharmacol Sci 34:243–253

29. Dara L, Ji C, Kaplowitz N (2011) The contribution of endoplasmic reticulum stress to liver diseases. Hepatology 53:1752–1763

30. Win S, Than TA, Fernandez-Checa J et al (2014) JNK interaction with Sab mediates ER stress induced inhibition of mitochondrial respiration and cell death in primary mouse hepatocytes. Cell Death Dis 5:e989

31. Fiorese C, Haynes C (2017) Integrating the UPRmt into the mitochondrial maintenance network. Crit Rev Biochem Mol Biol 52:304–313

32. Chen Y, Dorn G (2013) PINK-1 phosphorylated mitofusin 2 is a parkin receptor for culling damaged mitochondria. Science 340:471–475

33. Ni H, Bockus A, Boggess N et al (2012) Activation of autophagy protects against acetaminophen-induced hepatotoxicity. Hepatology 55:222–232

34. Grove J, Aithal G (2015) Human leukocyte antigen genetic risk factors of drug-induced liver toxicology. Expert Opin Drug Metab Toxicol 11:395–409

35. Chen M, Borlak J, Tong W (2013) High lipophilicity and high daily dose of oral medications are associated with significant risk for drug-induced liver injury. Hepatology 58: 388–396

36. Bell L, Chalasani N (2009) Epidemiology of idiosyncratic drug-induced liver injury. Semin Liver Dis 29:337–347

37. Lucena MI, Andrade RJ, Kaplowitz N et al (2009) Phenotypic characterization of idiosyncratic drug-induced liver injury: the influence of age and sex. Hepatology 49:2001–2009

38. Aithal G, Ramsay L, Daly A et al (2004) Hepatic adducts, circulating antibodies, and cytokine polymorphisms in patients with diclofenac hepatotoxicity. Hepatology 39:1430–1440

39. Russmann S, Jetter A, Kullak-Ublick G (2010) Pharmacogenetics of drug-induced liver injury. Hepatology 52:748–761

40. Megherbi R, Kiorpelidou E, Foster B et al (2013) Role of protein haptenation in triggering maturation events in the dendritic cell surrogate cell line THP-1. Toxicol Appl Pharmacol 238:120–132

41. Monshi M, Faulkner L, Gibson A (2013) Human leukocyte antigen (HLA)-B*57:01-restricted activation of drug-specific T cells provides the immunological basis for flucloxacillin-induced liver injury. Hepatology 57:727–739

42. Pichler W (2002) Pharmacological interaction of drugs with antigenspecific immune receptors: the p-i concept. Curr Opin Allergy Clin Immunol 2:301–305

43. Wuillemin N, Adam J, Fontana R et al (2013) HLA haplotype determines hapten or p-i T cell reactivity to flucloxacillin. J Immunol 190: 4956–4964

44. Illing P, Vivian J, Dudek N et al (2012) Immune self-reactivity triggered by drugmodified HLA-peptide repertoire. Nature 486: 554–558

45. Ostrov D, Grant B, Pompeu Y et al (2012) Drug hypersensitivity caused by alteration of the MHC-presented self-peptide repertoire. Natl Acad Sci 109:9959–9964

46. Roth R, Maiuri A, Ganey P (2017) Idiosyncratic drug-induced liver injury: is drug-cytokine interaction the linchpin? J Pharmacol Exp Ther 360:461–470

47. Li A (2002) A review of the common properties of drugs with idiosyncratic hepatotoxicity and the 'multiple determinant hypothesis' for the manifestation of idiosyncratic drug toxicity. Chem Biol Interact 142:7–23

48. Ulrich R (2007) Idiosyncratic toxicity: a convergence of risk factors. Annu Rev Med 58:17–34

49. Dugan C, MacDonald A, Roth R (2010) A mouse model of severe halothane hepatitis based on human risk factors. J Pharmacol Exp Ther 333:364–372

50. Deng X, Luyendyk J, Ganey P et al (2009) Inflammatory stress and idiosyncratic hepatotoxicity: hints from animal models. Pharmacol Rev 61:262–282

51. Knolle P, Schlaak J, Uhrig A et al (1995) Human Kupffer cells secrete IL-10 in response to lipopolysaccharide (LPS) challenge. J Hepatol 22:226–229

52. Huang L, Soldevila G, Leeker M et al (1991) The liver eliminates T cells undergoing antigen-triggered apoptosis in vivo. Immunity 1: 741–749

53. Gorczynki R (1994) Adoptive transfer of unresponsiveness to allogeneic skin grafts with hepatic gamma delta + T cells. Immunology 81:27–35

54. Chalasani N, Bonkovsky H, Fontana R et al (2015) Features and outcomes of 899 patients with drug-induced liver injury: the DILIN prospective study. Gastroenterology 148: 1340–1352

55. Clayton T, Baker D, Lindon J et al (2009) Pharmacometabonomic identification of a significant hostmicrobiome metabolic interaction affecting human drug metabolism. Proc Natl Acad Sci 106:14728–14733

56. Thaiss C, Levy M, Korem T et al (2016) Microbiota diurnal rhythmicity programs host transcriptome oscillations. Cell 167:1495–1510

57. Chakraborty M, Fullerton A, Semple K et al (2015) Drug-induced allergic hepatitis develops in mice when myeloid-derived suppressor cells are depleted prior to halothane treatment. Hepatology 62:546–557

58. Metushi I, Hayes M, Uetrecht J et al (2015) Treatment of PD-1(−/−) mice with amodiaquine and anti-CTLA4 leads to liver injury similar to idiosyncratic liver injury in patients. Hepatology 61:1332–1342

59. Uetrecht J, Kaplowitz N (2015) Inhibition of immune tolerance unmasks drug-induced allergic hepatitis. Hepatology 62(346–8):2015

Part II

In Silico and Modeling Approaches

Chapter 2

Detection, Elimination, Mitigation, and Prediction of Drug-Induced Liver Injury in Drug Discovery

Francois Pognan

Abstract

Despite being among the most efficiently detected and managed toxicity during preclinical drug development, drug-induced liver injury (DILI) remains a major hurdle and is recognized to be a major cause of drug attrition and market withdrawal. DILI impacts many different sectors of society including patients, public health systems, health insurers and the pharmaceutical industry. Animal models are very efficient at detecting direct, dose-dependent and species-independent toxicity to the liver, the so-called intrinsic DILI. Compounds inducing mild liver signals can be developed as drugs if they exhibit a positive therapeutic benefit and are deemed to be superior to the currently available standard of care/medications. These cases are well managed as opposed to the unpredictable, dose-independent, individual-specific idiosyncratic toxicities, which are typically not detected in preclinical phases of drug development. Considerable efforts are dedicated to the detection and understanding of idiosyncratic DILI, and to the prediction of intrinsic DILI. Ever more complex and biologically relevant in vitro models are emerging for compound prescreening purposes. These data are also being used to the development of in silico algorithms which, when combined with compound chemical properties, in vivo observations and human-based post-marketing data, yield analytical and potentially predictive systems. In addition, the recent emergence of viable humanized liver animal models should bring forth a new battery of assays for accurately predicting compound-induced intrinsic liver toxicity in patients, and may also pave the way toward a better understanding of idiosyncratic DILI reactions.

Key words Drug-induced liver injury (DILI), In silico hepatotoxicity, In vitro hepatotoxicity, In vivo hepatotoxicity, Predictive toxicology, Intrinsic DILI; idiosyncratic DILI, Preclinical safety

1 Introduction

It is commonly recognized that drug-induced liver injury (DILI) remains one of the primary causes of drug development attrition and market withdrawal [1–5]. However, the overall detection and elimination of potentially hepatotoxic compounds during preclinical phases is somewhat effective [1, 6, 7]. Liver toxicity events represent one of the most common adverse side effects observed in both animal and human studies, most likely due to the high concentrations of xenobiotics to which liver is exposed and its

Minjun Chen and Yvonne Will (eds.), *Drug-Induced Liver Toxicity*, Methods in Pharmacology and Toxicology,
https://doi.org/10.1007/978-1-4939-7677-5_2, © Springer Science+Business Media, LLC, part of Springer Nature 2018

detoxifying role in the body. Direct and dose-proportional hepato-toxicity, also known as intrinsic DILI (Table 1), is the most common type of liver toxicity [8]. Intrinsic DILI is efficiently detected in preclinical studies and thus there are only very rare exceptions of human-specific intrinsic DILI cases. This is to be opposed to idio-syncratic DILI which is not dose dependent or operates through a direct action of the compounds to cells, but is rather the result of a unique combination of events usually involving the immune system leading to delayed and sometimes severe liver injury [9] (Table 1). Idiosyncratic DILI is very poorly translatable from one species to another, if at all. So far, there are no animal models that can be routinely used to uncover such events in preclinical development phases. These idiosyncratic reactions specific to human and consequential to a combination of uncommon conditions are not predictable in regulated preclinical animal studies [1, 9, 10]. Hence, despite an efficient elimination of most of hepatotoxic compounds during animal studies, some are being progressed and will induce liver events serious enough in humans to preclude the clinical development of otherwise very promising drug candidates. More infrequently, compounds can reach the drug status, i.e., being marketed after demonstrating an acceptable safety profile and successfully fulfilling all other criteria, and may trigger extremely rare but devastating idiosyncratic DILI when used within larger populations. Such cases may require organ transplant and may sometimes lead to a fatal outcome [11]. Beyond the dramatic impact on those patients, such adverse idiosyncratic DILI events waste vast amounts of money and time for the pharma industry, erode public trust into drugs in general, damage the reputation of the pharma industry, have a detrimental financial impact on public health systems, and most importantly delay patient access to new treatment options.

The necessity of eliminating these rare clinical DILI cases, either human-specific intrinsic or idiosyncratic, is imperative for all involved. Large efforts within the industry, in academic institutions, or addressed in private–public partnerships, are currently undertaken on a large scale of contributors and funding to match the height of the challenge. In addition, and most certainly more easily, in vitro and in silico detection of direct hepatotoxic compounds that would be detected in animal studies, will directly benefit from these efforts. The effects of such methods will be to eliminate poor drug candidates either before animals testing, hence having a real impact on 3Rs (refine, reduce, replace), or early in preclinical safety, refining candidate quality and avoiding potential accidents in human clinical trials (Fig. 1).

Table 1
Main differences between intrinsic and idiosyncratic drug-induced liver injury

Intrinsic DILI		Idiosyncratic DILI	
In vivo			
Predictable		Unpredictable	
High incidence		Very low incidence	
Dose dependent		Dose independent	
Direct mechanism of action, rapid tox development		Indirect MoA, usually involving the immune system, delayed tox events	
Mostly sex, species and individual-independent; external conditions may aggravate the DILI		Individual-specific with a concordance of various external conditions necessary for DILI	
Metabolic variations may introduce some sex and species differences		Metabolism involved in reactive metabolites, triggering immune reactions	
Severe DILI	Mild DILI	Severe DILI	Mild DILI
⬇	⬇	⬇	⬇
Compound stopped	May be progressed under certain conditions	Drug withdrawal	Mostly undiagnosed or unnoticed
Humanized animal models			
Predictable, useful for human specific metabolism-bound toxicities not linked to immune system		Hope in future dual humanized models: liver + bone marrow	
In vitro			
If mechanism known, toxicity can be recreated and used for screening and prediction		Models irrelevant	
In silico			
May predict with enough accurate and relevant data		May help the understanding and perhaps prediction in the future with enough relevant data	

This chapter reviews (1) the challenges faced by the pharma industry for the early detection of potential intrinsic hepatotoxic compounds and the associated opportunities for better and accelerated development of new drugs, (2) the current progresses of in silico, in vitro and in vivo approaches for predicting intrinsic DILI, (3) the difficulties and intricacies to address idiosyncratic DILI, (4) the current progress of in vitro and in silico approaches for understanding mechanisms of liver toxicity and species specificity, and (5) a brief mention of the challenges and promises borne by general public health-related big data collection.

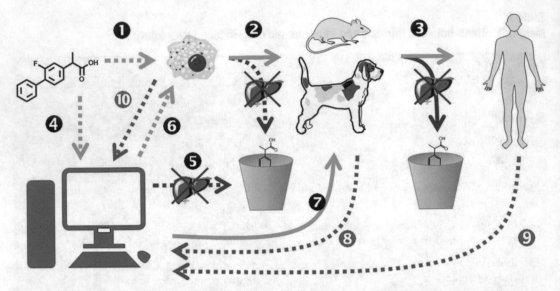

Fig. 1 Overall steps of compound elimination and learning feedback into in silico expert systems. New compounds may be tested in vitro in cell systems (❶) and eliminated before being tested in animals when hitting predefined criteria for suspicion of potential liver toxicity (❷; dotted red arrow) or progressed into in vivo testing (❷; plain green arrow). After testing in two different species, rodent and nonrodent, compounds showing unacceptable toxicity or with a too low safety margin are eliminated (❸; plain red arrow) or progressed into human healthy volunteers if fulfilling all preclinical safety criteria (❸; plain green arrow). Alternatively or in addition to early in vitro testing, in silico assessment may be performed (❹), and structures that are not passing predefined criteria may be either rejected (❺) or eventually tested in vitro for confirmation or invalidation of toxicity (❻) and follow steps 2 and 3 as previously. When there is enough confidence into predictive algorithms, compounds may skip the in vitro step, but will obligatory be tested in animals (❼) before being tested in humans (❸). All experimental data and knowledge acquired through actual testing can be used to refine and retrain the early in silico models (❽❾❿) that should constantly improve in sensitivity and specificity, that is in predictivity. Green arrows indicate positive progresses, red arrows symbolize rejection of potentially hazardous compounds, blue arrows represent knowledge feedback, and dotted arrows represent optional steps

2   Review

2.1   Preclinical In Vivo Detection of Intrinsic Hepatotoxicity Signals in Drug Development

Drug-induced liver toxicity is still a major hurdle for drug development and is considered as a major cause of attrition as well as of market drug-withdrawal [1, 8], despite a relatively good detection rate in preclinical toxicology [6, 7]. In animal studies, liver ranks as the top target organ for the occurrence of findings as obtained from the eTOX consortium database (Fig. 2a). The eTOX database comprises about 8000 extracted study reports from 13 participating pharmaceutical companies and represent a wide array of small chemical compounds, either stopped during development or progressed to the market (http://www.e-tox.net) [12–14]. One of the difficulties of translation of preclinical findings to human resides in part of the nature of the hepatotoxicity observed in animals. For example, Fig. 2b shows that hypertrophy, which can be adaptive or adverse, is the first type of finding and known to be

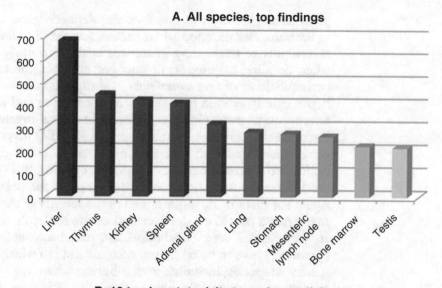

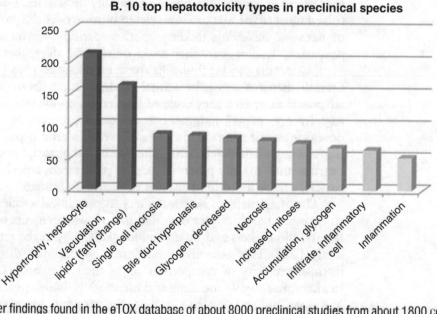

Fig. 2 Liver findings found in the eTOX database of about 8000 preclinical studies from about 1800 compounds and drugs. These studies include various routes of administration and a wide range of dosing duration, from 5 days to 2 years, with 28 days studies being the most represented. (a) Top ten findings for all preclinical species in the DB (mostly rat, followed by dog, monkey, rabbit, mouse, …). Liver is ranking first with close to 700 compounds recorded with at least one treatment-related hepatotoxicity event. (b) Top ten type of treatment-related hepatotoxicity findings for all species. Hypertrophy ranking first can only be detected by histopathology and usually does not lead to release of biomarkers in bloodstream

poorly detectable by classical blood-borne biomarkers [15]. Next finding in line, fat vacuoles in hepatocytes, follows more or less the same principle. Such a finding in isolation would not stop the development of a compound, especially if the safety margin [16] between the lowest dose inducing hepatocyte hypertrophy and the pharmacological dose is comfortable, depending on the disease indication. The duration of treatment foreseen in clinic and the reversibility of the finding in animals is also extremely important when deciding to progress or not. For example, the exaggerated accumulation of phospholipids (phospholipidosis—PLD) in hepatocyte lysosomes is both relatively common and not seen as adverse on its own. However, if found in several organs or in key organs such as brain or heart at high density, PLD may create concerns. Associated with liver enzyme elevation but without other noticeable adverse events like hepatocyte necrosis, PLD would create debates about its relevance and danger potential, or lack thereof. Again the therapeutic index as well as the severity of the indication may grant a continued development of the molecule or not [16]. In addition, all drug metabolism and pharmacokinetic (DMPK) parameters have to be taken into account and can widely vary from species to species, including within human where the genetic heterogeneity introduces further predictability difficulties. DMPK has solved most of the metabolism-related hurdles over the past couple of decades, including tackling species-specific liver metabolism, potentially leading to either toxic or reactive drug metabolites. Further details can be found in these excellent reviews [17–20]. Overall, hepatotoxicity in animal studies ranges from clear cut adverse toxicity to a grey zone of borderline events which require case by case expert judgment in order to progress or stop the development of compounds. Hence, even if a mild hepatotoxicity signal is indeed detected during the preclinical phases, a compound bearing some toxicity potential may be progressed, especially if the toxicity can be monitored and/or mitigated in human.

The assessment of hepatotoxicity in preclinical species is routinely evaluated through a combination of measurements of plasma hepatic biomarkers and by tissue histopathology at the end of the study [21]. This assessment efficiently detects the direct (i.e., intrinsic) toxicity of compounds or of their metabolites. If biomarkers are roughly the same and identifying similar toxicity types in human and in animals [22], there are very few opportunities to directly assess morphological alterations in human biopsies. This is somehow hindering the ability to learn from clinical cases and makes the systematic assessment of human relevance very difficult. Nonetheless, this intrinsic toxicity of compounds to liver (e.g., to hepatocytes—necrosis, apoptosis, phospholipidosis, steatosis, hypertrophy, hyperplasia, preneoplastic transformations; to Kupffer cells—necrosis, senescence, downregulation; to sinusoidal cells— necrosis, apoptosis, proliferation; to cholangiocytes and the hepatobiliary system—intrahepatic and extrahepatic cholestasis, hypertrophy, hyperplasia; to stellate cells—activation and fibrosis induction) is thoroughly managed during preclinical and clinical development. The search for new biomarkers of hepatotoxicity, more translatable, more sensitive, more specific or prodromal is now yielding a whole array of possibilities [21, 23], from which the micro RNA 122 (miR122) is one of the most promising [24]. However, currently only the classical Liver Biochemical Tests are routinely used, but are known to be neither specific, nor sensitive, nor prodromal. Alanine aminotransferase (ALT) for example can be released by a large number of other organs than liver [25] or its plasma concentration even increased by reduced Kupffer cell clearance unrelated to any toxicity event [26, 27]. Thus, even well established and validated liver biomarkers cannot be fully trusted.

When only one out of two preclinical toxicology species shows signs of hepatotoxicity, the question of species-specific mechanisms and human relevance needs to be asked, often supported by investigative studies [28], eventually allowing some compounds to progress despite being associated with liver safety signals. In addition, it is not infrequent to observe liver signals out of one animal in a group of ten, leading to statistically nonsignificant variations. Besides, these odd cases are not always in the highest dose group rendering its relationship to treatment questionable. This kind of case is always puzzling and broadly ignored until and unless some events in clinic may force one to reconsider the significance of isolated single animal signals in preclinical studies. These may be just meaningless coincidences or represent a hint of idiosyncratic-like toxicity. The paucity of the literature regarding possible links between human idiosyncratic DILI and individual animal sensitivity to a compound tends to highlight the lack of possibility to extrapolate from one to the other.

These considerations are true for both small chemical and biological entities. For the latter however, the choice of the preclinical species is of particular importance since the target specificity of biologics is usually very high and may lack efficacy in classical rodent and nonrodent species (ICH S6 guidance; www.fda.gov/downloads/drugs/guidancecomplianceregulatoryinformation/guidances/ucm074957.pdf).

In summary, compounds inducing frank intrinsic liver toxicity (biomarkers elevation combined with histopathological findings proportional to dose exposure) in preclinical animal species are readily eliminated and not progressed further. However, there are multiple case configurations where the whole data package generated in preclinical studies and overall expert assessments (in vitro off-target profiles, in vitro cellular assays, in vivo toxicology and DMPK studies, consideration about reversibility of findings, monitorability of toxicity in clinical trials, indication severity, unmet medical needs and safety margins) are necessary to take decision about further progression of compounds. All these parameters are necessary to reply to the five key questions as defined by Kramer et al. [29]: (1) what is the safety margin, (2) is the toxicity reversible, (3) is there a biomarker, (4) what is the mechanism, and (5) what is the relevance of the finding to humans. Finally, absence of any signal in preclinical species certainly increases the chances of dealing with a safe future drug, but does not guarantee its innocuousness in human.

2.2 Prediction In Silico and Screening Out Intrinsic Hepatotoxicity In Vitro

Ideally, drug developers would prefer to eliminate compounds bearing intrinsic DILI before animal studies in order to increase compound selection quality and concentrate as early as possible on "liver-optimized" chemical series. Identifying potential toxicity liabilities before actually testing compounds in vivo can arguably be called predictive toxicology. According to the Webster dictionary, to predict means "to declare or tell in advance." The same dictionary also tells us that "prophesy" is synonymous to "prediction," but takes care to differentiate the terms. "Prophesy usually means to predict future events by the aid of divine or supernatural inspiration," while "To predict is usually to foretell with precision of calculation, knowledge or shrewd inference from facts or experience." The latter definition is precisely what predictive toxicology is about and acquisition of large amount of high quality data (knowledge and facts) is necessary for prediction (precision of calculation), as well as the expert knowledge for interpretation of data by experienced toxicologists (knowledge and shrewd inference). In actuality, "prediction" in this context is more about determining the rank order probability for one compound to induce a specific event, compared to a number of other chemicals belonging to the same chemical space. Two different approaches are used and developed: (1) compilation of data and/or knowledge into in silico algorithms to predict potential toxicity, and (2) the use of cellular assays in vitro to predict in vivo toxicity and eventually to feed in silico algorithms with standardized numerical data.

Several in silico approaches can be used to establish predictive algorithms, and not being exhaustive here, further details can be found in these thorough didactic reviews [30, 31]. Compound pattern recognition using publicly available data [32], structural alerts based on structure similarities and known in vivo outcomes [33], and quantitative structure–activity relationship (QSAR) [34], are likely the most popular. The one common ground to all approaches is the necessity of obtaining standardized good quality data in large quantity enough to both ensure the specificity of the prediction (enough training data set within the chemical space of the query) and accuracy (correct data details within that chemical space). This is undeniably an issue for several reasons: first, publicly available data are not standardized, each laboratory using their own internal procedures, always ever so slightly differing from the next institution; second, published data are not systematically quality checked in a thorough way leading to an alarming lack of reproducibility [35] and therefore to questioning of the accuracy or even worst, the legitimacy of the data; and third, data in the public domain are mostly not in the current druggable chemical space that the pharma industry is using. To palliate some of these lacks, the outcomes of some welcomed initiatives are now accessible, like the SWEETLEAD database (https://simtk.org/home/sweetlead) [36]. This repository contains curated data of chemical structures, e.g., a number of accurate chemical descriptors of marketed drugs and of a good amount of chemicals classified as nontoxic. Associated toxicology data are not in this chemical structure repository and these have to be found elsewhere and reassociated to each structure. This next step would be a colossal endeavor as corresponding accessible in vivo data would have to be fetched from various sources, mostly within summaries of published clinical trials available through various health authorities websites, either directly reachable or upon request for a specific project [37–39]. In any case, the most standardized in vivo data, run under Good Laboratory Practices (GLP) are the privately owned preclinical animal toxicology study reports, hence not available to the public scientific community. Fortunately, under the aegis of the European Innovative Medicine Initiative (IMI—www.imi.europa.eu), the eTOX consortium has collected undisclosed preclinical data of about 1800 chemical structures with a mix of compound stopped during preclinical and clinical phases, as well as of marketed and withdrawn drugs. This database has the advantage of getting together chemical structures and toxicology data overlapping with the druggable chemical space (World Drug Index database), ascertaining its relevance for drug development (Fig. 3). Unfortunately, the eTOX database is far from being exhaustive compared to all drugs ever marketed and even less compared to all compounds ever tested in animals, but is nonetheless most likely the largest database of its kind. Using these relevant data after normalization of terms (ontology-related issues to be found here [40]) for the building of predictive algorithms should yield the most trustable algorithms, but will still need to pass a number of validations before being accepted [41].

In summary, the few in silico algorithms existing for the prediction of liver toxicity are not routinely used in the pharma industry for all the reasons said above. Algorithms for "simpler" calculation, like hERG inhibition, are demonstrating the possibility of their use in drug development, but more complex predictions are not yet ready for application. Even if all conditions, including large amount of reliable quality data were available, the last and perhaps worst hurdle would remain: knowing that a compound will be liver toxic (however defined) is just not enough; a safety margin above the pharmacological dose is the essential knowledge to take a formal decision to stop or progress a compound. Consequently, in vitro assays where a therapeutic index, i.e., the efficacious dose in a cell system versus the toxic dose in the same or a similar cell assay, can be calculated have largely been privileged so far to eliminate the "bad" compounds.

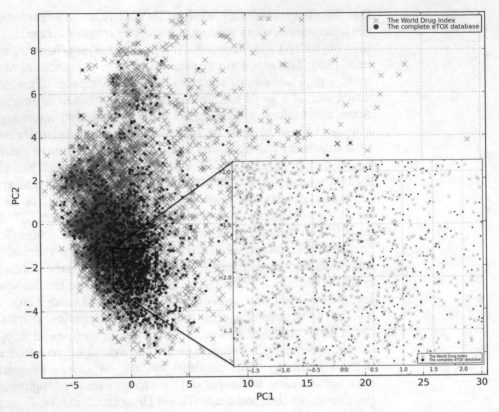

Fig. 3 The eTOX chemical space coverage overlapping the World Drug Index (WDI—www.daylight.com/products/wdi.html) which contains the structures of all marketed drugs worldwide (about 80,000 compounds). PCA plot using above 100 chemical descriptors representation, with a zoom-in in the most populated area. Blue crosses: WDI structures, red dots: eTOX structures

However, in vitro assays to eliminate those compounds that would directly hit hepatocytes have been used with more (acute toxicity) or mostly less success (chronic toxicity—the one of greatest interest). Until recently such in vitro assays were as straightforward as measuring cytotoxicity concentration 50 (CC_{50}) on cells lines easy to cultivate like HepG2, with the hope that such a simplistic approach would somehow reflect in vivo hepatotoxicity potential [42]. Increasing the complexity of the endpoints for measuring cytotoxicity, like calling upon mitochondrial swelling or lysosomal mass or any other cellular features consequential to cell death, is only adding to data analysis difficulties, but does not improve the irrelevance of the final endpoint: cytotoxicity. There are multiple reasons why this did not work and cannot work, ranging from the difficulty to extrapolate in vitro drug concentration and exposure in vivo, to lack of cell-, organ-, humoral- and hormonal-interactions, and mostly, lack of proper hepatocyte biology. Many more reasons have been largely discussed elsewhere [43–47], but it should finally be kept in mind that isolated hepatocytes do not constitute a liver. Refined assays have been developed over the years, either using less aberrant cells than HepG2s, e.g., HepaRG, primary hepatocytes or stem-cell derived hepatocyte-like cells in various culture configurations [46–50]. There is still no strong evidence that more elaborate systems would actually be able to predict intrinsic DILI, but there is certainly an impressive weight of evidence that combination of cocultures (e.g., with Kupffer cells, endothelial vascular cells or any nonparenchymal cell combination), addition of extracellular matrices, 3D configuration and fluidics movement of medium, all greatly improves the functional biology of hepatocytes in culture, and perhaps brings such systems closer to an in vivo liver [48, 51–58]. A number of functional assays which endpoints can be assessed or quantified by high content imaging are possible and already used for mechanistic understanding of cell toxicity [59, 60]. It is quite clear that compounds inducing cholestasis in vivo would not be detected by a cytotoxicity test in vitro, but rather by a functional assay in hepatocytes looking at the inhibition of canaliculi transporters. It is therefore quite possible that optimizing conditions for proper hepatic biology with elaborated and functional endpoints may lead toward in vitro assays that will be at least in part able to identify compounds with potential hepatic toxicity. It is still too early to assert if any of these elaborate functional liver-like systems will be used for safety assessment and if decisions can be made from them without running ulterior in vivo studies [61] as can already be done for skin irritancy [62]. Certainly a level of standardization for comparison of performance and reproducibility from one laboratory to the next, will be necessary. Here again, consortia like MIP-DILI running under the IMI umbrella should help defining which bunch of assays is the most adapted to drug development needs and what level of standardization needs to be achieved [63].

Human primary cell sources will remain a practical limitation for extensive use in safety assessment. Also, donor to donor variations introduce the need to test compounds not just once in technical replicates but also with multiple donors to assess the biological variations, or the "responsiveness" of various donors. This is both an advantage and disadvantage since it increases the quality of the assessment but also the workload and associated costs. Another avenue which may help these hurdles is the development of iPS-derived and/or adult stem cells-derived hepatocytes which could fix both the lot-to-lot variations and provide abundant cells supply. However, currently such cells are derived from an embryonic-like phase and do retain fetal characteristics which can be gradually improved with culture conditions and duration [64, 65], which may or not be of importance. Nonetheless, this approach can also open the door to screen compounds for certain genetic conditions by using diseased rather than healthy donors [66–68]. In addition, some cellular amplification can be obtained through liver-humanized mice [69]. This may not be quite the whole requirements for idiosyncratic investigations, but is certainly getting closer to real life conditions.

2.3   Idiosyncratic Hepatotoxicity

As opposed to intrinsic liver toxicity which is dose and time dependent, hits all individuals, and is often predictable from one species to the next, idiosyncrasy results from a unique combination of genetic background, gender, ethnicity, age, lifestyle and hygiene, diversity of microbiome, environmental stress and pollution, preexisting diseases and comedications [9, 11, 23, 70]. The category "genetic background" is a collection of physiological traits such as endogenous metabolism, xenobiotic metabolism, polymorphism, genetic mutations, genetic variations such as SNPs, and of course the variability of the immune system and the various haplotypes susceptible to react to neoantigens [11, 70]. Clearly, such cases cannot be tracked in classical animal studies with homogeneous, inbred, young, healthy animals with an equilibrated food regimen and standardized "lifestyle". Developing approaches where either old animals, diseased animal models, outbred species, increasing to a very large number of animals per group or any other ways to mimic patient diversity is laudable but unrealistic in a screening mode. Unambiguously, the multiplicity of combination is just too large for tempting reproducing all the possibilities and would cost too much time, number of animals, resources and compound volume needed for testing and would engender endless model validations. In addition, the clinical identification of idiosyncratic DILI is not straightforward, leaving the build of corresponding preclinical models somewhat challenging. The link of causality involving a drug to a liver abnormality in a diseased population often largely medicated, cannot be always clearly established [10, 23]. It cannot be ignored that a large number of unexpected DILI also comes from "traditional" herbal remedies [10] that patients may take as self-comedication and forget to make mention of it to their physicians. This and other factors, like underreporting alcohol consumption, may lead to difficult data interpretation, rendering preclinical strategies to address idiosyncratic DILI particularly difficult. Normalizations of intrinsic and idiosyncratic DILI diagnostics have been established such as the RUCAM causality assessment [10]. These kinds of initiatives will help better characterization and learning out of DILI, enabling efficient classification of liver toxicity events, and perhaps reverse translatability to animal data.

Currently, the pharma industry does not possess the means to evaluate, detect and eliminate compounds with idiosyncratic DILI potential. Therefore, until a practical solution(s) is found for the prediction of such cases, there will be new cases of idiosyncratic toxicities with future new drugs. However, large efforts are made in this direction, either in large consortia, in private institutions or in biotechs. Approaches taken are multiple, from in silico algorithms to complex in vitro systems, to humanized liver animal models. In vitro cellular assays are akin to those described in Sect. 2.2, but entirely dedicated to human systems and their peculiarities. However, recreating circumstances needed to generate idiosyncratic conditions seems very unlikely if not simply impossible. In silico algorithms greedy of large volume of accurate information cannot rely on such in vitro systems suspected of being irrelevant as an information source, and therefore will need to feed on sparse identified human cases. Consequently, it will likely require many more years of data collection and idiosyncrasy understanding before being truly applicable. Hence, some hopes are turning to humanized animal models. Indeed, relatively recent and remarkable technical breakthroughs have allowed the creation of mice bearing humanized liver [71–74]. Several methodologies have emerged permitting mice to support up to 95% of human hepatocytes in replacement of their own, and may remain alive for many months [75]. This is needed for chronic treatment from which most liver toxicities are dependent, and particularly the immune-mediated ones. Such models allow the detection of human-specific liver toxicity with the advantage of producing in vivo and in situ human specific metabolites and follow human liver biology. As a consequence, any human-specific intrinsic DILI not detected in classical animal studies should be sizeable in these humanized animals [76]. However, despite the advantages of this human compartment, everything else remains murine and particularly the immune system, or what is left of it since all models use immuno-compromised animals in order to tolerate the human cells [71–73]. On the other hand, humanized mice for immune cells already exist [74, 77] and it is only matter of time before usable mouse models combining both humanized liver and immune system emerge. Some attempts in that direction are already published [72, 78], but difficulties remains substantial, particularly if one wants both cell compartments from the same or compatible donors [72, 79]. Thorough validation of their predictive value will have to be done before triggering a large use in the pharma industry. In addition, the current cost associated with the use of these mice remains far too high to use in routine screening and can be used only for mechanistic investigations for the time being. With time and larger use, the cost may fall but the production rate of these complex models may then become limiting.

In summary, the idiosyncratic toxicity detection problem is unlikely to be quickly solved by using wet experimental approaches. Likewise, dry or in silico methodologies using knowledge from the understanding of how these cases happen in human, seem possible but still remote. Extensive additional knowledge will be necessary before it becomes reality, some of it potentially coming from "big data" collection (see Sect. 2.5).

2.4 Understanding Mechanisms of Hepatotoxicity

In vitro "black box" systems like measuring cytotoxicity without knowing why or how cells are dying and if it may correspond to anything possible in vivo, does not yield much added value. Even if a serendipitous statistical correlation happens between the CC_{50} ranking order of a chemical series and the in vivo hepatotoxicity potency, the lack of understanding of how this statistical correlation could translate into a biological relationship, very certainly means a one-off lucky outcome that may never repeat. Only the understanding of mechanisms of toxicity may allow the conception of better, more functional assays incorporating the right conditions to let emerge a cellular alteration similar to those observed in vivo. An astute reader would argue that therefore, a prior in vivo knowledge, or at least a detailed description of in vivo hepatotoxicity, is needed before building a mechanistic in vitro system. Henceforth, such assays would not be able to predict toxicity, but only mimic it after the knowledge has already been generated. In addition, if a compound has already been tested in vivo, it seems superfluous to test it in a less relevant and somewhat artifactual in vitro arrangement. This is certainly right, but absolutely necessary to progress efficacious management of preclinical toxicities. Efforts have to be conceded by drug makers to elaborate afterward in vitro mechanistic assays that will help both the understanding of in vivo findings and the building of predictive screening for future chemical series. In vitro assays that recapitulate at least in part a relevant biology trait can be used to identify future compounds affecting this feature. It is only by understanding how drugs can induce cholestasis in vivo that in vitro cholestatic-like assays can be elaborated. Therefore prior in vivo knowledge is applied to in vitro assays for future screening out potential cholestatic drugs. Likewise, when a lead compound is displaying hepatotoxicity in vivo and an assay can be devised to mimic this toxicity, backup compounds may be triaged in vitro, using the lead compound as positive control and benchmark for the selection of the best backup [28]. This methodology which could be called "transparent-box assay strategy," leads however to an unavoidable difficulty which is the multiplicity of assays, each corresponding to optimized conditions for each specific type of identified liver toxicities. This is again conducting to high resources demands if used routinely, especially since this scheme cannot be limited to liver only.

This line of attack also means sizeable investments to characterize and unravel in vivo toxicity mechanisms. Indeed, the simple description of a toxicity event as thorough as it can be, is not enough to determine if it is linked to on- or off-target, what cellular compartment would be the initial culprit or victim, what would be the initiating molecular event and the whole cascade conducting to an adverse outcome. For a number of years, both individual initiatives and consortium organizations have produced large amounts of data, mostly using gene expression analysis [80], but also using various tools to knock-down/out or knockin specific genes [81–83], run large genetic-linked analyses in human [84], and more recently studying the important role of epigenetics imprinting [85, 86]. Compilation, organization and visualization of these large amount of data is also key for a proper use and several open access resources are now available such as the FDA Liver Toxicity Knowledge Base (LTKB) [87], knowledge-based like the OECD-driven Adverse Outcome Pathways initiative (AOP—http://aopkb.org), or epigenome data like the International Human Epigenome Consortium Data Portal (IHEC—http://epigenomesportal.ca/ihec) [88]. To a large extent, this has yielded novel insights into toxicity mechanisms, as well as hints for the molecular basis of species specificity [89, 90], which are key for assessing the translatability of data. In a way, this also often leads to a more relevant choice of nonrodent second species for the in vivo assessment of drug candidates.

Data generated in transparent-box assays in vitro can be used for elaborating predictive algorithms based on biological understanding and not just on statistical correlations. There are still no evidences that such algorithms are predictive, but if they turn out to be, one can argue that they will be predictive of in vitro assays and not of real in vivo findings. That is why algorithms that combine both in vitro and in vivo data should have more chances to achieve a good predictivity [91, 92].

Overall, mechanistic toxicology is an area that necessitate a fair investment but also yields indispensable knowledge for the build of both in silico algorithm and relevant in vitro cellular assays for the selection of best lead compounds [28].

2.5 Big Data

As seen earlier, one of the main issues for predictive toxicology is the collection and access to enough relevant and quality data into the drug able chemical space and associated preclinical and clinical data, to ensure prediction with precision of calculation, knowledge or shrewd inference from facts and experience. Therefore, the recent advent of the possibility to collect a very large amount of health-related data should be a great opportunity for predictive toxicology [93, 94]. Three broad different categories of these data can be defined: (1) scientific, (2) post-marketing safety, and (3) general population sports-like data.

The stunning technology progresses in scientific data generation such as gene and RNA sequencing, and epigenetic profiling of large human population samples is creating on its own a category of big data, that will influence our knowledge and how we will have to handle personalized medicine and safety [93, 95]. This type of data is only starting to amass, but it is expected to very rapidly grow exponentially. These data will have to be turned into knowledge which is done by expert scientists with the support of ever more innovative bioinformatics tools. Some time will be needed to have a positive impact on predictive toxicology, but there are little doubts that it will happen and may change the future of personalized safety assessment [96].

Post-marketing safety and health data collections are of another nature and represent a large and yet still underused sources of potential knowledge for the understanding human-specific DILI biological mechanisms [97]. Each country has arranged large public health records collections. Exploiting these data is delicate as a lot of various data types are gathered, sometimes not fully organized or standardized, as well as with a fair amount of background noise that will be very strenuous to sort afterward [98, 99]. Various systems are being used not only from one institution to another, but also within the same organization leading to a great lack of interoperability [100]. In addition a number of ethical issues may hinder data access [98, 101, 102]. Nonetheless, considering that these health records are from real situations, i.e., human populations treated on a large scale with marketed drugs and facing all the diversity met in real life conditions, these data sources should be in the heart of data collection and analysis for the good sake, among many others aspects [103–105], of predictive safety [103, 106]. Indeed some attempts of cross-country harmonization are on their way [107, 108].

The large use of public health trackers devices, such as connected watches and other such contraptions permanently monitoring "health" data, is generating exponential data volume that theoretically, should bring undefined additional knowledge about the impact of medication on human health. The main issue using these data will be triaging out the yet undetermined volume of polluting background noise intertwined into the informative figures [109, 110]. On one hand, these devices record "health" data in real and continuous time, and at an ever growing rate fulfilling the need for human related data in very large amount. On the other hand, this is done in an uncontrolled manner, accumulating tremendous amount of unwanted background noise. It is still unknown how these data can and will be used, misused or abused [111].

3   Conclusion and Future Directions

Compound-induced intrinsic liver toxicity is readily detected in animal preclinical studies at a reasonable high rate. Some cases of human-specific intrinsic toxicity may be missed in animal studies, especially with biological drugs, but should be detectable in more elaborated in vitro human cell-based assays. Altogether, in vitro animal and human cellular assays should be able to identify compounds bearing potential liver toxicity before running animal studies and therefore have a true impact on the 3Rs. However, in some cases compounds with liver signals can be knowingly progressed especially when beneficiating from a large safety margin, reliable toxicity biomarkers, reversibility of adverse events, or evidence for adaptive rather than adverse outcomes. In other words, some intrinsic liver toxicity can be managed and mitigated when identified and relatively well characterized. Prediction of how these compounds will behave in human should be in theory relatively easy from data and knowledge generated in vitro and in vivo before moving into clinic. This intrinsic toxicity even if human specific, is not so much of an issue as opposed to idiosyncratic toxicity which is basically by definition, unpredictable. New types of data, coming from:

- In vitro physiologically relevant cellular assays,
- In vivo humanized models,
- Systematic genetic and epigenetic information, especially the one related to the immune system variations,
- Yet underused sources of information like electronic health records
- New sources of data like the "big data" collected from public use of connected health monitors despite its messiness,

should allow the elaboration of in silico algorithms usable in drug development. Overall, if not yet in systematic use in the pharma industry for all the abovementioned issues, in silico algorithms should constitute the spearhead of toxicity prediction. Possibly, elaborated humanized animal models will, in some undefined future, allow the detection of the most common of the uncommon idiosyncratic toxicities.

The following chapters of this book will go into further details about approaches for developing predictive algorithms, "transparent-box cellular assays" development and use, emerging liver biomarkers in clinic, the difficulties to establish the causal relationship drug-liver toxicity in clinical trials and many more aspects of DILI. All these following chapters illustrate one of the most difficult tasks to come for in silico predictive algorithm moving forward. This will be to transition from the paucity of relevant and usable information of the recent past, to the ability to gather, sort and use overwhelming volumes of pertinent but heterogeneous data in the very near future.

Acknowledgments

Dr. Jonathan Moggs is warmly thanked for his thorough and insightful review of the manuscript.

References

1. Regev A (2014) Drug-induced liver injury and drug development: industry perspective. Semin Liver Dis 34(2):227–239. https://doi.org/10.1055/s-0034-1375962
2. van Tonder JJ, Steenkamp V, Gulumi M (2013) Pre-clinical assessment of the potential intrinsic hepatotoxicity of candidate drugs. In: Gowder S (ed) New insights into toxicity and drug testing. InTech, London, pp 3–28. https://doi.org/10.5772/54792
3. Galie N, Hoeper MM, Gibbs JS, Simonneau G (2011) Liver toxicity of sitaxentan in pulmonary arterial hypertension. Eur Respir J 37(2):475–476. https://doi.org/10.1183/09031936.00194810
4. Jaeschke H (2007) Troglitazone hepatotoxicity: are we getting closer to understanding idiosyncratic liver injury? Toxicol Sci 97(1):1–3. https://doi.org/10.1093/toxsci/kfm021
5. Watkins PB (2005) Insight into hepatotoxicity: the troglitazone experience. Hepatology 41(2):229–230. https://doi.org/10.1002/hep.20598
6. Olson H, Betton G, Stritar J, Robinson D (1998) The predictivity of the toxicity of pharmaceuticals in humans from animal data—an interim assessment. Toxicol Lett 102–103:535–538
7. Olson H, Betton G, Robinson D, Thomas K, Monro A, Kolaja G, Lilly P, Sanders J, Sipes G, Bracken W, Dorato M, Van Deun K, Smith P, Berger B, Heller A (2000) Concordance of the toxicity of pharmaceuticals in humans and in animals. Regul Toxicol Pharmacol 32(1):56–67. https://doi.org/10.1006/rtph.2000.1399
8. van Tonder JJ, Steenkamp V, Gulumian M (2013) Pre-clinical assessment of the potential intrinsic hepatotoxicity of candidate drugs. In: Gowder S (ed) New insights into toxicity and drug testing. InTech, London, pp 3–28. https://doi.org/10.5772/54792
9. Kaplowitz N (2005) Idiosyncratic drug hepatotoxicity. Nat Rev Drug Discov 4(6):489–499. https://doi.org/10.1038/nrd1750
10. Chalasani NP, Hayashi PH, Bonkovsky HL, Navarro VJ, Lee WM, Fontana RJ, Gastroenterol AC (2014) ACG clinical guideline: the diagnosis and management of idiosyncratic drug-induced liver injury. Am J Gastroenterol 109(7):950–966. https://doi.org/10.1038/ajg.2014.131
11. Chen MJ, Suzuki A, Borlak J, Andrade RJ, Lucena MI (2015) Drug-induced liver injury: interactions between drug properties and host factors. J Hepatol 63(2):503–514
12. Briggs K, Cases M, Heard DJ, Pastor M, Pognan F, Sanz F, Schwab CH, Steger-Hartmann T, Sutter A, Watson DK, Wichard JD (2012) Inroads to predict in vivo toxicology-an introduction to the eTOX Project. Int J Mol Sci 13(3):3820–3846. https://doi.org/10.3390/ijms13033820
13. Cases M, Briggs K, Steger-Hartmann T, Pognan F, Marc P, Kleinoder T, Schwab CH, Pastor M, Wichard J, Sanz F (2014) The eTOX data-sharing project to advance in silico drug-induced toxicity prediction. Int J Mol Sci 15(11):21136–21154. https://doi.org/10.3390/ijms151121136
14. Steger-Hartmann T, Pognan F (2017) The eTOX Consortium: to improve the safety assessment of new drug candidates. Pharm Med 19(1):4–13
15. Hall AP, Elcombe CR, Foster JR, Harada T, Kaufmann W, Knippel A, Kuttler K, Malarkey DE, Maronpot RR, Nishikawa A, Nolte T, Schulte A, Strauss V, York MJ (2012) Liver hypertrophy: a review of adaptive (adverse and non-adverse) changes—conclusions from the 3rd international ESTP expert workshop. Toxicol Pathol 40(7):971–994. https://doi.org/10.1177/0192623312448935
16. Muller PY, Milton MN (2012) The determination and interpretation of the therapeutic index in drug development. Nat Rev Drug Discov 11(10):751–761. https://doi.org/10.1038/nrd3801
17. Yengi LG, Leung L, Kao J (2007) The evolving role of drug metabolism in drug discovery and development. Pharm Res 24(5):842–858. https://doi.org/10.1007/s11095-006-9217-9
18. Pelkonen O, Turpeinen M, Uusitalo J, Rautio A, Raunio H (2005) Prediction of drug metabolism and interactions on the basis of in vitro investigations. Basic Clin Pharmacol 96(3):167–175. https://doi.org/10.1111/j.1742-7843.2005.pto960305.x
19. Park BK, Boobis A, Clarke S, Goldring CEP, Jones D, Kenna JG, Lambert C, Laverty HG, Naisbitt DJ, Nelson S, Nicoll-Griffith DA, Obach RS, Routledge P, Smith DA, Tweedie DJ, Vermeulen N, Williams DP, Wilson ID, Baillie TA (2011) Managing the challenge of chemically reactive metabolites in drug development. Nat Rev Drug Discov 10(4):292–306. https://doi.org/10.1038/nrd3408
20. Kirchmair J, Goller AH, Lang D, Kunze J, Testa B, Wilson ID, Glen RC, Schneider G (2015) Predicting drug metabolism:

experiment and/or computation? Nat Rev Drug Discov 14(6):387–404. https://doi.org/10.1038/nrd4581

21. Corsini A, Ganey P, Ju C, Kaplowitz N, Pessayre D, Roth R, Watkins PB, Albassam M, Liu BL, Stancic S, Suter L, Bortolini M (2012) Current challenges and controversies in drug-induced liver injury. Drug Saf 35(12):1099–1117

22. Weiler S, Merz M, Kullak-Ublick GA (2015) Drug-induced liver injury: the dawn of biomarkers? F1000Prime Rep 7:34. 10.12703/P7-34

23. Fontana RJ (2014) Pathogenesis of idiosyncratic drug-induced liver injury and clinical perspectives. Gastroenterology 146(4):914–U437. https://doi.org/10.1053/j.gastro.2013.12.032

24. Thakral S, Ghoshal K (2015) miR-122 is a unique molecule with great potential in diagnosis, prognosis of liver disease, and therapy both as miRNA mimic and antimir. Curr Gene Ther 15(2):142–150. https://doi.org/10.2174/1566523214666141224095610

25. Yang RZ, Park S, Reagan WJ, Goldstein R, Zhong S, Lawton M, Rajamohan F, Qian K, Liu L, Gong DW (2009) Alanine aminotransferase isoenzymes: molecular cloning and quantitative analysis of tissue expression in rats and serum elevation in liver toxicity. Hepatology 49(2):598–607. https://doi.org/10.1002/hep.22657

26. Radi ZA, Koza-Taylor PH, Bell RR, Obert LA, Runnels HA, Beebe JS, Lawton MP, Sadis S (2011) Increased serum enzyme levels associated with kupffer cell reduction with no signs of hepatic or skeletal muscle injury. Am J Pathol 179(1):240–247. https://doi.org/10.1016/j.ajpath.2011.03.029

27. Wang T, Papoutsi M, Wiesmann M, DeCristofaro M, Keselica MC, Skuba E, Spaet R, Markovits J, Wolf A, Moulin P, Pognan F, Vancutsem P, Petryk L, Sutton J, Chibout SD, Kluwe W (2011) Investigation of correlation among safety biomarkers in serum, histopathological examination, and toxicogenomics. Int J Toxicol 30(3):300–312. https://doi.org/10.1177/1091581811401920

28. Moggs J, Moulin P, Pognan F, Brees D, Leonard M, Busch S, Cordier A, Heard DJ, Kammuller M, Merz M, Bouchard P, Chibout SD (2012) Investigative safety science as a competitive advantage for Pharma. Expert Opin Drug Metab Toxicol 8(9):1071–1082. https://doi.org/10.1517/17425255.2012.693914

29. Kramer JA, Sagartz JE, Morris DL (2007) The application of discovery toxicology and pathology towards the design of safer pharmaceutical lead candidates. Nat Rev Drug Discov 6(8):636–649. https://doi.org/10.1038/nrd2378

30. Raies AB, Bajic VB (2016) In silico toxicology: computational methods for the prediction of chemical toxicity. Wiley Interdiscip Rev Comput Mol Sci 6(2):147–172. https://doi.org/10.1002/wcms.1240

31. Combes RD (2012) In silico methods for toxicity prediction. Adv Exp Med Biol 745:96–116. https://doi.org/10.1007/978-1-4614-3055-1

32. Zhang C, Cheng FX, Li WH, Liu GX, Lee PW, Tang Y (2016) In silico prediction of drug induced liver toxicity using substructure pattern recognition method. Mol Inform 35(3–4):136–144. https://doi.org/10.1002/minf.201500055

33. Hewitt M, Enoch SJ, Madden JC, Przybylak KR, Cronin MTD (2013) Hepatotoxicity: a scheme for generating chemical categories for read-across, structural alerts and insights into mechanism(s) of action. Crit Rev Toxicol 43(7):537–558. https://doi.org/10.3109/10408444.2013.811215

34. Combes RD (2011) Challenges for computational structure-activity modelling for predicting chemical toxicity: future improvements? Expert Opin Drug Metab Toxicol 7(9):1129–1140

35. Baker M (2016) 1,500 scientists lift the lid on reproducibility. Nature 533(7604):452–454. https://doi.org/10.1038/533452a

36. Novick PA, Ortiz OF, Poelman J, Abdulhay AY, Pande VS (2013) SWEETLEAD: an in silico database of approved drugs, regulated chemicals, and herbal isolates for computer-aided drug discovery. PLoS One 8(11):ARTN e79568. https://doi.org/10.1371/journal.pone.0079568

37. Lo B (2015) Sharing clinical trial data: maximizing benefits, minimizing risk. JAMA 313(8):793–794. https://doi.org/10.1001/jama.2015.292

38. Goldacre B, Gray J (2016) OpenTrials: towards a collaborative open database of all available information on all clinical trials. Trials 17:ARTN 164. https://doi.org/10.1186/s13063-016-1290-8

39. Bonini S, Eichler HG, Wathion N, Rasi G (2014) Transparency and the European Medicines Agency—sharing of clinical trial data. N Engl J Med 371(26):2452–2455. https://doi.org/10.1056/NEJMp1409464

40. Ravagli C, Pognan F, Marc P (2016) OntoBrowser: a collaborative tool for curation of ontologies by subject matter experts. Bioinformatics. https://doi.org/10.1093/bioinformatics/btw579

41. Hewitt M, Ellison CM, Cronin MT, Pastor M, Steger-Hartmann T, Munoz-Muriendas J, Pognan F, Madden JC (2015) Ensuring confidence in predictions: a scheme to assess the scientific validity of in silico models. Adv Drug Deliv Rev. https://doi.org/10.1016/j.addr.2015.03.005

42. Lin Z, Will Y (2012) Evaluation of drugs with specific organ toxicities in organ-specific cell lines. Toxicol Sci 126(1):114–127. https://doi.org/10.1093/toxsci/kfr339

43. Atienzar FA, Blomme EA, Chen MJ, Hewitt P, Kenna JG, Labbe G, Moulin F, Pognan F, Roth AB, Suter-Dick L, Ukairo O, Weaver RJ, Will Y, Dambach DM (2016) Key challenges and opportunities associated with the use of in vitro models to detect human DILI: integrated risk assessment and mitigation plans. Biomed Res Int 2016:ARTN 9737920. https://doi.org/10.1155/2016/9737920

44. Hartung T, Daston G (2009) Are in vitro tests suitable for regulatory use? Toxicol Sci 111(2):233–237. https://doi.org/10.1093/toxsci/kfp149

45. Yoon M, Campbell JL, Andersen ME, Clewell HJ (2012) Quantitative in vitro to in vivo extrapolation of cell-based toxicity assay results. Crit Rev Toxicol 42(8):633–652. https://doi.org/10.3109/10408444.2012.692115

46. Astashkina A, Mann B, Grainger DW (2012) A critical evaluation of in vitro cell culture models for high-throughput drug screening and toxicity. Pharmacol Therapeut 134(1):82–106. https://doi.org/10.1016/j.pharmthera.2012.01.001

47. Allen DD, Caviedes R, Cardenas AM, Shimahara T, Segura-Aguilar J, Caviedes PA (2005) Cell lines as in vitro models for drug screening and toxicity studies. Drug Dev Ind Pharm 31(8):757–768. https://doi.org/10.1080/03639040500216246

48. Peck Y, Wang DA (2013) Three-dimensionally engineered biomimetic tissue models for in vitro drug evaluation: delivery, efficacy and toxicity. Expert Opin Drug Deliv 10(3):369–383. https://doi.org/10.1517/17425247.2013.751096

49. Csobonyeiova M, Polak S, Danisovic L (2016) Toxicity testing and drug screening using iPSC-derived hepatocytes, cardiomyocytes, and neural cells. Can J Physiol Pharmacol 94(7):687–694. https://doi.org/10.1139/cjpp-2015-0459

50. Horvath P, Aulner N, Bickle M, Davies AM, Del Nery E, Ebner D, Montoya MC, Ostling P, Pietiainen V, Price LS, Shorte SL, Turcatti G, von Schantz C, Carragher NO (2016) Screening out irrelevant cell-based models of disease. Nat Rev Drug Discov 15(11):751–769. https://doi.org/10.1038/nrd.2016.175

51. Bale SS, Geerts S, Jindal R, Yarmush ML (2016) Isolation and co-culture of rat parenchymal and non-parenchymal liver cells to evaluate cellular interactions and response. Sci Rep UK 6:ARTN 25329. https://doi.org/10.1038/srep25329

52. Bhatia SN, Ingber DE (2014) Microfluidic organs-on-chips. Nat Biotechnol 32(8):760–772. https://doi.org/10.1038/nbt.2989

53. Edmondson R, Broglie JJ, Adcock AF, Yang LJ (2014) Three-dimensional cell culture systems and their applications in drug discovery and cell-based biosensors. Assay Drug Dev Technol 12(4):207–218. https://doi.org/10.1089/adt.2014.573

54. Esch MB, Prot JM, Wang YI, Miller P, Llamas-Vidales JR, Naughton BA, Applegate DR, Shuler ML (2015) Multi-cellular 3D human primary liver cell culture elevates metabolic activity under fluidic flow. Lab Chip 15(10):2269–2277. https://doi.org/10.1039/c5lc00237k

55. Fatehullah A, Tan SH, Barker N (2016) Organoids as an in vitro model of human development and disease. Nat Cell Biol 18(3):246–254

56. Fennema E, Rivron N, Rouwkema J, van Blitterswijk C, de Boer J (2013) Spheroid culture as a tool for creating 3D complex tissues. Trends Biotechnol 31(2):108–115. https://doi.org/10.1016/j.tibtech.2012.12.003

57. Griffith LG, Swartz MA (2006) Capturing complex 3D tissue physiology in vitro. Nat Rev Mol Cell Biol 7(3):211–224. https://doi.org/10.1038/nrm1858

58. Pampaloni F, Reynaud EG, Stelzer EHK (2007) The third dimension bridges the gap between cell culture and live tissue. Nat Rev Mol Cell Biol 8(10):839–845. https://doi.org/10.1038/nrm2236

59. Germano D, Uteng M, Pognan F, Chibout SD, Wolf A (2015) Determination of liver specific toxicities in rat hepatocytes by high content imaging during 2-week multiple treatment. Toxicol In Vitro 30(1 Pt A):79–94. https://doi.org/10.1016/j.tiv.2014.05.009

60. Uteng M, Germano D, Balavenkatraman K, Pognan F, Wolf A (2014) High content imaging approaches for in vitro toxicology. In: Bal-Price A, Jennings P (eds) In vitro toxicol systems. Methods in pharmacology and toxicology. Springer, New York, NY, pp 377–397

61. Stierum R, Aarts J, Boorsma A, Bosgra S, Caiment F, Ezendam J, Greupink R, Hendriksen P, Soeteman-Hernandez LG, Jennen D, Kleinjans J, Kroese D, Kuper F, van

Loveren H, Monshouwer M, Russel F, van Someren E, Tsamou M, Groothuis G (2014) Assuring safety without animal testing concept (ASAT). Integration of human disease data with in vitro data to improve toxicology testing. Toxicol Lett 229:S4–S4. https://doi.org/10.1016/j.toxlet.2014.06.041

62. Aeby P, Ashikaga T, Bessou-Touya S, Schepky A, Gerberick F, Kern P, Marrec-Fairley M, Maxwell G, Ovigne JM, Sakaguchi H, Reisinger K, Tailhardat M, Martinozzi-Teissier S, Winkler P (2010) Identifying and characterizing chemical skin sensitizers without animal testing: Colipa's research and method development program. Toxicol In Vitro 24(6):1465–1473. https://doi.org/10.1016/j.tiv.2010.07.005

63. Sison-Young RL, Lauschke VM, Johann E, Alexandre E, Antherieu S, Aerts H, Gerets HHJ, Labbe G, Hoet D, Dorau M, Schofield CA, Lovatt CA, Holder JC, Stahl SH, Richert L, Kitteringham NR, Jones RP, Elmasry M, Weaver RJ, Hewitt PG, Ingelman-Sundberg M, Goldring CE, Park BK (2017) A multicenter assessment of single-cell models aligned to standard measures of cell health for prediction of acute hepatotoxicity. Arch Toxicol 91(3):1385–1400. https://doi.org/10.1007/s00204-016-1745-4

64. Gieseck RL, Hannan NRF, Bort R, Hanley NA, Drake RAL, Cameron GWW, Wynn TA, Vallier L (2014) Maturation of induced pluripotent stem cell derived hepatocytes by 3D-culture. PLoS One 9(1):ARTN e86372. https://doi.org/10.1371/journal.pone.0086372

65. Song ZH, Cai J, Liu YX, Zhao DX, Yong J, Duo SG, Song XJ, Guo YS, Zhao Y, Qin H, Yin XL, Wu C, Che J, Lu SC, Ding MX, Deng HK (2009) Efficient generation of hepatocyte-like cells from human induced pluripotent stem cells. Cell Res 19(11):1233–1242. https://doi.org/10.1038/cr.2009.107

66. Yi F, Qu J, Li M, Suzuki K, Kim NY, Liu GH, Belmonte JC (2012) Establishment of hepatic and neural differentiation platforms of Wilson's disease specific induced pluripotent stem cells. Protein Cell 3(11):855–863. https://doi.org/10.1007/s13238-012-2064-z

67. Eggenschwiler R, Loya K, Sgodda M, Andre F, Cantz T (2011) Hepatic differentiation of murine disease-specific induced pluripotent stem cells allows disease modelling in vitro. Stem Cells Int 2011:924782. https://doi.org/10.4061/2011/924782

68. Ghodsizadeh A, Taei A, Totonchi M, Seifinejad A, Gourabi H, Pournasr B, Aghdami N, Malekzadeh R, Almadani N, Salekdeh GH, Baharvand H (2010) Generation of liver disease-specific induced pluripotent stem cells along with efficient differentiation to functional hepatocyte-like cells. Stem Cell Rev 6(4):622–632. https://doi.org/10.1007/s12015-010-9189-3

69. Ohshita H, Tateno C (2017) Propagation of human hepatocytes in uPA/SCID mice: producing chimeric mice with humanized liver. Methods Mol Biol 1506:91–100. https://doi.org/10.1007/978-1-4939-6506-9_6

70. Uetrecht J, Naisbitt DJ (2013) Idiosyncratic adverse drug reactions: current concepts. Pharmacol Rev 65(2):779–808. https://doi.org/10.1124/pr.113.007450

71. Strom SC, Davila J, Grompe M (2010) Chimeric mice with humanized liver: tools for the study of drug metabolism, excretion, and toxicity. Methods Mol Biol 640:491–509. https://doi.org/10.1007/978-1-60761-688-7_27

72. Walsh NC, Kenney LL, Jangalwe S, Aryee KE, Greiner DL, Brehm MA, Shultz LD (2017) Humanized mouse models of clinical disease. Annu Rev Pathol 12:187–215. https://doi.org/10.1146/annurev-pathol-052016-100332

73. Grompe M, Strom S (2013) Mice with human livers. Gastroenterology 145(6):1209–1214. https://doi.org/10.1053/j.gastro.2013.09.009

74. Ito R, Takahashi T, Katano I, Ito M (2012) Current advances in humanized mouse models. Cell Mol Immunol 9(3):208–214. https://doi.org/10.1038/cmi.2012.2

75. Tateno C, Kawase Y, Tobita Y, Hamamura S, Ohshita H, Yokomichi H, Sanada H, Kakuni M, Shiota A, Kojima Y, Ishida Y, Shitara H, Wada NA, Tateishi H, Sudoh M, Nagatsuka S, Jishage K, Kohara M (2015) Generation of novel chimeric mice with humanized livers by using hemizygous cDNA-uPA/SCID mice. PLoS One 10(11):ARTN e0142145. https://doi.org/10.1371/journal.pone.0142145

76. Foster JR, Jacobsen M, Kenna G, Schulz-Utermoehl T, Morikawa Y, Salmu J, Wilson ID (2012) Differential effect of troglitazone on the human bile acid transporters, MRP2 and BSEP, in the PXB hepatic chimeric mouse. Toxicol Pathol 40(8):1106–1116. https://doi.org/10.1177/0192623312447542

77. Shultz LD, Brehm MA, Garcia-Martinez JV, Greiner DL (2012) Humanized mice for immune system investigation: progress, promise and challenges. Nat Rev Immunol 12(11):786–798. https://doi.org/10.1038/nri3311

78. Wilson EM, Bial J, Tarlow B, Bial G, Jensen B, Greiner DL, Brehm MA, Grompe M

(2014) Extensive double humanization of both liver and hematopoiesis in FRGN mice. Stem Cell Res 13(3):404–412. https://doi.org/10.1016/j.scr.2014.08.006

79. Qi ZP, Li L, Wang XF, Gao X, Wang X, Wei HM, Zhang J, Sun R, Tian ZG (2014) Bone marrow transplantation concurrently reconstitutes donor liver and immune system across host species barrier in mice. PLoS One 9(9):ARTN e106791. https://doi.org/10.1371/journal.pone.0106791

80. Hirode M, Omura K, Kiyosawa N, Uehara T, Shimuzu T, Ono A, Miyagishima T, Nagao T, Ohno Y, Urushidani T (2009) Gene expression profiling in rat liver treated with various hepatotoxic-compounds inducing coagulopathy. J Toxicol Sci 34(3):281–293

81. Mohr SE, Smith JA, Shamu CE, Neumuller RA, Perrimon N (2014) RNAi screening comes of age: improved techniques and complementary approaches. Nat Rev Mol Cell Biol 15(9):591–600. https://doi.org/10.1038/nrm3860

82. Housden BE, Muhar M, Gemberling M, Gersbach CA, Stainier DYR, Seydoux G, Mohr SE, Zuber J, Perrimon N (2017) Loss-of-function genetic tools for animal models: cross-species and cross-platform differences. Nat Rev Genet 18(1):24–40. https://doi.org/10.1038/nrg.2016.118

83. Doyle A, McGarry MP, Lee NA, Lee JJ (2012) The construction of transgenic and gene knockout/knockin mouse models of human disease. Transgenic Res 21(2):327–349. https://doi.org/10.1007/s11248-011-9537-3

84. Ott J, Wang J, Leal SM (2015) Genetic linkage analysis in the age of whole-genome sequencing. Nat Rev Genet 16(5):275–284. https://doi.org/10.1038/nrg3908

85. Watson RE, Goodman JI (2002) Epigenetics and DNA methylation come of age in toxicology. Toxicol Sci 67(1):11–16

86. Miousse IR, Currie R, Datta K, Ellinger-Ziegelbauer H, French JE, Harrill AH, Koturbash I, Lawton M, Mann D, Meehan RR, Moggs JG, O'Lone R, Rasoulpour RJ, Pera RAR, Thompson K (2015) Importance of investigating epigenetic alterations for industry, and regulators: an appraisal of current efforts by the Health and Environmental Sciences Institute. Toxicology 335:11–19. https://doi.org/10.1016/j.tox.2015.06.009

87. Chen M, Zhang J, Wang Y, Liu Z, Kelly R, Zhou G, Fang H, Borlak J, Tong W (2013) The liver toxicity knowledge base: a systems approach to a complex end point. Clin Pharmacol Ther 93(5):409–412. https://doi.org/10.1038/clpt.2013.16

88. Bujold D, Morais DAD, Gauthier C, Cote C, Caron M, Kwan T, Chen KC, Laperle J, Markovits AN, Pastinen T, Caron B, Veilleux A, Jacques PE, Bourque G (2016) The international human epigenome consortium data portal. Cell Syst 3(5):496. https://doi.org/10.1016/j.cels.2016.10.019

89. Braeuning A, Gavrilov A, Brown S, Wolf CR, Henderson CJ, Schwarz M (2014) Phenobarbital-mediated tumor promotion in transgenic mice with humanized CAR and PXR. Toxicol Sci 140(2):259–270. https://doi.org/10.1093/toxsci/kfu099

90. Terranova R, Vitobello A, Del Rio EA, Wolf CR, Schwartz M, Thomson J, Meehan R, Moggs J (2017) Progress in identifying epigenetic mechanisms of xenobiotic-induced non-genotoxic carcinogenesis. Curr Opin Toxicol 3:626–670

91. Sanz F, Carrio P, Lopez O, Capoferri L, Kooi DP, Vermeulen NPE, Geerke DP, Montanari F, Ecker GF, Schwab CH, Kleinoder T, Magdziarz T, Pastor M (2015) Integrative modeling strategies for predicting drug toxicities at the eTOX Project. Mol Inform 34(6–7):477–484. https://doi.org/10.1002/minf.201400193

92. Low YS, Sedykh AY, Rusyn I, Tropsha A (2014) Integrative approaches for predicting in vivo effects of chemicals from their structural descriptors and the results of short-term biological assays. Curr Top Med Chem 14(11):1356–1364. 10.14573/altex.1603091

93. Hartung T (2016) Making big sense from big data in toxicology by read-across. Altex-Altern Anim Ex 33(2):83–93

94. Miyamoto SW, Henderson S, Young HM, Pande A, Han JJ (2016) Tracking health data is not enough: a qualitative exploration of the role of healthcare partnerships and mHealth technology to promote physical activity and to sustain behavior change. Jmir Mhealth Uhealth 4(1):44–55. https://doi.org/10.2196/mhealth.4814

95. Alemayehu D, Berger ML (2016) Big data: transforming drug development and health policy decision making. Health Serv Outcome 16(3):92–102. https://doi.org/10.1007/s10742-016-0144-x

96. Soroushmehr SMR, Najarian K (2016) Transforming big data into computational models for personalized medicine and health care. Dialogues Clin Neurosci 18(3):339–343

97. Raschi E, De Ponti F (2015) Drug- and herb-induced liver injury: progress, current challenges and emerging signals of post-marketing

risk. World J Hepatol 7(13):1761–1771. https://doi.org/10.4254/wjh.v7.i13.1761

98. Menachemi N, Collum TH (2011) Benefits and drawbacks of electronic health record systems. Risk Manag Healthc Policy 4:47–55. https://doi.org/10.2147/RMHP.S12985

99. Maciejewski M, Lounkine E, Whitebread S, Farmer P, DuMouchel W, Shoichet BK, Urban L, (2017) Reverse translation of adverse event reports paves the way for de-risking preclinical off-targets. eLife 6

100. Outcome Sciences I, A Quintiles Company, Cambridge, MA (2014) Interfacing registries with electronic health records. In: Gliklich RE, Dreyer NA, Leavy MB (eds) Registries for evaluating patient outcomes: a user's guide, 3rd edn. AHRQ methods for effective health care, 3rd edn. AHRQ, Rockville, MD

101. Luo J, Wu M, Gopukumar D, Zhao Y (2016) Big data application in biomedical research and health care: a literature review. Biomed Inform Insights 8:1–10. https://doi.org/10.4137/BII.S31559

102. Kruse CS, Goswamy R, Raval Y, Marawi S (2016) Challenges and opportunities of big data in health care: a systematic review. JMIR Med Inform 4(4):e38. https://doi.org/10.2196/medinform.5359

103. Zhao J, Henriksson A, Asker L, Bostrom H (2015) Predictive modeling of structured electronic health records for adverse drug event detection. BMC Med Inform Decis Mak 15(Suppl 4):S1. https://doi.org/10.1186/1472-6947-15-S4-S1

104. Blumenthal D, Tavenner M (2010) The "Meaningful Use" regulation for electronic health records. New Engl J Med 363(6):501–504. https://doi.org/10.1056/NEJMp1006114

105. Lin C, Karlson EW, Dligach D, Ramirez MP, Miller TA, Mo H, Braggs NS, Cagan A, Gainer V, Denny JC, Savova GK (2015) Automatic identification of methotrexate-induced liver toxicity in patients with rheumatoid arthritis from the electronic medical record. J Am Med Inform Assn 22(E1):E151–E161. https://doi.org/10.1136/amiajnl-2014-002642

106. Miotto R, Li L, Kidd BA, Dudley JT (2016) Deep patient: an unsupervised representation to predict the future of patients from the electronic health records. Sci Rep 6:26094. https://doi.org/10.1038/srep26094

107. Auffray C, Balling R, Barroso I, Bencze L, Benson M, Bergeron J, Bernal-Delgado E, Blomberg N, Bock C, Conesa A, Del Signore S, Delogne C, Devilee P, Di Meglio A, Eijkemans M, Flicek P, Graf N, Grimm V, Guchelaar HJ, Guo YK, Gut IG, Hanbury A, Hanif S, Hilgers RD, Honrado A, Hose DR, Houwing-Duistermaat J, Hubbard T, Janacek SH, Karanikas H, Kievits T, Kohler M, Kremer A, Lanfear J, Lengauer T, Maes E, Meert T, Muller W, Nickel D, Oledzki P, Pedersen B, Petkovic M, Pliakos K, Rattray M, Mas JRI, Schneider R, Sengstag T, Serra-Picamal X, Spek W, Vaas LAI, van Batenburg O, Vandelaer M, Varnai P, Villoslada P, Vizcaino JA, Wubbe JPM, Zanetti G (2016) Making sense of big data in health research: towards an EU action plan. Genome Med 8:ARTN 71. https://doi.org/10.1186/s13073-016-0323-y

108. Coloma PM, Schuemie MJ, Trifiro G, Gini R, Herings R, Hippisley-Cox J, Mazzaglia G, Giaquinto C, Corrao G, Pedersen L, van der Lei J, Sturkenboom M, Consortium E-A (2011) Combining electronic healthcare databases in Europe to allow for large-scale drug safety monitoring: the EU-ADR Project. Pharmacoepidemiol Drug Saf 20(1):1–11. https://doi.org/10.1002/pds.2053

109. Chiauzzi E, Rodarte C, DasMahapatra P (2015) Patient-centered activity monitoring in the self-management of chronic health conditions. BMC Med 13:ARTN 77. https://doi.org/10.1186/s12916-015-0319-2

110. Redmond SJ, Lovell NH, Yang GZ, Horsch A, Lukowicz P, Murrugarra L, Marschollek M (2014) What does big data mean for wearable sensor systems? contribution of the IMIA wearable sensors in healthcare WG. Yearb Med Inform 9:135–142. 10.15265/IY-2014-0019

111. Schukat M, McCaldin D, Wang K, Schreier G, Lovell NH, Marschollek M, Redmond SJ (2016) Unintended consequences of wearable sensor use in healthcare. Contribution of the IMIA wearable sensors in healthcare WG. Yearb Med Inform 1:73–86. 10.15265/IY-2016-025

Chapter 3

Drug-Induced Liver Injury (DILI) Classification and Its Application on Human DILI Risk Prediction

Shraddha Thakkar, Minjun Chen, Huixiao Hong, Zhichao Liu, Hong Fang, and Weida Tong

Abstract

Drug-induced liver injury (DILI) is one of the primary reasons for drugs being terminated in premarket studies or being withdrawn from the market after approval. Many new methodologies have been examined to improve DILI prediction, including high-throughput/high-content screening assays, in silico approaches and toxicogenomics, all of which rely on a truth set of drugs with well-defined DILI potential. However, defining a drug's DILI risk is on varying interpretations, leading to differing classification schemes. Even when the same drug list is employed, variability in scheme affects predictive variables and models which lead to disparate risk prediction. Each model imbeds truth and knowledge in a different manner and context. An integrative approach melding models and variables should yield a system with enhanced prediction accuracy and better characterized mechanisms of action. Toward such an integrative predictor, we present four different classification schemes, i.e., an FDA labeling data-based approach (DILIrank dataset), a clinical evidence-based approach (LiverTox dataset), literature-based approaches (Greene and Xu datasets), and a registry-based approach (Suzuki dataset). Comparative analyses showed good general agreement between these approaches, with the most substantial difference observed between in silico models for drug-centric classification methods (i.e., drug-labeling and literature based approaches) versus clinical evidence-based methods (i.e., case reports and registry based approaches). The results suggest that substantial benefits can be obtained by consolidating various classification schemes to generate a larger dataset imbedding more diverse knowledge, and especially the new data streams from emerging technologies.

Key words Drug-induced liver injury, Risk assessment, DILI classification, Rule-of-two model, DILIscore model

1 Introduction

Safety contributes significantly to drug attrition [1, 2]. Safety issues in both preclinical and clinical stages of drug development are a formidable challenge, especially at the lead optimization and the early clinical development stages [3]. DILI (Drug-Induced Liver Injury) is one of the key drug safety issues, which is a frequent cause of regulatory action such as "Black Box Warning" or denial

Minjun Chen and Yvonne Will (eds.), *Drug-Induced Liver Toxicity*, Methods in Pharmacology and Toxicology, https://doi.org/10.1007/978-1-4939-7677-5_3, © Springer Science+Business Media, LLC, part of Springer Nature 2018

in approval [1]. Currently animal models are not effective enough in prediction of DILI risk in humans, evident by the fact that close to 50% of drugs failed in the clinical trials due to hepatotoxicity are not detected by these animal models [4]. Therefore, significant efforts are needed to bridge the gap and to reduce DILI risk for humans and improve upon early detection of DILI.

Meanwhile, recent changes in toxicology discipline reveal a paradigm shift in increasing the efforts to develop alternative methods with emerging technologies for safety assessment. These include high throughput in vitro methodologies, in silico approaches and toxicogenomics, which provide a better understanding of mechanism of action and enhances safety related assessments [5]. Several large-scale studies made in this regard are Tox21 [6], ToxCast [7], and EU activities under the REACH initiative [5] that aim to evaluate the utility of the emerging technologies for the toxicity assessment. In vitro techniques use both high-throughput and high-content screening methodologies to record the cellular responses of multiple drugs and chemicals. In silico methods have been developed to predict potential toxicity based on the chemical structures of compounds. Toxicogenomics examines the gene activities following chemical exposure to understand the molecular mechanisms of toxicity. These methodologies usually involve a training-validation process. Specifically, a predictive model is constructed first based on a list of compounds (training set) with known outcomes (e.g., DILI-positive and DILI-negative), which is followed by a validation step where the model is challenged using an independent list of compounds (test set) with known outcomes to assess its validity. As depicted in Fig. 1, a reference list with a large number of compounds with known outcomes was used as a foundation to successfully employ these in vitro and in silico methods. Therefore, a reference drug list with clear and well-defined DILI classification is important for the development of predictive models utilizing emerging technologies.

DILI classification is to divide drugs into either binary (e.g., DILI-positive or DILI-negative) groups or ordinal classes (most-, less-, and no-DILI-concern). However, assigning a drug as either positive or negative for liver injury is a challenge [6]. This is largely due to the fact that DILI is often associated with a low incidence (particularly in the study of marketed drugs) but with a wide range of severity and different injury patterns. In addition, causality of liver injury (i.e., incriminating the drug for DILI) is frequently difficult to ascertain due to multiple reasons, e.g., comedication, alcohol consumption, preexisting liver disease etc. Therefore, determining the extent of DILI risk for a drug is somewhat subjective and often based on how we weigh frequency (i.e., how many incidences deemed significant?), causality (what is the likelihood of incriminating a drug for DILI?), and severity (how serious the liver

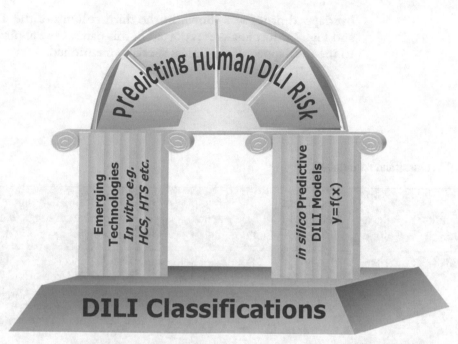

Fig. 1 Development and performance of a predictive model for assessing the human DILI risk depends heavily upon the accuracy and consistency of the DILI classification. DILI classification differentiates drugs as DILI positive (drugs that can cause liver injury) and DILI negative (drugs that have not revealed signs of liver injury), and used to identify mechanistic parameters using emerging methodologies for DILI prediction. Emerging technologies used for DILI prediction included, but are not limited to, in vitro methods (e.g., High Content Screening and High Throughput Screening assays), and in silico methodologies

injury is?) [8]. Using different data sources, (e.g., the number of case reports [8–12] or FDA approved-drug labeling [8, 13]) and weighing differently on each of these factors could vary the assignment of DILI classification to the same drugs. In this paper, we first summarize the four different DILI classifications within five reported large DILI datasets ($n > 200$). We then conducted comparative analysis between these classification schemas and demonstrated the variability in classification on the model prediction by applying our DILIscore model (a quantitative predictive model for DILI severity).

2   DILI Classifications

Table 1 summarizes five DILI classification datasets for human hepatotoxicity including >200 drugs. The DILI classification of all the datasets was for DILI severity assessments (not for injury patterns or disease types). DILIrank has the largest size, which overlapped significantly with other four datasets; the number of overlapped drugs was shown in the third column of the Table 1 and Fig. 2. Most analyses reported in this paper were applied only to the overlapped drugs unless specially mentioned.

Table 1
Various DILI classification datasets

DILI classification datasets[a]	No. of drugs	No. of drugs overlap with DILIrank[b]	DILI evidence information	DILI classification scheme (the number of drugs in each category)[c]
DILIrank [8]	1036	1036	FDA drug labeling and DILI causality evidence	Four DILI-concern groups: • [v]No-DILI-concern (312) • [v]Less-DILI-concern (278) • [v]Most-DILI-concern (192) • Ambiguous DILI-concern (254)
LiverTox [14]	663	493 (74%)	Human DILI case reports	Five DILI likelihood levels: • Category A (36); most likely • Category B (68) • Category C (87) • Category D (108) • Category E (195); least likely
Xu et al. [12, 15]	532	343 (64%)	Literature evidence and DILI case reports	Two categories: • DILI positive (196) • DILI negative (147)
Greene et al. [9]	1266	325[d] (26%)	Literature evidence and DILI case reports	Three categories • Human hepatotoxicity (189) • Weak evidence (50) • No evidence (86)
Suzuki et al. [16]	385[e]	287[e] (75%)	Case reports collected by large DILI registries	Three categories: • General liver injury (157) • Acute liver failure (87) • Withdrawn or suspension for DILI (43)

[a]The DILI classification datasets were complied from the supplemental tables associated with the original publications, including DILIrank [8], LiverTox [14], Xu et al. [12, 15], Greene et al. [9] and Suzuki et al. [16]
[b]The number of drugs reported from each classification reflect only human data and that were approved from FDA before 2010
[c]The number of drugs reported in each categories of all the classification are only the DILIrank subset
[d]Does not contanin the compounds tested on animals
[e]Reported list of drug that are hepatotoxic

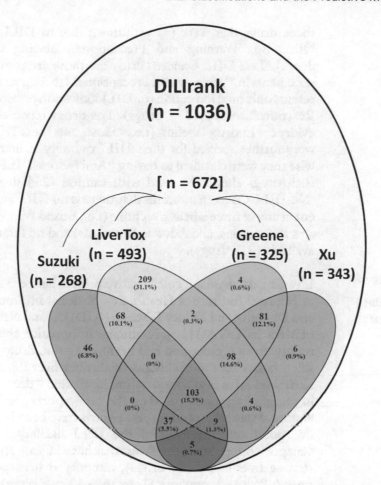

Fig. 2 DILIrank data set was generated using FDA drug labeling and DILI causality approach and contains the drugs approved by the US FDA before 2010. It also contains number of drugs from the other type of DILI classifications that are overlapped with DILIrank such as Greene (325 drugs), Suzuki (268 drugs), LiverTox (493 drugs), and Xu (343 drugs). This analysis was done to understand the coverage of drugs from each database and overlapping with others. However, this analysis is independent of DILI classification assigned by each dataset. Besides DILIrank, other four datasets follow different approaches to identify DILI positive and DILI negative drugs and there is very little overlap (15.3%) between them. Greene and Xu classifications used similar approach and thus with the largest overlap (47.5%) while Suzuki's and LiverTox method contain unique list of DILI drugs and non-DILI drugs (Those drugs were not identified by any other classification system)

2.1   DILIrank: A Drug Labeling Based Approach

The DILIrank dataset contained 1036 drugs approved by the FDA before 2010 with classified DILI categories [8]. This classification was based on the FDA drug labeling documents and in addition, it also accounted for DILI causality evidence in literature. DILI categories were classified for the drugs as ᵛNo-, ᵛLess-, or ᵛMost-DILI-Concerns while the drugs that could not be categorized in the above classification for the DILI concern was classified as "Ambiguous-DILI-Concern." ᵛMost-DILI-concern drugs are those drugs that were (a) withdrawn due to DILI, or (b) have "Black-Box Warning and Precautions" labeling section (192 drugs). ᵛLess-DILI-Concern drugs are those drugs that have DILI statements in "Warning and Precautions" labeling section that represents only mild indications or DILI indication present in "Adverse Reactions" section (278 drugs). For drugs recorded with DILI evidences in drug labeling (i.e., ᵛMost- and ᵛLess-DILI-Concern) were further verified for their DILI causality in literature, otherwise they were classified as having "Ambiguous-DILI-Concern" as such drugs should be used with caution (254 drugs); whereas ᵛNo-DILI-Concern indicates that there is no DILI indication present in any of three labeling sections (i.e., Boxed Warning, Warnings and Precautions, and Adverse Reactions) and no litrature evidence available (312 drugs).

2.2   LiverTox: A Clinical Evidence Based Approach

LiverTox database is a collaborative project between two institutes of National Institute of Health, i.e., National Institute of Diabetes and Digestive and Kidney Diseases (NIDDK) and National Library of Medicine (NLM) [17]. It contains information about DILI case reports from prescription and nonprescription drugs and are classified based on the likelihood of causing liver injury [14]. This likelihood takes into consideration how often a drug is responsible in causing liver injury based on the case-reports obtained from literature. Multiple individual case reports have been used to develop five point categorization of the DILI likelihood scores [14]. Category A represents the drugs that has >50 case reports demonstrating liver injury (36 drugs), category B between 12 and 50 cases (68 drugs), category C less than 12 case reports (87 drugs), and category D three or less case reports per drug (108 drugs). Category E represents the list of drugs that does not indicate sign of liver injury even after multiple years of usage (109 drugs). Since the categories were defined by number of cases, there are more patients reporting DILI related issues for drugs from category A in comparison with drugs from category D. Thus drug listed in the category A will have more chances of DILI likelihood in comparison with the other categories.

2.3   Greene Classification: A Literature Based Approach

This dataset consists of DILI information from both human and animal studies, but only human data were used in this paper (shown in Table 1 column 3 and 5). The number of case reports in conjunction with literature based evidence were used for human DILI classification of 325 drugs in Greene classification [9]. Drugs are classified into human hepatotoxicity (189 drugs) with weak evidence (50 drugs) or no evidence (86 drugs) for DILI.

2.4   Suzuki Classification: A Registry Based Approach

Classification from Suzuki [16] has consolidated the DILI information from major DILI registries, including the Spanish DILI registry, the Swedish adverse reaction databases and the DILI network from USA. This classification system has identified 157 drugs with general liver injury and 87 drugs with acute liver failure. Additionally, 43 drugs were identified as withdrawn or suspended due to concern for DILI.

2.5 Xu Classification: A Literature Based Approach

Xu et al. [15] have classified 343 drugs based on the case reports and information available in the various literature. The drugs were classified as either DILI positive or negative. There were 196 drugs identified as DILI positive and 147 drugs identified as DILI negative.

3 Comparative Analysis Between Various DILI Classification Schemes

Each classification system mentioned above follows a set of approaches to identify drugs that have potential to cause liver injury or not. Specifically, DILIrank classifies the drugs based on the DILI information that was gathered during preclinical development, clinical trials, approval, and postmarket study. The LiverTox classification is based on the clinical observation and consolidates the likelihood to cause the liver injury based on the frequency and severity of clinical observation. Both Greene and Xu classifications are based on literature evidences and Suzuki is a registry based approach. Thus, comparative analysis from the various classification schemes was made to evaluate the variability across these five datasets.

The analyses were specifically focused on only those drugs from the four datasets that were present in the DILIrank. As shown in Fig. 2, the overlap of DILIrank with the other four datasets was in the following order of Suzuki (75%) > LiverTox (74%) > Xu (64%) > Greene (26%). The analysis was done to understand the overlap of the drugs across various databases and it was independent of their DILI classification. The result indicates that combining all these five datasets could generate the largest reference list to support DILI studies.

As shown in Fig. 3a, concordance between DILIrank and LiverTox databases was consistent only for those drugs that overlap in the following categories (a) ᵛMost-DILI-Concern of DILIrank and Category A of LiverTox (b) ᵛLess-DILI-Concern of DILIrank and Category D of LiverTox (c) ᵛNo-DILI-Concern of DILIrank and Category E of LiverTox. For example, 29 out of 36 drugs (81%) are most likely to cause liver injury (Category A, >50 Cases) as determined by LiverTox were also the ᵛMost-DILI-Concern drugs in DILIrank. Similarly, 87 out of 108 drugs (81%) with lower likelihood to cause liver injury (Category D, 1–3 cases) by LiverTox were the ᵛLess-DILI-Concern drugs by DILIrank. Additionally, LiverTox also identified the drugs which have been used extensively and does not contain any reported DILI case reports, of which 90 of 100 drugs (90%) were also identified as ᵛNo-DILI-Concern drugs by DILIrank. The general trend of

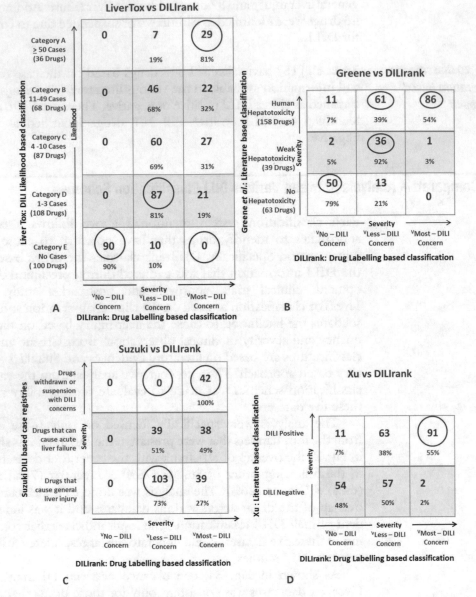

Fig. 3 (**a**) Comparison of DILIrank with LiverTox database (i.e., the labeling based classification against the clinical report based classification). (**b**) Comparison of DILIrank with Greene classification (i.e., the labeling based classification against a literature based approach). (**c**) Comparison of DILIrank with Suzuki classification (i.e., the labeling based classification against the clinical report based classification). (**d**) Comparison of DILIrank with Xu classification (i.e., the labeling based classification against the literature based classification)

overlap by DILI severity is apparent between the two databases. The comparisons of DILIrank dataset with the Greene dataset reveal concordance (Fig. 3b). There were overlap in the following categories (a) ᵛMost-DILI-Concern and ᵛLess-DILI-Concern of DILIrank compared to Human Hepatotoxicity of Greene (b)

^{v}Less-DILI-Concern of DILIrank compared to weak hepatotoxicity of Greene (c) ^{v}No-DILI-Concern of the DILIrank compared to no hepatotoxicity of Greene. For example, 50 out of 63 drugs (79%) have no evidence of causing liver injury were also found to be in the category of no-DILI-Concern drugs in DILIrank. Similarly, 36 out of 39 drugs (92%) with weak evidence of hepatotoxicity based on literature evidence are also defined as ^{v}Less-DILI-Concern by DILIrank. The Human hepatotoxicity classification of Greene, demonstrated the overlap with ^{v}Less-DILI-Concern category (39%) as well as ^{v}Most-DILI-Concern category (54%). Of note, Greene classification reports that all the drugs are hepatotoxic to humans in the human hepatotoxicity category, irrespective of the severity of the classification. However, majority of drugs from Human Hepatotoxicity category (86 out of 158 drugs) were the ^{v}Most-DILI-Concern drugs. Thus, Greene classification shows concordance in data of the general trend in comparison with the DILIrank dataset.

A similar trend was observed for Xu dataset which is also a literature-based approach (Fig. 3d), where 55% of the drugs belong to the DILI positive categories by Xu are represented in the ^{v}Most-DILI-Concern category of DILIrank.

The Suzuki dataset is derived from the DILI information based on the case registry, which divided the dataset into three categories based on severity and liver injury risk to humans. Suzuki dataset contains information related to human hepatotoxicity and it does not contain the list of drugs that does not cause liver injury. As depicted in Fig. 3c, all the drugs that are either withdrawn or suspended due to DILI on Suzuki's are represented in the ^{v}Most-DILI-Concern category of DILIrank. Additionally, 73% of the drugs that cause general liver injury in Suzuki dataset belong to the ^{v}Less-DILI-Concern category of DILIrank.

By comparing DILIrank with other four classification schemes for the drugs overlapped, there is an apparent trend between these classification schemes (highlighted as red circles). However, differences were also observed between data sets, which could affect the performance of predictive models. Therefore, a predictive model developed using one classification scheme would not necessary converge when using a different classification scheme.

4 DILI Classification and Its Influence on Model Development

Various bioinformatics approaches have been employed for the development of DILI predictive model [18–22] . For example, to understand the structure and toxicity relationship [21, 23], we developed a DILI prediction system (called DILIps) [18]. In addition, we have also developed a "Rule of Two" model (RO2) to identify drugs that are likely cause of DILI risk in humans [20], which specified that an oral medication having high lipophilicity [24] and high daily dose [25], is statistically significantly associated with DILI risk in humans [24]. Here, the threshold logP (measured by its $\log P \geq 3$) [26] [27] and daily dose of ≥ 100 mg/day [24] were determined according to the recommendations from literature.

By realizing that the reactive metabolites play a major role in the development of drug toxicity, we incorporated the reactive metabolite formation into RO2, which yielded a DILIscore model that allows quantitative assessment of DILI risk [28]. Specifically, a mathematically derived equation inferred from the analysis of a dataset including $N = 192$ FDA approved drugs as given below was established in DILIscore to quantitatively assess DILI risk based on the daily dose, lipophilicity, and the formation of reactive metabolite [29].

$$DILIscore = 0.608 \times \log(daily\ dose\ /\ mg) + 0.227 \times \log P + 2.833 \times RM.$$

Here, log (daily dose/mg) is a natural log or equivalent to ln (daily dose/mg), and the numerical value of 1 or 0 was given to drugs either producing reactive metabolites or not. In DILIscore, the score ≥ 7 were concomitant with severe clinical outcome. The DILIscore ≥ 3 are associated with the moderate liver injury. DILIscore of <3 were rarely found to be related to severe liver injury.

We calculated the scores for each drug shown in Fig. 2 using DILIscore model, and then generated the density plots of score from each classification scheme. In an idea situation, for each classification, the plot should show a complete separation between different severity groups defined by a classification scheme. However, the purpose of this analysis was to examine the influence of various DILI classification systems. If two plots bear similarity, it implies that the two classification schemes corresponding to these two plots have the similar performance in the context of the DILI score model.

Evidently, DILIrank, Greene, and Xu datasets had similar distribution patterns, indicating that these three classification schemes are consistent. Most sever DILI drugs in these data sets (i.e., [V]Most-DILI-Concern drugs in DILIrank, Human Hepatotoxic drug in Greene and DILI positive drugs in Xu) had the score of ~7 while DILI negative drugs have lower DILIscore (i.e., [V]No-DILI-Concern drugs in DILIrank ~2.5, no Hepatotoxic drug in Greene ~2.5 and DILI negative drugs in Xu ~4) in Fig. 4. On the contrary, the separation between different severity groups in both LiverTox and Suzuki classification was less clean, highlighting the impact of the classification scheme on the performance of predictive model. Thus, a predictive model using one classification scheme should be used in the right context and it might not be applicable to other classification schemes.

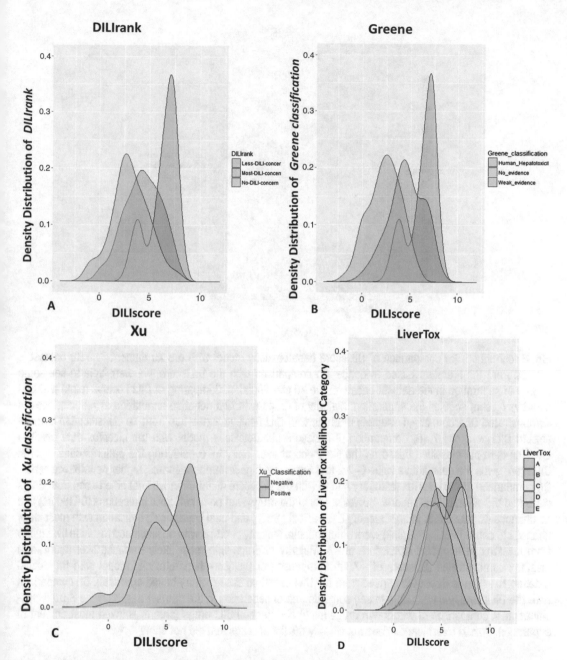

Fig. 4 (**a**) Comparison of DILIscore hepatotoxicity model with the DILIrank dataset. The DILIrank dataset classified drugs based on drug labeling. In comparison of DILIrank with the DILIscore, we could demonstrate some degree of separation in the dataset. The vNo-DILI-Concern drugs (green) and vMost-DILI concern drugs (pink) showed most amount of separation. Most of the vNo-DILI-Concern drugs (green) had the DILIscore of ~2.5 and most of the vMost-DILI-Concern drugs with the DILIscore of ~7. Weak Hepatotoxic drugs demonstrated the average DILIscore of ~4. (**b**) Comparison of DILIscore hepatotoxicity model with the Greene dataset. The Greene dataset classified drugs based on the literature evidence. On comparison with the DILIscore, we were able to see some degree of separation in the dataset based on the DILIscore. However, comparing the No Hepatotoxicity evidence drugs (green) and Human Hepatotoxicity drugs (pink) showed most amount of separation. Most of the no DILI evidence drugs had the DILIscore of ~2.5 and most of the Human Hepatotoxicity drugs with the DILIscore of ~7. Weak Hepatotoxic drugs demonstrated the average DILIscore of ~5.

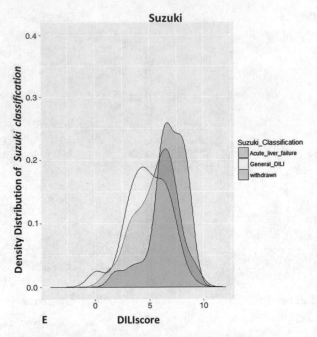

E   DILIscore

Fig. 4 (continued) (**c**) Comparison of DILIscore hepatotoxicity model with the Xu dataset. The Xu dataset is derived from the literature based evidence. On comparison with the DILIscore, we were able to see some degree of separation in the dataset based on the Xu classification. Comparing of DILI Positive (pink) and DILI negative (green) showed the separation. Majority of drugs with DILI negative annotation at Xu classification demonstrated DILIscore of ~4. Majority of drugs with DILI Positive annotation from Xu classification demonstrated DILIscore of ~7. (**d**) Comparison of DILIscore hepatotoxicity model with the LiverTox data set. The LiverTox data set classified based on the likelihood of liver injury by considering the patients case reports. DILIscore gives the quantitative value (−1.9 to 8.64) where higher number denotes, higher hepatotoxicity risk. On comparison of the LiverTox (category A to E) with the DILIscore distribution was not able to separate drugs classified based on clinical reports. However, few of the drugs with no hepatotoxic indications (DILIScore) and no chances (to cause liver injury category E (LiverTox) (green) and fatal hepatotoxic indication with most likely chances to cause liver injury (pink) were differentiable. Majority of drugs with no likelihood to cause liver injury from LiverTox demonstrated DILIscore of ~4. Majority of drugs with most likely to cause liver injury from LiverTox demonstrated DILIscore of ~7. (**e**) Comparison of DILIscore hepatotoxicity model with the Suzuki dataset. The Suzuki dataset is derived from the DILI based on case registry based approach. On comparison with the DILIscore, we were able to see some degree of separation in the dataset based on the Suzuki classification. A comparison of withdrawn drugs (pink) and general DILI drugs (cream) showed most amount of separation. Suzuki classification does not classify the list of drugs that did not show

A comparative analysis was conducted to understand the influence of various DILI classification systems in the DILIscore prediction (Fig. 4). DILIscore quantitatively models the hepatotoxicity risk in the LiverTox classification, and the drugs are classified based on the clinical reports and measures the likelihood showed good concordance with DILIrank data set. Overall comparison of the DILIscore distribution from LiverTox and Greene classification raise an important issue that the observed variability is brought by the classification data set based on its source of the information. However, the concordance is demonstrated by comparison of the quantitative DILIscore's average quantitative values at few categories in both classifications. For example, category D of LiverTox with the Weak Hepatotoxicity evidence of Greene and ᵛLess-DILI-Concern of DILIrank demonstrated the average DILIscore of ~5. Likewise, Category A of LiverTox with the Human Hepatotoxicity evidence of Greene and ᵛMost-DILI-Concern of DILIrank demonstrated the average DILIscore of ~7. Suzuki and Xu classification also demonstrated the degree of separation in the on comparison with the DILIscore (Fig. 4a–e).

Even though the model is sufficient enough to differentiate DILI with ᵛNo-DILI-Concern drugs, variation brought by the source of the data can modulate the quality of the prediction and eventually, the reliability and reproducibility for the prediction model.

5 Conclusion

With the advent of the emerging technologies (e.g., high-throughput and high-content screening assays) and in silico methodologies widely adopted in toxicity studies, it is important to have a reference list of compounds with accurate DILI classification to develop biomarkers with these technologies. Such a list could be derived from different classification schemes. We found that different classification system using different sources of information can vary in assigning a drug for DILI and which can also affect the model performance. A robust predictive model is heavily dependent on dataset size, class prevalence (e.g., data set size, distribution of Active/Inactive) and the signal/noise strength for class determination [30]. This study evaluated and compared five large datasets (>200 drugs) whose classification was derived from four different approaches. This analysis offers an opportunity to integrate these methods to combine these datasets into one consolidated list that covers most of the drug classes for DILI prediction. This consolidated information has potential to cover the landscape of DILI information. Using this comprehensive DILI dataset, the predictive models using the new data stream from emerging technologies can be robust enough to identify drug potentially causing DILI at earlier stage and can reduce the liver injury related attrition.

Disclaimer

The views presented in this chapter do not necessarily reflect current or future opinion or policy of the US Food and Drug Administration. Any mention of commercial products is for clarification and not intended as an endorsement.

References

1. Chen M, Bisgin H, Tong L, Hong H, Fang H, Borlak J, Tong W (2014) Toward predictive models for drug-induced liver injury in humans: are we there yet? Biomarkers 8(2):201–213

2. Kola I, Landis J (2004) Can the pharmaceutical industry reduce attrition rates? Nat Rev Drug Discov 3(8):711–716

3. Brody T (2016) Clinical trials: study design, endpoints and biomarkers, drug safety, and FDA and ICH guidelines. Academic Press, Cambridge, MA

4. Olson H, Betton G, Robinson D, Thomas K, Monro A, Kolaja G, Lilly P, Sanders J, Sipes G, Bracken W et al (2000) Concordance of the toxicity of pharmaceuticals in humans and in animals. Regul Toxicol Pharmacol 32(1):56–67

5. Raunio H (2011) In silico toxicology-nontesting methods. Front Pharmacol 2:33

6. Collins FS, Gray GM, Bucher JR (2008) Transforming environmental health protection. Science (New York, NY) 319(5865):906

7. Dix DJ, Houck KA, Martin MT, Richard AM, Setzer RW, Kavlock RJ (2007) The ToxCast program for prioritizing toxicity testing of environmental chemicals. Toxicol Sci 95(1):5–12

8. Chen M, Suzuki A, Thakkar S, Yu K, Hu C, Tong W (2016) DILIrank: the largest reference drug list ranked by the risk for developing drug-induced liver injury in humans. Drug Discov Today 21(4):648–653

9. Greene N, Fisk L, Naven RT, Note RR, Patel ML, Pelletier DJ (2010) Developing structure–activity relationships for the prediction of hepatotoxicity. Chem Res Toxicol 23(7):1215–1222

10. Guo JJ, Wigle PR, Lammers K, Vu O (2005) Comparison of potentially hepatotoxic drugs among major US drug compendia. Res Social Adm Pharm 1(3):460–479

11. Gustafsson F, Foster AJ, Sarda S, Bridgland-Taylor MH, Kenna JG (2014) A correlation between the in vitro drug toxicity of drugs to cell lines which express human P450s and their propensity to cause liver injury in humans. Toxicol Sci 137:189–211

12. Xu JJ, Henstock PV, Dunn MC, Smith AR, Chabot JR, de Graaf D (2008) Cellular imaging predictions of clinical drug-induced liver injury. Toxicol Sci 105(1):97–105

13. Chen M, Vijay V, Shi Q, Liu Z, Fang H, Tong W (2011) FDA-approved drug labeling for the study of drug-induced liver injury. Drug Discov Today 16(15):697–703

14. Björnsson ES, Hoofnagle JH (2016) Categorization of drugs implicated in causing liver injury: Critical assessment based on published case reports. Hepatology 63(2):590–603

15. Ekins S, Williams AJ, Xu JJ (2010) A predictive ligand-based Bayesian model for human drug-induced liver injury. Drug Metab Dispos 38(12):2302–2308

16. Suzuki A, Andrade RJ, Bjornsson E, Lucena MI, Lee WM, Yuen NA, Hunt CM, Freston JW (2010) Drugs associated with hepatotoxicity and their reporting frequency of liver adverse events in VigiBase™. Drug Saf 33(6):503–522

17. Hoofnagle JH, Serrano J, Knoben JE, Navarro VJ (2013) LiverTox: a website on drug-induced liver injury. Hepatology 57(3):873–874

18. Liu Z, Shi Q, Ding D, Kelly R, Fang H, Tong W (2011) Translating clinical findings into knowledge in drug safety evaluation-drug induced liver injury prediction system (DILIps). PLoS Comput Biol 7(12):e1002310

19. Yu K, Geng X, Chen M, Zhang J, Wang B, Ilic K, Tong W (2014) High daily dose and being a substrate of cytochrome P450 enzymes are two important predictors of drug-induced liver injury. Drug Metab Dispos 42(4):744–750

20. Chen M, Borlak J, Tong W (2013) High lipophilicity and high daily dose of oral medications are associated with significant risk for drug-induced liver injury. Hepatology 58(1):388–396

21. Chen M, Hong H, Fang H, Kelly R, Zhou G, Borlak J, Tong W (2013) Quantitative structure-activity relationship models for predicting drug-induced liver injury based on FDA-approved drug labeling annotation and using a large collection of drugs. Toxicol Sci 136(1):242–249

22. Chen M, Suzuki A, Borlak J, Andrade RJ, Lucena MI (2015) Drug-induced liver injury: interactions between drug properties and host factors. J Hepatol 63(2):503–514

23. Kaplowitz N (2013) Avoiding idiosyncratic DILI: two is better than one. Hepatology 58(1):15–17

24. Waring MJ (2009) Defining optimum lipophilicity and molecular weight ranges for drug candidates—molecular weight dependent lower logD limits based on permeability. Bioorg Med Chem Lett 19(10):2844–2851

25. Lammert C, Einarsson S, Saha C, Niklasson A, Bjornsson E, Chalasani N (2008) Relationship between daily dose of oral medications and idiosyncratic drug-induced liver injury: search for signals. Hepatology 47(6):2003–2009

26. Walgren JL, Mitchell MD, Thompson DC (2005) Role of metabolism in drug-induced idiosyncratic hepatotoxicity. Crit Rev Toxicol 35(4):325–361

27. Uetrecht J (2001) Prediction of a new drug's potential to cause idiosyncratic reactions. Curr Opin Drug Discov Devel 4(1):55–59

28. Chen M, Borlak J, Tong W (2016) A model to predict severity of drug-induced liver injury in humans. Hepatology 64(3):931–940

29. Stepan AF, Walker DP, Bauman J, Price DA, Baillie TA, Kalgutkar AS, Aleo MD (2011) Structural alert/reactive metabolite concept as applied in medicinal chemistry to mitigate the risk of idiosyncratic drug toxicity: a perspective based on the critical examination of trends in the top 200 drugs marketed in the United States. Chem Res Toxicol 24(9):1345–1410

30. Thakkar S, Chen M, Fang H, Liu Z, Roberts R, Tong W (2017) The liver toxicity knowledge base (LTKB) and drug-induced liver injury (DILI) classification for assessment of human liver injury. Expert Rev Gastroenterol Hepatol 9:1–8. https://doi.org/10.1080/17474124.2018.1383154

Chapter 4

Physicochemical Properties and Structural Alerts

Lilia Fisk, Nigel Greene, and Russ Naven

Abstract

Drug-induced liver injury (DILI) is one of the major reasons for the termination of drug candidates in the development and the withdrawal of drugs from the market. Significant efforts are being made to utilize existing knowledge of chemical and biological mechanisms that have been linked with causing DILI. These mechanisms are often varied and can include overt chemical reactivity or bioactivation to reactive metabolites; unintended interactions with cellular proteins such as transporters and nuclear receptors; or the disruption of cellular processes like mitochondrial function and oxidative stress. For DILI to be observed the chemical needs (1) to possess the required chemical features to disrupt biological processes and (2) to reach a certain concentration in the liver. Structure–activity relationships (SARs) are often used to determine whether a chemical possesses the required features to disrupt a biological process. Whereas the concentration of a drug in the liver is highly dependent on its physicochemical properties as these influence many pharmacokinetic characteristics. However, despite the ability to assess compounds for their potential to cause DILI using in silico methods in combination with a battery of in vitro assays, it is often difficult to accurately predict the risk for a specific compound as the efficacious concentration is often not truly known until it reaches the clinic and is tested in man. In addition, the complexities of mechanisms that can lead to hepatotoxicity make the accurate identification of liver toxicants a challenging task. This chapter summarizes the importance of the consideration of physicochemical properties while applying SARs for toxicity assessment.

Key words Structure–activity relationships, Hepatotoxicity, Reactivity, Physicochemical properties, Mitochondrial dysfunction

1 Introduction

The liver plays an important role in the normal function of the human body. It regulates the levels of most chemicals in the blood and excretes bile. Bile helps to break down fats, preparing them for further digestion and absorption. Drugs can be absorbed into the bloodstream from the stomach and intestines and then pass through the liver. One of the liver's functions is to remove unwanted chemicals from the blood through metabolism into forms that are easier for the body to excrete.

Minjun Chen and Yvonne Will (eds.), *Drug-Induced Liver Toxicity*, Methods in Pharmacology and Toxicology, https://doi.org/10.1007/978-1-4939-7677-5_4, © Springer Science+Business Media, LLC, part of Springer Nature 2018

Many drugs are administered orally, and as a consequence are absorbed through the gastrointestinal tract and pass through the liver. During metabolism, the parent drug often undergoes bioactivation into reactive species that are then conjugated with water soluble biomolecules such as glucuronic acid or glutathione to enable excretion. However, sometimes these activated species can potentially interact with the intracellular or extracellular apparatus causing adverse or undesired effects. For orally administered drugs, the liver is therefore exposed to both the parent drug and varying concentrations of drug metabolites, making it a primary target for toxicity.

To mitigate such eventualities, it is important to understand the various factors that can contribute to the potential risk for liver injury, and aim to minimize them. The two main considerations are: (1) does the drug have chemical features that have been linked to causing deleterious effects to the liver? and (2) will it reach the organ in sufficient quantities to cause that effect? Understanding the relationships between the chemical structure and these considerations for liver injury will ultimately enable the design of safer drug molecules. Chemical characteristics that can play a role in determining the manifestation of DILI include the physicochemical properties of the drug and the presence of known structural features that (1) are associated with causing liver injury; or (2) have been associated with affecting certain biological mechanisms thought to be involved in causing liver injury.

2   The Role of Physicochemical Properties in Liver Injury

2.1   Dose, Toxicology and Liver Injury

Toxicology is founded on the basic principle that the dose determines the poison. In other words, toxicity is intrinsic to the molecule, but the administered dose defines whether that toxicity will be observed. Therefore the expression of human (and mammalian) toxicity for the most part is predicated on the absorption, distribution, metabolism and elimination of the drug.

The amount and frequency of dosing of an oral drug is largely determined by the minimum concentration required to achieve efficacy along with its absorption, distribution, metabolism and excretion (ADME) properties [1]. In addition, the pharmacological interaction of a drug is driven by the unbound or free concentration of the drug in the body and so the degree of protein binding of a given drug will also play a key role in determining the dose. These ADME properties are heavily influenced by each compound's physicochemical properties and these are in turn determined by its molecular structure and therefore are an important consideration in drug design.

Several key physicochemical properties have been shown to affect the pharmacokinetic profile of a compound. These are:

1. Molecular size and shape
2. Lipophilicity
3. pKa
4. Hydrogen bonding

Probably the most important property of a drug molecule is its lipophilicity as this plays a role in many of the most important attributes of a good drug. Lipophilicity is most frequently characterized via the partition (P) or distribution (D) coefficients, which represent the ratio of concentrations of a given compound in the two phases of a mixture of two immiscible solvents at equilibrium. Quantified as log$P$ and log$D$, the former refers to the ratio of the concentration of compound in the lipid phase to the concentration of all species (ionized and unionized) in aqueous phase at a given pH, while the latter is defined as the logarithm of the ratio of unionized compound in each phase. Since log$D$ varies with the pH at which the measurement is made, the pH value is often specified. At biological pH, therefore log$D_{7.4}$ is most typically used.

Knowledge of the pK_a value is crucial for analyzing both lipophilicity and the solubility of ionizable compounds. Ionization equilibria also affect several pharmacokinetic parameters, such as absorption, membrane permeability, protein binding and certain metabolic transformations.

2.2 The Influence of Physicochemical Properties on Key ADME Properties

2.2.1 Oral Bioavailability

Oral bioavailability (F) is a product of fraction absorbed (Fa), fraction escaping gut-wall elimination (Fg), and fraction escaping hepatic elimination (Fh) [1, 2]. After conducting an analysis of the distribution of certain physicochemical properties across several thousand marketed drugs, Lipinski and coworkers [3] observed that the majority of oral drugs that have good oral bioavailability had a molecular weight (MW) <500; calculated LogP (cLog$P$) <5; number of hydrogen bond donor atoms (HBD) <5; and the number of hydrogen bond acceptor atoms (HBA) <10. This set of observations, dubbed the "rule of 5" has become a set of guiding principles for designing oral drugs with good absorption. Lipinski et al. observed that chemicals are less likely to have good oral absorption if they violate two or more of these guidelines. However, it should be noted that there are numerous examples of drugs, e.g., acyclovir, that adhere to these criteria yet have poor bioavailability in the region of less than 30% of the administered dose. Conversely, there are examples of drugs, e.g., cyclosporine, that are readily absorbed yet do not pass more than two of these criteria. Cyclosporine has an oral bioavailability of up to 60% and thus has reasonable absorption. The absorption of most drugs is predominated by passive diffusion across membrane barriers, however both uptake and efflux active transport mechanisms exist and these might explain some of the outliers in this analysis of bioavailability.

Varma et al. also looked at a trend analysis that clearly indicated molecular weight (MW), ionization state, lipophilicity, polar descriptors, and free rotatable bonds (RB) influence bioavailability [2]. They observed that higher MW significantly impacted Fa, while Fg and Fh decreased with increasing LogP. Whereas polar descriptors often gave parabolic trends for bioavailability where low and high values showed similar effects. The most interesting observation was that the number of free rotatable bonds had a negative effect on all three parameters, Fa, Fg, and Fh, leading to a pronounced effect on bioavailability. They concluded that physicochemical properties influence bioavailability with typically opposing effects on Fa and first-pass elimination.

2.2.2 Plasma Protein Binding

Drug molecules circulating in the blood stream of any in vivo system are either bound to proteins and lipids in plasma or to proteins and lipids in tissues, or are unbound (sometimes referred to as free) and diffuse among the aqueous environment of the blood and tissues [4]. Plasma protein binding (PPB), among other factors, can strongly influence volume of distribution and half-life of chemicals [5]. In turn, physicochemical properties such as $\log P$ and pKa can have a strong influence on the degree of PPB observed for a given drug. As a general trend, molecules with high lipophilicity will have a lower fraction unbound and acidic molecules will similarly have a greater degree of PPB than basic compounds [6].

2.2.3 Volume of Distribution

An important measure of compound distribution that has been demonstrated to have a link to toxicity in mammals is the concept of Volume of Distribution (Vd). This is defined as the theoretical volume that the total amount of administered drug would have to occupy (if it were uniformly distributed), to provide the same concentration as it currently is in plasma. A higher value of Vd shows that the drug is more diluted than it should be in the bloodstream implying that more of the chemical is distributed into the tissues. Drugs with high lipophilicity (nonpolar), not ionized at physiological pH, i.e., basic molecules, or have low plasma protein binding have higher volumes of distribution than drugs which are more polar, more highly ionized (i.e., acidic molecules) or exhibit high plasma protein binding [1]. Vd directly influences the half-life of a compound whereby large Vd leads to a longer half-life, i.e., prolongs the duration of exposure. In studies looking at properties that influence the lowest observable adverse effect level (LOAEL) in rodent studies, the Vd of a given compound was observed to have a strong influence on the LOAEL where a larger value for Vd results in a lower LOAEL [7].

2.2.4 Clearance
(Metabolism and Excretion)

Clearance (CL) is one of the most important of all pharmacokinetic parameters. It describes the relationship between the rate of elimination of chemical and its concentration in plasma. Total clearance describes the elimination of a chemical from the body without identifying the mechanisms involved in the process but most chemicals are eliminated primarily via the liver and/or kidney. CL is affected significantly by the binding of chemicals to serum proteins as only the free (unbound) fraction of a compound can undergo clearance mechanisms. In studies published the rate of clearance is heavily dependent on the lipophilicity of the molecule at pH 7.4 as expressed by the term $LogD_{7.4}$ which is ultimately related to the $LogP$ and pKa of a compound [8].

2.2.5 Elimination
Half-Life

The elimination half-life of a drug is the time it takes for a drug to lose half of its concentration in the blood plasma. The half-life of a drug is directly related to Vd and CL and so by inference, it is also heavily influenced by the same physicochemical properties of compounds as Vd and CL.

However, dose or plasma concentration alone does not directly cause toxicity. A drug molecule needs to have the ability to interact with the biological processes of the liver in a way that will lead to toxicity if severe or prolonged enough that the system is unable to restore or correct itself.

3   Structure–Activity Relationships Associated with DILI

3.1 Development
of SAs

A method to identify a drug's inherent liability leading to toxicity is to search for structural motifs or structural alerts that commonly occur in compounds known to cause a particular effect. These structural alerts can be simple correlations between common motifs and an observed biological response but often are supported by a plausible chemical or biological mechanism that would explain the expression of chemical toxicity.

A structural alert is the chemical representation of a structural feature that is associated with a specific biological event. In toxicology, the presence of a structural alert, sometimes referred to as a toxicophore, within a query compound is an indication that a particular toxicological event (or events) is more likely than if the feature was not present. The structural alert methodology is inherently conservative because they often do not take into account other structural features or physicochemical properties of the query molecule that could mitigate the observation of a toxicological event. As such, all identified structural alerts need to be investigated further to understand the relevance of both the structural and mechanistic rationale of the alert to the query compound.

There are a number of approaches for the identification of structural features within a toxicological dataset. Features can be identified statistically through the use of computer algorithms, such as in the application of quantitative structure–activity relationship (QSAR) techniques, pharmacophore modeling, and automated machine learning approaches. Features can also be identified through a visual analysis of the dataset by a human expert that is familiar with the endpoint being modeled, i.e., through the development of structure–activity relationships (SARs). An advantage of applying this expert methodology is the opportunity to link the toxicophore to a particular mechanism of toxicity, thereby reducing chance correlations that are more likely to be a reflection of structural bias within the dataset, rather than of the toxicological event itself. In addition to the ability to synthesize disparate, sparse or contradictory data into a coherent SAR, a human expert analysis can impart further knowledge that may be useful toward improving the applicability of a structural alert, such as ADME properties and additional structural features that may mitigate the toxicological event. One disadvantage of this approach, however, is that it is a time-consuming process and cannot be readily updated on the availability of new toxicological data. On the other hand, models based on a statistical analysis can often be built and updated quickly, but depending on the chemical descriptors used can lack the transparency that is associated with SAR systems.

An initial SAR study usually results in grouping of compounds with similar chemical features, followed by an analysis of the toxicological profile of each class. For those classes that are highly correlated with the toxicological activity under analysis, additional evidence is then collected to support the implementation of a structural alert. Such evidence may include a mechanistic rationale, similarities in the histopathological profile of liver damage and availability of any in vitro toxicological data that may be associated with the observed hepatotoxicity, such as metabolic activation, BSEP inhibition and/or mitochondrial liabilities. There is no strict rule on the number of compounds required to support an alert as the derivation of strong mechanistic rationale could warrant the alert being supported by only one or two compounds. In the ideal scenario the evaluation of these alerts should be carried out using data that was not used in the development of the alert and to take into account, if possible, the impact of exposure and species to species variability when assessing new datasets.

3.2 Published SARs for Drug-Induced Liver Injury (DILI)

One of the first reports of computationally derived structural alerts for liver toxicity was published by Egan et al. in 2004 [9]. The authors developed 74 alerts through the interrogation of a dataset of 244 compounds using an internal chemoinformatics platform at Vertex. Of the 74 alerts identified, 56 were based on the chemical features that had the potential to form reactive metabolites.

Unfortunately, neither the actual toxicophores nor an assessment of their predictive performance was published. The remaining 18 alerts were based on their high structural similarity to known hepatotoxic drugs where the toxicological mechanisms were not known or were not clear.

Subsequently, Greene et al. developed 38 structural alerts for hepatotoxicity which were implemented in the Derek for Windows (version 10) expert system [10]. To achieve this, the authors constructed a dataset of 1266 chemicals from public sources [11–13] where liver toxicity data for drugs and other chemicals in animals and humans were collected. Although animal data was included in the dataset, the main focus of the work was to derive SARs associated with liver damage in humans and for each alert to be supported by published toxicity data and mechanistic evidence. The updated custom Derek knowledge base was evaluated using a proprietary Pfizer dataset of 626 compounds that had liver toxicity data in both humans and animals. The evaluation showed that the updated Derek knowledge base had a sensitivity of 46% with a specificity of 73% against the external test set. The relatively low sensitivity in this case was explained by the focus on human-derived structural alerts and the desire to implement only those alerts that had sufficient mechanistic evidence and several supporting compounds.

In 2013, Hewitt and coworkers developed and published toxicophores for 16 hepatotoxicity structural alerts that were generated by the clustering of structurally similar chemicals in a hybrid approach that combined an automated method with human evaluation [14]. Compounds within each cluster were then used to search for data that would support a mechanistic rational for the hepatotoxic profile associated with each chemical class. The authors provided the detailed supporting evidence behind each alert and highlighted that some of these classes were likely to be associated with multiple mechanisms of liver damage.

Pizzo and coworkers described a similar study [15] in their attempt to create an in silico model for hepatotoxicity using rodent repeat-dose toxicity studies data that was extracted from the Hazard Evaluation Support System (HESS) database [16]. Nine structural features were selected based on the high levels performance for each class. The relevance of these features for hepatotoxicity was investigated using the public literature by way of mechanistic evidence and/or experimental data. For example, mechanism-related information was available for the bioactivation of halobenzenes, naphthalene containing compounds and para-alkylphenols, and experimental liver toxicity was identified in animals for the bisphenyl and bromomethane toxicophores. The authors did not report overall performance of their alerts for the training nor external sets; their intention, however, is to use these alerts for the identification and prioritization of potentially toxic substances.

In 2015, Liu and coworkers also identified 12 structural fragments that are statistically correlated to an increased risk of DILI from 606 drugs that have been annotated with respect to their hepatotoxicity profile [17]. Example classes include cyclopropyl amine and the commonly identified arylacetic acid. Studies such as these are useful for providing structural hypotheses, but it is essential that new toxicophores are investigated further to ensure mechanistic integrity. For example, isoflurane (a fluorinated anesthetic) and efavirenz (a nonnucleoside reverse transcriptase inhibitor) are classed together because they share a similar 2-atom structural feature, yet they are likely to have very different hepatotoxic mechanisms. Such statistical anomalies are thought to be the product of machine learning algorithms, but they can also be a property of some expert SAR studies too.

In 2016 Pizzo and coworkers carried out a second SAR study using a dataset of 950 compounds with human hepatotoxicity data that was compiled from various public sources [18]. In total 51 alerts were generated, 11 structural alerts were manually selected and 40 alerts were automatically generated from a computer algorithm. Two out of the 11 manually selected alerts were to identify nonhepatotoxic compounds (steroids backbone, and cephalosporin beta-lactam antibiotics). The authors created a structural alert decision tree which gave high levels of sensitivity (>80% for all the training and test sets), but relatively poor levels of specificity for the test sets (<33% each).

These results support the notion that it may be relatively simple to build a structural alert model that is predictive of the training set, but it is a challenge to retain predictive performance when robustly evaluating with external test sets. One of the reasons for this is the incorrect identification of the toxicophore associated with hepatotoxicity. Therefore, despite numerous publications describing the development of SARs for compounds with known hepatotoxicity profiles, the prediction of DILI potential for new chemicals using structural alerts remains a challenge.

3.3 Published Structural Alerts for Reactive Metabolites

A significant number of structural alerts for hepatotoxicity are based on chemical features that undergo bioactivation to generate reactive metabolites (RMs). For example, a well-known example of intrinsic, dose-dependent hepatotoxicity is acetaminophen. This compound has been shown to be converted to the highly reactive metabolite, N-acetyl p-benzoquinoneimine (NAPQI) [19]. At high doses, NAPQI will react with cellular components when the usual conjugation pathways are saturated (such as the formation of glutathione adducts), leading to disruption of cellular functions [20]. It is unlikely that this widely used painkiller would pass through the stringent testing in use today.

Although RMs have been shown to covalently bind to cellular nucleophiles and cause a significant reduction in the cellular antioxidant, glutathione, it is often a challenge to prove that these are the actual causative events that lead to hepatotoxicity. Furthermore, in some cases, the formation of a specific RM is a requirement for the intended pharmacological action of a parent drug, e.g., clopidogrel (and closely related analogues ticlopidine, prasugrel, and vicagrel) [21].

For example, tienilic acid was withdrawn from the market due to a high incidence of liver toxicity [22] and the proposed mechanism involves the bioactivation of the thiophene ring to form reactive metabolites that have been shown to covalently modify cellular proteins [23] (Fig. 1). As such, thiophene is considered a structural alert for hepatotoxicity.

However the activation of a RM-based structural alert does not necessarily mean that the feature will undergo bioactivation [21]. In some cases, metabolism may occur at another location on the molecule, reducing the likelihood that the toxicological events associated with the toxicophore may occur. Furthermore, even though cellular adducts may be detected in in vitro studies with human liver microsomes (HLM), the metabolic profile of a chemical in vivo could vary significantly owing to the presence of additional metabolic routes that are not represented in HLMs. As a consequence, the observation of RMs in vitro or the activation of a RM-based structural alert does not necessarily lead to the observation of toxicity. For example clopidogrel and olanzapine contain the thiophene ring system and yet are successfully marketed drugs.

Moreover the refinement of SARs for RMs could be achieved by including factors related to the probability of bioactivation of a specific chemical feature. Such an approach was successfully applied by Dang et al. for four structural alerts: furans, phenols, nitroaromatics, and thiophenes [24]. The authors used XenoSite to generate scores for the potential sites of metabolism and where a structural alert was colocated with a predicted site of metabolism, then it was considered likely that bioactivation could occur (conversely where an alert was present but predicted to be a site of metabolism, then bioactivation was considered unlikely).

As stated previously, another factor that may mitigate the toxicological impact of a structurally alerting group is the daily dose. A number of publications provide evidence for the link between exposure and toxicity potential [21, 25].

One of the most comprehensive reviews of the structural alert methodology was carried out by Stepan and coworkers in 2011 [26]. In this study, the authors investigated the difference in structural alert profiles between two sets of drugs, one set based on 68 drugs that have been withdrawn or have black box warnings (BBW), and the other based on 200 currently marketed drugs [26]. Although the majority of drugs in the withdrawn/BBW set

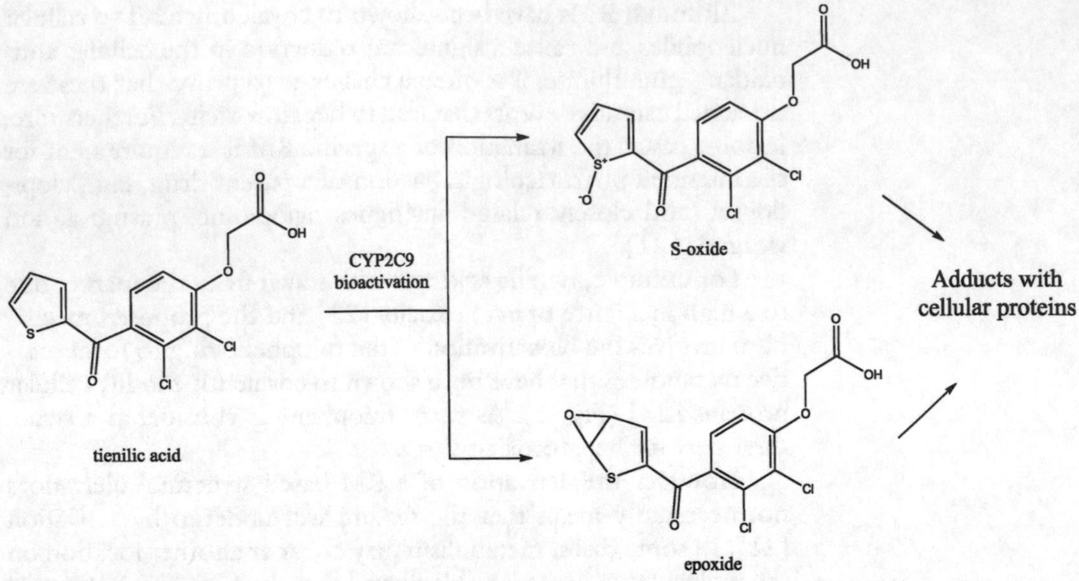

Fig. 1 Bioactivation of tienilic acid to S-oxide and/or epoxide that implicated in formation of adducts with cellular proteins

had structural alerts and/or evidence of RM formation, it was also noted that so do half of the set of market drugs. Additionally, no significant difference was observed between the physicochemical properties of each drug set. It was concluded that the majority of the toxic drugs (causing hepatotoxicity and other adverse effects) have high daily doses (100–2400 mg), giving an indication that the best de-risking strategy is to minimize exposure from structurally alerting candidates through improving pharmacokinetics and increasing intrinsic potency during pharmaceutical development.

One caveat of global analyses that evaluate the performance of structural alerts is that the limitations of the structural alert methodology are often acknowledged but not addressed during the analysis. For example, the class of phenols was included as a structural alert in the Stepan study [26] on the basis of their increased likelihood of oxidation to reactive quinoidal moieties. In the absence of an SAR study to understand which subgroup of phenols are more likely to oxidize and form RMs, then the inclusion of this broad class would inadvertently lead to a high false positive rate in any analysis. Therefore, what is often being assessed is the scientific rigor by which the applicability domain of a structural alert is derived and the amount of evidence that supports it.

Hepatotoxicity is often a result of two or more mechanisms which are frequently overlapping. This is illustrated with the thiazolidinedione antidiabetic drugs, troglitazone, pioglitazone, and rosiglitazone. Although these drugs all show a similar bioactivation profile of the thiazolidinedione ring [27] as well as being inhibitors of the bile salt export pump (BSEP) [28], only troglitazone has been withdrawn from the market for liver injury. It has also been shown to decrease mitochondrial membrane potential (MMP) [29] and is also a potent agonist of FXR (farnesoid X receptor) [30]. In addition, troglitazone has a relatively high daily dose (200–400 mg/day) in comparison to pioglitazone and rosiglitazone (15–45 and 2–8 mg/day respectively). In contrast, rosiglitazone has been withdrawn for cardiac toxicity and pioglitazone has been withdrawn in some markets for its link to causing bladder cancer. Therefore, the thiazolinedione structural alert may well be a useful alert for the identification of potential reactive metabolites, but more evidence is required before it can be used in the prediction of DILI.

4 Published Nonreactive SARs for DILI

The mechanism for reactive metabolites is largely dependent upon a compound's structural features and so the application of structural alert methodology is ideal for these classes of DILI-causing compounds. In contrast, hepatotoxicity that is derived from a pharmacological mechanism, such as FXR agonism or BSEP inhibition, is dependent upon the attainment of several, complex structural interactions that give rise to the pharmacological interaction with the protein. These drug-protein interactions can involve the formation of hydrogen and/or covalent bonds, electrostatic interactions, or hydrophobic bonds that can displace surface water molecules from the protein to gain entropic energy. As a consequence, lipophilicity can also play a role in determining whether or not a molecule will interact with unintended targets such as FXR and BSEP. There are many studies reported where the relative selectivity of a molecule is highly correlated to its $LogP$ value with lipophilic molecules being less selective, i.e., having pharmacological interactions with multiple receptors [31–33].

In most cases, it is the unbound fraction of molecules that interact with protein receptors to produce a pharmacological effect on the system. Chemicals that act via a pharmacological interaction with a protein receptor, such as the peroxisome proliferator-activated receptor (PPAR), that are also highly bound to plasma proteins will generally require higher doses to achieve the required free concentrations to elicit an equivalent response to a chemical that has a lower PPB level provided the rate and fraction absorbed for both are equivalent.

The chemical features that determine pharmacological activity may be challenging to capture as a structural alert with any reasonable levels of accuracy. However, the following examples reflect structural properties that have been investigated for various nonreactive mechanisms associated with DILI.

4.1 Redox Cycling

The presence of reactive oxygen species and the subsequent disruption of cellular redox homeostasis are believed to be a key driver of hepatotoxicity [34, 35]. Rana and coworkers modified a hydrogen-peroxide assay to identify structural features that correlate with the observation of redox cycling in the assay [36]. As expected, quinoidal-type compounds, such as the hepatotoxic compound menadione, were active in this assay and their ability to redox cycle has been reported [37]. In addition, the study identified other toxicophores that were linked to redox cycling, such as pyrimidine triazinediones and arylidenepyridenediones (Fig. 2).

The authors concluded that these observations support the hypothesis that extended "push–pull" pi-systems have a higher likelihood of redox cycling, which may contribute toward a hepatotoxic profile of any compound containing these toxicophores.

4.2 Mitochondrial Dysfunction

Many of the marketed drugs that have been withdrawn due to hepatotoxicity are able to inhibit mitochondrial respiration or are capable of disconnecting mitochondrial electron transport from the production of ATP (the so-called uncoupling of oxidative phosphorylation). A SAR study by Naven and coworkers demonstrated that lipophilicity and the presence of an acidic proton were essential for protonophoric uncoupling. In addition, they proposed that stabilization of the ionized protonophore through delocalization or intramolecular hydrogen bonding was a critical factor for potent uncoupling activity study [38]. As part of this study, 14 structural alerts were identified, 11 of which were highly associated with potent uncoupling activity.

As with the prediction of RMs, structural alert methodology is useful for the prediction of uncouplers because, ultimately, activity is largely dependent on one structural feature, the absence of which precludes activity. In contrast, inhibition of one of the complexes in the mitochondrial electron transport chain may involve so many molecular interactions that the development of SAR may be limited to whole molecules and their closely related structural analogues, rather than to specific functional groups. A comprehensive review of the compounds that are known to disrupt mitochondrial dysfunction has been published in the book chapter by Mehta et al. [39].

4.3 Disruption of Transporter Homeostasis

Inhibition of the bile salt export pump has been identified as a potential toxicological mechanism that contributes to the induction of DILI [40, 41]. To highlight the challenge of identifying SARs for such pharmacological mechanisms, a study conducted by Pedersen and coworkers found that only physicochemical features, such as lipophilicity, charge, and molecular size, were highly associated with BSEP inhibition and not specific functional groups [42]. This indicates that, at least for BSEP inhibition, one particular group by itself is not a useful predictive factor for activity. In support, a similar dependency of BSEP inhibition on molecular weight

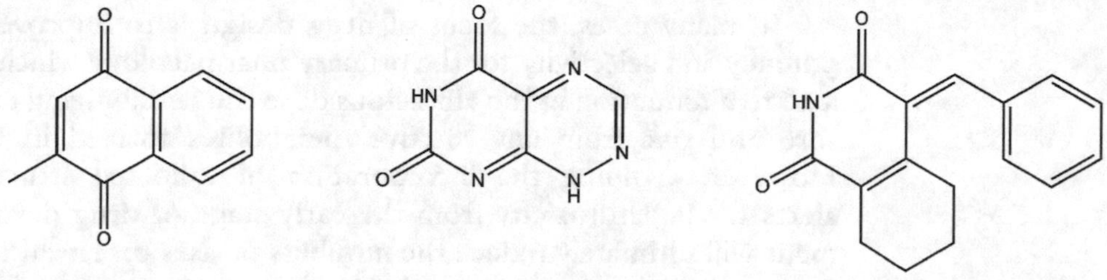

Menadione   Pyrimidinetriazinedione   Arylidenepyridenedione
                           toxicophore   toxicophore

Fig. 2 Toxicophores implicated in redox cycling

and lipophilicity was also found by Warner et al. [43]. In contrast, a structure-based QSAR study for the prediction of cholestasis identified 16 structural features that were associated with BSEP inhibition [44]. The activation of two or more features lead to a greater confidence in BSEP inhibition and this was supported by the known BSEP inhibitor and idiosyncratic hepatotoxicant, troglitazone, which activated four structural features in the model. In another study, Welch and coworkers identified structural features that were predictive of inhibition of both BSEP and MRP4, including those that correlated with noninhibition, such as the presence of a basic side chain [45]. It is important to note, however, that the authors of this study concluded that the predictive performance of the structure-based models could be improved by including a lipophilicity threshold below which a structural alert was considered not relevant.

These studies suggest that a statistical QSAR methodology based on physicochemical properties of chemicals and/or pharmacophore descriptors, rather than structural alerts, may be the best approach toward the prediction of these pharmacologically based mechanisms of hepatotoxicity.

5   Summary

Drug-induced liver injury is a complex endpoint, and the expression of DILI is dependent upon multiple factors of pharmacology, pharmacokinetics, physicochemical properties, metabolism, and genetic variability. As such, the ideal predictive in silico strategy would include a cumulative assessment of toxicological potential across multiple pharmacological, structural and physicochemical mechanisms as well as a consideration of liver exposure through the evaluation of several pharmacokinetic parameters. Structural alerts can play a key role in this strategy provided that they are derived from sufficient data that enables the development of an applicability domain and defined mechanism of action.

In many cases, the focus of drug design is to improve the potency and selectivity for the primary pharmacology which can lead to a reduction in the efficacious dose thus minimizing exposure and risk from any reactive metabolites formed in vivo. However, avoiding the incorporation of validated structural alerts for hepatotoxicity from the early stage of drug development will ultimately reduce the numbers of risks that need to be managed downstream. Drug design approaches that can incorporate all of the various aspects of compound liabilities (in addition to structural alerts and reactive metabolite formation), together with physicochemical properties, will ultimately lead to the avoidance of safety risks during the drug development process [46, 47]. However, some factors that link to individual variability (such as genetic polymorphism in major histocompatibility complex—MHC, human leukocytes antigen—HLA) are currently difficult to assess by conventional experiments, but the new in vitro approaches that can accommodate genetic population differences are being continuously investigated by academia and research organizations.

References

1. Grime KH, Barton P, McGinnity DF (2013) Application of in silico, in vitro and preclinical pharmacokinetic data for the effective and efficient prediction of human pharmacokinetics. Mol Pharm 10(4):1191–1206. https://doi.org/10.1021/mp300476z

2. Varma MV, Obach RS, Rotter C, Miller HR, Chang G, Steyn SJ, El-Kattan A, Troutman MD (2010) Physicochemical space for optimum oral bioavailability: contribution of human intestinal absorption and first-pass elimination. J Med Chem 53(3):1098–1108. https://doi.org/10.1021/jm901371v

3. Lipinski CA, Lombardo F, Dominy BW, Feeney PJ (1997) Experimental and computational approaches to estimate solubility and permeability in drug discovery and development settings. Adv Drug Deliv Rev 23(1–3):3–25. https://doi.org/10.1016/S0169-409X(96)00423-1

4. Smith DA, Di L, Kerns EH (2010) The effect of plasma protein binding on in vivo efficacy: misconceptions in drug discovery. Nat Rev Drug Discov 9(12):929–939. https://doi.org/10.1038/nrd3287

5. Hollosy F, Valko K, Hersey A, Nunhuck S, Keri G, Bevan C (2006) Estimation of volume of distribution in humans from high throughput HPLC-based measurements of human serum albumin binding and immobilized artificial membrane partitioning. J Med Chem 49(24):6958–6971. https://doi.org/10.1021/jm050957i

6. Vallianatou T, Lambrinidis G, Tsantili-Kakoulidou A (2013) In silico prediction of human serum albumin binding for drug leads. Expert Opin Drug Dis 8(5):583–595. https://doi.org/10.1517/17460441.2013.777424

7. Sutherland JJ, Raymond JW, Stevens JL, Baker TK, Watson DE (2012) Relating molecular properties and in vitro assay results to in vivo drug disposition and toxicity outcomes. J Med Chem 55(14):6455–6466. https://doi.org/10.1021/jm300684u

8. Zhivkova Z, Doytchinova I (2013) Quantitative structure–clearance relationships of acidic drugs. Mol Pharm 10(10):3758–3768. https://doi.org/10.1021/mp400251k

9. Egan WJ, Zlokarnik G, Grootenhuis PD (2004) In silico prediction of drug safety: despite progress there is abundant room for improvement. Drug Discov Today Technol 1(4):381–387. https://doi.org/10.1016/j.ddtec.2004.11.002

10. Greene N, Fisk L, Naven RT, Note RR, Patel ML, Pelletier DJ (2010) Developing structure-activity relationships for the prediction of hepatotoxicity. Chem Res Toxicol 23(7):1215–1222. https://doi.org/10.1021/tx1000865

11. Zimmerman HJ (1999) Hepatotoxicity: the adverse effects of drugs and other chemicals on

the liver. Lippincott Williams & Wilkins, Philadelphia, PA

12. Ludwig J, Axelsen R (1983) Drug effects on the liver. An updated tabular compilation of drugs and drug-related hepatic diseases. Dig Dis Sci 28(7):651–666

13. Lee WM (2003) Drug-induced hepatotoxicity. N Engl J Med 349(5):474–485. https://doi.org/10.1056/NEJMra021844

14. Hewitt M, Enoch SJ, Madden JC, Przybylak KR, Cronin MT (2013) Hepatotoxicity: a scheme for generating chemical categories for read-across, structural alerts and insights into mechanism(s) of action. Crit Rev Toxicol 43(7):537–558. https://doi.org/10.3109/10408444.2013.811215

15. Pizzo F, Gadaleta D, Lombardo A, Nicolotti O, Benfenati E (2015) Identification of structural alerts for liver and kidney toxicity using repeated dose toxicity data. Chem Cent J 9:62. https://doi.org/10.1186/s13065-015-0139-7

16. Sakuratani Y, Zhang HQ, Nishikawa S, Yamazaki K, Yamada T, Yamada J, Gerova K, Chankov G, Mekenyan O, Hayashi M (2013) Hazard Evaluation Support System (HESS) for predicting repeated dose toxicity using toxicological categories. SAR QSAR Environ Res 24(5):351–363. https://doi.org/10.1080/1062936X.2013 773375

17. Liu R, Yu X, Wallqvist A (2015) Data-driven identification of structural alerts for mitigating the risk of drug-induced human liver injuries. J Chem 7(1):4. https://doi.org/10.1186/s13321-015-0053-y

18. Pizzo F, Lombardo A, Manganaro A, Benfenati E (2016) A new structure-activity relationship (SAR) model for predicting drug-induced liver injury, based on statistical and expert-based structural alerts. Front Pharmacol 7:442. https://doi.org/10.3389/fphar.2016.00442

19. Corcoran GB, Mitchell JR, Vaishnav YN, Horning EC (1980) Evidence that acetaminophen and N-hydroxyacetaminophen form a common arylating intermediate, N-acetyl-p-benzoquinoneimine. Mol Pharmacol 18(3):536–542

20. Mitchell JR, Jollow DJ, Potter WZ, Gillette JR, Brodie BB (1973) Acetaminophen-induced hepatic necrosis. IV protective role of glutathione. J Pharmacol Exp Ther 187(1):211–217

21. Kalgutkar AS, Dalvie D (2015) Predicting toxicities of reactive metabolite-positive drug candidates. Annu Rev Pharmacol Toxicol 55:35–54. https://doi.org/10.1146/annurev-pharmtox-010814-124720

22. Dansette PM, Amar C, Valadon P, Pons C, Beaune PH, Mansuy D (1991) Hydroxylation and formation of electrophilic metabolites of tienilic acid and its isomer by human liver microsomes. Catalysis by a cytochrome P450 IIC different from that responsible for mephenytoin hydroxylation. Biochem Pharmacol 41(4):553–560

23. Manier JW, Chang WW, Kirchner JP, Beltaos E (1982) Hepatotoxicity associated with ticrynafen—a uricosuric diuretic. Am J Gastroenterol 77(6):401–404

24. Dang NL, Hughes TB, Miller GP, Swamidass SJ (2017) Computational approach to structural alerts: furans, phenols, nitroaromatics, and thiophenes. Chem Res Toxicol. https://doi.org/10.1021/acs.chemrestox.6b00336

25. Shah F, Leung L, Barton HA, Will Y, Rodrigues AD, Greene N, Aleo MD (2015) Setting clinical exposure levels of concern for drug-induced liver injury (DILI) using mechanistic in vitro assays. Toxicol Sci 147(2):500–514. https://doi.org/10.1093/toxsci/kfv152

26. Stepan AF, Walker DP, Bauman J, Price DA, Baillie TA, Kalgutkar AS, Aleo MD (2011) Structural alert/reactive metabolite concept as applied in medicinal chemistry to mitigate the risk of idiosyncratic drug toxicity: a perspective based on the critical examination of trends in the top 200 drugs marketed in the United States. Chem Res Toxicol 24(9):1345–1410. https://doi.org/10.1021/tx200168d

27. Alvarez-Sanchez R, Montavon F, Hartung T, Pahler A (2006) Thiazolidinedione bioactivation: a comparison of the bioactivation potentials of troglitazone, rosiglitazone, and pioglitazone using stable isotope-labeled analogues and liquid chromatography tandem mass spectrometry. Chem Res Toxicol 19(8):1106–1116. https://doi.org/10.1021/tx050353h

28. Morgan RE, Trauner M, van Staden CJ, Lee PH, Ramachandran B, Eschenberg M, Afshari CA, Qualls CW Jr, Lightfoot-Dunn R, Hamadeh HK (2010) Interference with bile salt export pump function is a susceptibility factor for human liver injury in drug development. Toxicol Sci 118(2):485–500. https://doi.org/10.1093/toxsci/kfq269

29. Masubuchi Y, Kano S, Horie T (2006) Mitochondrial permeability transition as a potential determinant of hepatotoxicity of antidiabetic thiazolidinediones. Toxicology 222(3):233–239. https://doi.org/10.1016/j.tox.2006.02.017

30. Kaimal R, Song X, Yan B, King R, Deng R (2009) Differential modulation of farnesoid X receptor signaling pathway by the thiazolidinediones. J Pharmacol Exp Ther 330(1):125–134. https://doi.org/10.1124/jpet.109.151233

31. Hughes JD, Blagg J, Price DA, Bailey S, Decrescenzo GA, Devraj RV, Ellsworth E, Fobian YM, Gibbs ME, Gilles RW, Greene N, Huang E, Krieger-Burke T, Loesel J, Wager T, Whiteley L, Zhang Y (2008) Physiochemical drug properties associated with in vivo toxicological outcomes. Bioorg Med Chem Lett 18(17):4872–4875. https://doi.org/10.1016/j.bmcl.2008.07.071

32. Leeson PD, Springthorpe B (2007) The influence of drug-like concepts on decision-making in medicinal chemistry. Nat Rev Drug Discov 6(11):881–890. https://doi.org/10.1038/nrd2445

33. Price DA, Blagg J, Jones L, Greene N, Wager T (2009) Physicochemical drug properties associated with in vivo toxicological outcomes: a review. Expert Opin Drug Metab Toxicol 5(8):921–931. https://doi.org/10.1517/17425250903042318

34. Tolosa L, Gómez-Lechón MJ, Pérez-Cataldo G, Castell JV, Donato MT (2013) HepG2 cells simultaneously expressing five P450 enzymes for the screening of hepatotoxicity: identification of bioactivable drugs and the potential mechanism of toxicity involved. Arch Toxicol 87(6):1115–1127. https://doi.org/10.1007/s00204-013-1012-x

35. Saito J, Okamura A, Takeuchi K, Hanioka K, Okada A, Ohata T (2016) High content analysis assay for prediction of human hepatotoxicity in HepaRG and HepG2 cells. Toxicol In Vitro 33:63–70. https://doi.org/10.1016/j.tiv.2016.02.019

36. Rana P, Naven R, Narayanan A, Will Y, Jones LH (2013) Chemical motifs that redox cycle and their associated toxicity. MedChemComm 4(8):1175–1180. https://doi.org/10.1039/C3MD00149K

37. Badr M, Yoshihara H, Kauffman F, Thurman R (1987) Menadione causes selective toxicity to periportal regions of the liver lobule. Toxicol Lett 35(2–3):241–246

38. Naven RT, Swiss R, Klug-Mcleod J, Will Y, Greene N (2013) The development of structure-activity relationships for mitochondrial dysfunction: uncoupling of oxidative phosphorylation. Toxicol Sci 131(1):271–278. https://doi.org/10.1093/toxsci/kfs279

39. Mehta R, Chan K, Lee O, Tafazoli S, O'Brien PJ (2008) Drug-associated mitochondrial toxicity. In: Wojtczak L (ed) Drug-induced mitochondrial dysfunction. John Wiley & Sons, Inc, Hoboken, NJ, pp 71–126. https://doi.org/10.1002/9780470372531.ch3

40. Aleo MD, Luo Y, Swiss R, Bonin PD, Potter DM, Will Y (2014) Human drug-induced liver injury severity is highly associated with dual inhibition of liver mitochondrial function and bile salt export pump. Hepatology 60(3):1015–1022. https://doi.org/10.1002/hep.27206

41. Dawson S, Stahl S, Paul N, Barber J, Kenna JG (2012) In vitro inhibition of the bile salt export pump correlates with risk of cholestatic drug-induced liver injury in humans. Drug Metab Dispos 40(1):130–138. https://doi.org/10.1124/dmd.111.040758

42. Pedersen JM, Matsson P, Bergström CAS, Hoogstraate J, Norén A, LeCluyse EL, Artursson P (2013) Early identification of clinically relevant drug interactions with the human bile salt export pump (BSEP/ABCB11). Toxicol Sci 136(2):328–343. https://doi.org/10.1093/toxsci/kft197

43. Warner DJ, Chen H, Cantin L-D, Kenna JG, Stahl S, Walker CL, Noeske T (2012) Mitigating the inhibition of human bile salt export pump by drugs: opportunities provided by physicochemical property modulation, in silico modeling, and structural modification. Drug Metab Dispos 40(12):2332–2341. https://doi.org/10.1124/dmd.112.047068

44. Sakurai A, Kurata A, Onishi Y, Hirano H, Ishikawa T (2007) Prediction of drug-induced intrahepatic cholestasis: in vitro screening and QSAR analysis ofdrugs inhibiting the human bile salt export pump. Expert Opin Drug Saf 6(1):71–86. https://doi.org/10.1517/14740338.6.1.71

45. Welch MA, Köck K, Urban TJ, Brouwer KLR, Swaan PW (2015) Toward predicting drug-induced liver injury: parallel computational approaches to identify multidrug resistance protein 4 and bile salt export pump inhibitors. Drug Metab Dispos 43(5):725–734. https://doi.org/10.1124/dmd.114.062539

46. Park BK, Boobis A, Clarke S, Goldring CE, Jones D, Kenna JG, Lambert C, Laverty HG, Naisbitt DJ, Nelson S, Nicoll-Griffith DA, Obach RS, Routledge P, Smith DA, Tweedie DJ, Vermeulen N, Williams DP, Wilson ID, Baillie TA (2011) Managing the challenge of chemically reactive metabolites in drug development. Nat Rev Drug Discov 10(4):292–306. https://doi.org/10.1038/nrd3408

47. Thompson RA, Isin EM, Ogese MO, Mettetal JT, Williams DP (2016) Reactive metabolites: current and emerging risk and hazard assessments. Chem Res Toxicol 29(4):505–533. https://doi.org/10.1021/acs.chemrestox.5b00410

Chapter 5

Quantitative Structure–Activity Relationship Models for Predicting Risk of Drug-Induced Liver Injury in Humans

Huixiao Hong, Jieqiang Zhu, Minjun Chen, Ping Gong, Chaoyang Zhang, and Weida Tong

Abstract

Drug-induced liver injury (DILI) risk in humans is a complicated safety concern due to diverse mechanisms, various severity levels, variation in population groups, and difficulty in annotation of drugs, especially for the drugs that have been on the market for a short period of time. DILI remains a challenge for the industry and regulatory agencies. Assessing DILI risk in humans is important to assist drug development for the industry and to inform decision making on safety evaluation of drug products in regulatory science. Though various experimental methods have been used in current practices for assessment of DILI risk, in silico methods have been adopted in the field as an alternative because the development and validation of in silico models are much faster and cheaper. Many quantitative structure–activity relationship (QSAR) DILI prediction models have been reported. To better understand the QSAR models reported and to foster development of more reliable QSAR models, this chapter provides an instruction to the principals and the components of QSAR modeling, a summary on some popular algorithms and tools for QSAR modeling, and a review of QSAR models developed for prediction of DILI.

Key words Drug-induced liver injury, DILI, Quantitative structure–activity relationship, QSAR, Prediction, Chemical descriptors, Algorithm, Drug, Safety

1 Introduction

Drug-induced liver injury (DILI) remains a challenge for pharmaceutical industry, clinicians, research scientists, and regulatory agencies [1]. DILI can be idiosyncratic or caused by specific intrinsic mechanisms (dose-dependent) [2]. There are a number of mechanisms (including alterations in bile acid homeostasis, mitochondrial dysfunction, reactive metabolite formation, and oxidative stress) that are known for hepatotoxicity of idiosyncratic and nonidiosyncratic DILI drugs [3]. A lot of research efforts have been carried out to eliminate drug candidates that might cause DILI. Therefore, predicting human DILI risk is an urgent need to

Minjun Chen and Yvonne Will (eds.), *Drug-Induced Liver Toxicity*, Methods in Pharmacology and Toxicology,
https://doi.org/10.1007/978-1-4939-7677-5_5, © Springer Science+Business Media, LLC, part of Springer Nature 2018

improve development of safer drugs and to facilitate safety evaluation of drug products.

Different methods have been developed to assess DILI risk in humans associated with drug products and candidates. Many in vitro and in vivo assays have been designed for evaluation of DILI risk of chemicals during drug development [4–15]. Additionally findings from retrospective studies and postapproval drug monitoring could be further used to assess DILI risk in humans [16–19]. Although in vitro and in vivo experimental data and observations in clinical investigations helped our understanding of DILI and improved our capability to assess human DILI risk of drug products and candidates, accurately predicting human DILI risk remains to be a challenge in drug development, regulatory science, and clinical practices. As new technologies such as mass spectrometry-based proteomics [20], microarray genotyping [21, 22], and next-generation sequencing [23–26] emerged in the scientific community to facilitate discovery and development of biomarkers [27], tremendous and concerted efforts were made to promote these technologies to identify sensitive and specific biomarkers for prediction of DILI risk [28]. However, most of the more recently identified DILI biomarkers such as microRNA biomarkers have not been translated into regulatory decision making and drug development [29–32].

Much more experimental studies and clinical investigations are needed to enhance predictive capability of assessing DILI risk in humans. Although in vitro experiments are much cheaper than time-consuming and at costly in vivo experiments and clinical investigations, in silico methods are attractive as an alternative approach for prediction of human DILI risk due to possibility to analyze a vast chemical space in timely manner. Many in silico models have been developed for predicting DILI risk [33–46]. Most of the developed in silico models were based on the principal of quantitative structure–activity relationship (QSAR) [33–42]. QSAR models not only demonstrated potential to predict human DILI risk but also gained a lot of attractions in the DILI field due to low costs at both time and money guiding further in vitro and in vivo studies. To advance development of more reliable QSAR models for predicting human DILI risk, this chapter introduces principal and technical components of QSAR models. Case studies of QSAR models for DILI prediction are reviewed and future perspectives for development of DILI prediction QSAR models are discussed.

2 QSAR

2.1 QSAR Rationale

QSAR is used to define the relationship between biological activity and chemical structures. A QSAR model is a mathematical function that is used to estimate the biological activity of a compound based on its chemical structure [47]. Mathematically, development of a QSAR model using a set of training chemicals is to determine a mathematical transformation that can be used to estimate the bioactivity data of the training chemicals using numerical descriptions of their structures so that the sum of errors between the estimated and the actual bioactivity data is optimized to a minimum as presented in Eq. (5.1).

$$\mathbf{A} = f(\mathbf{S}) + \varepsilon. \tag{5.1}$$

In Eq. (5.1), $\mathbf{A}$ is the vector of bioactivity data; $\mathbf{S}$ represents the matrix of numerical descriptions of structures of the training chemicals; f indicates the mathematical function that transforms the numerical description of structures into a vector for estimation of bioactivity; ε denotes the minimized error that consists of modeling error (bias) and experimental error or observational variability of the actual bioactivity data $\mathbf{A}$.

Bioactivity data $\mathbf{A}$ could be categorical (such as positive and negative) or continuous (numerical). For a QSAR model to predict categorical bioactivity of chemicals, the mathematical function f assigns categorical classes to the chemicals based on the description of their structures. This type of QSAR models is termed "Classification models." When a QSAR model is used to estimate continuous bioactivity, the mathematical function f transforms the description of a chemical structure to a numerical estimation of its bioactivity. They are termed "Regression models." Both classification and regression models are considered as supervised learning in the machine learning field [48], i.e., a model is determined by learning training chemicals with known bioactivity data obtained either in experiments or through calculations.

In order to develop a classification or regression QSAR model, chemical structures should be described numerically. A variety of methods have been used to describe chemical structures. The methods for numerical description of chemical structures can be divided into two major types depending at the way they are calculated: target structure based (or 3D QSAR) and small molecule based (or ligand based).

When the target protein is known for the bioactivity in a QSAR modeling, the structure of a chemical can be described using the interactions between the target and the chemical. Most of the protein structure-based QSAR models have been developed using molecular docking [49–53].

When the target protein is not known or multiple targets are involved in the bioactivity to be modeled, the structures of a set of chemicals that have been tested are used to train a QSAR model. This is the so-called ligand-based or small molecule-based QSAR modeling. The methods for ligand-based QSAR modeling can be divided into three types. The first type is structural alert, i.e., structural features that associated with toxic effects due to (1) chemical's intrinsic reactivity, (2) its bioactivation/metabolism to reactive species, or (3) interaction with proteins leading to disruption of cellular functions. For example steroid skeleton (any bond types), diethylstilbestrol skeleton (any bond type for the linker), and phenolic ring were demonstrated to be the good structural alerts for binding with the estrogen receptor [56]. In addition to a single structural alert, a structural alert could be a group of structural features and is termed as a combined structural alert. A pharmacophore is a combined structural alert that consists of steric and electronic features that are correlated with a specific biological activity. Pharmacophore modeling has been widely used in QSAR studies [57–59].

The second type of ligand-based methods for numerical description of compounds is molecular descriptor. Molecular descriptors are a large number (hundreds to thousands) of values for description of a chemical structure. Molecular descriptors can be classed as fingerprints and (numerical) descriptors. One of the well-known examples of numerical descriptors application is Lipinski's rule of five. This rule is a set of molecular properties that are important for a drug's pharmacokinetics (absorption, distribution, metabolism, and excretion—ADME) and used in drug development to screen compounds that would be orally active in humans [54, 55]. Number of hydrogen bond acceptors, number of hydrogen bond donors, molecular weight and $\log P$ (octanol–water partition coefficient) are criteria in Lipinski's rule of five. In some literature Lipinski's rule also referred as a structural alert. A fingerprint is a particular complex form of descriptors. It is an ensemble of a set of structural fragments that can be binary or numerical; but binary fingerprints are more popular as they are much more efficient in chemoinformatics. Examples of fingerprints and popular sources that can be used to calculate fingerprints are given in Table 1 [60–63]. General numerical descriptors are calculated to characterize the electronic, geometric, steric, and topological properties of a chemical compound. A few notable tools for molecular descriptors calculation are Mold2 [64], ADAT [65], CODESSA [66], BlueDesc (http://www.ra.cs.uni-tuebingen.de/software/bluedesc), OASIS [67], POLLY [68], CERIUS2 (www.accelrys.com), PaDEL [62], ChemAxon JChem (https://www.chemaxon.com/), CDK Descriptor Calculator (http://www.rguha.net/code/java/cdkdesc.html), DRAGON (www.talete.mi.it), MOLCONN-Z (http://www.edusoft-lc.com/molconn/mconprod.html), ADMEWORKS ModelBuilder (http://www.fqs.pl/chemistry_materials_life_science/products/admeworks_modelbuilder), CDK (http://cdk.github.io/cdk/), RDKit (http://sourceforge.net/projects/rdkit/), and Chemopy [61].

Table 1
Fingerprints and the tools for QSAR

Fingerprint	Description	Tools to calculate
FP2	A fingerprint records linear fragments of up to seven atoms in a molecular structure. Through path analysis, linear segments of length 1–7 atoms are identified. A path ends when the atoms form a ring. Only canonical fragments are recorded in the fingerprint which is a 1024 bit vector	Pybel (https://pypi.python.org/pypi/PyBEL/0.3.8) [60]
FP3	A set of functional groups based on 55 SMARTS patterns stored in patterns.txt from Open Babel	Pybel
FP4	A set of functional groups based on 55 SMARTS patterns stored in SMARTS_InteLigand.txt from Open Babel	Pybel; Chemopy (https://sourceforge.net/projects/chemopy/) [61]
MACCS	A set of substructure keys stored in MACCS.txt from Open Babel	Pybel; Chemopy; CDK (http://cdk.github.io/cdk/); RDKit (http://sourceforge.net/projects/rdkit/); PaDEL (http://padel.nus.edu.sg/software/padeldescriptor) [62]; JCompoundMapper (jcompoundmapper.sourceforge.net/) [63]
Daylight-like fingerprint	A daylight-like topological fingerprint based on hashing molecular subgraphs	Chemopy
E-state	A set of 79 E-state fragments	Chemopy; CDK; RDKit; PaDEL
Atom pairs	A set of counts for atom pairs	Chemopy; RDKit; PaDEL
Torsion fingerprint	A set of topological torsions	Chemopy; RDKit
Morgan fingerprint	Fingerprints calculated using Morgan algorithm	Chemopy; RDKit
CDK fingerprint	Fingerprints are one-dimensional bit arrays in which bits are used for particular structural features	CDK; PaDEL
PubChem fingerprint	A PubChem fingerprint is a set of 881 structural keys	CDK; PaDEL
CDK extended fingerprint	A fingerprint that extends the CDK fingerprint with additional bits describing ring features	CDK; PaDEL

(continued)

Table 1
(continued)

Fingerprint	Description	Tools to calculate
Klekota-Roth fingerprint	A fingerprint of 4860 SMARTS based substructures	CDK; PaDEL
GraphOnly fingerprint	A fingerprint that does not take bond orders into account	CDK; PaDEL
Hybridization fingerprint	A fingerprint that does not take into account of aromatic fragment; but takes into account of SP2 hybridization	CDK
Substructure fingerprint	A fingerprint for 307 substructures	CDK; PaDEL
RDK fingerprint	A Daylight-like topological fingerprint generated using an alternate (faster) hashing algorithm	RDKit
Layered fingerprint	A fingerprint that is calculated using a layer-based hashing algorithm	RDKit
Pattern fingerprint	A fingerprint that is generated using a series of predefined structural patterns	RDKit
DFS	A fingerprint of paths generated by a graph traversal with a modified depth first search	JCompoundMapper
ASP	DFS like, only paths that have shortest distances are recorded	JCompoundMapper
AP2D	A fingerprint that consists of atom types and the shortest paths between all pairs of atoms	JCompoundMapper
AP3D	Similar to AP2D. The difference is that the geometrical distance matrix is used for distance calculation	JCompoundMapper
CATS2D	A set of pairwise topological relationships of PPP (potential pharmacophore points) patterns	JCompoundMapper
CATS3D	Similar to CATS2D. The difference is that geometric relationships of PPP patterns are used	JCompoundMapper

The third type of ligand-based methods for numerical description of compounds is the force field-based description that needs three-dimensional (3D) structures of a set of small training chemicals with known activities. This type of methods is different from the second type of methods (molecular descriptors that are computed from scalar quantities such as energies, geometric parameters, some even need 3D structures). This methodology requires 3D structures of a set of training chemicals to be superimposed together for the calculation of force fields to describe the training chemicals for QSAR model development. The first QSAR modeling method based on force fields was proposed by Cramer et al. and was termed as Comparative Molecular Field Analysis [69]. In a CoMFA model, the electrostatic fields and the steric fields (shape of the molecule) are correlated with bioactivity data of the training chemicals by means of partial least square (PLS) derived from principal component analysis (PCA). CoMFA has been widely utilized in QSAR models for drug development and toxicological endpoint prediction [70, 71]. Molecular Similarity Indices in a Comparative Analysis (CoMSIA) is another QSAR modeling method based on field description of chemicals [72]. CoMFA mainly uses Lennard-Jones and Coulomb potentials that solely describe the energetic fields in ligand binding without consideration of entropic contributions. Because Lennard-Jones potential energy at grids changes dramatically, very small conformational changes or slight different superimposition of molecules can result in strong variations in the field description values. Different from CoMFA, CoMSIA uses a common probe atom to calculate similarity indices at regularly spaced grid points for each of the superimposed molecules of training chemicals. The distance between the probe atom and the atoms of a training chemical is used to determine the similarity indices. Any relevant physical chemical property such as steric, electrostatic, and hydrophobic properties could be used to calculate the field of similarity indices in CoMSIA. This method attracted applications in the QSAR field [73, 74].

Supervised machine learning requires input variables (descriptors) and an output variable (biological activity). Supervised learning algorithms could be further grouped into classification and regression problems. Classification QSAR models can be separated into two types: binary classification and multiclass classification. In a binary classification QSAR model, only two classes of samples are contained in the training set. A multiclass classification QSAR model assigns a chemical to one of multiple classes of bioactivity. Many classification methods have been used specifically for binary classification such as Decision Forest (DF) [75–80]. Therefore, one type of multiclass classification methods is to combine multiple binary classifiers such as multiclass DF [81]. Supervised machine learning algorithms are used to determine the mathematical function f by learning from a training data set for QSAR modeling

[82–86]. Theoretically all machine learning algorithms could be used for this purpose. Table 2 summarizes some popular machine learning algorithms used in QSAR modeling.

2.2 QSAR Model Development

The process for development of QSAR models is illustrated in Fig. 1. In order to develop a QSAR model, the bioactivity data and structures for a set of chemicals should be collected as the training set. Databases are designed for this purpose. The direct transformation of chemical structures to their biological activity using a mathematical function (the red arrow in Fig. 1) is difficult, if not impossible. Therefore, in the QSAR field, tools have been developed to generate numerical descriptions of the chemical structures (fingerprints or descriptors). Then machine learning algorithms are used to determine the mathematical function to convert the numerical descriptions of structures to the predicted biological activity as shown by the blue arrows in Fig. 1.

2.2.1 Databases

Many databases have been constructed to facilitate the development of QSAR models. In this chapter, we briefly introduce the FDA's liver toxicity knowledge base (LTKB) to demonstrate the importance of specialized databases for developing reliable QSAR models. LTKB was developed at FDA/NCTR to improve the understanding of DILI and to facilitate construction of DILI prediction QSAR models [46].

In the FDA's Advancing Regulatory Science initiative, many technologies including in silico modeling are embraced to help the extrapolation from preclinical findings to clinical practices. LTKB is a knowledgebase which serves as a resource of all types of data needed for safety evaluation in terms of liver toxicity. Figure 2 depicts the overall structure of the LTKB. Diverse types of data (e.g., in vitro test results, in vivo assays, toxicogenomics, histopathology, and adverse effects reports) have been curated from the literature or have been generated from experiments for most FDA-approved drugs in the database. The DILI risks of the drugs collected in LTKB were classified using the FDA-approved drug labeling as the primary source [87] and coupled with DILI severity [88].

DILI is considered a heterogeneous disease and could be affected by many factors. Using a single type of data sources or a single model to predict DILI could result in a high rate of incorrect predictions. Therefore, combination of diverse data to annotate DILI risk of drugs is vital for the success of QSAR models for predicting DILI. A "benchmark data set" that contains the drugs with well annotated DILI risks has been established in LTKB. This standard set of drugs has been made available to the scientific community to promote assay design and QSAR model development (https://www.fda.gov/ScienceResearch/BioinformaticsTools/LiverToxicityKnowledgeBase/ucm2024036.htm).

Table 2
Machine learning algorithms

Algorithm	Description	Tools[a]
Artificial neuro network	Definition of functions for connection weights of the architecture of neurons	R, Rapidminer, AZOrange, Annie, EasyNN, libF2N2, Neuroph, NetMaker
Decision forest	Consensus of multiple decision trees which are accurate (deep) using diverse descriptors	Decision Forest
Decision tree	A tree-like model of decisions and their possible consequences, including probabilities of a type or values of outcomes	R, ELKI, mlpy, MOA
Hidden Markov model	A connection of states with different probability distributions for transition between states	R, zipHMM, GHMM, SFIHMM
k-NN	K nearest neighbors are taken from a training set to determine the class (for classification) or the property value (for regression) of an unknown sample	R, Rapidminer,
Logistic regression	A regression model for categorical biological activity data	R, SAS, NCSS
Naïve Bayes	A probabilistic algorithm based on Bayes' theorem with strong (naive) independence assumptions between descriptors	R, Orange, Rapidminer, Weka, KNIME, Tanagra, jBNC, MOA
Random Forest	Consensus of many shallow decision trees using a subset of descriptors and a subset of samples	R, Orange, Rapidminer, Weka, AZOrange, Tanagra
Support Vector Machine	A hyperplane in a high-dimensional space that can be used separate samples for classification and regression	R, KNIME, LIBSVM, Dlib, Orange, Rapidminer, Weka, AZOrange, Tanagra, SVMlight, mlpy

[a]Tools: Annie (http://annie.sourceforge.net/); AZOrange (https://github.com/AZcompTox/AZOrange); Decision Forest (https://www.fda.gov/ScienceResearch/BioinformaticsTools/DecisionForest/ucm2006645.htm); Dlib (http://dlib.net/ml.html); EasyNN (http://www.easynn.com/); ELKI (https://elki-project.github.io/); GHMM (http://www.ghmm.org/); jBNC (http://jbnc.sourceforge.net/); KNIME (http://www.knime.org/), libF2N2 (http://libf2n2.sourceforge.net/); mlpy (http://mlpy.sourceforge.net/); LIBSVM (https://www.csie.ntu.edu.tw/~cjlin/libsvm/); MOA (http://moa.cms.waikato.ac.nz/); NCSS (https://www.ncss.com/); NetMaker (http://www.ire.pw.edu.pl/~rsulej/NetMaker/); Neuroph (http://neuroph.sourceforge.net/); Orange (http://orange.biolab.si/); R (https://www.r-project.org/); Rapidminer (https://rapidminer.com/); SAS (https://www.sas.com/); SFIHMM (http://tuvalu.santafe.edu/~simon/styled-8/); SVMlight (http://svmlight.joachims.org/); Tanagra (http://eric.univ-lyon2.fr/~ricco/tanagra/en/tanagra.html); Weka (http://www.cs.waikato.ac.nz/ml/weka/); zipHMM (http://birc.au.dk/software/zipHMM/)

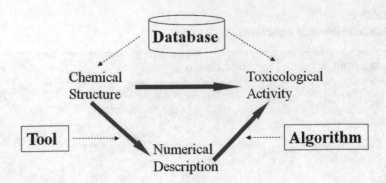

Fig. 1 Overview of QSAR model development

The DILI risk of a drug can be assessed by three factors: causality, incidence, and severity. The FDA-approved drug labels used in LTKB consider comprehensive information related to all of the three factors for drugs. The advantage of DILI risk annotation within LTKB is the unique characteristic of the FDA-approved drug labels that are the outcome of the consensus of opinions from many experts based on diverse preclinical and clinical data. Furthermore, the label of a drug would be revised if postmarket surveillance data showed evidence of DILI risk in patients. The drugs in LTKB have been annotated to have most-DILI, less-DILI, and no-DILI concern based on their FDA-approved drug labels [87, 88].

As shown in Fig. 2, LTKB contains a large number of FDA-approved drugs with comprehensive data, including physiochemical properties, in vitro data, chemical structures, toxicogenomic data, histopathological data, and adverse reactions collected from multiple resources. In addition to the data for QSAR modeling, a huge amount of toxicogenomic data have been curated in LTKB from the Japanese Toxicogenomics Project [89] and the DrugMatrix database of National Institute of Environmental Health Sciences (https://ntp.niehs.nih.gov/drugmatrix/).

2.2.2 Description of Chemical Structures

It is very difficult to directly use molecular structures in QSAR models. The common practice in QSAR modeling is the use of numerical descriptors to indirectly describe the chemical structures. Structural descriptors are numerical descriptions that describe the structural features. QSAR models correlate a set of molecular descriptors of chemicals with the biological activity of interest. Many structural descriptors have been developed. Mold2 [64] is taken as an example for discussion in this chapter.

In the early time of QSAR history, the empirical physical-chemical properties of chemicals such as partition coefficients, substituent constants, and various electronegativity-related parameters were used as molecular descriptors. With the increased calculation power and advances in computational chemistry, more and more

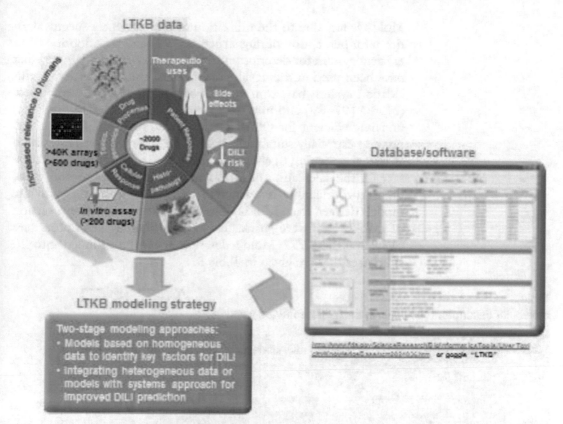

Fig. 2 LTKB structure and data types collected. LTKB has three components of LTKB: curation drug-elicited data curation, predictive DILI models construction, and database and related software development

numerical parameters are calculated from 2D- and 3D-structures as molecular descriptors for the development of QSAR models. The types of molecular descriptors used in the current QSAR modeling practices vary from the easily calculated constitutional and topological descriptors to sophisticatedly derived quantum chemical descriptors [90].

The debate on the superiority of 3D molecular descriptors over 2D molecular descriptors has been continuing for a long period of time in the QSAR community. However, no consensus has been reached. Similar performance of QSAR models constructed using 3D and 2D molecular descriptors was observed in the comparative studies [91–93], arguing that 2D molecular descriptors implicitly contain 3D structural information. Another drawback of 3D descriptors is the difficulty in determination of the bioactive conformations. Therefore, the best set of molecular descriptors may be indeterminable in the absolute sense.

A set of molecular descriptors were implemented in the Mold2 software package to be calculated from 2D chemical structures [64]. As a free software tool (http://www.fda.gov/ScienceResearch/BioinformaticsTools/Mold2/default.htm),

Mold2 is fast due to the utilization of the extremely speedy algorithm for perception of ring structures [94] and the adoption of an efficient system for description of chemical structures [95, 96] that have been used in the development of the chemical structure elucidation system based on analysis of nuclear magnetic resonance (NMR) [97–99] and infrared spectra [100]. Therefore, Mold2 is not only efficient for QSAR models based on small size data sets but also especially suitable for QSAR on large-sized data sets such as virtual screening of chemicals. The 3D structures are not necessary for the calculation of Mold2 molecular descriptors and, thus, high reproducibility is warranted to Mold2 descriptors and the models derived from Mold2 descriptors. Using the current version of Mold2 software package, 777 structural descriptors are calculated. The 777 Mold2 descriptors can be grouped into 20 subclasses that are given in Table 3.

Table 3
Molecular descriptors contained in the Mold2 software package

Class	Subclass	Number of descriptors	Example of descriptors
1D	Counts for atoms	105	Number of O atoms
	Chemical physical property	2	Molecular weight
2D	Counts for atoms	80	Number of ring tertiary C
	Counts for bonds	9	Number of rotatable bonds
	Counts for functional groups	104	Number of carboxylic (aromatic)
	Chemical physical property	16	$\log P$
	Structural features	13	Number of 5 member rings
	2D autocorrelation	96	Moran coefficient
	Balaban index	12	Normalized centric index
	Connectivity index	36	Randic connectivity index
	Detour index	24	Cyclicity index
	Distance (topological) index	73	Average atom eccentricity
	Eigen value based descriptors	88	Folding degree index
	Information content	45	Mean information content
	Kier index	14	Kier flexibility
	Molecular walk counts	13	Total walk count
	Schultz index	4	Reciprocal Schultz index
	Topological charge index	21	Mean topological charge
	Wiener index	17	Normalized Wiener index
	Zagreb index	5	Quadratic index

2.2.3 Algorithms

When biological activity data and numerical descriptions of a set of chemicals are ready to train a QSAR model, the training task is done by using a machine learning algorithm. A brief summary of some machine learning algorithms is given in Table 2. As an example, we give a detailed description of the novel machine learning algorithm DF [75, 76].

DF is a consensus modeling algorithm and combines a number of decision trees to make a consensus model so that the prediction performance is improved. DF algorithm generates deep decision trees ensuring each decision tree has a good prediction performance. Another feature of DF is the diversity of the member decision trees constructed using different molecular descriptors. The chemical diversity of member decision trees warrants that each member decision tree contributes to the consensus DF model in a complementary way. In brief, building a DF model consists of four steps: (1) train a decision tree model using a unique set of descriptors; (2) discard the used descriptors in the decision tree constructed; (3) repeat steps (1) and (2) until the improvement in prediction performance is less than a preset value by adding a decision tree; (4) ensemble of the results from all of the decision trees as the final prediction.

DF provides algorithms for both binary classification and multiclass classification. The binary classification DF algorithm is available online(http://www.fda.gov/ScienceResearch/BioinformaticsTools/DecisionForest/default.htm). The binary classification DF algorithm is a consensus modeling method in which a number of binary decision tree models are constructed separately. Figure 3a illustrates the principal of binary DF algorithm. A set of binary decision trees were constructed using diverse molecular descriptors. The probability values for a chemical to be positive from the binary decision tree models are averaged with equal weights. The result is used as the consensus probability value of the DF model for the chemical to be positive.

The rationale of the multiclass DF algorithm is depicted in Fig. 3B. In short, a binary classification DF model is built for each of the M classes by merging the rest M-1 classes of chemicals into one class. The probability values from the M binary classification DF models are used to predict the likelihood of a chemical to be the class modeled. The final prediction for the chemical from the multiclass DF model depends on the M probability values from the M binary classification DF models using the winner-take-all approach. If two or more winners are obtained for a chemical, assigning the chemical to only one class is not possible and, thus, the multiclass DF model predicts the chemical to be a new class of "unknown."

2.3 QSAR Model Validation

Similar to other scientific methods and experiments, QSAR modeling is not an error free approach. All QSAR models have errors, small or large. The source of errors in QSAR models are diverse

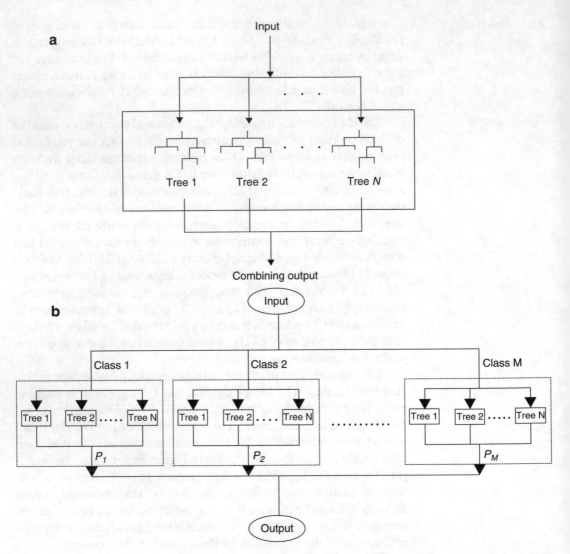

Fig. 3 DF algorithmic flowcharts. The flowchart for binary classification DF is illustrated in (**a**). Accurate decision tree models are constructed from training dataset using diverse molecular descriptors. Prediction of a chemical is the combination of predictions from the N decision tree models for the chemical. The average value of the probabilities from the N decision tree models is used as the consensus probability from DF for the chemical. The flowchart for multiclass DF is shown in (**b**). First, for each of the M classes, a binary classification DF model (all other classes are treated as another class) is built as illustrated in (**a**). The multiclass DF model is to compare the probabilities the M DF models. A chemical is predicted as the class with the largest probability value. If more two or more probability values are equally the largest for a chemical, a new class "unknown" is assigned to the chemical

and are summarized in the error term in Eq. (5.1). The errors could result from the biological activity data and/or the modeling process. Therefore, thorough validation of a QSAR model is vital for the consideration of potential regulatory applications of the model. To facilitate potential applications of QSAR models for regulatory purposes, OECD (Organization for Economic

Co-operation and Development) published the OECD principles for the validation, for regulatory purposes, of (quantitative) structure–activity relationship models (http://www.oecd.org/chemicalsafety/risk-assessment/37849783.pdf). The OECD principal no. 4, appropriate measures of goodness-of-fit, robustness and predictivity, is the core for validation of QSAR models and should be applied to all practices of QSAR models, both regulatory and scientific. This section will discuss the appropriate methods and procedures for validation of QSAR models.

<table>
<tr><td>2.3.1 Internal Validation</td><td>Validation methods can be divided into two types: internal and external validations. The use of the terms in the literature is not standardized and sometimes causes confusion to the readers. Special attention should be paid to the OECD definition of internal and external validations. The internal validation defined by the OECD's guidance document on the validation of (quantitative) structure–activity relationship [(Q)SAR] models (http://www.oecd.org/env/guidance-document-on-the-validation-of-quantitative-structure-activity-relationship-q-sar-models-9789264085442-en.htm) only estimates the goodness-of-fit of a QSAR model and is often equivalent to the training results reported in the literature.</td></tr>
</table>

We use the term of internal validation to represent the validation processes that use the data obtained from the same experimental protocol in the same laboratory that is used to generate the training data set. In this sense, the internal validation used in this chapter is equivalent to the external validation in the OECD guidance and reported in some scientific publications. The main purpose of internal validation is to estimate the robustness and predictive performance of the QSAR modeling that could be expected to perform on the data that have been obtained using the same protocol in the same laboratory. Alternatively, the errors in the bioactivity data for the QSAR are minimized so that the error terms of Eq. (5.1) observed in an internal validation is mainly caused by the modeling technique.

Three internal validation processes are used in the current QSAR practices. The first is leave-one-out cross-validation (LOOCV). LOOCV is an approach that estimates the performance of QSAR models generated by the QSAR modeling procedure, rather than that of a specific model. Basically, in LOOCV, each chemical in the training set is taken out to test the model generated from the rest of the chemicals. All prediction results are summed up as an estimation of the model built in the training set. Therefore, LOOCV result is a performance estimation of a generalized model constructed using the same modeling procedure on the training chemicals. Rather than choosing one model trained on all training chemicals, LOOCV is used to provide a slightly conservative estimation of the performance of the QSAR model that trained on all training chemicals.

The second internal validation scenario is k-fold cross-validation. A k-fold cross-validation is a procedure to estimate performance of QSAR models by partitioning a set of chemicals into a training set to build a QSAR model, and a test set to challenge the model. In a k-fold cross-validation, the chemicals are first randomly divided into k portions with equal or near equal sizes. One portion of chemicals is left out for testing the QSAR model trained using the remaining $k - 1$ portions of chemicals. The process is then repeated k times with each of the k portions used once and only once as the testing samples. The results from testing the k portions are finally averaged to make an estimation of model performance. Similar to LOOCV, the feature of this method is that all chemicals are used for both training and testing, and all chemicals are used for validation once (cross-validation).

The third internal validation is holdout validation. In a holdout validation, a portion of the original set of chemicals is holdout for testing the model constructed using the remaining chemicals. The prediction results are used to estimate the model performance. Theoretically, holdout validation can be considered as equivalent to partial result of k-fold cross-validation. Statistically speaking, k-fold cross-validation is better than holdout validation for estimation of generalization of models and robustness of the modeling procedure used. However, due to k-fold validation being usually computationally expensive the holdout set could be useful for initial validation of a model. One time of holdout validation is the estimate of goodness of the model on the holdout chemicals, while k-fold cross-validations and LOOCV are the estimate of robustness and generalization capability of the QSAR modeling procedure. Though holdout validation can be used for internal validation in QSAR, we have to note that there are many ways to draw a holdout set randomly from the original set of chemicals. The results from different holdout sets from the same original set of chemicals have a large variance (especially compared to the equivalent k-fold cross-validations). The best practice for holdout validation in QSAR is to run many holdout validations using different randomly splitting the original set of chemicals and to use the average model performance. This validation method is often referred to as repeated random sub-sampling or Monte Carlo cross-validation. It is worth to point out that holdout validation is often incorrectly used as external validation that needs an independent test set in the QSAR community.

2.3.2 External Validation

External validation is different from internal validation. Internal validation is used to validate a QSAR modeling procedure, while external validation is used for validation of a QSAR model. Though both validation methods are used to estimate the performance of the QSAR model constructed from a training set of chemicals, they emphasize different aspects of generalization of a QSAR model.

Internal validation measures robustness of the QSAR model and external validation focuses on extrapolation of the QSAR model.

External validation is the validation of a QSAR model using a set of chemicals that are not used in the training set with the experimental data for the same biological activity from different laboratories or different assays or generated after the model is developed. Using chemicals different from the training chemicals is the necessary condition (the same for internal validation) but not the sufficient condition of external validation. The experimental data used in external validation should be the one generated after the QSAR model is developed or obtained from other laboratories if the endpoint is the same with training set or the same biological data of different assays, depending at the validation purpose. Many external validation results are actually one type of internal validation without robustness measure (e.g., one holdout validation is reported as an external validation).

3   QSAR Models for DILI Prediction

Many QSAR models for predicting DILI risk have been developed using machine learning algorithms [33–37, 41, 42]. Here we review the QSAR models for predicting DILI risk in humans using DF [33].

To develop QSAR models for predicting DILI risk in humans, labeled data of a large set of FDA-approved drugs were used [33]. Drug labeling can be used to assess risk of human hepatotoxicity. The labels of FDA-approved drugs were used to categorize drugs into three groups: most-DILI-concern, less-DILI-concern, and no-DILI-concern [87]. The DILI risk groups were used as the dependent variable for the development of DILI prediction QSAR models. Three published data sets, including NCTR dataset [33], Greene et al. dataset [101], and Xu et al. dataset [37] were used as the independent external validation sets to estimate the prognostic performance of the QSAR model developed based on the training set [33, 101]. The molecular descriptors calculated by Mold2 software [64] were used to develop the QSAR models. The machine learning algorithm DF [75–80] was used to train the models. Tenfold cross-validations were used to measure robustness of the model performance. Permutation tests were conducted to determine predictive power of the models and to assess the chance correlation of the models. Figure 4 shows the overall strategy for developing and validating the DILI prediction QSAR model.

The average sensitivity, specificity and accuracy yielded from the 2000 repetitions of tenfold cross-validation were 57.8 ± 6.2% (standard deviation), 77.9 ± 3.0%, and 69.7 ± 2.9%, respectively. The low prediction accuracy of the permutation results (48.5%) indicated that the average prediction accuracy from the cross-validations (69.7%) was not obtained by mere chance correlations.

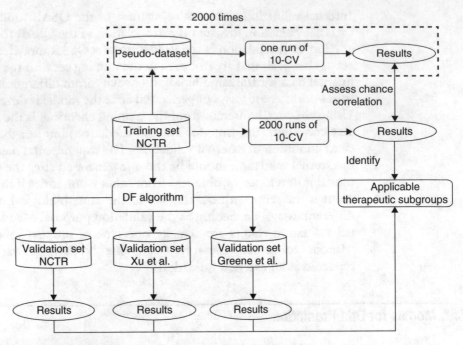

Fig. 4 Study design for the development of DILI prediction QSAR model

Three external data sets (NCTR, Greene, and Xu data sets) were used to estimate prediction performance of the QSAR model. The prediction accuracy, sensitivity, and specificity were 68.6%, 66.3%, and 70.8%, respectively, for 191 drugs (95 most-DILI-concern +96 no-DILI concern) in the NCTR data set; 61.6%, 58.4%, and 67.5% for 328 drugs (214 most-DILI-concern +114 no-DILI concern) in the Greene data set; 63.1%, 60.6%, and 66.1% for 241 drugs (132 most-DILI-concern +109 no-DILI concern) in the Xu data set.

We compared the QSAR model predictions for the drugs having consistent DILI annotations across the three external data sets with the drugs containing different DILI annotations. The results revealed that 70% of the drugs that were consistently annotated in NCTR and Greene data sets were predicted correctly using the QSAR model, however, only 58.8% of the drugs that were inconsistently annotated were predicted correctly. The same trend stands when comparing NCTR validation set with Xu data set and comparing Greene data set with Xu data set.

Predictive performance of the QSAR DILI model in the tenfold cross-validations on drugs that belong to different therapeutic subgroups was analyzed using the second level Anatomical Therapeutic Chemical (ATC) code. The results showed that the drugs in the 22 therapeutic subgroups were predicted more accurately than the rest drugs and were determined as the high-confidence subgroups; while the drugs in the remaining 18 therapeutic subgroups were more difficult to predict and were termed as the low-confidence subgroups. The results demonstrated that the QSAR model could be used for human DILI prediction, especially for the high-confidence therapeutic subgroups.

4 Perspectives

Appropriate annotation of DILI risk in humans is extremely important for the development of robust QSAR models for prediction of DILI risk in humans. Many DILI risk annotation (or classification) methods have been proposed and are based on different information such as case reports and the FDA approved drug labels. A better DILI risk annotation system for a large number of drugs is expected to improve the performance of QSAR models for DILI prediction, therefore we will see more efforts to develop comprehensive approaches for DILI risk annotation by integration of rich data on drugs such as causality, frequency, and severity of DILI observed in preclinical and clinical studies, case reports of postmarketing surveillances, and drug labels approved by the FDA. Challenges remain in annotation of DILI risk in humans due to the dynamic nature of DILI risk assessment. The DILI annotation for the same drugs may be changed after QSAR models are developed when new evidence is obtained to revise their DILI annotation.

Description of molecules in numerical way is critical for the success of development and application of QSAR models for DILI prediction. Training a DILI QSAR model is to define a mathematical function for converting the numerical description of drugs to their potential human DILI risk categories. Thus, the completeness in chemical space, information content, redundancy, and mixture of units of the numerical description of molecules play roles in the development of QSAR models. It is a huge challenge, if not impossible, to have the best and unique set of molecular descriptors for QSAR model development. Unlike shallow neuro networks that map numerical description of chemicals to their activity values, a deep learning QSAR model consists of many mapping units in a layered and hierarchical way to optimize accuracy of the model. A deep learning neuro network learns descriptions of the molecules in multiple levels of abstraction with the final layer mapping the last description to bioactivity values. Deep learning has shown success in QSAR modeling, especially for large data sets [37, 101]. It is expected that more deep learning algorithms will be developed for DILI QSAR modeling.

The most vital process in QSAR modeling is validation of the developed models. Cross-validation is used to measure the robustness and reliability of the models, while a holdout validation is used to measure the performance of a specific model on the holdout set. External validation is used to estimate how well a specific model can be generalized in predictions, and therefore wider use of the model.

Disclamier

The views expressed in this chapter do not necessarily represent those of the US Food and Drug Administration.

References

1. Raschi E, De Ponti F (2017) Drug-induced liver injury: towards early prediction and risk stratification. World J Hepatol 9(1):30–37. https://doi.org/10.4254/wjh.v9.i1.30

2. Hamilton LA, Collins-Yoder A, Collins RE (2016) Drug-induced liver injury. AACN Adv Crit Care 27(4):430–440. https://doi.org/10.4037/aacnacc2016953

3. Mosedale M, Watkins PB (2016) Drug-induced liver injury: advances in mechanistic understanding that will inform risk management. Clin Pharmacol Ther. https://doi.org/10.1002/cpt.564

4. Gustafsson F et al (2014) A correlation between the in vitro drug toxicity of drugs to cell lines that express human P450s and their propensity to cause liver injury in humans. Toxicol Sci 137:189–211. https://doi.org/10.1093/toxsci/kft223

5. Aleo MD et al (2014) Human drug-induced liver injury severity is highly associated with dual inhibition of liver mitochondrial function and bile salt export pump. Hepatology 60:1015–1022. https://doi.org/10.1002/hep.27206

6. Atienzar FA et al (2014) Predictivity of dog co-culture model, primary human hepatocytes and HepG2 cells for the detection of hepatotoxic drugs in humans. Toxicol Appl Pharmacol 275:44–61. https://doi.org/10.1016/j.taap.2013.11.022

7. Tomida T et al (2015) Multiparametric assay using HepaRG cells for predicting drug-induced liver injury. Toxicol Lett 236:16–24. https://doi.org/10.1016/j.toxlet.2015.04.014

8. Goldring C et al (2017) Stem cell-derived models to improve mechanistic understanding and prediction of human drug-induced liver injury. Hepatology 65(2):710–721. https://doi.org/10.1002/hep.28886

9. Goda K et al (2016) Usefulness of in vitro combination assays of mitochondrial dysfunction and apoptosis for the estimation of potential risk of idiosyncratic drug induced liver injury. J Toxicol Sci 41(5):605–615. https://doi.org/10.2131/jts.41.605

10. Tomida T, Okamura H, Yokoi T, Konno Y (2017) A modified multiparametric assay using HepaRG cells for predicting the degree of drug-induced liver injury risk. J Appl Toxicol 37(3):382–390. https://doi.org/10.1002/jat.3371

11. Bell CC et al (2016) Characterization of primary human hepatocyte spheroids as a model system for drug-induced liver injury, liver function and disease. Sci Rep 6:25187. https://doi.org/10.1038/srep25187

12. Wu Y et al (2016) The HepaRG cell line, a superior in vitro model to L-02, HepG2 and hiHeps cell lines for assessing drug-induced liver injury. Cell Biol Toxicol 32(1):37–59. https://doi.org/10.1007/s10565-016-9316-2

13. Hirashima R, Itoh T, Tukey RH, Fujiwara R (2017) Prediction of drug-induced liver injury using keratinocytes. J Appl Toxicol. https://doi.org/10.1002/jat.3435

14. Zhang M, Chen M, Tong W (2012) Is toxicogenomics a more reliable and sensitive biomarker than conventional indicators from rats to predict drug-induced liver injury in humans? Chem Res Toxicol 25:122–129. https://doi.org/10.1021/tx200320e

15. Hill A et al (2012) Comparisons between in vitro whole cell imaging and in vivo zebrafish-based approaches for identifying potential human hepatotoxicants earlier in pharmaceutical development. Drug Metab Rev 44:127–140. https://doi.org/10.3109/03602532.2011.645578

16. Chalasani N, Regev A (2016) Drug-induced liver injury in patients with preexisting chronic liver disease in drug development: how to identify and manage? Gastroenterology 151(6):1046–1051. https://doi.org/10.1053/j.gastro.2016.10.010

17. Lu RJ et al (2016) Clinical characteristics of drug-induced liver injury and related risk factors. Exp Ther Med 12(4):2606–2616. https://doi.org/10.3892/etm.2016.3627

18. Friedrich ME et al (2016) Drug-induced liver injury during antidepressant treatment: results of AMSP, a Drug Surveillance Program. Int J Neuropsychopharmacol 19(4):pii:pyv126. https://doi.org/10.1093/ijnp/pyv126

19. Baekdal M, Ytting H, Skalshøi Kjær M (2017) Drug-induced liver injury: a cohort study on patients referred to the Danish transplant

center over a five year period. Scand J Gastroenterol 52(4):450–454. https://doi.org/10.1080/00365521.2016.1267790

20. Hong H et al (2005) Quality control and quality assessment of data from surface-enhanced laser desorption/ionization (SELDI) time-of-flight (TOF) mass spectrometry (MS). BMC Bioinformatics 6(Suppl 2):S5. https://doi.org/10.1186/1471-2105-6-S2-S5

21. Hong H et al (2008) Assessing batch effects of genotype calling algorithm BRLMM for the Affymetrix GeneChip Human Mapping 500 K array set using 270 HapMap samples. BMC Bioinformatics 9(Suppl 9):S17. https://doi.org/10.1186/1471-2105-9-S9-S17

22. Hong H et al (2012) Technical reproducibility of genotyping SNP arrays used in genome-wide association studies. PLoS One 7(9):e44483. https://doi.org/10.1371/journal.pone.0044483

23. Liu J, Jennings SF, Tong W, Hong H (2011) Next generation sequencing for profiling expression of miRNAs: technical progress and applications in drug development. J Biomed Sci Eng 4(10):666–676. https://doi.org/10.4236/jbise.2011.410083

24. Hong H et al (2013) Critical role of bioinformatics in translating huge amounts of next-generation sequencing data into personalized medicine. Sci China Life Sci 56(2):110–118. https://doi.org/10.1007/s11427-013-4439-7

25. Hong H, Goodsaid F, Shi L, Tong W (2010) Molecular biomarkers: a US FDA effort. Biomark Med 4(2):215–225. https://doi.org/10.2217/bmm.09.81

26. Zhang W et al (2014) Whole genome sequencing of 35 individuals provides insights into the genetic architecture of Korean population. BMC Bioinformatics 15(Suppl 11):S6. https://doi.org/10.1186/1471-2105-15-S11-S6

27. Zhang W et al (2015) Quality control metrics improve repeatability and reproducibility of single-nucleotide variants derived from whole-genome sequencing. Pharmacogenomics J 15(4):298–309. https://doi.org/10.1038/tpj.2014.70

28. Hong H, Tong W (2014) Emerging efforts for discovering new biomarkers of liver disease and hepatotoxicity. Biomark Med 8(2):143–146. https://doi.org/10.2217/bmm.13.156

29. Koturbash I et al (2015) microRNAs as pharmacogenomic biomarkers for drug efficacy and drug safety assessment. Biomark Med 9(11):1153–1176. https://doi.org/10.2217/bmm.15.89

30. Wang Y et al (2015) Molecular regulation of miRNAs and potential biomarkers in the pro-gression of hepatic steatosis to NASH. Biomark Med 9(11):1189–1200. https://doi.org/10.2217/bmm.15.70

31. Hong H, Slikker W Jr (2015) Advancing translation of biomarkers into regulatory science. Biomark Med 9(11):1043–1046. https://doi.org/10.2217/bmm.15.104

32. Antoine DJ, Dear JW (2017) Transformative biomarkers for drug-induced liver injury: are we there yet? Biomark Med 11(2):103–106. https://doi.org/10.2217/bmm-2016-0338

33. Chen M et al (2013) Quantitative structure-activity relationship models for predicting drug-induced liver injury based on FDA-approved drug labeling annotation and using a large collection of drugs. Toxicol Sci 136:242–249. https://doi.org/10.1093/toxsci/kft189

34. Liu Z et al (2011) Translating clinical findings into knowledge in drug safety evaluation-drug induced liver injury prediction system (DILIps). PLoS Comput Biol 7:e1002310. https://doi.org/10.1371/journal.pcbi.1002310

35. Huang SH et al (2015) Developing a QSAR model for hepatotoxicity screening of the active compounds in traditional Chinese medicines. Food Chem Toxicol 78:71–77. https://doi.org/10.1016/j.fct.2015.01.020

36. Zhang H et al (2016) Predicting drug-induced liver injury in human with Naïve Bayes classifier approach. J Comput Aided Mol Des 30:889–898. https://doi.org/10.1007/s10822-016-9972-6

37. Xu Y et al (2015) Deep learning for drug-induced liver injury. J Chem Inf Model 55:2085–2093. https://doi.org/10.1021/acs.jcim.5b00238

38. Dragovic S et al (2016) Evidence-based selection of training compounds for use in the mechanism-based integrated prediction of drug induced liver injury in man. Arch Toxicol 90(12):2979–3003. https://doi.org/10.1007/s00204-016-1845-1

39. Longo DM et al (2016) Elucidating differences in the hepatotoxic potential of tolcapone and entacapone with DILIsym®, a mechanistic model of drug-induced liver injury. CPT Pharmacometrics Syst Pharmacol 5(1):31–39. https://doi.org/10.1002/psp4.12053

40. Xi L et al (2017) The in silico identification of human bile salt export pump (ABCB11) inhibitors associated with cholestatic drug-induced liver injury. Mol BioSyst 13(2):417–424. https://doi.org/10.1039/c6mb00744a

41. Toropova AP, Toropov AA (2017) CORAL: binary classifications (active/inactive) for drug-induced liver injury. Toxicol Lett 268:51–57. https://doi.org/10.1016/j.toxlet.2017.01.011

42. Pizzo F, Lombardo A, Manganaro A, Benfenati E (2016) A new structure-activity relationship (SAR) model for predicting drug-induced liver injury, based on statistical and expert-based structural alerts. Front Pharmacol 7:442. https://doi.org/10.3389/fphar.2016.00442

43. Mulliner D et al (2016) Computational models for human and animal hepatotoxicity with a global application scope. Chem Res Toxicol 29:757–767. https://doi.org/10.1021/acs.chemrestox.5b00465

44. Chen M, Borlak J, Tong W (2013) High lipophilicity and high daily dose of oral medications are associated with significant risk for drug-induced liver injury. Hepatology 58:388–396. https://doi.org/10.1002/hep.26208

45. Chen M, Borlak J, Tong W (2016) A model to predict severity of drug-induced liver injury in humans. Hepatology 64(3):931–940. https://doi.org/10.1002/hep.28678

46. Ivanov S et al (2017) In silico identification of proteins associated with drug-induced liver injury based on the prediction of drug-target interactions. Mol Inform. https://doi.org/10.1002/minf.201600142

47. Woodhead JL et al (2017) The role of quantitative systems pharmacology modeling in the prediction and explanation of idiosyncratic drug-induced liver injury. Drug Metab Pharmacokinet 32(1):40–45. https://doi.org/10.1016/j.dmpk.2016.11.008

48. Hong H, Chen M, Ng HW, Tong W (2016) QSAR models at the US FDA/NCTR. Methods Mol Biol 1425:431–459. https://doi.org/10.1007/978-1-4939-3609-0_18

49. Alpaydin E (2010) Introduction to machine learning. The MIT Press, London. ISBN 978-0-262-01243-0

50. Luo H, Mattes W, Mendrick DL, Hong H (2016) Molecular docking for identification of potential targets for drug repurposing. Curr Top Med Chem 16(30):3636–3645

51. Ng HW et al (2015) Estrogenic activity data extraction and in silico prediction show the endocrine disruption potential of bisphenol A replacement compounds. Chem Res Toxicol 28(9):1784–1795. https://doi.org/10.1021/acs.chemrestox.5b00243

52. Luo H et al (2015) Molecular docking to identify associations between drugs and class I human leukocyte antigens for predicting idiosyncratic drug reactions. Comb Chem High Throughput Screen 18(3):296–304

53. Ng HW et al (2014) Competitive molecular docking approach for predicting estrogen receptor subtype α agonists and antagonists. BMC Bioinformatics 15(Suppl 11):S4. https://doi.org/10.1186/1471-2105-15-S11-S4

54. Shen J et al (2013) Homology modeling, molecular docking, and molecular dynamics simulations elucidated α-fetoprotein binding modes. BMC Bioinformatics 14(Suppl 14):S6. https://doi.org/10.1186/1471-2105-14-S14-S6

55. Lipinski CA, Lombardo F, Dominy BW, Feeney PJ (2001) Experimental and computational approaches to estimate solubility and permeability in drug discovery and development settings. Adv Drug Deliv Rev 46(1–3):3–26. https://doi.org/10.1016/S0169-409X(00)00129-0

56. Lipinski CA (2004) Lead- and drug-like compounds: the rule-of-five revolution. Drug Discov Today Technol 1(4):337–341. https://doi.org/10.1016/j.ddtec.2004.11.007

57. Hong H et al (2002) Prediction of estrogen receptor binding for 58,000 chemicals using an integrated system of a tree-based model with structural alerts. Environ Health Perspect 110(1):29–36

58. Hong H et al (1997) Discovery of HIV-1 integrase inhibitors by pharmacophore searching. J Med Chem 40(6):930–936. https://doi.org/10.1021/jm960754h

59. Neamati N et al (1998) Salicylhydrazine-containing inhibitors of HIV-1 integrase: implication for a selective chelation in the integrase active site. J Med Chem 41(17):3202–3209. https://doi.org/10.1021/jm9801760

60. Hong H et al (1998) Identification of HIV-1 integrase inhibitors based on a four-point pharmacophore. Antivir Chem Chemother 9(6):461–472. https://doi.org/10.1177/095632029800900602

61. O'Boyle NM et al (2011) Open Babel: an open chemical toolbox. J Cheminform 3:33. https://doi.org/10.1186/1758-2946-3-33

62. Cao DS, Xu QS, Hu QN, Liang YZ (2013) ChemoPy: freely available python package for computational biology and chemoinformatics. Bioinformatics 29(8):1092–1094. https://doi.org/10.1093/bioinformatics/btt105

63. Yap CW (2011) PaDEL-descriptor: an open source software to calculate molecular descriptors and fingerprints. J Comput Chem 32(7):1466–1474. https://doi.org/10.1002/jcc.21707

64. Hinselmann G et al (2011) jCompoundMapper: an open source Java library and command-line tool for chemical fingerprints. J Cheminform 3:3. https://doi.org/10.1186/1758-2946-3-3

65. Hong H et al (2008) Mold2, molecular descriptors from 2D structures for chemoinformatics and toxicoinformatics. J Chem Inf Model 48(7):1337–1344. https://doi.org/10.1021/ci800038f

66. Jurs PC, Chou JT, Yuan M (1979) Computer-assisted structure-activity studies of chemical carcinogens. A heterogeneous data set. J Med Chem 22(5):476–483. https://doi.org/10.1021/jm00191a004

67. Katritzky AR, Lobanov VS, Karelson M (1995) QSPR: the correlation and quantitative prediction of chemical and physical properties from structure. Chem Soc Rev 24:279–287. https://doi.org/10.1039/CS9952400279

68. Mekenyan O, Karabunarliev S, Bonchev D (1990) The microcomputer OASIS system for predicting the biological activity of chemical compounds. Comp Chem 14:193–200. https://doi.org/10.1016/0097-8485(90)80046-5

69. Basak SC, Magnuson VR, Niemi GJ, Regal RR (1988) Determining structural similarity of chemicals using graph-theoretic indices. Disc Appl Math 19:17–44. https://doi.org/10.1016/0166-218X(88)90004-2

70. Cramer RD, Patterson DE, Bunce JD (1988) Comparative molecular field analysis (CoMFA). 1. Effect of shape on binding of steroids to carrier proteins. J Am Chem Soc 110(18):5959–5967. https://doi.org/10.1021/ja00226a005

71. Hong H et al (2005) Comparative molecular field analysis (CoMFA) model using a large diverse set of natural, synthetic and environmental chemicals for binding to the androgen receptor. SAR QSAR Environ Res 14(5–6):373–388. https://doi.org/10.1080/10629360310001623962

72. Cramer RD (2015) Template CoMFA generates single 3D-QSAR models that, for twelve of twelve biological targets, predict all ChEMBL-tabulated affinities. PLoS One 10(6):e0129307. https://doi.org/10.1371/journal.pone.0129307

73. Klebe G, Abraham U, Mietzner T (1994) Molecular similarity indices in a comparative analysis (CoMSIA) of drug molecules to correlate and predict their biological activity. J Med Chem 37(24):4130–4146. https://doi.org/10.1021/jm00050a010

74. Punkvang A, Hannongbua S, Saparpakorn P, Pungpo P (2016) Insight into the structural requirements of aminopyrimidine derivatives for good potency against both purified enzyme and whole cells of M. tuberculosis: combination of HQSAR, CoMSIA, and MD simulation studies. J Biomol Struct Dyn 34(5):1079–1091. https://doi.org/10.1080/07391102.2015.1068711

75. Mouchlis VD et al (2012) Molecular modeling on pyrimidine-urea inhibitors of TNF-α production: an integrated approach using a combination of molecular docking, classification techniques, and 3D-QSAR CoMSIA. J Chem Inf Model 52(3):711–723. https://doi.org/10.1021/ci200579f

76. Tong W et al (2003) Decision forest: combining the predictions of multiple independent decision tree models. J Chem Inf Comput Sci 43(2):525–531. https://doi.org/10.1021/ci020058s

77. Hong H et al (2005) An in silico ensemble method for lead discovery: decision forest. SAR QSAR Environ Res 16(4):339–3347. https://doi.org/10.1080/10659360500203022

78. Ng HW et al (2015) Development and validation of decision forest model for estrogen receptor binding prediction of chemicals using large data sets. Chem Res Toxicol 28(12):2343–2351. https://doi.org/10.1021/acs.chemrestox.5b00358

79. Hong H et al (2016) Consensus modeling for prediction of estrogenic activity of ingredients commonly used in sunscreen products. Int J Environ Res Public Health 13(10):pii E958

80. Hong H et al (2016) Experimental data extraction and in silico prediction of the estrogenic activity of renewable replacements for bisphenol A. Int J Environ Res Public Health 13(7):pii: E705. https://doi.org/10.3390/ijerph13070705

81. Hong H et al (2016) A rat α-fetoprotein binding activity prediction model to facilitate assessment of the endocrine disruption potential of environmental chemicals. Int J Environ Res Public Health 13(4):372. https://doi.org/10.3390/ijerph13040372

82. Hong H et al (2004) Multiclass decision forest—a novel pattern recognition method for multiclass classification in microarray data analysis. DNA Cell Biol 23(10):685–694. https://doi.org/10.1089/dna.2004.23.685

83. Mansouri K et al (2016) CERAPP: collaborative estrogen receptor activity prediction project. Environ Health Perspect 124(7):1023–1033. https://doi.org/10.1289/ehp.1510267

84. Hong H et al (2009) The accurate prediction of protein family from amino acid sequence by measuring features of sequence fragments. J Comput Biol 16(12):1671–1688. https://doi.org/10.1089/cmb.2008.0115

85. Huo H et al (2015) Machine learning methods for predicting HLA-peptide binding activity. Bioinform Biol Insights 9(Suppl 3):21–29. https://doi.org/10.4137/BBI.S29466

86. Liu J et al (2015) Predicting hepatotoxicity using ToxCast in vitro bioactivity and chemical structure. Chem Res Toxicol 28(4):738–751. https://doi.org/10.1021/tx500501h

87. Chen M et al (2013) The liver toxicity knowledge base: a systems approach to a complex end point. Clin Pharmacol Ther 93(5):409–412. https://doi.org/10.1038/clpt.2013.16

88. Chen M et al (2011) FDA-approved drug labeling for the study of drug-induced liver injury. Drug Discov Today 16(15–16):697–703. https://doi.org/10.1016/j.drudis.2011.05.007

89. Chen M et al (2016) DILIrank: the largest reference drug list ranked by the risk for developing drug-induced liver injury in humans. Drug Discov Today 21:648–453. https://doi.org/10.1016/j.drudis.2016.02.015

90. Igarashi Y, Nakatsu N, Yamashita T, Ono A, Ohno Y, Urushidani T, Yamada H (2015) Open TG-GATEs: a large-scale toxicogenomics database. Nucleic Acids Res 43(Database issue):D921–D927. https://doi.org/10.1093/nar/gku955

91. Arulmozhiraja S, Morita M (2004) Structure-activity relationships for the toxicity of polychlorinated dibenzofurans: approach through density functional theory-based descriptors. Chem Res Toxicol 17:348–356. https://doi.org/10.1021/tx0300380

92. Brown RD, Martin YC (1997) The information content of 2D and 3D structural descriptors relevant to ligand-receptor binding. J Chem Inf Comput Sci 37:1–9. https://doi.org/10.1021/ci960373c

93. Matter H, Potter T (1999) Comparing 3D pharmacophore triplets and 2D fingerprints for selecting diverse compound subsets. J Chem Inf Comput Sci 39:1211–1225. https://doi.org/10.1021/ci980185h

94. Hong H, Xin X (1992) ESSESA: an expert system for structure elucidation from spectra analysis. 2. A novel algorithm of perception of the linear independent smallest set of smallest rings. Anal Chim Acta 262:179–191

95. Hong H, Xin X (1992) ESSESA: an expert system for structure elucidation from spectra analysis. 3. LNSCS for chemical knowledge representation. J Chem Inf Comput Sci 32:116–120

96. Hong H, Xin X (1994) ESSESA: an expert system for structure elucidation from spectra analysis. 4. Canonical representation of structures. J Chem Inf Comput Sci 34:730–734

97. Hong H, Xin X (1994) ESSESA: an expert system for structure elucidation from spectra analysis. 5. Substructure constraints from from analysis of first-order 1H-NMR spectra. J Chem Inf Comput Sci 34:1259–1266

98. Hong H, Han Y, Xin X, Shi Y (1995) ESSESA: an expert system for structure elucidation from spectra. 6. Substructure constraints from analysis of 13C-NMR spectra. J Chem Inf Comput Sci 35(6):979–1000

99. Masui H, Hong H (2006) Spec2D: a structure elucidation system based on 1H NMR and H-H COSY spectra in organic chemistry. J Chem Inf Model 46:775–787. https://doi.org/10.1021/ci0502810

100. Hong H, Xin X (1990) ESSESA: an expert system for structure elucidation from spectra analysis. 1. The knowledge base of infrared spectra and analysis and interpretation program. J Chem Inf Comput Sci 30:203–210

101. Greene N et al (2010) Developing structure-activity relationships for the prediction of hepatotoxicity. Chem Res Toxicol 23(7):1215–1222. https://doi.org/10.1021/tx1000865

Chapter 6

An Introduction to DILIsym® Software, a Mechanistic Mathematical Representation of Drug-Induced Liver Injury

Christina Battista, Brett A. Howell, Scott Q. Siler, and Paul B. Watkins

Abstract

Drug-induced liver injury (DILI) is one of the primary reasons why a new drug candidate may fail during development. To address this challenge, a mathematical representation, DILIsym®, has been developed as a result of an ongoing public-private partnership involving scientists from industry, academia, and the FDA. DILIsym employs mathematical representations of mechanistic interactions and events from drug administration through the progression of liver injury and regeneration to the release of traditional and novel serum biomarkers. The model parameters are varied to recreate population variation in DILI susceptibility. Using in vitro data to represent potential mitochondrial dysfunction, bile acid transporter inhibition, and/or reactive oxygen species generation, DILIsym has been able to predict the in vivo liver safety profile in individuals and in simulated populations for a growing list of drugs. DILIsym is being increasingly used to assist in decision making throughout the development pipeline, from predicting interspecies differences and their hepatotoxicity potential to aiding in the design of dosing regimens to minimize hepatotoxicity when this liability is identified. Furthermore, DILIsym's incorporation of the release and clearance kinetics of traditional and emerging serum biomarkers can improve interpretation of potential liver safety signals. This chapter outlines the interactions and toxicity mechanisms included in DILIsym and the process of representing a compound in the software. Examples of toxicity profile predictions and biomarker interpretations are included along with future directions for the software.

Key words Drug-induced liver injury (DILI), DILIsym, Mechanistic modeling, Quantitative systems toxicology, Quantitative systems pharmacology, Hepatotoxicity predictions

1 Introduction

Currently, drug development is an expensive, lengthy process with rising research costs and an abundance of regulatory requests, most of which require longer clinical studies. These are some of the challenges facing the pharmaceutical industry, coincident with fewer drug candidates available in the pipeline. One possible method to increase pharmaceutical efficiency is to improve drug safety early on in development, thereby avoiding problematic safety signals during clinical trials. While this is easier said than done, retrospective analyses of adverse event drug withdrawals or drugs

Minjun Chen and Yvonne Will (eds.), *Drug-Induced Liver Toxicity*, Methods in Pharmacology and Toxicology,
https://doi.org/10.1007/978-1-4939-7677-5_6, © Springer Science+Business Media, LLC, part of Springer Nature 2018

terminated during development have demonstrated that there is potential to select not only better compounds but also to increase preclinical attrition rates [1].

Given the complexity of seeing a drug through the development process to the market, pharmaceutical companies are addressing safety concerns from different approaches such as cell-free and cell-based assays, animal experiments, animal models, and computational models [2–7]. This chapter outlines one such computational approach, DILIsym, which is software containing a mathematical model aimed at improving liver safety in drug development by simulating the mechanistic interactions and events from dosing through the progression of liver injury and regeneration. Development of the DILIsym software has been supported by the DILI-sim Initiative, a consortium consisting of pharmaceutical companies whose prevailing voices guide development to ensure that the model is of maximum utility as it is developed within their respective organizations.

2   Method and Materials

2.1   The DILIsym Software

The DILIsym software is designed to provide an enhanced understanding of the DILI hazard posed by an individual molecule during drug development. The software also provides deeper insight into the mechanisms that contribute to observed DILI responses at various stages throughout the development process.

DILIsym (version 5A) is built in the MATLAB (The MathWorks, Natick, MA) computing platform, enabling users to work directly with the MATLAB code or use the graphical user interface (GUI). Within the GUI, the user has the ability to specify new experiments, including but not limited to compound, dose, dosing frequency and duration, toxicity mechanism(s), and species (Fig. 1). The software can run simulations for individuals or populations and utilizes parallel computing for quicker results when applicable. The GUI allows users to visualize results within MATLAB or export results to a spreadsheet where further analysis can be performed using the software of choice.

2.2   DILIsym Design Principles

DILIsym is constructed using a "middle-out," multiscale approach which involves mechanistic modeling of detailed, essential processes in liver physiology together with the molecular and systemic levels necessary to capture key mechanisms or qualitative outcomes, respectively. The model consists of a number of differential and algebraic equations, parameters, and a hefty reference library list which has been used to support model decisions (Table 1). It includes key liver cell populations, e.g., hepatocytes and Kupffer cells, intracellular biochemical systems, e.g., mitochondrial bioenergetics, and whole body dynamics, e.g., drug distribution and

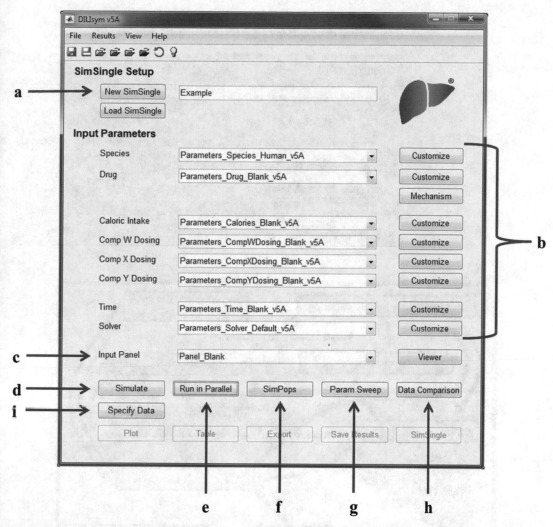

Fig. 1 DILIsym graphical user interface (GUI): (**a**) SimSingle saves all parameter sets under a user-defined name that can be reloaded or shared between computers; (**b**) User-defined parameter sets pertaining to species, drug, caloric intake, dosing scheme, simulation time, and solver settings; (**c**) Input Panel which can save all values (default) or just user-specified values for quicker computation; (**d**) Simulate in one individual; (**e**) Run in Parallel to simulate multiple SimSingles simultaneously; (**f**) SimPops feature; (**g**) Parameter Sweep feature; (**h**) Data Comparison feature; (**i**) Specify Data feature

metabolism, to predict DILI in mice, rats, dogs, and humans. Mechanistic representation of preclinical species and humans allows for the extrapolation of preclinical data to prospective predictions of hepatotoxicity in humans. The model is organized into smaller submodels, where the submodels are mathematically integrated to simulate an organism level response. An overview of DILIsym and its submodels is shown in Fig. 2. These submodels are integrated to generate liver outcome predictions, heavily dependent on hepatocyte death and regeneration (the hepatocyte life cycle) and the release and clearance of serum biomarkers. Brief descriptions of submodels are given in Table 2.

Table 1
Quantitative descriptors of the DILIsym model (version v5A)

Model descriptor	Count
Ordinary differential equations	588
Algebraic expressions	1200
Parameters characterizing the species (mouse, rat, human, dog)	616
Parameters characterizing the caloric intake	14
Parameters characterizing the drug	841
Parameters characterizing the dosing quantity, dynamics, and route	206
References library entries	5510

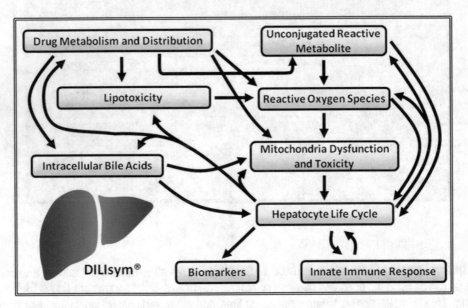

Fig. 2 DILIsym overview showing qualitative interactions between submodels. Reprinted with permission from [68]

DILIsym includes baseline animals and humans to provide insight about DILI responses in the average individual, but DILIsym also predicts outcomes on a population level by varying key model parameters in simulated populations, or SimPops™. Alternate parameterizations of the model with distribution constraints are used to account for inter-individual variability and generate SimPops. Important model parameters that are varied in SimPops include baseline glutathione levels, cellular response to oxidative stress, hepatocellular stress recovery speed, and inflammation, among others. Literature was used to identify mean and range values along with the distribution for a given parameter.

Table 2
Brief descriptions of the DILIsym submodels

Submodel	Description
PBPK (drug distribution and metabolism)	Describes the disposition of the parent compound and its major metabolites, including absorption, distribution, metabolism, and excretion
Unconjugated reactive metabolite	Describes the link between unconjugated reactive metabolites and ROS production
Lipotoxicity	Describes the link between saturated fatty acids and ROS production
Reactive oxygen/nitrogen species (ROS/RNS)	Describes the rates of ROS/RNS production plus any contribution from parent compound or metabolites
Intracellular bile acids	Describes the uptake and efflux of bile acids into and out of hepatocytes, including competitive or noncompetitive inhibition of relevant transporters
Mitochondrial dysfunction and toxicity	Describes glycolytic function, the production of ATP, and any dysfunction in ATP synthesis due to ETC inhibition, mitochondrial uncoupling, or direct inhibition of ATP synthesis
Hepatocyte life cycle	Includes apoptosis, necrosis, and proliferation rates for hepatocytes based on compound-mediated effects. When fewer hepatocytes are available, this submodel has the ability to impact drug disposition
Innate immune response	Includes life cycle models for liver macrophages and LSECs, along with their respective mediator production in response to inflammatory signals
Biomarkers	Models the dynamics of traditional biomarkers (ALT, AST, TBIL, prothrombin time) and some emerging biomarkers (HMGB1, miR-122, SDH, etc.) as functions of liver injury

This process was repeated for other parameters and then specific parameter values were combined to create unique individuals, with most SimPops consisting of 100–300 individuals. However, the range of parameters employed within these SimPops should reflect population heterogeneity existing in far larger real life populations. Specific SimPops have been constructed to model the effects of drugs in a normal healthy volunteer population, a type II diabetes population, a nonalcoholic fatty liver disease (NAFLD) population, as well as smaller cohorts of simulated individuals from each population who are particularly susceptible to certain mechanisms of toxicity. Additional SimPops are added as necessary to model relevant target populations and can be constructed to account for variability in drug disposition by including variability in metabolism and distribution parameters. SimPops have been used to explore the risk of methapyrilene toxicity across species [8] and to assess the effectiveness of varying courses of NAC treatment in humans [9]. DILIsym also contains SimPops for rats, mice, and dogs, akin to those for human populations.

Since the first version release in 2012, DILIsym has incorporated many additional features by utilizing scientific literature, novel experiments, clinical trials and reports, expert opinions, and basic scientific principles to optimize and validate the software. The submodels have been built, refined, validated, and tested by a number of exemplar compounds whose outcomes were known and whose quantitative data sets have been included within the software. To facilitate review of these data sets, DILIsym's Data Comparisons feature (Fig. 1h) displays comparisons of simulation results with these data.

2.2.1 Submodels Within DILIsym

Cellular processes essential to mathematical modeling of DILI have been explored and are included in DILIsym, and Fig. 2 is a summary of these processes and their interactions. For instance, drug metabolism and distribution provides predictions of the hepatic exposure of the parent compound and/or metabolite with the potential to interact with mechanistic pathways associated with hepatotoxicity: inhibition of bile acid transporters, generation of reactive metabolites, disturbances in reactive oxygen species, mitochondrial toxicity, and lipotoxicity. These submodels interact with each other and, together or individually, can disrupt the hepatocyte life cycle by inducing apoptosis and/or necrosis. Furthermore, there is the potential for an interaction with the innate immune system which can either exacerbate or ameliorate injury and provide support for hepatocellular regeneration post-injury. DILIsym also includes a submodel that captures the dynamics for serum biomarkers of hepatocellular injury, comparable to what can be measured in the clinic. While Fig. 2 displays the qualitative interactions, quantitative biochemical and cellular relationships between submodels have been determined through basic biochemical and physiological concepts/data and by exemplar drugs of hepatotoxicity. Exemplars for reactive metabolite-based hepatotoxicity include acetaminophen [8–10], methapyrilene [8], furosemide, and carbon tetrachloride. Buprenorphine and etomoxir were some of the exemplar compounds used to quantify mitochondrial toxicity, and for bile acid-mediated toxicity, bosentan and telmisartan [11] were used. Additionally, there have been exemplars with combinations of mechanisms such as CP-724,714 [11]. For each new compound, DILIsym predicts injury solely based on features of that compound in comparison to the aforementioned exemplars [12–15]. Moreover, DILIsym has utilized pairs of compounds such as tolcapone and entacapone [14] or troglitazone and pioglitazone [12] to show its capability to predict "toxic" or "clean" for each drug in the pair, designating these positive and negative controls as "clean/toxic" pairings.

Reactive Oxygen Species and Reactive Metabolite Submodels

Compounds and their stable or reactive metabolites can increase the production of reactive oxygen/nitrogen species (ROS/RNS) in hepatocytes by proposed mechanisms such as reduction in cellular antioxidants or direct reactive metabolite-membrane interactions. Modest increases in ROS/RNS can lead to activation of caspase enzymes, triggering caspase-mediated hepatocellular apoptosis. Greater increases in ROS/RNS can cause reductions of hepatocellular ATP, which in turn disrupts other cellular processes and can result in necrosis (see "Mitochondrial Toxicity Submodel" section).

Within DILIsym, ROS/RNS can be generated in any zone of the liver and spread to directly adjacent zones through a gradient driven, first-order process. The parameters describing the spreading across the zones are based on the overall liver ROS/RNS data for mice and rats [16–19] and detailed images of gap junction-mediated spreading in [20]. Because no liver ROS/RNS data were available for humans or dogs following acute liver injury, exploration from the rodents was combined with endpoint dose-response data in humans and dogs to determine the appropriate parameter values. Many of the parameters pertaining to downstream injury, such as those defining how ROS/RNS affects ATP production and how ATP levels induce necrosis, were held constant across the species.

Mitochondrial Toxicity Submodel

Disruptions in mitochondrial function can easily contribute to DILI, being that mitochondria are responsible for the majority of cellular ATP synthesis. A disruption in ATP synthesis leads to lower ATP levels which can trigger disturbances in other cellular processes and ultimately result in necrotic cell death [21]. Parent compounds or their metabolites can disrupt ATP production in a number of ways, namely reduction in the mitochondrial proton gradient via uncoupling, inhibition of the electron transport chain (ETC) flux, or direct inhibition of ATP synthesis. Changes in ROS/RNS (as discussed previously) can also decrease ATP synthesis.

DILIsym includes the above pathways by representing plasma glucose, glycolysis, and dynamic regulation of the mitochondria ETC activity, substrate utilization, and the proton gradient. A companion software, MITOsym®, also made up of differential equations and representing in vitro mitochondrial function, was developed alongside DILIsym to address the transition from in vitro data to in vivo predictions [22]. The cellular parameters included are oxygen consumption rate (OCR) and extracellular acidification rate (ECAR), which are used to determine changes in

ETC activity and glycolytic function. Experimental data from HepG2, primary human hepatocytes, and primary rat hepatocytes treated with exemplar ATP disruptors—rotenone (ETC inhibitor), oligomycin (ATP synthesis inhibitor), and FCCP (uncoupling agent)—were used to optimize MITOsym [22–25]. The quantitative relationships in these pathways were than translated from MITOsym to DILIsym to predict in vivo effects. While MITOsym includes many mitochondrial contributions found within DILIsym, DILIsym represents additional contributions to mitochondrial function, such as fatty acids and mitochondrial biogenesis.

Bile Acid Homeostasis Submodel

Bile acids are crucial regulatory molecules regulating lipid and glucose homeostasis. However, bile acids can wield toxic effects when they accumulate in hepatocytes [26], and the toxicity of bile acids correlate with their hydrophobicity [27]. Inhibition of the hepatic efflux transporters, bile salt export pump (BSEP) and multidrug resistance-associated protein (MRP3 and MRP4), by drugs may result in supraphysiological concentrations of toxic bile acids, leading to hepatotoxicity [28–31].

Bile acids are transported from sinusoidal blood across the basolateral membranes into hepatocytes and across the canalicular membranes into bile. They are taken up from the sinusoidal blood into hepatocytes mainly by sodium taurocholate cotransporting polypeptide (NTCP) transporters, although organic anion transporting polypeptides (OATPs) can also transport bile acids into hepatocytes. Once bile acids enter hepatocytes, they are metabolized and excreted into the bile predominantly via BSEP in an ATP-dependent matter [32]. They can also be excreted into the sinusoidal blood via MRP3, MRP4, or organic solute transporter (OST-) α/β [33–35]. After secretion into bile, bile acids undergo enterohepatic recirculation with about 90–95% of the bile acids being reabsorbed from the intestinal lumen by apical sodium-dependent bile acid transporter (ASBT) or by passive diffusion. Bile acid homeostasis is tightly regulated through multiple nuclear receptors, namely the farnesoid X receptor (FXR), the constitutive androstane receptor (CAR), and the liver X receptor (LXR) [36–38].

DILIsym represents the synthesis, metabolism, transport, and enterohepatic recirculation of lithocholic acid (LCA), chenodeoxycholic acid (CDCA), and their respective conjugates in addition to a bulk bile acid pool to account for the rest of the bile acid species [39]. LCA and CDCA are known to be hydrophobic and cytotoxic, commanding their specific inclusion in DILIsym [27]. Additionally, LCA and CDCA conjugates are reported to be potent activators of FXR [38], which downregulates bile acid synthesis enzymes, downregulates uptake transporters, and upregulates efflux transporters at both the canalicular and basolateral membranes.

Hepatic bile acid transport processes are represented using saturable Michaelis-Menten kinetics whose K_m values were obtained from available literature and V_{max} values were optimized to known bile acid profiles in humans, dogs, and rats [40, 41]. Inhibition of any of the hepatic transporters can be simulated as competitive or noncompetitive, based on the available data, and with inhibition constants (i.e., K_i or IC_{50}) for the parent compound and its metabolite(s). The type of transporter inhibition can have profound effects on the bile acid mediated hepatotoxicity [11]. If no data are available to determine competitive or noncompetitive inhibition of a particular transporter, the DILIsym developers recommend assuming competitive inhibition with $\alpha = 5$ but also recommend performing additional sensitivity analysis simulations to probe this assumption. In addition, the efflux transporters are ATP-dependent functions; depletion of hepatic ATP results in impaired transporter function. Increased accumulation of bile acids in hepatocytes inhibits hepatic ATP synthesis, thereby decreasing intracellular ATP concentrations, ultimately leading to necrotic cell death. This results in elevations in serum biomarkers of hepatocellular injury and function.

Innate Immune Submodel

The innate immune system has been shown to contribute to APAP hepatotoxicity, and thus, parts of the innate immune system have been incorporated into DILIsym. The submodel currently includes liver macrophages (Kupffer cells), liver sinusoidal endothelial cells (LSECs), tumor necrosis factor alpha (TNF-α), interleukin-10 (IL-10), acetylated high mobility group box protein (acHMGB1), and hepatocyte growth factor (HGF). The submodel was constructed in such a way that additional elements can easily be incorporated in the future, e.g., neutrophils.

The cell population life cycles for macrophages and LSECs include recruitment, maturation/differentiation, local proliferation, and apoptosis [42]. Mature cells can be activated by cell death or inflammatory signals and drive mediator release. The mediators—TNF-α, IL-10, acHMGB1, and HGF—can modulate hepatocyte cell death and proliferation/regeneration, exacerbating injury or ameliorating it, respectively. Mediators also upregulate or downregulate production of other mediators, e.g., IL-10 inhibits HMGB1 and TNF-α production [43] while TNF-α upregulates its own production as well as that of the other mediators [44–47].

Biomarkers in DILIsym

DILIsym includes classic serum biomarkers such as alanine aminotransferase (ALT), aspartate aminotransferase (AST), total bilirubin (TBIL), and prothrombin time, but it also incorporates emerging biomarkers of DILI such as HMGB1, cytokeratin 18 (K18), sorbitol dehydrogenase (SDH), Arginase-1 (Arg-1), and micro-RNA 122 (miR-122.) A list of the biomarkers and their implications are given in Table 3.

Table 3
Biomarkers of DILIsym with corresponding category of injury

Marker	Category	References
Alanine aminotransferase (ALT)	Necrosis	[69–73]
Total bilirubin (TBIL)	Function/cholestasis	[70, 71, 74]
Aspartate aminotransferase (AST)	Necrosis	[69–73]
Prothrombin time	Function	[70, 73]
High mobility group box protein 1 (HMGB1)	Necrosis/apoptosis	[73, 75]
Full length cytokeratin-18 (FL-K18)	Necrosis	[73]
Cleaved cytokeratin-18 (cK-18)	Apoptosis	[73]
Sorbitol dehydrogenase (SDH)	Necrosis	[72, 73]
Arginase-1 (Arg-1)	Necrosis	[76]
Liver-derived mRNA and miRNA	Necrosis	[77, 78]

Bilirubin

In DILIsym, serum levels of both conjugated and unconjugated bilirubin in the model are regulated by changes in clearance, mediated by glucuronidation and transport of bilirubin out of hepatocytes. These rates can be further regulated by cellular ATP levels, mimicking liver injury severity as described in the bile acid submodel. The enzyme- and transporter-mediated hepatobiliary disposition of bilirubin enables simulations of drug-induced hyperbilirubinemia mediated by either the inhibition of the bilirubin conjugating enzyme (UGT1A1) or transporters in the absence of overt liver injury [15].

Both plasma and liver bilirubin pools consist of unconjugated and conjugated bilirubin, where OATP1B1/B3 facilitates hepatic uptake of unconjugated bilirubin and hepatic reuptake of conjugated bilirubin [48–50]. UGT1A1 mitigates the conversion of unconjugated bilirubin in the liver [51], and conjugated bilirubin is excreted into the bile via MRP2 or MRP3 [52, 53]. Any of these processes can be inhibited by compounds or their metabolites, leading to hyperbilirubinemia.

Emerging Biomarkers
in DILIsym

HMGB1 is a damage-associated molecular pattern (DAMP) molecule capable of activating immune cells. Many forms of HMGB1 are found within DILIsym: an active, nonacetylated form representing the disulfide and fully reduced forms released directly from hepatocytes undergoing primary necrosis; an active, acetylated form representing HMGB1 secreted by active immune cells; and an inactive, nonacetylated form representing the sulfonyl form generated by caspase-mediated cell death [54–60]. Levels of active, nonacetylated HMGB1 are driven by hepatocyte necrotic flux, whereas levels of inactive, nonacetylated HMGB1 are driven by apoptotic flux and subsequent secondary necrosis triggered by high rates of apoptosis. Acetylated HMGB1 is driven by macrophage activation and the number of mature macrophages. Together with TNF-α, active nonacetylated HMGB1 positively regulates macrophage activation and the subsequent release of pro- and anti-inflammatory cytokines.

Cytokeratin 18 (K18) has two forms in DILIsym: full-length (FL-K18) and caspase-cleaved (cK-18). The former is released into serum when hepatocyte necrosis occurs, while the latter is produced when apoptosis occurs. During apoptosis, a fraction of the K18 within hepatocytes is cleaved [61–63]. When necrosis and apoptosis occur simultaneously, FL-K18 is released from necrosis and high levels of apoptosis, and cK18 is released from high levels of apoptosis (or secondary necrosis).

SDH, Arg-1, and miR-122 levels are likewise driven by the rates of hepatocyte necrosis and apoptosis in DILIsym. Much like ALT and AST, hepatocyte death due to necrosis is assumed to leak cellular SDH, Arg-1, and miR-122 into circulation. However, the release of these biomarkers from apoptotic hepatocytes is more complex; they are not released when the rate of hepatocyte apoptosis occurs at very low levels. At low levels of apoptosis, the cleanup of cellular debris is assumed to be very efficient such that cellular contents are not leaked into circulation during phagocytosis. However, at high levels of apoptosis, macrophages become saturated, cell cleanup becomes inefficient, and cellular contents, i.e., biomarkers such as ALT, AST, SDH, Arg-1, and miR-122, are leaked into circulation.

While not biomarkers, DILIsym represents many other critical model outputs that help to assess the level of liver injury such as the fraction of viable hepatocytes, liver levels of adenosine triphosphate (ATP) and glutathione (GSH), and other various PK outputs. The fraction of viable hepatocytes, reflecting net loss and regeneration, is computed over time and can be directly viewed as an output. Thus, for a given ALT profile, DILIsym can be used to predict hepatocyte loss. An example of this will be discussed later in the chapter.

2.3 Representing a Compound in DILIsym

Simulating each compound in DILIsym can be somewhat unique depending on the compound characteristics, but the same general flow follows for all compounds. First, a physiologically-based pharmacokinetic (PBPK) model must be constructed or adapted from an existing model. Data for constructing the PBPK model can generally be found in literature or from early stages of drug development. Alternatively, an existing PBPK model produced in another software platform can be adapted to the DILIsym PBPK submodel inputs or the outputs of the already-existing model, i.e., drug and metabolite concentrations in the liver, can be specified within

DILIsym using the Specify Data feature (Fig. 1i). Constructing the PBPK model within DILIsym requires optimization of relevant compound-specific parameters found by iteratively comparing simulated results to experimental data until the determined accuracy is achieved. For certain compounds, this requires also modeling the major metabolites, particularly if they are thought to have hepatotoxic liabilities.

In vitro experiments relating to DILIsym's three major mechanisms of toxicity, i.e., ROS production, mitochondrial dysfunction, and bile acid transporter inhibition, are then used to identify and activate the relevant toxicity submodels within DILIsym. The data must be quantified and translated to the appropriate DILIsym parameter values. For mitochondrial toxicity parameters, this is sometimes achieved using DILIsym's sister software, MITOsym [22]. Parameters relating to ROS production can be determined within DILIsym, and IC_{50} or K_i values for bile acid transporter inhibition can be directly input into the software.

Once the disposition and toxicity mechanisms of the parent compound and any of its major metabolites have been included in DILIsym, simulations can be performed across multiple drug levels with various dosing schemes to characterize simulated outcome measures and alterations in the underlying biology. Simulations in the baseline individual/subject give insight into a compound's effect on the average representative of that species. Further analysis can be performed by simulating a normal, healthy population or a diseased population (if applicable/available) with existing SimPops. This provides a better prediction for toxicity outcomes associated with a larger population sample. Additional examples of DILIsym's capabilities will be discussed in the next section.

3   Results

The most evident uses of DILIsym may be to predict liver toxicity outcomes in a population, or to optimize a dosing scheme to minimize toxicity signals. However, DILIsym, as with most computational tools, can serve multiple purposes. DILIsym can predict other outcomes, such as viable liver mass, or test hypotheses that otherwise cannot be tested. The following examples display the predictive power of DILIsym to date.

3.1   Troglitazone

Troglitazone (TGZ), the first thiazolidinedione drug approved in worldwide markets for the treatment of type II diabetes, caused delayed, life-threatening DILI in some patients but was not found to be hepatotoxic in rats. Fourteen years after TGZ had been withdrawn from the market, TGZ was represented in DILIsym, as well as its major metabolite, TGZ sulfate (TS). In vitro vesicular transport assays suggested that TGZ and TS alter bile acid homeostasis

[12] by inhibiting BSEP, MRP4, and NTCP. DILIsym was used to evaluate the in vivo hepatotoxic potential of TGZ using inhibition constants determined by in vitro data. To test the role that bile acid accumulation had on hepatotoxicity of TGZ, other potential mechanistic contributors to DILI were not included in these simulations.

The disposition of TGZ and TS were represented in DILIsym, the bile acid toxicity mechanism was activated and quantified, and human and rat SimPops with variability in bile acid homeostasis parameters were used to predict ALT elevations in both species. Multiple dose levels were evaluated for each species, and DILIsym accurately predicted outcomes; no hepatotoxicity was predicted for the rat population, and some ALT elevations >3× the upper limit of normal (ULN) were predicted in the human population as shown in Fig. 3. These results were in line with the previously reported results from preclinical experiments and clinical trials. Had these simulations been performed in advance of the clinical trials, this risk in humans would have been highlighted, and clinical trials might have been designed differently.

DILIsym not only captures differences in species ALT elevations, but it can also be used to address "what if" scenarios. With TGZ, the model was used to investigate how each bile acid transporter contributed to the predicted toxicity. By performing simulations where inhibition of a single transporter is turned off, the effect of inhibition of that particular transporter becomes apparent (Table 4). Pertaining to 600 mg/day dosing for a month, TGZ- and TS-mediated toxicity decreases to virtually no ALT elevations when BSEP or MRP4 inhibition is removed. However, when NTCP inhibition is no longer active, an increase in toxicity is observed, corresponding to an increase in the uptake of bile acids into the hepatocyte followed by subsequent inhibition of efflux transporters. This type of investigation is possible through computational modeling but would otherwise be extremely difficult to explore.

3.2 Entolimod

Entolimod, a Toll-like receptor 5 agonist, produced marked elevations in serum ALT exceeding 1000 U/L in some healthy volunteers, but the duration of the elevations were noted to be quite brief. DILIsym simulations were used to estimate the percentage of total hepatocytes that underwent necrosis in these subjects [64]. This was accomplished by first optimizing DILIsym to produce the liver enzyme profiles observed during the study, and then the level of hepatocyte loss predicted by the model to produce the ALT profiles was assessed.

ALT release from hepatocytes is driven by necrosis and apoptosis (secondary necrosis) rates. By studying the serum ALT levels associated with potential liver toxicity, the loss of hepatocytes can be inferred based on this dynamic ALT level. Furthermore, the

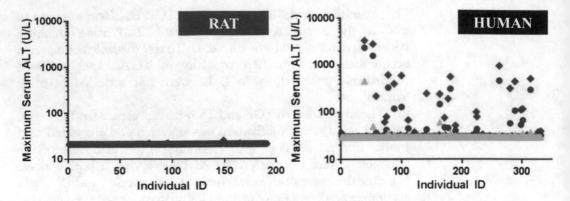

Fig. 3 DILIsym predicts species differences in troglitazone hepatotoxicity. (Left) No rat hepatotoxicity is predicted with oral doses of 5 (blue circle) or 25 (red diamond) mg/kg/day for 6 months, in line with preclinical experiments. (Right) Human ALT elevations >3× ULN predicted in 0.3%, 3.0%, and 5.1% of the simulated population after oral doses of 200 (green triangle), 400 (blue circle), or 600 (red diamond) mg/day for 6 months, respectively. Reprinted with permission from [12]

Table 4
Simulations with TGZ and TS bile acid transporter inhibition to investigate the contribution each transporter has on predicted toxicity

Transporter	Simulation I	Simulation II	Simulation III	Simulation IV
BSEP inhibition	Active	Inactive	Active	Active
MRP4 inhibition	Active	Active	Inactive	Active
NTCP inhibition	Active	Active	Active	Inactive
ALT > 3× ULN	3.6% (12/331)	0.3% (1/331)	0.3% (1/331)	5.1% (17/331)
TBIL > 2× ULN	0.6% (2/331)	0% (0/331)	0% (0/331)	1.2% (4/331)
Death	0.3% (1/331)	0% (0/331)	0% (0/331)	0.3% (1/331)

Results from individuals dosed 600 mg/day for a month

relationship between distribution of patients within a predicted ALT range and probability of severe liver injury can be deduced, such as was done with Entolimod.

Figure 4a shows serum ALT time course data from healthy volunteers after receiving a single dose of Entolimod. DILIsym was used to capture three ALT time courses corresponding to the maximum peak ALT observed, the upper 95th percentile peak ALT observed, and the median peak ALT observed (Fig. 4b). From these profiles, the maximum hepatocyte loss was determined (Fig. 4c). For the majority of volunteers receiving Entolimod, the predicted hepatocyte loss was less than 0.5% of their baseline value. The maximum responder whose ALT peak was greater than 1000 U/L was predicted to have lost at most 3.5% of their

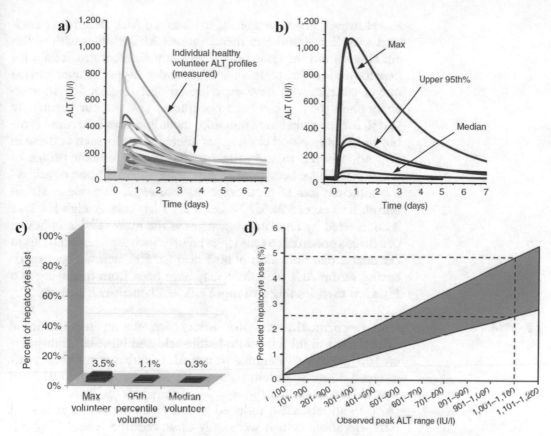

Fig. 4 DILIsym estimates the viable liver mass based on ALT signals for Entolimod. (**a**) ALT profiles for healthy volunteers. (**b**) The maximum ALT value observed (black line) was used along with the time-course dynamics for ALT to optimize DILIsym simulations (red line.) Also shown are the upper 95th percentile and median ALT observations with their respective DILIsym simulated ALT profiles. (**c**) Estimated maximum level of hepatocyte loss after Entolimod dosing in the DILIsym model corresponding to the maximum, 95th percentile, and median peak ALT responses measured in the clinical trial. (**d**) Range of predicted hepatocyte loss (% of baseline) as a function of observed peak ALT range in healthy volunteers. The dashed lines indicate the predicted range of hepatocyte loss associated with the observed maximum ALT level in normal healthy volunteers dosed with Entolimod. Reprinted with permission from [64]

hepatocytes. Although the observed and modeled serum ALT levels seem severe, a minimal fraction of hepatocytes were lost.

A SimPops was constructed with variability in key parameters related to ALT production, e.g., ALT content per hepatocyte, and clearance to simulate potential inter-individual variation in the relationship between serum ALT time-course profiles and loss of hepatocyte mass (Fig. 4d). Figure 4d functions as a look-up table for ALT time-course profiles exhibited by Entolimod responders. For example, a maximum observed ALT response of 1001–1100 U/L corresponds to an estimated 2.6–4.9% loss of hepatocytes.

However, Fig. 4d is specific to observed ALT elevations associated with Entolimod treatment; various ALT profiles with different kinetics and the same peak have vastly different predictions for hepatocyte loss [64]. Because of extensive biopsy studies carried out in patients who have experienced liver injuries due to acetaminophen [65], it has been possible to link percent hepatocyte loss to loss of global liver function, including rises in serum bilirubin and INR (a blood clotting parameter). Results such as those in Fig. 4d, tailored to the drug-specific time dependent profile of serum ALT, have been used to determine the likelihood of achieving sufficient loss of hepatocyte mass to result in a rise in serum bilirubin to exceed 2× ULN, i.e., a Hy's law case. A Hy's law case is considered by regulatory agencies as the most reliable indicator of a drug's potential to cause liver failure. Such analyses in DILIsym can enable determination of how near (or far) each subject experiencing serum ALT elevations may have been from qualifying as a Hy's law case, leading to a more efficient benefit-risk analysis.

3.3 CKA

CKA, a chemokine receptor antagonist, was an investigational drug shown to inhibit multiple bile acid and bilirubin transporters [66]. It caused minimal serum ALT increases in humans but induced dose-dependent serum ALT increases in rats. DILIsym was able to capture the species differences in hepatotoxicity [67]. In all rats, CKA induced hyperbilirubinemia, regardless of ALT elevations which were only observed in a subset (Fig. 5). This suggests that factors other than liver injury contributed to bilirubin increases, and DILIsym was used to investigate this hypothesis [15].

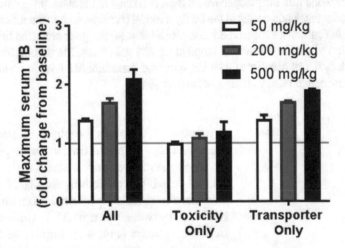

Fig. 5 DILIsym determines whether observed increases in bilirubin are due to liver damage or inhibition of bilirubin transporters by CKA. Maximum serum TBIL fold-change from baseline for increasing doses of CKA simulated with combined effects of hepatotoxicity and bilirubin transporter inhibition, hepatotoxicity only, or bilirubin transporter inhibition only. Reprinted with permission from [15]

Initial simulations incorporating CKA disposition, hepatotoxicity mechanisms (ROS generation, bile acid transporter inhibition, and mitochondrial dysfunction), and bilirubin transporter inhibition in rats predicted average TBIL increases of 1.4-, 1.7-, and 2.1-fold at respective single doses of 50, 200, and 500 mg/kg. When the same dosing protocols were simulated without inhibition of bilirubin transporters, TBIL levels changed minimally: 1.0-, 1.1-, and 1.2-fold change. However, when all toxicity mechanisms were deactivated and only bilirubin transport inhibition was included with CKA disposition, TBIL levels predicted 1.4-, 1.7-, and 1.9-fold changes. This indicates that the main contributor to simulated TBIL increases was inhibition of bilirubin transporters and not overt liver injury.

4   Conclusion and Future Directions

Although DILI has a variety of clinical presentations and can be mediated by multiple mechanisms, accurate predictions of the hepatotoxic potential of drug candidates have been demonstrated by DILIsym. By quantitatively characterizing perturbations in the biological system and integrating their effects with drug exposure, DILIsym has been able to predict in vivo hepatotoxicity in a number of species. The aforementioned applications of DILIsym showed how systems pharmacology modeling can be useful to predict the hepatotoxic potential of novel compounds based on in vitro and in vivo data, which show how the compound interacts with the biological pathways represented within the various submodels. As shown with Entolimod and CKA, biomarker elevations can be used to estimate the hepatocyte loss and gauge liver damage, serious or otherwise, and in cases similar to troglitazone, DILIsym can be used to predict species differences and test experimental conditions that would otherwise be unfeasible.

Future directions extend DILIsym into other related areas. One such example is NAFLDsym™, a novel quantitative systems pharmacology (QSP) representation of nonalcoholic fatty liver disease (NAFLD). Despite substantial worldwide prevalence of the disease, NAFLD currently has few available treatment options. NAFLDsym has been developed to help accelerate clinical development by reducing the number of required experiments. NAFLDsym mechanistically represents many of the key components of steatosis and lipotoxicity, in addition to innate immune responses, hepatocyte turnover, and biomarkers. NAFLDsym also includes a distinct set of simulated population of patients with varying degrees of NAFLD pathophysiology and clinical presentation. This SimPops can be used to evaluate the efficacious potential for NAFLD targets and compounds in support of the clinical development of NAFLD treatments.

QSP or quantitative systems toxicology (QST) models, while useful in predicting many outcomes, do have some limitations. These computational tools must be continually maintained and updated as new science emerges, allowing the mathematical framework to develop over time. Additional mechanisms and pathways supported by available data must be incorporated. In this way, current gaps do exist within all in silico models, and DILIsym is no exception; for instance, work is currently being devoted into developing a mechanistic model of the adaptive immune response as it is likely to be a final mediator of many idiosyncratic drug reactions. At the same time, QSP/QST models help to facilitate and identify key areas where data gaps exist, guiding further experimentation. The iterative process of science pushes the computational model and experimental methods forward, expanding the current knowledge and improving the ability to predict and prevent future instances of DILI.

References

1. Olson H, Betton G, Robinson D et al (2000) Concordance of the toxicity of pharmaceuticals in humans and in animals. Regul Toxicol Pharmacol 32:56–67. https://doi.org/10.1006/rtph.2000.1399

2. Dixit R, Boelsterli UA (2007) Healthy animals and animal models of human disease(s) in safety assessment of human pharmaceuticals, including therapeutic antibodies. Drug Discov Today 12:336–342. https://doi.org/10.1016/j.drudis.2007.02.018

3. Valerio LG Jr (2009) In silico toxicology for the pharmaceutical sciences. Toxicol Appl Pharmacol 241:356–370. https://doi.org/10.1016/j.taap.2009.08.022

4. Greer ML, Barber J, Eakins J, Kenna JG (2010) Cell based approaches for evaluation of drug-induced liver injury. Toxicology 268:125–131. https://doi.org/10.1016/j.tox.2009.08.007

5. Sugiyama Y, Yamashita S (2011) Impact of microdosing clinical study – why necessary and how useful? Adv Drug Deliv Rev 63:494–502. https://doi.org/10.1016/j.addr.2010.09.010

6. Astashkina A, Mann B, Grainger DW (2012) A critical evaluation of in vitro cell culture models for high-throughput drug screening and toxicity. Pharmacol Ther 134:82–106. https://doi.org/10.1016/j.pharmthera.2012.01.001

7. LeCluyse EL, Witek RP, Andersen ME, Powers MJ (2012) Organotypic liver culture models: meeting current challenges in toxicity testing. Crit Rev Toxicol 42:501–548. https://doi.org/10.3109/10408444.2012.682115

8. Howell BA, Yang Y, Kumar R et al (2012) In vitro to in vivo extrapolation and species response comparisons for drug-induced liver injury (DILI) using DILIsym™: a mechanistic, mathematical model of DILI. J Pharmacokinet Pharmacodyn 39:527–541. https://doi.org/10.1007/s10928-012-9266-0

9. Woodhead JL, Howell BA, Yang Y et al (2012) An analysis of N-acetylcysteine treatment for acetaminophen overdose using a systems model of drug-induced liver injury. J Pharmacol Exp Ther 342:529–540. https://doi.org/10.1124/jpet.112.192930

10. Howell BA, Siler SQ, Watkins PB (2014) Use of a systems model of drug-induced liver injury (DILIsym(®)) to elucidate the mechanistic differences between acetaminophen and its less-toxic isomer, AMAP, in mice. Toxicol Lett 226:163–172. https://doi.org/10.1016/j.toxlet.2014.02.007

11. Woodhead JL, Yang K, Siler SQ et al (2014) Exploring BSEP inhibition-mediated toxicity with a mechanistic model of drug-induced liver injury. Front Pharmacol 5:240. https://doi.org/10.3389/fphar.2014.00240

12. Yang K, Woodhead JL, Watkins PB et al (2014) Systems pharmacology modeling predicts delayed presentation and species differences in bile acid-mediated troglitazone hepatotoxicity. Clin Pharmacol Ther:589–598. https://doi.org/10.1038/clpt.2014.158

13. Yang K, Woodhead J, Morgan R, et al (2015) Mechanistic modeling with DILIsym® predicts dose-dependent clincial hepatotoxicity of AMG 009 that involves bile acid (BA) transporter inhibition. J Pharmacokinet Pharmacodyn. Springer, New York, NY

14. Longo DM, Yang Y, Watkins PB et al (2016) Elucidating differences in the hepatotoxic potential of tolcapone and entacapone with DILIsym(®), a mechanistic model of drug-induced liver injury. CPT Pharmacomet Syst Pharmacol 5:31–39. https://doi.org/10.1002/psp4.12053

15. Yang K, Battista C, Woodhead JL et al (2017) Systems pharmacology modeling of drug-induced hyperbilirubinemia: differentiating hepatotoxicity and inhibition of enzymes/transporters. Clin Pharmacol Ther. https://doi.org/10.1002/cpt.619

16. Bhattacharyya D, Pandit S, Mukherjee R et al (2003) Hepatoprotective effect of Himoliv, a polyherbal formulation in rats. Indian J Physiol Pharmacol 47:435–440

17. Song Z, McClain CJ, Chen T (2004) S-Adenosylmethionine protects against acetaminophen-induced hepatotoxicity in mice. Pharmacology 71:199–208. https://doi.org/10.1159/000078086

18. Valentovic M, Terneus M, Harmon RC, Carpenter AB (2004) S-Adenosylmethionine (SAMe) attenuates acetaminophen hepatotoxicity in C57BL/6 mice. Toxicol Lett 154:165–174. https://doi.org/10.1016/j.toxlet.2004.07.010

19. Chen Y-H, Lin F-Y, Liu P-L et al (2009) Antioxidative and hepatoprotective effects of magnolol on acetaminophen-induced liver damage in rats. Arch Pharm Res 32:221–228. https://doi.org/10.1007/s12272-009-1139-8

20. Patel SJ, Milwid JM, King KR et al (2012) Gap junction inhibition prevents drug-induced liver toxicity and fulminant hepatic failure. Nat Biotechnol 30:179–183. https://doi.org/10.1038/nbt.2089

21. Nieminen AL, Saylor AK, Herman B, Lemasters JJ (1994) ATP depletion rather than mitochondrial depolarization mediates hepatocyte killing after metabolic inhibition. Am J Phys 267:C67–C74

22. Yang Y, Nadanaciva S, Will Y et al (2014) MITOsym®: a mechanistic, mathematical model of hepatocellular respiration and bioenergetics. Pharm Res. https://doi.org/10.1007/s11095-014-1591-0

23. Zahno A, Brecht K, Morand R et al (2011) The role of CYP3A4 in amiodarone-associated toxicity on HepG2 cells. Biochem Pharmacol 81:432–441. https://doi.org/10.1016/j.bcp.2010.11.002

24. Mullen PJ, Zahno A, Lindinger P et al (2011) Susceptibility to simvastatin-induced toxicity is partly determined by mitochondrial respiration and phosphorylation state of Akt. Biochim Biophys Acta 1813:2079–2087. https://doi.org/10.1016/j.bbamcr.2011.07.019

25. Nadanaciva S, Rana P, Beeson GC et al (2012) Assessment of drug-induced mitochondrial dysfunction via altered cellular respiration and acidification measured in a 96-well platform. J Bioenerg Biomembr 44:421–437. https://doi.org/10.1007/s10863-012-9446-z

26. Yang K, Guo C, Woodhead JL et al (2016) Sandwich-cultured hepatocytes as a tool to study drug disposition and drug-induced liver injury. J Pharm Sci 105:443–459. https://doi.org/10.1016/j.xphs.2015.11.008

27. Perez M-J, Briz O (2009) Bile-acid-induced cell injury and protection. World J Gastroenterol 15:1677–1689

28. Maillette-de-Buy-Wenniger L, Beuers U (2010) Bile salts and cholestasis. Dig Liver Dis 42:409–418. https://doi.org/10.1016/j.dld.2010.03.015

29. Dawson SE, Stahl S, Paul N et al (2011) In vitro inhibition of the bile salt export pump correlates with risk of cholestatic drug induced liver injury in man. Drug Metab Dispos Biol Fate Chem. https://doi.org/10.1124/dmd.111.040758

30. Morgan RE, van Staden CJ, Chen Y et al (2013) A multifactorial approach to hepatobiliary transporter assessment enables improved therapeutic compound development. Toxicol Sci Off J Soc Toxicol 136:216–241. https://doi.org/10.1093/toxsci/kft176

31. Pedersen JM, Matsson P, Bergström CAS et al (2013) Early identification of clinically relevant drug interactions with the human bile salt export pump (BSEP/ABCB11). Toxicol Sci Off J Soc Toxicol 136:328–343. https://doi.org/10.1093/toxsci/kft197

32. Meier PJ, Stieger B (2002) Bile salt transporters. Annu Rev Physiol 64:635–661. https://doi.org/10.1146/annurev.physiol.64.082201.100300

33. Akita H, Suzuki H, Hirohashi T et al (2002) Transport activity of human MRP3 expressed in Sf9 cells: comparative studies with rat MRP3. Pharm Res 19:34–41

34. Rius M, Hummel-Eisenbeiss J, Hofmann AF, Keppler D (2006) Substrate specificity of human ABCC4 (MRP4)-mediated cotransport of bile acids and reduced glutathione. Am J Physiol Gastrointest Liver Physiol 290:G640–G649. https://doi.org/10.1152/ajpgi.00354.2005

35. Jackson JP, Freeman KM, Friley WW et al (2016) Basolateral efflux transporters: a potentially important pathway for the prevention of cholestatic hepatotoxicity. Appl Vitro Toxicol 2:207–216. https://doi.org/10.1089/aivt.2016.0023

36. Uppal H, Saini SPS, Moschetta A et al (2007) Activation of LXRs prevents bile acid toxicity and cholestasis in female mice. Hepatology 45:422–432. https://doi.org/10.1002/hep.21494

37. Beilke LD, Aleksunes LM, Holland RD et al (2009) Constitutive androstane receptor-mediated changes in bile acid composition contributes to hepatoprotection from lithocholic acid-induced liver injury in mice. Drug Metab Dispos Biol Fate Chem 37:1035–1045. https://doi.org/10.1124/dmd.108.023317

38. Jonker JW, Liddle C, Downes M (2012) FXR and PXR: potential therapeutic targets in cholestasis. J Steroid Biochem Mol Biol 130:147–158. https://doi.org/10.1016/j.jsbmb.2011.06.012

39. Woodhead JL, Yang K, Brouwer KLR et al (2014) Mechanistic modeling reveals the critical knowledge gaps in bile acid-mediated DILI. CPT Pharmacomet Syst Pharmacol 3:e123. https://doi.org/10.1038/psp.2014.21

40. Trottier J, Caron P, Straka RJ, Barbier O (2011) Profile of serum bile acids in noncholestatic volunteers: gender-related differences in response to fenofibrate. Clin Pharmacol Ther 90:279–286. https://doi.org/10.1038/clpt.2011.124

41. García-Cañaveras JC, Donato MT, Castell JV, Lahoz A (2012) Targeted profiling of circulating and hepatic bile acids in human, mouse, and rat using a UPLC-MRM-MS-validated method. J Lipid Res 53:2231–2241. https://doi.org/10.1194/jlr.D028803

42. Shoda LKM, Battista C, Siler SQ, et al. (2017) Mechanistic modelling of drug-induced liver injury: investigating the role of innate immune responses. Gene Regul Syst Biol. 11:1177625017696074. http://doi.org/10.1177/1177625017696074

43. Fiorentino D, Zlotnik A, TR M et al (2016) IL-10 inhibits cytokine production by activated macrophages. J Immunol 197:1539–1546

44. Smith D, Lackides G, Epstein L (1990) Coordinated induction of autocrine tumor necrosis factor and interleukin 1 in normal human monocytes and the implications for monocyte-mediated cytotoxicity. Cancer Res 50:3146–3153

45. Shnyra A, Brewington R, Alipio A et al (1998) Reprogramming of lipopolysaccharide-primed macrophages is controlled by a counterbalanced production of IL-10 and IL-12. J Immunol (Baltim, MD, 1950) 160:3729–3736

46. Bonaldi T, Talamo F, Scaffidi P et al (2003) Monocytic cells hyperacetylate chromatin protein HMGB1 to redirect it towards secre-

tion. EMBO J 22:5551–5560. https://doi.org/10.1093/emboj/cdg516

47. Chen G, Li J, Ochani M et al (2004) Bacterial endotoxin stimulates macrophages to release HMGB1 partly through CD14- and TNF-dependent mechanisms. J Leukoc Biol 76:994–1001. https://doi.org/10.1189/jlb.0404242

48. Cui Y, Konig J, Leier I et al (2001) Hepatic uptake of bilirubin and its conjugates by the human organic anion transporter SLC21A6. J Biol Chem 276:9626–9630. https://doi.org/10.1074/jbc.M004968200

49. Briz O, Serrano M, MacIas R (2003) Role of organic anion-transporting polypeptides, OATP-A, OATP-C and OATP-8, in the human placenta-maternal liver tandem excretory pathway for foetal bilirubin. Biochem J 905:897–905

50. Keppler D (2014) The roles of MRP2, MRP3, OATP1B1, and OATP1B3 in conjugated hyperbilirubinemia. Drug Metab Dispos 42:561–565. https://doi.org/10.1124/dmd.113.055772

51. Ritter JK, Chen F, Sheen YY et al (1992) A novel complex locus UGT1 encodes human bilirubin, phenol, and other UDP-glucuronosyltransferase isozymes with identical carboxyl termini. J Biol Chem 267:3257–3261

52. Kamisako T, Leier I, Cui Y et al (1999) Transport of monoglucuronosyl and bisglucuronosyl bilirubin by recombinant human and rat multidrug resistance protein 2. Hepatology (Baltim, MD) 30:485–490. https://doi.org/10.1002/hep.510300220

53. Lee Y-MA, Cui Y, König J et al (2004) Identification and functional characterization of the natural variant MRP3-Arg1297His of human multidrug resistance protein 3 (MRP3/ABCC3). Pharmacogenetics 14:213–223

54. Kazama H, Ricci J-E, Herndon JM et al (2008) Induction of immunological tolerance by apoptotic cells requires caspase-dependent oxidation of high-mobility group box-1 protein. Immunity 29:21–32. https://doi.org/10.1016/j.immuni.2008.05.013

55. Yang R, Zhang S, Cotoia A et al (2012) High mobility group B1 impairs hepatocyte regeneration in acetaminophen hepatotoxicity. BMC Gastroenterol 12:45. https://doi.org/10.1186/1471-230X-12-45

56. Venereau E, Casalgrandi M, Schiraldi M et al (2012) Mutually exclusive redox forms of HMGB1 promote cell recruitment or proinflammatory cytokine release. J Exp Med 209:1519–1528. https://doi.org/10.1084/jem.20120189

57. Lu B, Nakamura T, Inouye K et al (2012) Novel role of PKR in inflammasome activation and HMGB1 release. Nature 488:670–674. https://doi.org/10.1038/nature11290

58. Nyström S, Antoine DJ, Lundbäck P et al (2013) TLR activation regulates damage-associated molecular pattern isoforms released during pyroptosis. EMBO J 32:86–99. https://doi.org/10.1038/emboj.2012.328

59. Antoine DJ, Harris HE, Andersson U et al (2014) A systematic nomenclature for the redox states of high mobility group box (HMGB) proteins. Mol Med (Camb, MA) 20:135–137. https://doi.org/10.2119/molmed.2014.00022

60. Lu B, Antoine DJ, Kwan K et al (2014) JAK/STAT1 signaling promotes HMGB1 hyper-acetylation and nuclear translocation. Proc Natl Acad Sci U S A 111:3068–3073. https://doi.org/10.1073/pnas.1316925111

61. Caulín C, Salvesen GS, Oshima RG (1997) Caspase cleavage of keratin 18 and reorganization of intermediate filaments during epithelial cell apoptosis. J Cell Biol 138:1379–1394

62. Kramer G, Erdal H, Mertens HJMM et al (2004) Differentiation between cell death modes using measurements of different soluble forms of extracellular cytokeratin 18. Cancer Res 64:1751–1756

63. Linder S, Olofsson MH, Herrmann R, Ulukaya E (2010) Utilization of cytokeratin-based biomarkers for pharmacodynamic studies. Expert Rev Mol Diagn 10:353–359. https://doi.org/10.1586/erm.10.14

64. Howell BA, Siler SQ, Shoda LKM et al (2014) A mechanistic model of drug-induced liver injury AIDS the interpretation of elevated liver transaminase levels in a phase I clinical trial. CPT Pharmacomet Syst Pharmacol 3:e98. https://doi.org/10.1038/psp.2013.74

65. Portmann B, Talbot IC, Day DW et al (1975) Histopathological changes in the liver following a paracetamol overdose: correlation with clinical and biochemical parameters. J Pathol 117:169–181. https://doi.org/10.1002/path.1711170307

66. Ulloa JL, Stahl S, Yates J et al (2013) Assessment of gadoxetate DCE-MRI as a biomarker of hepatobiliary transporter inhibition. NMR Biomed 26:1258–1270. https://doi.org/10.1002/nbm.2946

67. Battista C, Yang K, Mettetal JT et al (2016) Mechanistic modeling with DILIsym® predicts species differences in CKA via multiple hepatotoxic mechanisms. J Pharacokinet Pharmacodyn 43:15

68. Woodhead JL, Watkins PB, Howell BA et al (2017) The role of quantitative systems pharmacology modeling in the prediction and explanation of idiosyncratic drug-induced liver injury. Drug Metab Pharmacokinet 32:40–45. https://doi.org/10.1016/j.dmpk.2016.11.008

69. Horn KD, Wax P, Schneider SM et al (1999) Biomarkers of liver regeneration allow early prediction of hepatic recovery after acute necrosis. Am J Clin Pathol 112:351–357

70. Giannini EG, Testa R, Savarino V (2005) Liver enzyme alteration: a guide for clinicians. Can Med Assoc J 172:367–379. https://doi.org/10.1503/cmaj.1040752

71. Lewis JH (2006) "Hy's law,' the "Rezulin Rule," and other predictors of severe drug-induced hepatotoxicity: putting risk-benefit into perspective. Pharmacoepidemiol Drug Saf 15:221–229. https://doi.org/10.1002/pds.1209

72. Ozer J, Ratner M, Shaw M et al (2008) The current state of serum biomarkers of hepatotoxicity. Toxicology 245:194–205. https://doi.org/10.1016/j.tox.2007.11.021

73. Antoine DJ, Mercer AE, Williams DP, Park BK (2009) Mechanism-based bioanalysis and biomarkers for hepatic chemical stress. Xenobiotica 39:565–577. https://doi.org/10.1080/00498250903046993

74. Antoine DJ, Williams DP, Kipar A et al (2009) High-mobility group box-1 protein and keratin-18, circulating serum proteins informative of acetaminophen-induced necrosis and apoptosis in vivo. Toxicol Sci Off J Soc Toxicol 112:521–531. https://doi.org/10.1093/toxsci/kfp235

75. Harrill AH, Roach J, Fier I et al (2012) The effects of heparins on the liver: application of mechanistic serum biomarkers in a randomized study in healthy volunteers. Clin Pharmacol Ther 92:214–220. https://doi.org/10.1038/clpt.2012.40

76. Murayama H, Ikemoto M, Fukuda Y, Nagata A (2008) Superiority of serum type-I arginase and ornithine carbamyltransferase in the detection of toxicant-induced acute hepatic injury in rats. Clin Chim Acta Int J Clin Chem 391:31–35. https://doi.org/10.1016/j.cca.2008.01.023

77. Wetmore BA, Brees DJ, Singh R et al (2010) Quantitative analyses and transcriptomic profiling of circulating messenger RNAs as biomarkers of rat liver injury. Hepatol Baltim Md 51:2127–2139. https://doi.org/10.1002/hep.23574

78. Yang X, Greenhaw J, Shi Q et al (2012) Identification of urinary microRNA profiles in rats that may diagnose hepatotoxicity. Toxicol Sci Off J Soc Toxicol 125:335–344. https://doi.org/10.1093/toxsci/kfr321

Part III

In Vitro Technologies

Chapter 7

Prediction of Human Liver Toxicity Using In Vitro Assays: Limitations and Opportunities

Franck A. Atienzar and Jean-Marie Nicolas

Abstract

This chapter provides a short review of the current challenges to predict the risk for drug-induced liver injury (DILI) in humans using in vitro assays. Simple single cell-type in vitro cytotoxicity assays may fail to predict complex in vivo interconnected mechanism-based toxicities. Additionally, the lack of standardization of in vitro assays complicates data interpretation and makes assay comparison difficult. The selection of a given assay may depend on the DILI mechanism to be explored, short-term versus long-term culture, and the ability to study the toxicity of parent compounds or metabolites. Indeed, a single model is unlikely to address all the relevant mechanisms that can lead to liver toxicity. A better implementation of preclinical data as well as harmonization of current, emerging and novel in vitro systems should help to better predict human DILI. Case studies are also provided to illustrate how the in vitro assays can help to derisk preclinical in vivo toxicity findings and to better predict clinical human liver toxicity outcomes. Opportunities in the DILI field are also discussed, in particular the need to use more relevant in vitro models to better mimic the in vivo situation (e.g., pathological state, long term exposure, integration of inflammatory components), as well as the access to in vitro models from multiple species. Finally the use of relevant technologies (e.g., label free approach), in silico approaches integrating data from new chemical spaces, and the setting up of a preclinical DILI guidance from the scientific community and authorities are also important steps which should help the scientific community to improve DILI prediction.

Key words In vitro DILI assays, Limitations, Opportunities, Promises, Predictivity, In vitro–in vivo correlation, Technology, Guidance

1 Introduction

The prediction of intrinsic DILI has tremendously improved during the last decades in term of development of new technologies and hazard identification. Nevertheless, numerous challenges remain, especially with respect to the detection of idiosyncratic DILI, whose incidence is very low (e.g., 1–2 cases per million prescriptions for diclofenac [1]), and which involves multiple factors, e.g., genetic, environmental, and physiological [2].

Minjun Chen and Yvonne Will (eds.), *Drug-Induced Liver Toxicity*, Methods in Pharmacology and Toxicology, https://doi.org/10.1007/978-1-4939-7677-5_7, © Springer Science+Business Media, LLC, part of Springer Nature 2018

2   Challenges and Drawbacks of In Vitro Models

2.1   Single Cell-Type In Vitro Cytotoxicity Assays Versus Multiple Mechanism-Based Toxicity In Vivo

Various well-established in vitro assays are routinely used at early stages of drug development to identify compounds devoid of genotoxicity [3] and cardiotoxicity [4] risks. This contrasts with the in vitro prediction of DILI which remains far more challenging for the pharmaceutical industry. The understanding of the patho-physiological basis of DILI is still very rudimentary and involves multiple mechanisms and cell types. As a result, up to now, no consensus has been reached yet on the ideal set of predictive in vitro tools to detect and investigate DILI.

The structure of the liver is complex as illustrated in Fig. 1. It is composed of 60% hepatocytes and 40% of nonparenchymal cells including stellate cells, Kupffer cells, sinusoidal endothelial cells, biliary epithelial cells and immune cells [5]. Single cell-type

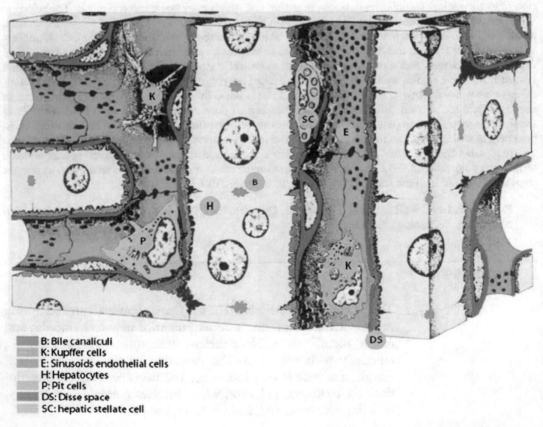

B: Bile canaliculi
K: Kupffer cells
E: Sinusoids endothelial cells
H: Hepatocytes
P: Pit cells
DS: Disse space
SC: hepatic stellate cell

Fig. 1 Cellular composition and architecture of the liver. Hepatocytes have two basolateral sides that face the sinusoidal blood vessels. The apical side consists of invaginations of the plasma membrane of adjacent hepatocytes. These invaginations form the strongly interconnected bile canaliculi. Tight junctions separate the apical compartments from the basolateral compartment. For more details, please refer to [5]. Figure reproduced with permission

assays measuring a few markers of late stage events in the cell injury process were firstly used to study liver toxicity [6]. These measured markers typically relate to cytolysis (e.g., LDH leakage), apoptosis (e.g., caspase activation), loss of critical macromolecules (e.g., ATP and GSH depletion), major metabolic dysfunction (e.g., neutral red uptake, MTT reduction), or antiproliferative effects [7–9]. Retrospective analysis of marketed pharmaceuticals revealed that such basal in vitro cytotoxic assays were poorly predictive of DILI [8]. Assays designed to detect acute late stage cell damage may miss hepatotoxic drugs that impair liver function without causing cell mortality. Thus, implementation of more subtle sub-lethal markers that better account for the hepatic side effects observed in vivo should be given high priority [8]. In addition, hepatocyte damages usually trigger secondary responses that involve several types of nonparenchymal cells or immune cells and potentially amplify the DILI reactions. As a consequence, in vitro assays focusing only on one cell type (i.e., hepatocytes) are unlikely to offer the optimal approach and nonparenchymal cells should be considered [5, 10–12].

Basic in vitro cytotoxicity assays are unlikely to accurately reproduce the whole range of interconnected processes underlying the hepatotoxic reactions observed in vivo [13]. The complexity of DILI responses is illustrated by the catechol-O-methyltransferase inhibitor tolcapone which is associated with liver enzyme elevation and some rare but life-threatening cases of fulminant hepatitis [14, 15]. This triggered a black-box warning in the USA, a temporary withdrawal in EU, and a definitive withdrawal in some other countries. Subsequent investigative studies demonstrated that multiple mechanisms were potentially involved in tolcapone-induced hepatotoxicity [16]. Tolcapone causes mitochondrial dysfunction by uncoupling the mitochondria proton gradient which ultimately impairs ATP synthesis and increases oxygen consumption [17]. Additionally, tolcapone might induce hepatobiliary toxicity by causing the accumulation of bile acids through inhibition of the efflux transporters bile salt export pump (BSEP) and Multidrug Resistance related Proteins (MRPs) [17]. Other studies suggested that tolcapone-induced hepatotoxicity might originate from the oxidation of the known metabolites M1 and M2 into reactive species forming covalent adducts to hepatic proteins [18]. Patients with variants of UGT1A9, the glucuronidation enzyme primarily involved in tolcapone elimination, appear to be more exposed to the drug and thus more susceptible to its hepatic side effects [19]. Finally, some authors argued that tolcapone produces an increase in catecholamine levels through excessive adrenergic stimulation, which in turn could potentiate the hepatotoxic effects [20]. Almost all the drugs associated with DILI are characterized by such multiple and interindependent toxicological mechanisms, often simultaneously involving mitochondrial impairment, reactive metabolites, hepato-biliary dysfunction, and immune responses [21].

The complexity and the interconnection of the DILI responses are also illustrated by the liver findings observed with a new anti-epileptic drug candidate in dog toxicity studies [22]. An exhaustive panel of assays including histopathological examinations, ex-vivo biochemical assays, mass spectrometry measurements, and metab-olite profiling led to the identification of the mechanisms underly-ing the formation of the brown pigment inclusions observed in the liver of treated animals. Briefly, in dog, the drug transforms into a reactive metabolite that alkylates the prosthetic heme of cyto-chrome CYP2B11. The alkylated heme, after iron atom removal, is released and converts to N-alkylprotoporphyrin which inhibits fer-rochelatase, the final enzyme in heme biosynthesis. As a result, the substrate of ferrochelatase, protoporphyrin IX, accumulates result-ing in liver deposits and liver impairment. In addition, the drug was found to induce hepatic CYP2B11 with increased reactive metabolite formation, depletion of hepatic heme reserve and acti-vation of the heme biosynthetic cascade; all these findings being likely to exacerbate the deposit formation. Although not investi-gated, other mechanisms such as hepatic transporter disruption might also contribute to the observed liver changes [23, 24]. Of notice, protoporphyrin IX accumulation and N-alkylprotoporphyrin formation could not be reproduced in vitro in cultured hepato-cytes. The lack of sensitive in vitro assays has been already reported for other porphyrinogenic agents with similar mode of action [25]. This case study further illustrates the multiplex nature of DILI, the tight regulation between the various mechanisms, the variety of assays and endpoints required, and the potential sensitivity issues associated with some in vitro approaches. For obvious reasons, recapitulating all these processes and their interplay in a "one-fits-all" in vitro assay represents a major challenge.

Many different in vitro models are available to investigate DILI mechanisms (Fig. 2). Models have been significantly refined in order to increase their physiological relevance (Fig. 2) with the overall aim to better predict human DILI. In most assays, cells are exposed to relatively high concentrations of compound for a short duration. Such approach may not facilitate the detection of DILI reactions that occur only after chronic exposure to the drug [26]. Primary human hepatocytes (PHHs) remain the gold standard model for metabolism and liver toxicity studies [26] as they more closely mimic the in vivo situation with regard to liver functions. However, in vitro hepatocyte assays suffer from a number of limita-tions including cell availability, interindividual variability, limited batch size, reduced life span, and cost. The rapid decline in CYP expression and activity, within 24 h of culture, is certainly a key issue given the central role of drug metabolism (e.g., reactive metabolite formation) in DILI events [27]. Consequently, some

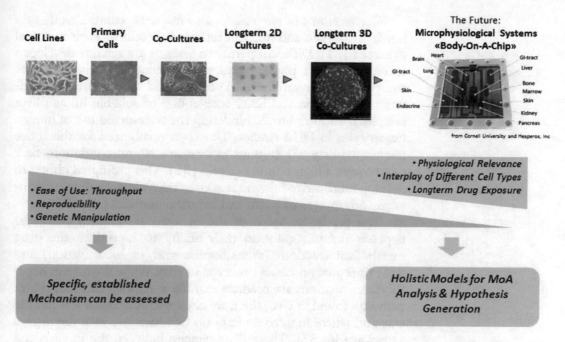

Fig. 2 Overview of some of the in vitro models available to predict human DILI. For more details, please refer to [89]. Figure reproduced with permission

alternative models have been proposed such as immortalized liver-derived cell lines (e.g., human hepatocellular carcinoma HepG2). Despite their unlimited availability, and phenotypic stability, cell lines have their own limitations such as low metabolism activity [28] and maintained cell proliferation even after confluency has been reached [29]. Cells such as HepaRG provide some advantages (better time frame for DILI studies, improved reproducibility, and easy access) but do not entirely mimic yet primary hepatocyte phenotype [27]. To reconstitute a more physiological microenvironment, different culture conditions have been investigated (e.g., sandwich cultures, spheroids, 3D cultures) [5]. These approaches bring some undeniable benefits but none are entirely satisfactory and no consensus has been reached yet about the optimal cell culture conditions. Furthermore, cocultures of hepatocytes with non-parenchymal cells are being investigated using different formats [30–32] with data suggesting a better maintained phenotype and an organotypic environment closer to the in vivo conditions [12]. Finally, liver slices have been proposed as an alternative model with the promise of maintained three dimensional liver structure and cell-cell interactions [33]. Unfortunately, liver slice technology has still to be improved to overcome the tissue necrosis that occurs after few days of culture, and the rapid loss of metabolic activity, both conferring a limited timeframe for suitable toxicity studies.

Conventional in vitro assays also use static conditions that do not favor oxygen and nutrient diffusion or cellular environmental dynamics [34]. Different perfusion systems are actually developed to create a more physiological environment and simultaneously overcome the limitations of 2D culture and static incubation conditions [35]. The restricted accessibility of suitable human liver samples is another hurdle hindering the widespread use of human hepatocytes in DILI studies. This is especially true for the above mentioned new 3D cultures in bioreactors and continuous flow that require a high number of cells [35]. This prompted efforts to develop miniaturized methods such as microfluidic culture systems taking advantages of micro and nanotechnologies [12, 35].

The predictive value of the in vitro DILI assay platforms depends unequivocally on their ability to reproduce the drug metabolism reactions (detoxification and/or bioactivation) and drug transport processes observed in vivo. While short term hepatocyte incubations are predictive of the metabolic and transporter pathways found in vivo, there are circumstances where it is not the case and where in vitro findings do not correlate with the in vivo situation [36, 37]. These discrepancies between the in vitro and in vivo drug disposition, e.g., CYP metabolism, should be scrutinized as it has a major impact on the overall predictivity of the DILI assays.

2.2 Lack of Standardization of In Vitro DILI Assays

As the use of in vitro DILI assays is increasing rapidly, there is an urgent need to standardize assay conditions. Some authors define standard conditions allowing them to better compare the predictivity of different in vitro DILI models [28, 38, 39] as illustrated in Table 1. A careful standardization of the assay conditions is mandatory to investigate and compare assay performances and, ultimately, to get regulatory acceptance for the selected assays [40]. Assay standardization and good practices should consider some important parameters:

2.2.1 Compound Management

Data from different studies indicate that some compounds were classified differently (e.g., tacrine classified as nonhepatotoxic, moderately hepatotoxic, or highly hepatotoxic; buspirone reported to be either nonhepatotoxic or mildly hepatotoxic in different studies) as already illustrated in Atienzar et al. [13]. One has to acknowledge as well that the DILI classification of a given chemical may progress with time as new data become available. It is of primary importance to rely on recently updated databases associated with a consistent, robust and transparent way of chemical classification. Consequently, it is recommended to use databases such as the Liver Toxicity Knowledge Base (LTKB) developed by the FDA with the specific objective of enhancing our understanding of liver toxicity [41, 42]. The LTKB uses data for marketed drugs at various level of biological organization including for instance

Table 1
Example of in vitro studies comparing multiple in vitro models to predict DILI

In vitro studies	Cellular models	Number of compounds	Concentrations tested	Cutoffs	Specificity (%)	Sensitivity (%)
[28]	HepG2	21 (5−, 16+)	Fixed concentrations: 0.1, 1, 10, 100 μM	− if TC_{50} > 10 μM + if TC_{50} < 10 μM	100 (5/5)	6.3 (1/16)
	Primary human hepatocytes				100 (5/5) (3 don.)	Don. 1: 31.3 (5/16) Don. 2: 50 (8/16) Don. 3: 43.8 (7/16)
	HepaRG				100 (5/5)	12.5 (2/16)
[38]	HepG2	51 (11−, 40+)	Multiple of Cmax: in the range 3, 6 or 12.5 up to 100 fold	− if the TC_{50} values of all the multiplexed assays >100-fold Cmax	36.4 (4/11)	82.1 (32/39)
	Primary human hepatocytes				45.5 (5/11)	82.5 (33/40)
	Dog-coculture			+ if the TC_{50} value of at least one of the multiplexed assays <100-fold Cmax	72.7 (8/11)	77.5 (31/40)
[39]	Human-coculture	49 (11−, 38+)			81.8 (9/11)	76.3 (29/38)

For more details please refer to the publications reported in the Table
− nonhepatotoxic compound, + hepatotoxic compound, TC_{50} concentration needed to produce 50% inhibition of the cellular response, *Don.* Donor

toxicogenomics, in vitro assays, histopathology, therapeutic uses, and clinical management of side effects.

A second important feature is that most sets of compounds that are used to validate in vitro DILI models contain a broad range of diverse molecules that vary in the severity of their hepatotoxic effects, in their incidence, in their mechanisms of toxicity (e.g., intrinsic versus idiosyncratic toxicity; immune versus nonimmune reactions) and in their physiopathological patterns (hepatocellular, cholestatic, mixed) [43]. Consequently, this brings confounding factors in the evaluation of the true predictive power of these assays. It would be advisable to separate drugs based on their incidence of injury [43]. The scientific community needs to increase the sharing of incidence data and to agree on a set of compounds to use as DILI and non-DILI compounds with ranges of concentrations to use. In an ideal scenario, drugs to be tested should cover a wide range of structures and pharmacological targets [13].

Finally, over the last decades, new discovery paradigms have been put in place with high-throughput ADME, early metabolite profiling and exploration of new chemical entities (e.g., external chemical libraries and combinatorial chemistry). As a result, the new drug candidates showed less pharmacokinetic failures in clinical development [44]. However, at the same time, drugs move to new physicochemical spaces [45] while showing a higher propensity to fail because of safety issues [46]. Consequently, it is critical that validation dataset consider the physicochemical and pharmacokinetic profile of the newer drugs, which may differ substantially from the profile of the historical compounds used for DILI investigations (e.g., acetaminophen, amiodarone, and diclofenac). As an example, drugs developed nowadays are associated with low metabolic clearance making metabolites including reactive metabolites more difficult to measure in vitro in conventional hepatocyte short-term culture systems [47].

2.2.2 Concentrations and Cutoffs

Predictivity of in vitro assays is evaluated by measuring assay performance in terms of sensitivity (true positive rate) and specificity (true negative rate). Table 1 provides some predictivity data obtained with in vitro models of different complexity. It has to be stressed that the assay predictivity strongly depends on the range of drug concentrations tested as well as on the cutoff values used to discriminate between hepatotoxic and nonhepatotoxic compounds (Table 1) [13]. Various strategies have been envisaged and many proposals have been reported; however, so far, no agreed standard has emerged yet. The drug concentrations to be tested can be selected as fixed multiples of the concentrations found active in in vitro and in vivo preclinical pharmacological assays (e.g., EC_{50} in vitro or in plasma; Table 1). In vitro and animal pharmacokinetic studies can also be used to better translate the preclinical data to the clinical settings and thus better understand the concentrations to be assessed in in vitro toxicology tests. It remains that all these approaches are still associated with a certain degree of uncertainty which actually limits the translatability and predictivity of the DILI assays [13, 35]. If clinical data are available, human exposure data should be taken into account to define the best range of concentrations to test under in vitro conditions. Xu and collaborators reported that the 100-fold Cmax cutoff is a rational threshold to differentiate non-DILI and DILI drugs [48]. However, plasma Cmax data can be misleading in case of significant drug accumulation in the liver, or toxicity linked to overall exposure (e.g., Area Under the Curves (AUC)) rather than peak plasma concentration (Cmax). This can be potentially addressed using physiologically based pharmacokinetic (PBPK) modeling. Although in its early days, PBPK has the potential to predict liver concentrations and the time-course of exposure based on the physicochemical properties of the drug and various other input parameters (please see Chap. 6 for more details).

2.2.3 *Endpoint Selection*

DILI may occur via many different mechanisms (necrosis, apoptosis, mitochondrial toxicity, chemically reactive metabolites, immune activation, hepatobiliary dysfunction, transporter/CYP inhibition, and so on) requiring a wide range of potential endpoints for evaluation (Fig. 3). The endpoints should be properly selected as they will ultimately affect the propensity of the DILI assay to generate false positive and negative responses. Based on the literature, a large number of endpoints (e.g., ATP, LDH, impedance, GSH, mitochondrial toxicity, albumin, urea, phospholipidosis, transport inhibition, and high content analysis) have been used in in vitro DILI studies [13] and one might question their respective predictivity. A study reported that, in micropatterned coculture models, albumin secretion (noninvasive endpoint) was the most sensitive parameter (10/10), followed by urea secretion (noninvasive endpoint), ATP levels (9/10) and GSH levels (7/10) [49]. As discussed earlier, the relevance of measuring general cytotoxicity markers (cell survival or cell lethality) may also be questioned in comparison to more mechanistic endpoints which may better reflect the in vivo conditions. It is recommended to select endpoints that cover many mechanisms leading to DILI based on the hypothesis illustrated by Thompson et al. [50]. Protocols evaluating a battery of assays and considering exposure show promising performance with respect to DILI prediction [50, 51].

Hepatobiliary disruption and cholestasis occur in about 50% of the reported cases of DILI [52]. Bile salt export pump (BSEP) inhibition and the resulting accumulation of bile acids ultimately resulting in apoptosis and necrosis have been proposed as the key mechanisms for drug-induced cholestasis. As a result, high throughput screening for BSEP inhibition and the accompanying QSAR have been proposed as important tools in DILI assessment [53, 54]. The homeostasis of bile acids, highly regulated by many mechanisms, beyond direct BSEP inhibition, may account for bile acid accumulation [55]. As example, chlorpromazine induces intrahepatic cholestasis through reactive oxygen species formation, mitochondrial toxicity, disruption of the pericanalicular distribution of F-actin, decreased messenger RNA expression of the two main canalicular bile transporters (BSEP and multidrug resistance protein 3) [56]. A number of protective mechanisms are concomitantly activated to partially reduce the intrahepatic accumulation of bile acid, which includes inhibition of Na+ dependent taurocholic cotransporting polypeptide, induction of multidrug resistance-associated protein 4, and CYP8B1 inhibition. From that example it is clear that a simple BSEP inhibition assay does not account for the complexity of some drug-induced cholestasis reactions and is likely to provide false responses. Sandwich human hepatocyte cultures have been developed to restore functional bile canaliculi (absent in standard monolayer arrangement) and to preserve the disposition pathways as well as cellular functions involved in bile

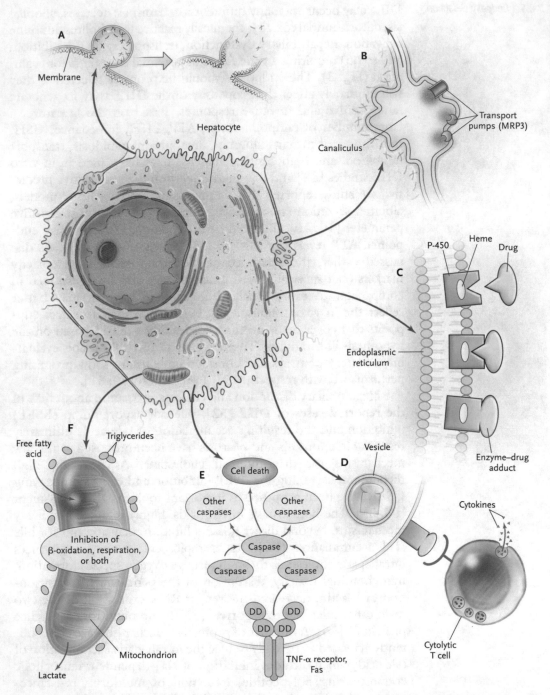

Fig. 3 Example of mechanisms (**A–F**) leading to liver injury. The mode of actions described refer to disruption of intracellular calcium homeostasis, cholestasis, inhibition of transport pumps, metabolite activation through heme-containing cytochrome P-450 system, covalent binding of drug to enzymes, immune response, activation of apoptotic pathways, inhibition of mitochondrial function, and formation of reactive oxygen species. For more details, please refer to [52]. Figure reproduced with permission

acid homeostasis [57–59]. Recent in vitro studies demonstrated that such model provides a more reliable identification of drug candidates with cholestatic DILI risk [60].

2.2.4 *Culture Conditions*   Minor changes in culture conditions may have a significant impact on the assay readout. For instance, the use of serum may allow long-term culturing but could potentially decrease the free drug concentration as a result of increased protein binding. Compounds that have the ability to alter culture medium composition may lead to unexpected effects. For instance, iron is an important factor for cellular proliferation; compounds that have the property to strongly chelate iron may result in iron depletion leading to cell cycle arrest and apoptosis [61]. In addition, most of the standard media used contain high level of glucose. Consequently, the preferred way to synthetize ATP is through the glycolytic path, not mitochondrial ATP synthase. As a consequence, hepatotoxicants acting through mitochondria impairment remain undetected because of this nonphysiological culture conditions [62, 63]. To detect drug-induced mitochondrial effects, cell lines should be cultured in presence of galactose rather than glucose to force them to produce ATP via mitochondrial oxidative phosphorylation rather than glycolysis [63].

2.2.5 *Validation of New Developed In Vitro Models*   In drug screening and discovery paradigm, 70% of the tests settled are cell-based assays [64]. In the last decade, much effort has been produced to generate three dimensional and dynamic, microphysiological models which may represent more physiological conditions principally in terms of structure of the organs and blood flow to test compounds. It is key to demonstrate that the new developed cellular models are carefully validated with superior predictivity compared to traditional cellular models. Interesting relatively new cellular models include for instance organ-on-a-chip [65], coculture model constituted of hepatocytes and mouse fibroblasts [66], human induced pluripotent stem cells [67] and 3D cellular models [68]. Nevertheless, some of the new models also need to tackle a certain number of technical limitations particularly in relation to level of oxygenation as hypo/hyper oxygenation may lead to toxic effects [69]. In addition, most of the recently developed models are not entirely validated yet. One needs to consider a multilevel validation as illustrated in Table 2, covering the biochemical and cellular processes, the technical aspects, the assay predictivity and its translation to the clinical/human situation. Examples are provided with coculture models associated with some relevant literature data. To allow detailed comparison with in vivo data, in vitro models need to be developed using multiple animal species as well as human cells. Although promising, the new 3D models, for the time being, suffer from an incomplete validation when compared to other in vitro models. Nevertheless, one has to

Table 2
Example of validation studies using coculture models

Level of validations	Investigations	Coculture models (HepatoPac® and/or HµREL™ models)
1. Biology	Phase I, II and transporter activities, expression of some functional endpoints (albumin, urea), metabolite formation rates and bile canaliculi formation	Evaluation of metabolite formation rates of 11 diverse phase I and phase II enzyme markers determined in HepatoPac®, HµREL™ and other in vitro models [97]
		Retained activities of several CYP450s, and phase II enzymes for several weeks. Monitoring of canalicular transport and bile canaliculi formation in HepatoPac® [66]
		Metabolite profile, activity and gene expression data measured at three different timepoints in HµREL™ [38]
		Viability, cell polarity (actin microfilaments, bile canaliculi), and functions (albumin, urea, Phase I/II enzymes, transporters) of fresh and cryopreserved rat hepatocytes studied up to 4 weeks in HepatoPac® [84]
		Study of compounds known to produce human-unique metabolites through CYP2C9, UGT1A4, aldehyde oxidase, or N-acetyltransferase that were poorly covered or not detected at all in the selected preclinical species [98]
		Gene expression of CYP 3A4, 1A2, 2C19, UGT; monitoring of bile camiculi and evaluation of metabolite formation rates using HµREL™ [99]
2. Technical validations	Technical validations: reproducibility inter intra laboratories reproducibility of negative and positive compounds over time	Evaluation of reproducibility of the dog coculture model exposed to three pairs of structurally related drugs in HµREL™ [38]
		Reproducibility of HepatoPac® with six prototypical compounds (two separate sets of human cultures): viability, GSH content, albumin and urea [49]

3. Predictivity of the assay	Evaluation of predictivity (sensitivity and specificity) with reference compounds	Human HepatoPac®: Specificity: 90% (9/10), Sensitivity: 65.7% (23/35) [49]; Sensitivity: 100% (19 compounds with severe DILI using two donors, [49]); Specificity: 81.8% (9/11), Sensitivity: 76.3% (29/38) [39]; model using induced pluripotent stem cell-derived human hepatocyte-like cells: Specificity: 100% (10/10), Sensitivity: 65% (24/37) [100] Dog-coculture (HμREL™): Specificity: 72.7 (8/11), Sensitivity: 76.3 (29/38) [38]
	Evaluation of predictivity with proprietary compounds (covering different chemical spaces)	Roche: Use of the well-stirred model with HepatoPac®. For 6/8 compounds, the predicted versus observed fold errors was on average close to 1 using the direct scaling appraoch. For the remaining two compounds, a >6-fold underprediction or overprediction was reported [97] Boehringer Ingelheim Pharmaceuticals: Test of faldaprevir (hepatitis C virus protease inhibitor associated with liver enrichment in rats) in HepatoPac®: liver enrichment values averaged 34-fold and were consistent with rat quantitative whole-body autoradiography (26.8-fold) and in vivo data (42-fold) [101]. In another study, human HepatoPac cultures provided valuable insights into the metabolism and disposition of faldaprevir in humans [102]
	Prediction of specific parameters (e.g., clearance, drug disappearance, and metabolic profiles)	Similar performance between hepatocyte in suspension and HepatoPac® system for medium to high clearance drugs (CYP-mediated) but superior predictivity of coculture model for the majority of the high metabolically stable compounds (within a twofold error) [97] Drug disappearance in dog coculture model (HμREL™) exposed to nine references compounds [38] Evaluation of 17 reference compounds with low to intermediate clearance (<12 mL/min/kg) using HepatoPac® [103] Study of 26 drugs in HepatoPac® that exhibit a wide range of turnover rates in vivo (0.05–19.5 mL/min/kg) [104] 27 compounds of diverse chemical structure and subject to a range of drug biotransformation reactions were assessed for metabolite profiles in the HepatoPac® human model [105] Evaluation of nine compounds with high, medium, and low clearance values in different in vitro systems (e.g., HμREL™) including flow based and static cultures in the presence and absence of nonparenchymal cells [99]
4. In vitro/in vivo translation	Mechanistic investigation	In vitro data using rat and human hepatocyte coculture models (HepatoPac®) correlated well with in vivo findings in rats and human [73] Evaluation of a perfusion-based hepatocyte coculture system (HepatoPac®) as platform to study CYP induction, drug metabolism, and resultant toxicity. Good correlation between rat in vivo acetaminophen toxicity and zonal drug toxicity in rat HepatoPac® model [106]

For more details please refer to the publications reported in the Table

recognize that these new assays are not yet fully optimized. As a final word, understanding the advantages and limitations of each assay is critical for its appropriate applications to study DILI. The selection of a particular model may be guided by the DILI mechanisms to investigate, the duration of exposure (acute versus chronic), and the aptitude to study the toxicity of parent compounds or metabolites [70] as a given model is unlikely to address all the relevant mechanisms leading to DILI.

3 Promises of In Vitro Models

Although still associated with some knowledge gaps and needs for further technological improvement and validation, in vitro DILI assays have been already successfully applied to the design and/or understanding of the potential liability associated with new drug candidates.

3.1 Using In Vitro DILI Assays to Investigate the Translatability to Animal Toxicological Data

Together with the early screening of new drug candidates, DILI approaches can also be used to derisk toxicological findings observed in regulatory animal toxicology studies. In the previously mentioned example, a new antiepileptic drug was found to produce liver toxicity in dog, but not in rodents [22]. The key question was to determine whether the adverse findings in dogs were relevant to human. Detailed in vitro investigations allowed understanding the mechanisms underlying the DILI reactions observed in dogs showing a central role for the bioactivation of the drug into a metabolite with porphyrinogenic potential. The investigations also identified precipitating factors (e.g., concomitant CYP induction, as well as surrogate endpoints such as CYP inactivation). In a second step, in vitro metabolism assays demonstrated that the causative metabolite was neither produced in rodents (in line with the absence of liver toxicity in that species) nor in humans. The predicted low risk of liver toxicity in humans was reinforced by the absence of CYP induction or CYP inactivation in human hepatocytes. In summary, these investigations allowed to derisk the dog findings and to progress the compounds to clinical stages and to drug approval.

3.2 Human In Vitro DILI Assays More Predictive Than Animal In Vivo Toxicological Studies

Fialuridine (FIAU), a second generation nucleoside analog, was developed for the treatment of hepatitis B. Preclinical toxicological studies in multiple species including rodents (mice and rats) as well as dog and monkey failed to detect induced liver injury adverse effects up to 1000-fold the human therapeutic dose [71]. However, during clinical investigations, seven treated patients (receiving 0.10 or 0.25 mg kg/day FIAU for 24 weeks) with chronic hepatitis B experienced life-threatening hepatotoxicity (five fatalities and two subjects survived following liver transplantation) [72]. DILI was associated with progressive lactic acidosis, jaundice, and hepatic synthetic malfunction likely due to mitochondrial damage [72]. In vitro experiments using hepatocyte coculture models indicated that FIAU was more toxic to human hepatocytes (IC_{50}: ~5 µM) as compared to rat hepatocytes (IC_{50} > 100 µM), while its diastereo-isomer was not toxic (IC_{50} > 100 µM) in either species [73]. Maximum human blood concentration (0.64 µM [60]) was in the range of the cytotoxic concentrations observed in human cocul-ture models. This example illustrates that in vivo preclinical toxi-cology studies do not always predict clinical outcome particularly for DILI [74], and well-validated human in vitro models could potentially be a relevant alternative.

3.3 In Vitro and In Vivo Data Integration to Increase Human DILI Prediction

Substantial progress has been made to develop newer approaches better describing the complexity of the DILI reactions. In vitro platforms are evolving toward dynamic 3D cultures, induced pluripotent stem cell cultures, multiorgan models, high content screening with imaging endpoints [75]. While in vivo animal toxicological studies suffer from a number of limitations (e.g., questionable translatability to human, low throughput, ethical pressure), they are still widely used to support regulatory sub-missions. As discussed earlier the in vitro and in vivo endpoints to consider evolved from monoparametric cytotoxicity mea-surements to a panel of more intertwined subtle changes in cell functions and cell-cell interactions. With this respect, omics technologies (e.g., array platform, new mass spectrometry tech-niques) have the potential to identify novel DILI markers that could help to improve prediction of human DILI [76]. Finally, in silico modeling has been proposed as a complementary method to link the structural properties of the drugs to liver toxicity end-points [77]. As the DILI assays are expanding, there is an increas-ing need for quantitative system biology tools to integrate the large dataset generated, comparing them with existing databases, dissecting-out the affected pathways and mathematically linking them to DILI events [78]. As example, the DILIsym® software has been developed in the MATLAB computing platform for this purpose. It integrates in vitro and in vivo data, considers the key liver cell populations (beyond parenchymal cells), the intracellular biochemical pathways, the drug disposition, the physiology of the organism, and the dynamics of the various processes (Fig. 4). For more details, please refer to Chap. 6. The software is aimed at building a mechanistic model to quantitatively predict the DILI reactions in animal species as well as humans and better inform decisions (e.g., experimental design, biomarker selection, and dosing regimen selection). Although in its early days, DILIsym® has been successfully used to understand the life-threatening DILI reported in some patients receiving troglitazone [79]. The model also accounts for the species difference in troglitazone

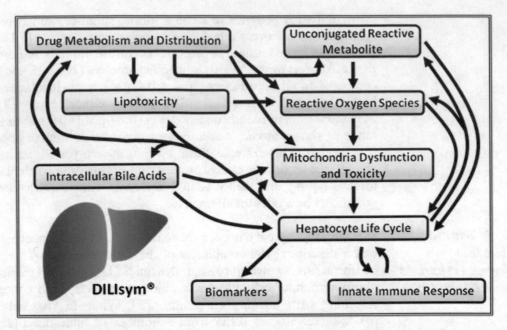

Fig. 4 Overview of multiscale representation of drug-induced liver injury using the DILIsym® modeling software. DILIsym® is designed to increase DILI understanding by providing insight into potential mechanisms leading to toxicity. The system extrapolates in vitro, in vivo data, translates preclinical results to clinical trial protocol design, and takes into account patient variability. Figure reproduced with permission. For more details please refer to http://www.dilisymservices.com/technology.html

hepatotoxicity and the improved safety profile of the analog pioglitazone. The model was built incorporating drug/metabolite disposition, pathways driving bile acid homeostasis, DILI biomarkers, and liver physiology. The previously discussed tolcapone-induced DILI was also successfully described in a DILIsym® model that revealed patient-related risk factors, and provide a rationale for the safer profile of the analog entacapone [17]. DILIsym® was proactively used to derisk the occasional elevated serum aminotransferase levels observed in healthy volunteers during the early clinical development of the Toll-like receptor 5 agonist Entolimod [80]. The number of hepatocytes entering necrosis in the responsive subjects was described in a mechanistic multiscale model, showing that the hepatocyte loss with Entolimod was low enough for not causing a liver dysfunction or a safety issue. In another study, the difference in the liver toxicity between acetaminophen and its isomer 3′-hydroxyacetanilide was investigated using DILIsym® [80]. Four plausible hypotheses were described in mathematical models and challenged against an array of toxicity endpoints collected in treated mice. A difference in reactive metabolite formation was found to be the key driver for the lower toxicity of 3′-hydroxyacetanilide.

4   The Path Forward

As evoked earlier, sustained efforts are needed to refine the DILI assays, focusing on developing more sensitive endpoints and more integrated models, at standardizing the assay conditions, at defining strict hepatotoxicant classification and at building robust knowledge databases.

4.1   Considering the Effects of Pathology Disease States and Genetic Diversity

The limited predictivity of animal studies could be due in part to the use of healthy animals with reduced genetic diversity as well as to species differences in biochemical and physiopathological processes [38]. Other complicating elements include environmental factors, physical activity, genetic predisposition, underlying diseases, age, gender, comedications, nutritional status, and activation of the innate immune system [81]. As for in vivo animal studies, the use of in vitro models could be of reduced value because of the use of healthy cells with reduced genetic diversity. Liang et al. demonstrated that human induced pluripotent stem cells cardiomyocytes (hiPSC-CMs), derived from healthy volunteers and patients suffering from diverse genetic cardiac diseases, were able to detect drug-induced cardiac toxicity more accurately than the classical preclinical assays required by the authorities [82]. These data using iPSCs highlight the usefulness of these models for safety testing at early stages of drug development and illustrate the concept of personalized medicine using in vitro assays, which takes into account genetic diversity among patients to better predict clinical outcomes [13]. In future drug development paradigms, the use of human in vitro models considering the influence of pathological state (and the other factors listed above) will undoubtedly allow to better predict DILI risk in humans. In particular, as already illustrated with the study of Liang and collaborators [82], the use of hiPSC-derived hepatocytes from healthy volunteers and DILI patients, using human dermal fibroblasts, could help the scientific community not only to better predict hepatotoxicity in humans but also to understand the role played by genetic predisposition. Nevertheless, it is clear that a few technical challenges still need to be sorted out particularly the generation of mature and fully functional hiPSC-derived hepatocytes with relevant metabolic capacities [83].

4.2   Developing Longer In Vitro Incubations to Better Mimic the Chronic Exposure Experienced in Clinics

Short-term, single exposure, and high dose approaches have been widely used to perform in vitro toxicology investigations. Such approach may not be suited to detect hepatotoxic drugs in humans occurring after months of exposure [26]. In vitro DILI assay designs have been refined allowing to incubate test compounds for a few weeks with the media renewed during the incubation period [38, 49, 84]. These refinements have been applied to various in vitro models including the hepatocyte cocultures and 3D cultures and were proven to improve the assay performances. For instance, it was reported that higher sensitivity (i.e., more hepatotoxic compounds detected) when compounds are incubated with human hepatocyte cocultures for 9 days (with medium renewed four times) when compared to a 5 day incubation (with two medium renewals) [49].

4.3 Integrating the Inflammatory Components

As previously discussed, DILI can occur via a large number of mechanisms among which inflammation might play a central role. The release of pro-inflammatory factors, reactive oxygen species and chemokines by specialized macrophages (e.g., Kupffer cells) is playing a key role in the cytotoxic response. The inflammatory response is also associated with the down regulation of major liver-specific metabolizing enzymes and transporters, which in turn also influence the DILI reaction (e.g., decreased detoxification by decreased metabolism or decreased active efflux). Unfortunately, most of the commonly used in vitro DILI models are not equipped to incorporate the inflammatory components. The inclusion of immune and liver stromal cell types, such as stellate cells, sinusoidal endothelial cells and Kupffer macrophages is likely to improve DILI predictions. Recently, micropatterned primary hepatocytes and fibroblasts were supplemented with primary Kupffer cells to better model inflammation-mediated hepatotoxicity. The HepatoMune triculture model developed by Ascendance/Hepregen is viable for a minimum 10 days while maintaining both Kupffer and hepatocyte cell functionality. Shaw and collaborators [85] demonstrated that DILI observed with trovafloxacin derived from its interaction with TNF through different mechanisms including the induction of different cytokines and sensitizing effects. Although promising, it still needs to be demonstrated if the newer cellular models are better suited to detect hepatotoxic compounds acting via inflammation using a larger set of validation compounds.

4.4 Developing Noninvasive Label-Free Endpoints

As indicated previously, longer exposure may be needed to better mimic in vivo conditions particular when DILI occur after long term treatment. In this context, noninvasive endpoints (e.g., albumin, and urea secretion) are likely to be preferred over invasive endpoints (e.g., ATP). In addition, if cells are exposed to compounds for a few weeks it would be even recommended to monitor cells continuously using label-free platforms based on acoustic resonance, electrical impedance, microcantilevers, nanowires, and differential calorimetry [86]. The main advantages of label-free detection include the use of a nondestructive approach, kinetic measurement, reduced time for assay optimization, and format available for medium throughput screening. For example, real-time cell analyzer (RTCA), a label-free technology based on impedance measurement, can be used to generate information on cell migration, mortality, proliferation, as well as receptor-mediated signaling including calcium modulators, nuclear receptor, antimitotic and DNA damaging agents [87, 88].

4.5   In Silico Approaches to Better Predict Human DILI

The mass of DILI-related data generated by the pharmaceutical industry is significant, as a result of the lead generation and drug optimization paradigms, as well as the use of high throughput screening technologies. Consequently, it is of primary importance to develop in silico models that will take advantage of these numerous data and the identified quantitative structure–activity relationships (QSAR) to predict DILI from the very early phases (i.e., virtual screening). However, there are a number of hurdles that should be taken into account. Firstly, hepatotoxicity is complex as it may occur through many different mechanisms of actions (Fig. 3) [21] and most of the in silico approaches use a relative small number of compounds with defined DILI potential and known DILI mechanism in man [89]. Secondly, in silico models depend on the quality and predictivity of in vitro models that need to be improved [90]. Thirdly, there is still a lack of sensitive and specific DILI markers leading to a scarcity of reliable hepatotoxic data [77]. A recent review paper provides perspectives on how to improve DILI prediction and focuses on the efforts to provide to develop predictive models from diverse data sources for potential use in detecting human DILI [91]. In silico models rely either on sub-chemical structures or on QSAR models using complex machine-learning methodologies. Recently, Mulliner and coworkers developed a DILI in silico model associated with 68% sensitivity and very high specificity (95%) based on an internal validation set of 221 compounds [90]. Another study has also focused on the development of in silico tools to detect mitochondrial toxicity [92]. Finally, there are an ongoing efforts to make these in silico DILI models more translatable by incorporating genetic and environmental factors [77] and by considering the multiplicity and the dynamics of various processes involved, as illustrated with the DILIsym® software already discussed earlier [93].

4.6   DILI Guidelines from the Scientific Field and Authorities

Many knowledge and technological gaps have been discussed in the present review. Increased scientific knowledge is required to better understand the underlying mechanisms and the specific histopathological and biochemical hallmarks associated with the hepatic lesions. There is also a need for clarity and consensus about the reference drugs to be used for the DILI assay validations, including recommendations around range of concentrations to test as well as cutoff criteria for interpreting the data. Successful examples could be taken from other disciplines. For instance, in the field of in vitro genotoxicity testing, a 2-day workshop was hosted and sponsored by the European Centre for the Validation of Alternative Methods (ECVAM) in 2006 to discuss assay performances and how to better address the high rate of false positive results [94]. The experts recommended to use cell systems that are p53 competent, with relevant metabolic capacities, and to reduce the top concentrations and the maximum level of cytotoxicity to reach [94]. A few years later, Kirkland et al. [95] published recommendations on reference chemicals to use to evaluate the predictivity of new/modified mammalian cell genotoxicity tests, in particular to reduce false positive results.

In order to assess the DILI risks for many new drugs submitted for approval, the FDA is currently using a program called "evaluation of drug-induced serious hepatotoxicity" (eDISH) which takes into account patient characteristics and liver test results [96]. In 2009, an FDA guidance was published to assist the pharmaceutical industry to assess the potential for a drug causing severe liver injury (i.e., irreversible liver failure that is fatal or requires liver transplantation, https://www.fda.gov/downloads/Drugs/GuidanceComplianceRegulatoryInformation/Guidances/UCM174090.pdf). The guidance focuses on clinical data and traditional markers of DILI (e.g., alanine aminotransferase and aspartate aminotransferase); multiple of the upper limits of normal (ULN) is provided for each biomarker to consider the compounds under investigation as hepatotoxic or nonhepatotoxic in human. Nevertheless, the guidance does not address issues of preclinical evaluation for signals of DILI, nor the detection and assessment of DILI after drug approval and marketing. There is a need to develop nonclinical DILI guidance, at early stages of drug development, combining safety, DMPK (including reactive metabolite evaluation) disciplines in order to help the pharmaceutical industry to develop compounds with reduced risk of DILI in animals and human.

References

1. Purcell P, Henry D, Melville G (1991) Diclofenac hepatitis. Gut 32(11):1381–1385
2. Leise MD, Poterucha JJ, Talwalkar JA (2014) Drug-induced liver injury. Mayo Clin Proc 89(1):95–106. https://doi.org/10.1016/j.mayocp.2013.09.016
3. Tilmant K, Gerets HH, De Ron P, Cossu-Leguille C, Vasseur P, Dhalluin S, Atienzar FA (2013) The automated micronucleus assay for early assessment of genotoxicity in drug discovery. Mutat Res 751(1):1–11. https://doi.org/10.1016/j.mrgentox.2012.10.011
4. Yu HB, Zou BY, Wang XL, Li M (2016) Investigation of miscellaneous hERG inhibition in large diverse compound collection using automated patch-clamp assay. Acta Pharmacol Sin 37(1):111–123. https://doi.org/10.1038/aps.2015.143
5. Godoy P, Hewitt NJ, Albrecht U, Andersen ME, Ansari N, Bhattacharya S, Bode JG, Bolleyn J, Borner C, Bottger J, Braeuning A, Budinsky RA, Burkhardt B, Cameron NR, Camussi G, Cho CS, Choi YJ, Craig Rowlands J, Dahmen U, Damm G, Dirsch O, Donato MT, Dong J, Dooley S, Drasdo D, Eakins R, Ferreira KS, Fonsato V, Fraczek J, Gebhardt R, Gibson A, Glanemann M, Goldring CE, Gomez-Lechon MJ, Groothuis GM, Gustavsson L, Guyot C, Hallifax D, Hammad S, Hayward A, Haussinger D, Hellerbrand C, Hewitt P, Hoehme S, Holzhutter HG, Houston JB, Hrach J, Ito K, Jaeschke H, Keitel V, Kelm JM, Kevin Park B, Kordes C,

Kullak-Ublick GA, LeCluyse EL, Lu P, Luebke-Wheeler J, Lutz A, Maltman DJ, Matz-Soja M, McMullen P, Merfort I, Messner S, Meyer C, Mwinyi J, Naisbitt DJ, Nussler AK, Olinga P, Pampaloni F, Pi J, Pluta L, Przyborski SA, Ramachandran A, Rogiers V, Rowe C, Schelcher C, Schmich K, Schwarz M, Singh B, Stelzer EH, Stieger B, Stober R, Sugiyama Y, Tetta C, Thasler WE, Vanhaecke T, Vinken M, Weiss TS, Widera A, Woods CG, JJ X, Yarborough KM, Hengstler JG (2013) Recent advances in 2D and 3D in vitro systems using primary hepatocytes, alternative hepatocyte sources and non-parenchymal liver cells and their use in investigating mechanisms of hepatotoxicity, cell signaling and ADME. Arch Toxicol 87(8):1315–1530. https://doi.org/10.1007/s00204-013-1078-5

6. Garcia-Canaveras JC, Castell JV, Donato MT, Lahoz A (2016) A metabolomics cell-based approach for anticipating and investigating drug-induced liver injury. Sci Rep 6:27239. https://doi.org/10.1038/srep27239

7. Zhang SZ, Lipsky MM, Trump BF, Hsu IC (1990) Neutral red (NR) assay for cell viability and xenobiotic-induced cytotoxicity in primary cultures of human and rat hepatocytes. Cell Biol Toxicol 6(2):219–234

8. Xu JJ, Diaz D, O'Brien PJ (2004) Applications of cytotoxicity assays and pre-lethal mechanistic assays for assessment of human hepatotoxicity potential. Chem Biol Interact 150(1):115–128. https://doi.org/10.1016/j.cbi.2004.09.011

9. Gomez-Lechon MJ, Lahoz A, Gombau L, Castell JV, Donato MT (2010) In vitro evaluation of potential hepatotoxicity induced by drugs. Curr Pharm Des 16(17):1963–1977

10. Kmiec Z (2001) Cooperation of liver cells in health and disease. Adv Anat Embryol Cell Biol 161(III–XIII):1–151

11. Roberts RA, Ganey PE, Ju C, Kamendulis LM, Rusyn I, Klaunig JE (2007) Role of the Kupffer cell in mediating hepatic toxicity and carcinogenesis. Toxicol Sci 96(1):2–15. https://doi.org/10.1093/toxsci/kfl173

12. Bale SS, Vernetti L, Senutovitch N, Jindal R, Hegde M, Gough A, McCarty WJ, Bakan A, Bhushan A, Shun TY, Golberg I, DeBiasio R, Usta OB, Taylor DL, Yarmush ML (2014) In vitro platforms for evaluating liver toxicity. Exp Biol Med (Maywood) 239(9): 1180–1191. https://doi.org/10.1177/1535370214531872

13. Atienzar FA, Blomme EA, Chen M, Hewitt P, Kenna JG, Labbe G, Moulin F, Pognan F, Roth AB, Suter-Dick L, Ukairo O, Weaver RJ, Will Y, Dambach DM (2016) Key chal-lenges and opportunities associated with the use of in vitro models to detect human DILI: integrated risk assessment and mitigation plans. Biomed Res Int 2016:9737920. https://doi.org/10.1155/2016/9737920

14. Borges N (2005) Tolcapone in Parkinson's disease: liver toxicity and clinical efficacy. Expert Opin Drug Saf 4(1):69–73

15. Lees AJ, Ratziu V, Tolosa E, Oertel WH (2007) Safety and tolerability of adjunctive tolcapone treatment in patients with early Parkinson's disease. J Neurol Neurosurg Psychiatry 78(9):944–948. https://doi.org/10.1136/jnnp.2006.097154

16. Haasio K (2010) Toxicology and safety of COMT inhibitors. Int Rev Neurobiol 95:163–189. https://doi.org/10.1016/B978-0-12-381326-8.00007-7

17. Longo DM, Yang Y, Watkins PB, Howell BA, Siler SQ (2016) Elucidating differences in the hepatotoxic potential of tolcapone and enta-capone with DILIsym®, a mechanistic model of drug-induced liver injury. CPT Pharmacometrics Syst Pharmacol 5(1):31–39. https://doi.org/10.1002/psp4.12053

18. Smith KS, Smith PL, Heady TN, Trugman JM, Harman WD, Macdonald TL (2003) In vitro metabolism of tolcapone to reactive intermediates: relevance to tolcapone liver toxicity. Chem Res Toxicol 16(2):123–128. https://doi.org/10.1021/tx025569n

19. Martignoni E, Cosentino M, Ferrari M, Porta G, Mattarucchi E, Marino F, Lecchini S, Nappi G (2005) Two patients with COMT inhibitor-induced hepatic dysfunction and UGT1A9 genetic polymorphism. Neurology 65(11):1820–1822. https://doi.org/10.1212/01.wnl.0000187066.81162.70

20. Rojo A, Fontan A, Mena MA, Herranz A, Casado S, de Yebenes JG (2001) Tolcapone increases plasma catecholamine levels in patients with Parkinson's disease. Parkinsonism Relat Disord 7(2):93–96

21. Dragovic S, Vermeulen NP, Gerets HH, Hewitt PG, Ingelman-Sundberg M, Park BK, Juhila S, Snoeys J, Weaver RJ (2016) Evidence-based selection of training compounds for use in the mechanism-based integrated prediction of drug-induced liver injury in man. Arch Toxicol 90(12):2979–3003. https://doi.org/10.1007/s00204-016-1845-1

22. Nicolas JM, Chanteux H, Mancel V, Dubin GM, Gerin B, Staelens L, Depelchin O, Kervyn S (2014) N-alkylprotoporphyrin formation and hepatic porphyria in dogs after administration of a new antiepileptic drug candidate: mechanism and species specificity. Toxicol Sci 141(2):353–364. https://doi.org/10.1093/toxsci/kfu131

23. Lin YH, Chang HM, Chang FP, Shen CR, Liu CL, Mao WY, Lin CC, Lee HS, Shen CN (2013) Protoporphyrin IX accumulation disrupts mitochondrial dynamics and function in ABCG2-deficient hepatocytes. FEBS Lett 587(19):3202–3209. https://doi.org/10.1016/j.febslet.2013.08.011

24. Hagiwara S, Nishida N, Park AM, Sakurai T, Kawada A, Kudo M (2015) Impaired expression of ATP-binding cassette transporter G2 and liver damage in erythropoietic protoporphyria. Hepatology 62(5):1638–1639. https://doi.org/10.1002/hep.27871

25. Wong SG, Marks GS (1999) Formation of N-alkylprotoporphyrin IX after interaction of porphyrinogenic xenobiotics with rat liver microsomes. J Pharmacol Toxicol Methods 42(3):107–113

26. Guillouzo A, Guguen-Guillouzo C (2008) Evolving concepts in liver tissue modeling and implications for in vitro toxicology. Expert Opin Drug Metab Toxicol 4(10):1279–1294. https://doi.org/10.1517/17425255.4.10.1279

27. Soldatow VY, Lecluyse EL, Griffith LG, Rusyn I (2013) In vitro models for liver toxicity testing. Toxicol Res (Camb) 2(1):23–39. https://doi.org/10.1039/C2TX20051A

28. Gerets HH, Tilmant K, Gerin B, Chanteux H, Depelchin BO, Dhalluin S, Atienzar FA (2012) Characterization of primary human hepatocytes, HepG2 cells, and HepaRG cells at the mRNA level and CYP activity in response to inducers and their predictivity for the detection of human hepatotoxins. Cell Biol Toxicol 28(2):69–87. https://doi.org/10.1007/s10565-011-9208-4

29. Masters JR (2000) Human cancer cell lines: fact and fantasy. Nat Rev Mol Cell Biol 1(3):233–236. https://doi.org/10.1038/35043102

30. Nguyen TV, Ukairo O, Khetani SR, McVay M, Kanchagar C, Seghezzi W, Ayanoglu G, Irrechukwu O, Evers R (2015) Establishment of a hepatocyte-kupffer cell coculture model for assessment of proinflammatory cytokine effects on metabolizing enzymes and drug transporters. Drug Metab Dispos 43(5):774–785. https://doi.org/10.1124/dmd.114.061317

31. Pfeiffer E, Kegel V, Zeilinger K, Hengstler JG, Nussler AK, Seehofer D, Damm G (2015) Featured article: isolation, characterization, and cultivation of human hepatocytes and non-parenchymal liver cells. Exp Biol Med (Maywood) 240(5):645–656. https://doi.org/10.1177/1535370214558025

32. Bale SS, Geerts S, Jindal R, Yarmush ML (2016) Isolation and co-culture of rat parenchymal and non-parenchymal liver cells to evaluate cellular interactions and response. Sci Rep 6:25329. https://doi.org/10.1038/srep25329

33. Hadi M, Westra IM, Starokozhko V, Dragovic S, Merema MT, Groothuis GM (2013) Human precision-cut liver slices as an ex vivo model to study idiosyncratic drug-induced liver injury. Chem Res Toxicol 26(5):710–720. https://doi.org/10.1021/tx300519p

34. Martinez I, Nedredal GI, Oie CI, Warren A, Johansen O, Le Couteur DG, Smedsrod B (2008) The influence of oxygen tension on the structure and function of isolated liver sinusoidal endothelial cells. Comp Hepatol 7:4. https://doi.org/10.1186/1476-5926-7-4

35. Bachmann A, Moll M, Gottwald E, Nies C, Zantl R, Wagner H, Burkhardt B, Sanchez JJ, Ladurner R, Thasler W, Damm G, Nussler AK (2015) 3D cultivation techniques for primary human hepatocytes. Microarrays (Basel) 4(1):64–83. https://doi.org/10.3390/microarrays4010064

36. Hallifax D, Foster JA, Houston JB (2010) Prediction of human metabolic clearance from in vitro systems: retrospective analysis and prospective view. Pharm Res 27(10):2150–2161. https://doi.org/10.1007/s11095-010-0218-3

37. Naritomi Y, Terashita S, Kagayama A, Sugiyama Y (2003) Utility of hepatocytes in predicting drug metabolism: comparison of hepatic intrinsic clearance in rats and humans in vivo and in vitro. Drug Metab Dispos 31(5):580–588

38. Atienzar FA, Novik EI, Gerets HH, Parekh A, Delatour C, Cardenas A, MacDonald J, Yarmush ML, Dhalluin S (2014) Predictivity of dog co-culture model, primary human hepatocytes and HepG2 cells for the detection of hepatotoxic drugs in humans. Toxicol Appl Pharmacol 275(1):44–61. https://doi.org/10.1016/j.taap.2013.11.022

39. Irrechukwu O, Delatour C, Gerets H, Tilmant K, Kanchagar C, Ungell AL, Moore A, Dhalluin S, Khetani SR, Ukairo O, Atienzar FA (2017) Assessment of drug induced liver injury and metabolite formation in engineered human micropatterned hepatocyte cocultures. SOT, Baltimore, MD, 12–16 Mar Poster 136

40. Balls M (1995) In vitro methods in regulatory toxicology: the crucial significance of validation. Arch Toxicol Suppl 17:155–162

41. Chen M, Vijay V, Shi Q, Liu Z, Fang H, Tong W (2011) FDA-approved drug labeling for the study of drug-induced liver injury. Drug Discov Today 16(15-16):697–703. https://doi.org/10.1016/j.drudis.2011.05.007

42. Chen M, Suzuki A, Shraddha T, Yu K, Hu C, Tong W (2016) DILIrank – the largest reference drug list ranked by the risk for developing drug-induced liver injury in humans. Drug Discov Today. https://doi.org/10.1016/j.drudis.2016.1002.1015

43. Thompson D (2016) Lack of adequate classification of hepatotoxicants hinders development of predictive in vitro screening assays. Annual meeting abstract supplement, society of toxicology, abstract no. 2017

44. Di L, Feng B, Goosen TC, Lai Y, Steyn SJ, Varma MV, Obach RS (2013) A perspective on the prediction of drug pharmacokinetics and disposition in drug research and development. Drug Metab Dispos 41(12):1975–1993. https://doi.org/10.1124/dmd.113.054031

45. Keseru GM, Makara GM (2009) The influence of lead discovery strategies on the properties of drug candidates. Nat Rev Drug Discov 8(3):203–212. https://doi.org/10.1038/nrd2796

46. Waring MJ, Arrowsmith J, Leach AR, Leeson PD, Mandrell S, Owen RM, Pairaudeau G, Pennie WD, Pickett SD, Wang J, Wallace O, Weir A (2015) An analysis of the attrition of drug candidates from four major pharmaceutical companies. Nat Rev Drug Discov 14(7):475–486. https://doi.org/10.1038/nrd4609

47. Di L, Obach RS (2015) Addressing the challenges of low clearance in drug research. AAPS J 17(2):352–357. https://doi.org/10.1208/s12248-014-9691-7

48. Xu JJ, Henstock PV, Dunn MC, Smith AR, Chabot JR, de Graaf D (2008) Cellular imaging predictions of clinical drug-induced liver injury. Toxicol Sci 105(1):97–105

49. Khetani SR, Kanchagar C, Ukairo O, Krzyzewski S, Moore A, Shi J, Aoyama S, Aleo M, Will Y (2012) The use of micropatterned co-cultures to detect compounds that cause drug induced liver injury in humans. Toxicol Sci 132(1):107–117

50. Thompson RA, Isin EM, Li Y, Weidolf L, Page K, Wilson I, Swallow S, Middleton B, Stahl S, Foster AJ, Dolgos H, Weaver R, Kenna JG (2012) In vitro approach to assess the potential for risk of idiosyncratic adverse reactions caused by candidate drugs. Chem Res Toxicol 25(8):1616–1632. https://doi.org/10.1021/tx300091x

51. Schadt S, Simon S, Kustermann S, Boess F, McGinnis C, Brink A, Lieven R, Fowler S, Youdim K, Ullah M, Marschmann M, Zihlmann C, Siegrist YM, Cascais AC, Di Lenarda E, Durr E, Schaub N, Ang X, Starke V, Singer T, Alvarez-Sanchez R, Roth AB, Schuler F, Funk C (2015) Minimizing DILI risk in drug discovery – a screening tool for drug candidates. Toxicol In Vitro 30(1 Pt B):429–437. https://doi.org/10.1016/j.tiv.2015.09.019

52. Lee WM (2003) Drug-induced hepatotoxicity. N Engl J Med 349(5):474–485. https://doi.org/10.1056/NEJMra021844

53. Hirano H, Kurata A, Onishi Y, Sakurai A, Saito H, Nakagawa H, Nagakura M, Tarui S, Kanamori Y, Kitajima M, Ishikawa T (2006) High-speed screening and QSAR analysis of human ATP-binding cassette transporter ABCB11 (bile salt export pump) to predict drug-induced intrahepatic cholestasis. Mol Pharm 3(3):252–265. https://doi.org/10.1021/mp060004w

54. Xi L, Yao J, Wei Y, Wu X, Yao X, Liu H, Li S (2017) The in silico identification of human bile salt export pump (ABCB11) inhibitors associated with cholestatic drug-induced liver injury. Mol Biosyst 13(2):417–424. https://doi.org/10.1039/c6mb00744a

55. Rodrigues AD, Lai Y, Cvijic ME, Elkin LL, Zvyaga T, Soars MG (2014) Drug-induced perturbations of the bile acid pool, cholestasis, and hepatotoxicity: mechanistic considerations beyond the direct inhibition of the bile salt export pump. Drug Metab Dispos 42(4):566–574. https://doi.org/10.1124/dmd.113.054205

56. Antherieu S, Bachour-El Azzi P, Dumont J, Abdel-Razzak Z, Guguen-Guillouzo C, Fromenty B, Robin MA, Guillouzo A (2013) Oxidative stress plays a major role in chlorpromazine-induced cholestasis in human HepaRG cells. Hepatology 57(4):1518–1529. https://doi.org/10.1002/hep.26160

57. Swift B, Pfeifer ND, Brouwer KL (2010) Sandwich-cultured hepatocytes: an in vitro model to evaluate hepatobiliary transporter-based drug interactions and hepatotoxicity. Drug Metab Rev 42(3):446–471. https://doi.org/10.3109/03602530903491881

58. De Bruyn T, Chatterjee S, Fattah S, Keemink J, Nicolai J, Augustijns P, Annaert P (2013) Sandwich-cultured hepatocytes: utility for in vitro exploration of hepatobiliary drug disposition and drug-induced hepatotoxicity. Expert Opin Drug Metab Toxicol 9(5):589–616. https://doi.org/10.1517/17425255.2013.773973

59. Germano D, Uteng M, Pognan F, Chibout SD, Wolf A (2014) Determination of liver specific toxicities in rat hepatocytes by high content imaging during 2-week multiple treatment. Toxicol In Vitro. https://doi.org/10.1016/j.tiv.2014.05.009

60. Oorts M, Baze A, Bachellier P, Heyd B, Zacharias T, Annaert P, Richert L (2016)

Drug-induced cholestasis risk assessment in sandwich-cultured human hepatocytes. Toxicol In Vitro 34:179–186. https://doi.org/10.1016/j.tiv.2016.03.008

61. Yu Y, Gutierrez E, Kovacevic Z, Saletta F, Obeidy P, Suryo Rahmanto Y, Richardson DR (2012) Iron chelators for the treatment of cancer. Curr Med Chem 19(17):2689–2702

62. Marroquin LD, Hynes J, Dykens JA, Jamieson JD, Will Y (2007) Circumventing the Crabtree effect: replacing media glucose with galactose increases susceptibility of HepG2 cells to mitochondrial toxicants. Toxicol Sci 97(2):539–547. https://doi.org/10.1093/toxsci/kfm052

63. Gohil VM, Sheth SA, Nilsson R, Wojtovich AP, Lee JH, Perocchi F, Chen W, Clish CB, Ayata C, Brookes PS, Mootha VK (2010) Nutrient-sensitized screening for drugs that shift energy metabolism from mitochondrial respiration to glycolysis. Nat Biotechnol 28(3):249–255. https://doi.org/10.1038/nbt.1606

64. Kirstein SL, Atienza JM, Xi B, Zhu J, Yu N, Wang X, Xu X, Abassi YA (2006) Live cell quality control and utility of real-time cell electronic sensing for assay development. Assay Drug Dev Technol 4(5):545–553. https://doi.org/10.1089/adt.2006.4.545

65. Caplin JD, Granados NG, James MR, Montazami R, Hashemi N (2015) Microfluidic organ-on-a-chip technology for advancement of drug development and toxicology. Adv Healthc Mater 4(10):1426–1450. https://doi.org/10.1002/adhm.201500040

66. Khetani SR, Bhatia SN (2008) Microscale culture of human liver cells for drug development. Nat Biotechnol 26(1):120–126. https://doi.org/10.1038/nbt1361

67. Gomez-Lechon MJ, Tolosa L (2016) Human hepatocytes derived from pluripotent stem cells: a promising cell model for drug hepatotoxicity screening. Arch Toxicol 90(9):2049–2061. https://doi.org/10.1007/s00204-016-1756-1

68. Lauschke VM, Hendriks DF, Bell CC, Andersson TB, Ingelman-Sundberg M (2016) Novel 3D culture systems for studies of human liver function and assessments of the hepatotoxicity of drugs and drug candidates. Chem Res Toxicol 29(12):1936–1955. https://doi.org/10.1021/acs.chemrestox.6b00150

69. Anada T, Fukuda J, Sai Y, Suzuki O (2012) An oxygen-permeable spheroid culture system for the prevention of central hypoxia and necrosis of spheroids. Biomaterials 33(33):8430–8441. https://doi.org/10.1016/j.biomaterials.2012.08.040

70. Mueller SO, Guillouzo A, Hewitt PG, Richert L (2015) Drug biokinetic and toxicity assessments in rat and human primary hepatocytes and HepaRG cells within the EU-funded Predict-IV project. Toxicol In Vitro 30(1 Pt A):19–26. https://doi.org/10.1016/j.tiv.2015.04.014

71. Honkoop P, Scholte HR, de Man RA, Schalm SW (1997) Mitochondrial injury. Lessons from the fialuridine trial. Drug Saf 17(1):1–7

72. McKenzie R, Fried MW, Sallie R, Conjeevaram H, Di Bisceglie AM, Park Y, Savarese B, Kleiner D, Tsokos M, Luciano C et al (1995) Hepatic failure and lactic acidosis due to fialuridine (FIAU), an investigational nucleoside analogue for chronic hepatitis B. N Engl J Med 333(17):1099–1105. https://doi.org/10.1056/NEJM199510263331702

73. Lebron JLL, Kulkarni S. et al (2015) Differential effects of FIAU, FIRU and DDC on functional and DNA content endpoints in HepatoPac andHuh-7 cells in proceedings of the 54th annual meeting of the society of toxicology, abstract 621

74. Olson H, Betton G, Robinson D, Thomas K, Monro A, Kolaja G, Lilly P, Sanders J, Sipes G, Bracken W, Dorato M, Van Deun K, Smith P, Berger B, Heller A (2000) Concordance of the toxicity of pharmaceuticals in humans and in animals. Regul Toxicol Pharmacol 32(1):56–67. https://doi.org/10.1006/rtph.2000.1399

75. Bale SS, Moore L, Yarmush M, Jindal R (2016) Emerging in vitro liver technologies for drug metabolism and inter-organ interactions. Tissue Eng Part B Rev 22(5):383–394. https://doi.org/10.1089/ten.TEB.2016.0031

76. Van den Hof WF, Ruiz-Aracama A, Van Summeren A, Jennen DG, Gaj S, Coonen ML, Brauers K, Wodzig WK, van Delft JH, Kleinjans JC (2015) Integrating multiple omics to unravel mechanisms of cyclosporin A induced hepatotoxicity in vitro. Toxicol In Vitro 29(3):489–501. https://doi.org/10.1016/j.tiv.2014.12.016

77. Przybylak KR, Cronin MT (2012) In silico models for drug-induced liver injury—current status. Expert Opin Drug Metab Toxicol 8(2):201–217. https://doi.org/10.1517/17425255.2012.648613

78. Noor F (2015) A shift in paradigm towards human biology-based systems for cholestatic-liver diseases. J Physiol 593(23):5043–5055. https://doi.org/10.1113/JP271124

79. Yang K, Woodhead JL, Watkins PB, Howell BA, Brouwer KL (2014) Systems pharmacology modeling predicts delayed presentation and species differences in bile acid-mediated troglitazone hepatotoxicity. Clin Pharmacol

Ther   96(5):589–598.   https://doi.org/10.1038/clpt.2014.158

80. Howell BA, Siler SQ, Watkins PB (2014) Use of a systems model of drug-induced liver injury (DILIsym®) to elucidate the mechanistic differences between acetaminophen and its less-toxic isomer, AMAP, in mice. Toxicol Lett   226(2):163–172.   https://doi.org/10.1016/j.toxlet.2014.02.007

81. Ulrich RG (2007) Idiosyncratic toxicity: a convergence of risk factors. Annu Rev Med 58:17–34.   https://doi.org/10.1146/annurev.med.58.072905.160823

82. Liang P, Lan F, Lee AS, Gong T, Sanchez-Freire V, Wang Y, Diecke S, Sallam K, Knowles JW, Wang PJ, Nguyen PK, Bers DM, Robbins RC, JC W (2013) Drug screening using a library of human induced pluripotent stem cell-derived cardiomyocytes reveals disease-specific patterns of cardiotoxicity. Circulation 127(16):1677–1691.   https://doi.org/10.1161/CIRCULATIONAHA.113.001883

83. Lu J, Einhorn S, Venkatarangan L, Miller M, Mann DA, Watkins PB, LeCluyse E (2015) Morphological and functional characterization and assessment of iPSC-derived hepatocytes for in vitro toxicity testing. Toxicol Sci 147(1):39–54.   https://doi.org/10.1093/toxsci/kfv117

84. Ukairo O, Kanchagar C, Moore A, Shi J, Gaffney J, Aoyama S, Rose K, Krzyzewski S, McGeehan J, Andersen ME, Khetani SR, Lecluyse EL (2013) Long-term stability of primary rat hepatocytes in micropatterned cocultures. J Biochem Mol Toxicol 27(3):204–212. https://doi.org/10.1002/jbt.21469

85. Shaw PJ, Beggs KM, Sparkenbaugh EM, Dugan CM, Ganey PE, Roth RA (2009) Trovafloxacin enhances TNF-induced inflammatory stress and cell death signaling and reduces TNF clearance in a murine model of idiosyncratic hepatotoxicity. Toxicol Sci 111(2):288–301. https://doi.org/10.1093/toxsci/kfp163

86. Atienzar FA, Tilmant K, Gerets HH, Toussaint G, Speeckaert S, Hanon E, Depelchin O, Dhalluin S (2011) The use of real-time cell analyzer technology in drug discovery: defining optimal cell culture conditions and assay reproducibility with different adherent cellular models. J Biomol Screen 16(6):575–587. https://doi.org/10.1177/1087057111402825

87. Abassi YA, Xi B, Zhang W, Ye P, Kirstein SL, Gaylord MR, Feinstein SC, Wang X, Xu X (2009) Kinetic cell-based morphological screening: prediction of mechanism of compound action and off-target effects. Chem

Biol   16(7):712–723.   https://doi.org/10.1016/j.chembiol.2009.05.011

88. Atienzar FA, Gerets H, Tilmant K, Toussaint G, Dhalluin S (2013) Evaluation of impedance-based label-free technology as a tool for pharmacology and toxicology investigations. Biosensors 3(1):132–156. https://doi.org/10.3390/bios3010132

89. Funk C, Roth A (2017) Current limitations and future opportunities for prediction of DILI from in vitro. Arch Toxicol 91(1):131–142.   https://doi.org/10.1007/s00204-016-1874-9

90. Mulliner D, Schmidt F, Stolte M, Spirkl HP, Czich A, Amberg A (2016) Computational models for human and animal hepatotoxicity with a global application scope. Chem Res Toxicol   29(5):757–767.   https://doi.org/10.1021/acs.chemrestox.5b00465

91. Chen M, Bisgin H, Tong L, Hong H, Fang H, Borlak J, Tong W (2014) Toward predictive models for drug-induced liver injury in humans: are we there yet? Biomark Med 8(2):201–213.   https://doi.org/10.2217/bmm.13.146

92. Nelms MD, Mellor CL, Cronin MT, Madden JC, Enoch SJ (2015) Development of an in silico profiler for mitochondrial toxicity. Chem Res Toxicol 28(10):1891–1902. https://doi.org/10.1021/acs.chemrestox.5b00275

93. Watkins P (2015) The dili-sim initiative, integrated systems pharmacology modeling to explain and predict drug hepatotoxicity. Clin Ther 37 8S, e170

94. Kirkland D, Pfuhler S, Tweats D, Aardema M, Corvi R, Darroudi F, Elhajouji A, Glatt H, Hastwell P, Hayashi M, Kasper P, Kirchner S, Lynch A, Marzin D, Maurici D, Meunier JR, Muller L, Nohynek G, Parry J, Parry E, Thybaud V, Tice R, van Benthem J, Vanparys P, White P (2007) How to reduce false positive results when undertaking in vitro genotoxicity testing and thus avoid unnecessary follow-up animal tests: report of an ECVAM workshop. Mutat Res 628(1):31–55. https://doi.org/10.1016/j.mrgentox.2006.11.008

95. Kirkland D, Kasper P, Muller L, Corvi R, Speit G (2008) Recommended lists of genotoxic and non-genotoxic chemicals for assessment of the performance of new or improved genotoxicity tests: a follow-up to an ECVAM workshop. Mutat Res 653(1-2):99–108. https://doi.org/10.1016/j.mrgentox.2008.03.008

96. Willyard C (2016) Foretelling toxicity: FDA researchers work to predict risk of liver injury from drugs. Nat Med 22(5):450–451. https://doi.org/10.1038/nm0516-450

97. Kratochwil NA, Meille C, Fowler S, Klammers F, Ekiciler A, Molitor B, Simon S, Walter I, McGinnis C, Walther J, Leonard B, Triyatni M, Javanbakht H, Funk C, Schuler F, Lave T, Parrott NJ (2017) Metabolic profiling of human long-term liver models and hepatic clearance predictions from in vitro data using nonlinear mixed-effects modeling. AAPS J 19(2):534–550. https://doi.org/10.1208/s12248-016-0019-7

98. Ballard TE, Wang S, Cox LM, Moen MA, Krzyzewski S, Ukairo O, Obach RS (2016) Application of a micropatterned cocultured hepatocyte system to predict preclinical and human-specific drug metabolism. Drug Metab Dispos 44(2):172–179. https://doi.org/10.1124/dmd.115.066688

99. Novik E, Maguire TJ, Chao P, Cheng KC, Yarmush ML (2010) A microfluidic hepatic coculture platform for cell-based drug metabolism studies. Biochem Pharmacol 79(7):1036–1044. https://doi.org/10.1016/j.bcp.2009.11.010

100. Ware BR, Berger DR, Khetani SR (2015) Prediction of drug-induced liver injury in micropatterned co-cultures containing iPSC-derived human hepatocytes. Toxicol Sci 145(2):252–262. https://doi.org/10.1093/toxsci/kfv048

101. Ramsden D, Tweedie DJ, St George R, Chen LZ, Li Y (2014) Generating an in vitro-in vivo correlation for metabolism and liver enrichment of a hepatitis C virus drug, faldaprevir, using a rat hepatocyte model (HepatoPac). Drug Metab Dispos 42(3):407–414. https://doi.org/10.1124/dmd.113.055947

102. Ramsden D, Tweedie DJ, Chan TS, Taub ME, Li Y (2014) Bridging in vitro and in vivo metabolism and transport of faldaprevir in human using a novel cocultured human hepatocyte system, HepatoPac. Drug Metab Dispos 42(3):394–406. https://doi.org/10.1124/dmd.113.055897

103. Chan TS, Yu H, Moore A, Khetani SR, Tweedie D (2013) Meeting the challenge of predicting hepatic clearance of compounds slowly metabolized by cytochrome P450 using a novel hepatocyte model, HepatoPac. Drug Metab Dispos 41(12):2024–2032. https://doi.org/10.1124/dmd.113.053397

104. Lin C, Shi J, Moore A, Khetani SR (2016) Prediction of drug clearance and drug-drug interactions in microscale cultures of human hepatocytes. Drug Metab Dispos 44(1):127–136. https://doi.org/10.1124/dmd.115.066027

105. Wang WW, Khetani SR, Krzyzewski S, Duignan DB, Obach RS (2010) Assessment of a micropatterned hepatocyte coculture system to generate major human excretory and circulating drug metabolites. Drug Metab Dispos 38(10):1900–1905. https://doi.org/10.1124/dmd.110.034876

106. Allen JW, Khetani SR, Bhatia SN (2005) In vitro zonation and toxicity in a hepatocyte bioreactor. Toxicol Sci 84(1):110–119. https://doi.org/10.1093/toxsci/kfi052

Chapter 8

Use of Liver-Derived Cell Lines for the Study of Drug-Induced Liver Injury

Zhen Ren, Si Chen, Baitang Ning, and Lei Guo

Abstract

In vitro liver-derived cell lines have been used extensively in toxicity testing and related studies as alternatives and complements to primary hepatocytes. Multiple hepatocyte derived cellular carcinoma cell lines, such as HepG2, Huh7, and HepaRG cells, have been established over the years, and they display distinct characteristics regarding the expression and activity levels of drug-metabolizing enzymes and other hepatocyte-specific factors. These cell lines have become useful tools and the models based on cell lines showed promising value for screening risks of drug-induced liver injury (DILI) in the early stage of drug development, although they have deficiencies in metabolism-related investigations. Engineered cell lines, expressing drug-metabolizing enzymes or other hepatic genes either stably or transiently, have partially overcome these limitations. The liver-derived cell lines have contributed significantly to mechanistic studies of DILI, and various underlying signaling pathways and signatures of DILI have been identified. In this chapter, we first introduce the major hepatic lines (e.g., HepG2, Huh7, HepaRG, Hep3B, BC2, THLE, and Fa2N-4 cells), including their origins, characteristics, advantages, and disadvantages for application in toxicity studies. We next depict the development and application of various engineered cell lines. We then discuss the current understanding of major DILI mechanisms and the endpoints for in vitro tests. The chapter is closed with a brief discussion of the challenges and opportunities in the field.

Key words DILI, In vitro cell lines, HepG2 cells, HepaRG cells, Engineered hepatic cell lines, Mechanistic studies

1 Introduction

At present, both animal models and in vitro models are used in the toxicity testing of drugs. Partly due to the species-differences in hepatic metabolism pathways, animal models display insufficient power in predicting human DILI. In an analysis of 150 drug candidates with human toxicities, the concordance found between hepatotoxicity observed in animal studies and that in subsequent clinical trials was only 50% [1]. Human primary hepatocytes and hepatic cell lines provide options to address this limitation. Primary hepatocytes, either freshly isolated or cryopreserved, are more

Minjun Chen and Yvonne Will (eds.), *Drug-Induced Liver Toxicity*, Methods in Pharmacology and Toxicology,
https://doi.org/10.1007/978-1-4939-7677-5_8, © Springer Science+Business Media, LLC, part of Springer Nature 2018

physiologically relevant and considered as the "golden standard" of in vitro tests, but they lose the metabolic activity quickly with a short life span [2]. In addition, the limited availability of human primary hepatocytes and the considerably interdonor variability in drug-metabolizing enzymes [3, 4] further restrict their use in large-scale toxicity testing. In contrary, hepatocyte-derived cell lines provide a valuable alternative with long life span, ready availability, easy manipulation, and cost efficiency. All these traits enable them to be useful tools in preclinical screening of drug candidates, particularly at an early stage of drug development, and in research on the molecular and cellular mechanisms of DILI.

In this chapter, we first describe the characteristics of commonly used hepatic cell lines, followed by a discussion on the current development of engineered cells. The application of these cell lines in mechanistic studies of DILI in vitro is also presented. Current developments, limitations, and challenges in the field are explored at the end of the chapter. It is important to note the impact of the technical advances, such as 3D cultures and high-content screening, in in vitro studies using cell lines. In addition, immortalized and genetically modified human hepatocytes have overcome some of the traditional obstacles of using primary hepatocytes, and are receiving increasing research interests. Detailed discussions of these new technologies are described in the other chapters.

2   Human Liver-Derived Cell Lines

Over the years, a variety of immortalized liver-derived cell lines, including HepG2, Huh7, HepaRG, Hep3B, THLE, BC2, and Fa2N-4 cells, have been established and are broadly used. These cell lines have different origins and display distinct characteristics regarding the expression and activity of the hepatocyte-specific proteins. The most critical concern for their applications in toxicity study is their low endogenous levels of the drug-metabolizing enzymes and transporters (DMETs). Comprehensive examination of the expression and activity of the DMETs in most human hepatic cell lines, and their comparison with primary human hepatocytes, have been conducted and discussed in multiple publications (Table 1). The profiles of these drug-metabolizing enzymes, together with other characteristics, define the applicability of these cell lines in toxicity testing.

2.1   HepG2 Cells

The HepG2 cell line was established from a liver tumor biopsy obtained from a 15-year-old Caucasian male in the 1970s [5]. It is the most frequently used hepatoma cell line in the testing and research of DILI, especially during the early screening of drug development. HepG2 cells are well-differentiated hepatocarcinoma

Table 1
Relative abundance of selective drug-metabolizing genes expressed in hepatic cell lines compared with that in primary human hepatocytes

UniGene ID	Gene symbol	HepG2	Huh7	Hep3B	THLE2	Human hepatocytes
Phase I enzymes						
Hs.72912	CYP1A1	+	++	+++	−	Ref.
Hs.1361	CYP1A2	−	±	±	−	Ref.
Hs.154654	CYP1B1	−	++	+++	+++	Ref.
Hs.1360	CYP2B6	−	+	+	−	Ref.
Hs.282871	CYP2C8	−	±	−	−	Ref.
Hs.282624	CYP2C9	−	−	−	−	Ref.
Hs.511872	CYP2C18	−	−	−	−	Ref.
Hs.282409	CYP2C19	−	−	−	−	Ref.
Hs.648256	CYP2D6	±	+	+	±	Ref.
Hs.12907	CYP2E1	−	−	−	−	Ref.
Hs.272795	CYP2W1	+++	+++	+++	−	Ref.
Hs.654391	CYP3A4	−	−	−	−	Ref.
Hs.695915	CYP3A5	±	+	±		Ref.
Hs.111944	CYP3A7	++	++	++	−	Ref.
Hs.524528	CYP27B1	++	+++	++	++	Ref.
Phase II enzymes						
Hs.446309	GSTA1	±	+	−	−	Ref.
Hs.102484	GSTA3	−	−	−	−	Ref.
Hs.485557	GSTA4	++	+++	++	+	Ref.
Hs.390667	GSTK1	+	++	++	+	Ref.
Hs.279837	GSTM2	++	+++	++	++	Ref.
Hs.2006	GSTM3	+	++	+++	+	Ref.
Hs.348387	GSTM4	++	++	++	+	Ref.
Hs.523836	GSTP1	−	+++	+	+++	Ref.
Hs.268573	GSTT1	++	−	++	++	Ref.
Hs.389700	MGST1	±	++	±	+	Ref.
Hs.81874	MGST2	++	++	++	+	Ref.
Hs.191734	MGST3	+	++	++	+	Ref.
Hs.591847	NAT1	+	++	++	+	Ref.
Hs.2	NAT2	−	±	±	±	Ref.

(continued)

Table 1
(continued)

UniGene ID	Gene symbol	HepG2	Huh7	Hep3B	THLE2	Human hepatocytes
Hs.368783	NAT5	+	++	++	+	Ref.
Hs.406515	NQO1	+++	+++	+++	+++	Ref.
Hs.567342	SULT1A1	++	++	++	+	Ref.
Hs.460587	SULT1A3	++	++	++	++	Ref.
Hs.129742	SULT1B1	−	±	±	−	Ref.
Hs.479898	SULT1E1	+	++	+++	−	Ref.
Hs.515835	SULT2A1	++	++	−	−	Ref.
Hs.654499	UGT1A1	−	±	±	−	Ref.
Hs.654499	UGT1A3	−	±	±	−	Ref.
Hs.654499	UGT1A4	−	±	−	−	Ref.
Hs.654499	UGT1A6	−	±	±	−	Ref.
Hs.654499	UGT1A9	−	±	±	−	Ref.
Hs.654424	UGT2B7	+	+	++	−	Ref.
Phase III enzymes (transporters)						
Hs.489033	ABCB1	±	++	++	−	Ref.
Hs.658439	ABCB11	−	++	−	−	Ref.
Hs.368243	ABCC2	+	+	±	−	Ref.
Hs.463421	ABCC3	±	+	++	±	Ref.
Hs.508423	ABCC4	++	+++	++	++	Ref.
Hs.480218	ABCG2	+	++	+	±	Ref.
Hs.436893	SLC15A1	−	+	++	−	Ref.
Hs.518089	SLC15A2	++	+++	++	−	Ref.
Hs.117367	SLC22A1	−	±	±	−	Ref.
Hs.436385	SLC22A2	−	++	−	−	Ref.
Hs.485438	SLC22A7	±	++	±	−	Ref.
Hs.502772	SLC22A9	+	+++	++	±	Ref.
Hs.449738	SLCO1B1	±	±	±	−	Ref.
Hs.504966	SLCO1B3	+	++	±	+	Ref.
Hs.7884	SLCO2B1	+	++	±	±	Ref.

For a more comprehensive mRNA profiling of the drug-metabolizing enzymes, please refer to Guo et al. [3]. The table was reproduced with permission

− genes were not detected, ± genes were barely detectable with a relative abundance less than 5% of those in primary hepatocytes, + genes were modestly expressed with relative abundance at 6–29% of those in primary hepatocytes, ++ genes were similarly expressed with relative abundance at 30%–300% of those in primary hepatocytes, +++ genes were overexpressed with a relative high abundance at >300% of those in primary hepatocytes

cells, share the same morphological characteristics of liver parenchymal cells, and have been shown to retain liver-specific functions,
such as plasma protein synthesis and secretion [5, 6]. Seventeen
major plasma proteins have been detected in the HepG2 cells culture medium, including albumin and α-fetoprotein (AFP). In addition, no hepatitis B viral genome was detected in the HepG2 cells.
All these features facilitate the broad application of the cell line in
liver-related toxicological research. A recent analysis has shown
that HepG2 cells are more sensitive to the stress compared with
other liver-derived cell lines [7] and have significantly upregulated
genes with regard to hepatotoxicity processes and cell cycle [8],
which further promotes the usage of this cell line in mechanistic
studies and early stage drug-testing. However, in contrast to primary hepatocytes, HepG2 cells rely more on glycolysis, and less on
oxidative phosphorylation, for ATP production [9]. Therefore,
only by manipulating glucose in the culture environment, the
effect of drugs on mitochondrial function can be assessed using
this particular cell line [10]. The use of HepG2 cells for studying
mitochondrial toxicity is described in other chapter. Moreover,
O'Brien and colleagues suggested that HepG2 cells show high sensitivity and specificity in identifying hepatotoxic drugs [11]. A
study showed that the HepG2 cell line displayed a comparable performance with rat primary hepatocytes when used to evaluated a
limited set of compounds, although the conclusion needs to be
further confirmed [12].

One significant drawback of using HepG2 cells is the low
expression and activity levels of the drug-metabolizing enzymes.
Although some biotransformation activity has been demonstrated
in the cell line [13–15], overall HepG2 cells display limited metabolic capacity. A systematic examination of mRNAs indicated that
out of 84 Phase I genes, only 44 were expressed in HepG2 cells, as
compared with 69 genes expressed in primary human hepatocytes
[3]. Importantly, the mRNA levels of some major CYPs for metabolizing, including CYP1A2, CYP2B6, CYP2C9, CYP2D6, and
CYP3A4, are either undetectable or drastically lower than those in
primary human hepatocytes [3, 16–18]. Phase II enzymes and
transporters are also generally underexpressed in HepG2 cells with
a few notable exceptions, such as NAD(P)H quinone dehydrogenase 1 (NQO1), glutathione S-transferase Mu 3 (GSTM3), and
multidrug resistance protein 1 (MRP1) [3, 19, 20]. Proteomic
analyses and activity assays have further confirmed the drastic
reduction in the biotransformation capacity in HepG2 cells [9, 18,
19, 21, 22].

Notably, the expression levels and activities of the biotransformation enzymes in HepG2 cells were reported with considerable
variations among different labs. Many factors could contribute to
these variations, including but not limited to the culture conditions [23], culture time [24], sources of the cell line [15, 25], and

experiment protocols [26, 27]. Besides, some of the minor Phase I enzymes such as CYP27B1 and CYP2W1 are expressed at significantly elevated levels in this cell line compared with those in human hepatocytes, suggesting HepG2 cells can be a potential surrogate in investigating selective drug-metabolizing enzymes [3]. It was also reported that the activities of some major CYPs can be induced to some extent in HepG2 cells [19, 28].

Collectively, HepG2 cells serve as a useful tool in the initial screening of toxicity in drug testing and in mechanistic studies of DILI. However, due to its lack of metabolic capability, they may not be a suitable model in investigating metabolism-mediated toxicity without additional modification.

2.2 Huh7 Cells

Huh7 cells were established from a liver tumor of a 57-year-old Japanese man in 1982 [29]. As with other well differentiated hepatic carcinoma cells, Huh7 cells have epithelial features, grow in 2D monolayers, and can secret plasma proteins, including albumin. They also have tumor-generating properties when injected into nude mice. Huh7 cells are more commonly used in studies of viral infection, such as hepatitis C [30], but have also been applied to DILI study.

A systematic examination found that Huh7 cells display the DMET expression patterns most similar to the pooled primary human hepatocytes among different hepatic cell lines tested (HepG2, Hep3B, THLE2, SK-Hep-1, and Huh7), though the cell line still suffers the common drawback of a low capacity of the metabolizing enzymes under normal culture conditions [3]. The activity of some CYP enzymes, including CYP3A4, is higher in Huh7 cells than in HepG2 cells [28], and the GST activity reached a level comparable to primary human hepatocytes [22]. Evaluation of Phase III transporters showed that some of the ATP-binding cassette (ABC) transporters are expressed at comparable levels to those in primary hepatocytes, although other transporters are at much lower levels [31]. A direct comparison with HepG2 cells suggests that the mRNA level of P-glycoprotein, organic anionic transporter protein 1B1 (OATP1B1), and organic cationic transporter-1 (OCT1) is higher in Huh7 cells than that in HepG2 cells [32].

An interesting discovery in Huh7 cells is that when they are cultured in the presence of 1% of dimethyl sulfoxide (DMSO), the cell cycle is arrested, and the expression of some hepatocyte-specific genes increase to levels comparable to those in primary human hepatocytes [33]. Under this condition, the mRNA and activity levels of the Phase I and II enzymes are significantly elevated, although still lower than those in primary hepatocytes. The induction of these enzymes and the expression of related orphan nuclear receptors are increased as well [34, 35]. Similarly, confluent Huh7 cells display a higher expression level and activity of CYP3A4, suggesting the change may result from reduced proliferation of the cells [36, 37]. These findings brought new insights to the in vitro drug testing and research, but further evaluation and confirmation are still needed.

2.3 HepaRG Cells

HepaRG cells were established from a liver tumor of a woman in 2002 [38]. In the presence of DMSO, upon reaching confluency the cells undergo extensive differentiation and acquire hepatocyte-like phenotype with elevated expression of liver specific markers, including many drug-metabolizing related enzymes [38–40]. When seeded at high-density, the hepatocyte-like features are retained in the differentiated HepaRG cells. It is worth noting that HepaRG cells have a bipotent progenitor phenotype, and can differentiate into both hepatocyte-like and biliary-like cells. Even the differentiated hepatocyte-like cells retain the ability to transdifferentiate into the other cell type [41, 42].

A systematic analysis of the DMETs found that, at the mRNA level, the differences between HepaRG cells and primary human hepatocytes are comparable to the inter-donor variability in primary human hepatocytes. HepaRG cells show a significant advantage over HepG2 cells in both the basal expression level and the inducibility of major CYP enzymes (e.g., CYP1A2, CYP2B6, and CYP3A4) [19, 43–46]. In particular, CYP3A4 is highly abundant in differentiated HepaRG and can be even higher than the basal expression level observed in primary human hepatocytes, but some other CYPs, such as CYP1A2, CYP2C9, and CYP2D6, are still lower than those in human hepatocytes [21]. For most Phase II enzymes and Phase III transporters, the profile of expression and activity levels in HepaRG cells are comparable to primary hepatocytes, although a few exceptions exist, such as organic anion transporting polypeptide 1B3 (OATP1B3) [21, 44, 46–48]. Major nuclear receptors regulating CYP enzymes, including aryl hydrocarbon receptor (AhR), constitutive androstane receptor (CAR), peroxisome proliferator-activated receptor α (PPAR α), and pregnane X receptor (PXR), are also well maintained in HepaRG cells [44, 46]. Importantly, the expression and activity levels of these proteins are relative stable over a 4-week confluence period, which further suggests that the cell line can be used for long-term or repeated-dose studies [45, 49].

Because of these advantages, the HepaRG cell line has gained great popularity in drug testing and toxicological studies. Its metabolic competence enables the cell line to be used in drug metabolism assessment and in detecting the cytotoxicity of both the parent drugs and reactive metabolites [50]. HepaRG cells have demonstrated promising predictive power as an in vitro model to identify compounds with DILI risks [43, 51–54]. In addition, HepaRG cells have been used as a surrogate to primary hepatocytes in studying CYP enzyme induction particularly for CYP3A4, the major Phase I enzyme that involves in drug metabolism, and drug–drug interactions [55–57]. Similar studies using primary hepatocytes generally show low reproducibility due to inter-donor variability in CYP enzyme profiles. The polarized expression of drug transporters in HepaRG cells closely reassembles that of primary hepatocytes, suggesting the cell line can be used in hepatic uptake and disposition research [21, 48, 58].

Some concerns still remained despite increasing applications of HepaRG cells. One concern is the requirement for DMSO (approximately 2%) in the culture medium to maintain maximal expression level of the CYP enzymes. The presence of DMSO, particularly at a relatively high concentration, could interfere with hepatic functions, induce cytotoxic effects, and in turn affect the results of drug-testing processes. Another concern is the lower expressions of some drug metabolism-related genes in HepaRG cells than those in primary hepatocytes, such as CYP2D6, CAR, and bile salt export pump (BSEP) [44, 46, 59]. In addition, the cell line only represents the hepatic phenotype of a single donor. Other concerns include the long-term differentiation and the demanding culture requirements. Recently a cryopreserved format of differentiated HepaRG cells (cryo-HepaRG) has been developed and could further facilitate the widespread use of this cell model [60].

2.4 Other Liver-Derived Cell Lines

In addition to HepG2, Huh7, and HepaRG cells, a few other liver-derived cell lines exist but have not been extensively applied in drug toxicity testing and related research. Some cell lines are only evaluated in the laboratory that generated them. Furthermore, due to their less frequent use, most of them lack a broad spectrum analysis regarding the overall gene and protein expression in comparison with primary human hepatocytes [3]. Only the expression and activity of a few major Phase I and II enzymes, such as CYP1A2, CYP3A4, glutathione S-transferase (GST), and uridine 5′-diphospho-glucuronosyltransferase (UGT), have been tested in some of these cell lines, whereas little detailed information is available regarding other drug-metabolizing enzymes, transporters, and related nuclear receptors. Further comprehensive evaluations are necessary for their broad use in drug discovery and toxicological research.

2.4.1 Hep3B Cells

Hep3B cells were isolated from liver biopsy specimens of an 8-year-old black man who suffered primary hepatocellular carcinoma. These cells were established alongside with HepG2 cells, and the two cell lines are phenotypically similar in many aspects [5, 6]. One major difference is that Hep3B cells synthesize hepatitis B virus surface antigen, and it can induce tumor when injected into nude mice. Similar to HepG2 cells, Hep3B also displays low expression and activity levels of DMETs [3].

2.4.2 BC2 Cells

BC2 cell line was derived from a human hepatocarcinoma [61]. At confluency, the cells undergo spontaneous differentiation and can stay stable for several weeks in culture [62]. Differentiated BC2 cells express most major CYP450 enzymes (CYP1A1/2, CYP2A6, CYP2B6, CYP2C9, CYP2E1, and CYP3A4) and Phase II enzymes GST and UGT. The activities of the CYP enzymes in this cell line reach a maximum during 21–28 days in culture, although still much lower than those observed in primary human hepatocytes (>100-fold difference). The enzymes also show response to model inducers [62, 63]. BC2 cells maintain some of the drug transporters such as P-glycoprotein (P-Gp) [64].

One of the drawbacks of BC2 cells is the complete absence of CYP2D6 [62]. To date, the use of BC2 cells has been limited to the laboratory that generated them [63, 65]; further evaluation regarding other drug-metabolizing enzymes and related regulatory factors is still required.

2.4.3 THLE Cells

THLE-2 and THLE-3 cells were generated by immortalizing human liver epithelial cells, using a recombinant simian virus 40 large T antigen virus (SV40 T) [66]. One of the advantages of these two cell lines is that they are originated from normal cells instead of cancerous cells. THLE cells have been shown to express most of the Phase II enzymes, but the CYP enzymes are largely undetectable [66]. The use of the THLE cells in DILI studies and toxicological research is not as widespread as other cell lines, and most of the related research work has been done using modified THLE cells that express specific human CYP genes [67–69]. The use of modified THLE cells will be discussed in the next section.

2.4.4 Fa2N-4 Cells

Fa2N-4 cells were established by immortalization of the human hepatocytes from a 12-year-old female donor via SV40 T transfection [70]. Upon application of model inducers, CYP1A2, CYP2C9, CYP3A4, and multidrug resistance protein 1 (MDR1) were induced in Fa2N-4 cells at levels comparable to those in primary hepatocytes. A more systematic examination found that in this cell line, the basal expression level of CYP3A4 is similar to primary hepatocytes, but the levels of CYP1A1, CYP1A2, CYP2D6, and CYP2E1, and Phase II enzyme UGT1A1, UGT1A6, UGT2B15, and UGT2B4 are significantly lower (>10-fold) [71]. The major criticism for Fa2N-4 cell line is the low expression of CAR and some hepatic uptake transporters, which raises concerns regarding its application in drug cytotoxicity testing, particularly as an in vitro model for CYP3A4 induction as initially suggested [71, 72].

3 Engineered Cell Lines

To overcome the deficiencies of low biotransformation capacity of most in vitro cell lines, efforts have been made to express one or more drug-metabolizing enzymes in a specific cell line, either transiently or stably. It should be noted that the proper function of CYP enzymes also depends on electron transport partners, such as the NADPH-cytochrome CYP450 reductase and cytochrome b_5; therefore, the recipient cells should display hepatocyte-comparable level of these proteins. To date, most of these studies have been conducted with HepG2 cells and THLE cells, both of which express sufficient CYP450 reductase and are easy to manipulate.

THLE-based cell lines stably expressing major CYP enzymes including CYP1A2, CYP2A6, CYP2C9, CYP2C19, CYP2D6, and CYP3A4 have been established [67, 68]. These cell lines have been used to explore the role of individual CYP enzyme in drug metabolism, as well as in metabolite-related genotoxicity and cytotoxicity [73, 74]. CYP-expressing THLE cells, particularly THLE-3A4 cells, have also been applied in large scale tests to identify drugs with DILI potential [75–78]. However, a study on the DMETs gene expression profile suggested that the overall gene expression is low in both THLE-null and THLE-CYP cells; many drug-metabolizing enzymes and nuclear receptors are also considerably lower than those in primary human hepatocytes [69]. This finding may hinder the further application of this system.

More approaches have been used in modifying HepG2 cells, and the majority focused on modulating the level of Phase I enzymes. In addition to single cell lines generated in various laboratories, the systematic establishment of 10 (CYP1A1, CYP1A2, CYP2A6, CYP2B6, CYP2C8, CYP2C9, CYP2C19, CYP2D6, CYP2E1, and CYP3A4) or 14 (CYP1A1, CYP1A2, CYP1B1, CYP2A6, CYP2B6, CYP2C8, CYP2C9, CYP2C18, CYP2C19, CYP2D6, CYP2E1, CYP3A4, CYP3A5, and CYP3A7) stable cell lines overexpress individual subtype of CYP450 has been reported [79, 80]. These cell lines have shown promising results in activity assessment using known substrates of CYP enzymes, and have been applied to drug metabolism studies, toxicity tests, and drug–drug interaction studies. These systems have strength in identifying the major CYP enzymes in the metabolism of specific compounds, investigating the role of individual enzymes, and studying the cytotoxicity of related metabolites or drug–drug interactions [81–84].

Besides modulating individual CYP enzymes, approaches that simultaneously change the expression and activity levels of multiple CYP enzymes have also been conducted. One method is the stable transfection of orphan nuclear receptors, such as PXR and CAR, into HepG2 cells. The expression and inducibility of CYP2B6, CYP2C9, and CYP3A4 are elevated simultaneously in these engineered cells [85]. Similar results are achieved by transfection of the hepatocyte nuclear factor 4 (HNF4) gene, which regulates the constitutive expression of many hepatic genes [86]. The development of recombinant adenovirus transfection has enabled simultaneous expression of multiple CYP genes. Currently, HepG2-based cell models transiently coexpressing three (CYP1A2, CYP2C9, and CYP3A4) or five (CYP1A2, CYP2D6, CYP2C9, CYP2C19, and CYP3A4) major CYP enzymes involved in drug metabolism have been reported; the activities of the cotransfected enzymes are comparable to those in primary human hepatocyte, and can be maintained stable for a few days in cultures [87, 88]. Attempts to cotransfect both Phase I and Phase II enzymes into HepG2 cells to achieve a full capacity of biotransformation have also been reported [89, 90].

Engineered cell lines based on HepaRG cells have also been reported, such as the CAR overexpressing line (HepaRG-CAR) generated by lentiviral transduction, which displays increased sensitivity in toxicity analyses and maintains high level of metabolic capacity even in DMSO-free medium [91]. With Huh7 cells, a CYP1A2 expressing cell line has been stably established and applied in a screening of over 200 drugs for metabolism-mediated cytotoxicity [92].

Overall, engineered cells overcome certain limitations of cell lines, and can be used to assess drug metabolism and metabolite-mediated toxicity. Nonetheless, they still have mutagenic potency, and have the limitation of heterogeneous expression of DMETs, which may influence the uptake, processing, and elimination of the drugs. Interpreting results obtained from these cell lines should be cautious, particularly when extrapolating to clinical outcomes.

4   Cell Line Based Mechanistic Studies and Endpoints Measured

An in vitro toxicity screening/testing generally starts with assessment of the cytotoxicity in cell culture upon various exposure, followed by testing for more specific pathways for further information or research interest. It is important to note that most of the tests for toxicity should be done in a concentration- and time-response manner, instead of using one single exposure. This concentration- and time-response approach could reduce false positives, or artificial effects, during toxicity tests. In addition, for certain drugs different pathways could be activated at different concentrations, which could be easily missed in single exposures [93]. Currently there is no clear consensus regarding how to select the concentrations to be tested. A practical approach is to use multiples of the plasma maximum concentration (Cmax) of the investigated drugs. Most hepatotoxic drugs displayed significant cytotoxicity within the 100-fold Cmax range for short-term treatment [94]. Different cut-off thresholds could influence both the sensitivity and the specificity of the predictive power of the in vitro models tested [52]. Another consideration is the drug exposure time. It might be more physiological relevant if a low-concentration, long-term approach could be used, to mimic the characteristic of certain DILI observed in patients [95].

Certain molecular mechanisms of DILI have been identified, and methods have been established for the investigation of each mechanism and their relationship. At present, there is no agreement on the selection and the cut-off thresholds of parameters used to assess DILI risk. However, considering the complicated mechanisms of DILI, a multiparametric approach is suggested because individual endpoints have poor predictive powers [27, 52]. Toxicological studies using in vitro cell lines provide insight into the molecular mechanisms of DILI and identify related characteristics, therefore are critical for drug testing. It should also be emphasized that none of the mechanisms are isolated; extensive crosstalk exists between different mechanisms, and in many cases contribute collectively to the cytotoxicity of a certain compound [96–99].

Interestingly, the cell lines with highly limited metabolizing capacity, such as unmodified THLE and HepG2 cells, were also reported with promising predictive power in identifying DILI risk [11, 27, 78]. Nonetheless, these reports still need further validation because the set of drugs selected, the parameters chosen, and the cut-off values applied can affect the outcomes from these studies.

In the following sections, we will describe the current understanding of the mechanisms of DILI, and the approaches used in each mechanism for in vitro testing and studies. Selective publications on each mechanism, including review articles and original research paper, are listed in Table 2. Most of the studies used HepG2 cells or HepaRG cells, but these studies could be applied to other cell lines including genetically modified cell lines, or primary hepatocytes.

4.1 Necrosis and Apoptosis

DILI can lead to cell death through apoptosis or necrosis. The major differences between the two cell death modes are the integrity of cell plasma membrane, and the activation of caspases. In contrast to apoptosis, necrosis results in cytoplasmic swelling and rupture of the plasma membrane; however, generally it does not trigger caspase-related signaling pathways [100, 101].

Necrosis has been shown to be one of the underlying mechanisms of DILI caused by drugs and chemicals, including acetaminophen [102–104]. Propidium iodide (PI) staining is recognized as a classical method for detecting necrosis in cells. PI binds to DNA but is membrane impermeant; thus, it indicates the leakage of

Table 2
Selected publications on the mechanistic studies of DILI

Mechanisms	Type	Related drugs	References
Necrosis	Review/ methodology		Vanden et al. [100], Krysko et al. [101]
	Examples	Acetaminophen	Hinson et al. [102], Jaeschke et al. [103]
		Benzo[a]pyrene	Lin et al. [104]
Mitochondrial dysfunction	Review/ methodology		Brand et al. [115], Labbe et al. [113]
	Examples	Nefazodone	Dykens et al. [112]
		Sertraline	Li et al. [116]
		Troglitazone	Tirmenstein et al. [117]
ROS generation and oxidative stress	Review/ methodology		Wang et al. [123], Pereira et al. [122], Videla et al. [121]
	Examples	Usnic acid	Chen et al. [124]
		Streptozotocin	Raza et al. [125]
		Acetaminophen	Gao et al. [126]
		Tenofovir, Zidovudine	Nagiah et al. [98]
		Chlorpromazine	Antherieu et al. [127]
ER stress and calcium homeostasis	Review/ methodology		Chen et al. [130], Iurlaro et al. [131], Samali et al. [132], Oslowski et al. [133]
	Examples	Sertraline	Chen et al. [134]
		Nefazodone	Ren et al. [135]
		Usnic acid	Chen et al. [136]
		Acetaminophen	Uzi et al. [137]
		Cryptotanshinone	Park et al. [138]
DNA damage and cell cycle arrest	Review/ methodology		Yusuf et al. [141], Huang et al. [142], Darzynkiewicz et al. [143], Sharma et al. [144]
	Examples	Goldenseal	Chen et al. [145]
		Acetaminophen	Cover et al. [146]
		Trovafloxacin	Poulsen et al. [147]
Autophagy	Review/ methodology		Barth et al. [154], Mizushima et al. [155], Klionsky et al. [156]
	Examples	Usnic acid	Chen et al. [157]

cellular components. Lactate dehydrogenase (LDH) release, which measures the integrity of plasma membrane, is also regarded as a marker for necrosis [101, 105]. It is worthwhile to mention that apoptosis can trigger secondary necrosis as a downstream response; therefore, positive results from these tests can also be observed at a late stage of apoptosis.

Apoptosis leads to characteristic cell morphological changes, such as blebbing and cell shrinkage. Generally, two major pathways are involved in apoptosis: the mitochondria dysfunction-initiated intrinsic pathway and death receptor-mediated extrinsic pathway [106, 107]. The intrinsic apoptotic pathway is characterized by the disturbance of mitochondrial membrane potential and the release of cytochrome c from mitochondria to the cytosol [108]. The Bcl-2 family of proteins directly regulates the leakage of cytochrome c [109]. Once cytochrome c is released, it interacts with apoptotic protease activating factor (APAF-1) and pro-caspase-9 to create a protein complex. It then cleaves the pro-caspase-9 to its active form of caspase-9, which in turn actives the effector caspase-3 [110, 111]. The activation of extrinsic apoptotic pathway is recognized by the induction of active caspase-8, which eventually activates caspase-3 as well. Caspase-3 is the "executioner" of apoptosis resulting in cell death, and it has been used as a hallmark of apoptosis.

4.2 Mitochondrial Dysfunction

Mitochondrial impairment can be induced directly by drugs or triggered by other intracellular stress, and then activate the intrinsic apoptotic pathway. Mitochondrial dysfunction has been shown to underlie the cytotoxicity of an expanding list of drugs such as nefazodone and troglitazone, and is frequently tested during an early stage of drug discovery [112–117].

HepG2 cells have been used extensively in assessing drug-induced mitochondrial dysfunction. In particular, HepG2 cells cultured in medium containing galactose instead of glucose show higher sensitivity to mitotoxicants, an approach generally referred as glucose-galactose assay [10, 118] (Details are described in mitochondrial chapter). Moreover, the mitochondrial membrane potential can be examined by JC-1 staining, which emits distinct fluorescent color according to different membrane potentials [116].

Mitochondrial dysfunction can result in changes of the Bcl-2 family proteins, which trigger either prosurvival or proapoptotic responses, depending on individual drugs. Severe mitochondrial damage causes the release of cytochrome c from mitochondria to the cytosol, which activates downstream caspase-3 and other factors. Measurement of the expression level and subcellular distribution of these hallmark proteins is generally performed to confirm the presence of mitochondrial dysfunction [119, 120]. Due to the pivotal roles of mitochondria in drug testing, a variety of procedures has been developed and will be detailed in the mitochondrial chapter.

4.3 ROS Generation and Oxidative Stress

Reactive oxygen species (ROS) are produced during oxidative phosphorylation chain reactions, and thus are closely related to the function of mitochondria. Stressful cellular conditions, such as triggered by drugs with DILI potential (e.g., tenofovir, usnic acid, and acetaminophen), can disrupt the balance between ROS generation and antioxidants defenses, and result in oxidative stress. A variety of drugs has been shown to induce oxidative stress, as the underlying mechanism of their DILI potential [98, 121–127].

Examination of oxidative stress in vitro generally consists of two parts: the measurement of ROS production, and the measurement of antioxidant defenses. Importantly, the Nrf2 (nuclear factor erythroid 2-related factor 2)–Keap1 (Kelch-like ECH-associated protein 1) signaling pathway plays regulatory role in the antioxidant defensive systems [128, 129]. It is worth noting that both HepaRG and HepG2 cells have been shown to have high expression level of Nrf2 and related proteins, although it is not clear whether this affect the usage of these cell lines in studying cellular response to drug-induced stress [27]. When testing the antioxidant defense, both the levels of reduced glutathione (GSH) and oxidized glutathione (GSSC) are generally measured, and the ratio in between (GSH/GSSC) is calculated. A significant decrease in GSH level and GSH/GSSC ratio indicates depletion of antioxidants in cells. Additional antioxidant enzymes, such as superoxide dismutase (SOD) and catalase (CAT), can also be measured together with Nrf2 regulated genes [122].

The detection of ROS production largely relies on plasma membrane permeable nonfluorescent dyes that become fluorescent after oxidation by ROS, which can then be monitored using fluorescence-based techniques, such as a fluorescence plate reader, confocal microscopy, and flow cytometry. Modulation of ROS by N-acetylcysteine (NAC), which increases intracellular GSH levels, or other ROS scavengers, can further elucidate the role of ROS in drug-induced cytotoxicity [122].

4.4 ER Stress and Calcium Homeostasis

Increasing evidences suggest that endoplasmic reticulum (ER) stress contributes substantially to the pathogenesis of DILI (e.g., usnic acid, nefazodone, and sertraline) [130–138]. ER stress generally triggers upregulation of proteins in the unfolded protein response (UPR) pathway, including CHOP and ATF4, and the phosphorylation of eIF2a. Examination of the expression levels of these proteins is commonly used to detect ER stress. Splicing of the XBP1 mRNA is another marker of UPR activation. The role of ER stress in drug-induced cytotoxicity can be assessed by modulating ER stress with inhibitors, such as 4-phenylbutyric acid (4-PBA) or salubrinal [134, 139]. Chen and colleagues previously reported the establishment and validation of two stable HepG2-derived cell lines that use reporter assays to detect ER stress, which have showed promising results in research on multiple drugs [134, 135].

Ca^{2+} signaling is essential for many cellular functions; ER as an intracellular storage site of Ca^{2+} plays critical roles in the modulation of Ca^{2+}. Disruption of Ca^{2+} homeostasis, therefore, is frequently observed in combination with severe ER stress [99, 130]. An important approach to measure Ca^{2+} signaling is by labeling intracellular calcium with visible light-excitable calcium indicators, such as Fluo-4 and Fluo-3, which display fluorescent increase upon calcium binding [136]. Another approach to assess the involvement of Ca^{2+} signaling is achieved through application of aminoethoxydiphenyl borate (2-APB) to block Ca^{2+} release and examine the effect on cytotoxicity endpoints [136, 140]. One criticism for 2-APB approach is its lack of specificity, a drawback shared by most inhibitors. Therefore, alternative approaches, such as overexpressing or knockdown of critical genes in regulating Ca^{2+} homeostasis, should be used to confirm the findings. These procedures could be readily performed in established cell lines. An example is that knockdown of ORAI1 (calcium release-activated calcium channel protein 1) prevented drug-induced ER stress and decreased cell viability in HepG2 cells [136].

4.5 DNA Damage and Cell Cycle Arrest

In vitro cell lines have long been used for the detection of DNA damage and genotoxicity induced by drugs (e.g., goldenseal, acetaminophen) [141–147]. One important consideration in choosing the cell lines for related studies is the presence of functional p53, a central tumor suppressor that regulate many DNA-damage-response mechanisms [148]. HepG2 and THLE cells have been reported to have functional p53 and carry no p53 mutation [149, 150], suggesting DNA damage response and growth arrest can be activated properly in these cell lines, whereas the HepB3 cell line is p53-deficient and Huh7 cells carry a mutation in p53 [149, 151], limiting their usage in related mechanism studies.

The most critical evidence of DNA strand breaks can be attained through single-cell gel electrophoresis, or commonly known as the "Comet assay," in which the denatured DNA fragments migrate out of the cell and form a "tail" during electrophoresis [141]. Adjusting the conditions of the "Comet assay" permits the detection of both single- and double-strand breaks [141]. Another well-recognized marker for DNA damage is the phosphorylation of histone H2A.X (γH2A.X), which can be detected by immunoblotting or immunostaining assays and shows high sensitivity [144, 152, 153].

In response to DNA damage, cells generally exhibit growth cessation or cell cycle arrest, and promote DNA repair [142]. The cell cycle distribution can be directly analyzed by flow cytometry. Increased expression and activation of the genes involved in cell cycle checkpoints and DNA repair, including phosphorylated Chk1 and Chk2, as well as p53, are frequently observed together with DNA damage [145]. An additional mechanism of DNA damage is the reduction of DNA topoisomerases (Topo I and Topo II), which play a critical role in regulating DNA strand breakage.

Many compounds have been shown to induce DNA damage through inhibition of topoisomerase activities [124, 143].

4.6 Autophagy

Multiple cellular stress, such as ROS, ER stress, and DNA damage, can trigger autophagy, an intrinsic pathway for degradation of dysfunctional cytoplasmic components. Increasing evidence has suggested that autophagy is one of the underlying mechanisms of DILI [154–157], and research has been performed using HepG2 or other hepatic cells. Detection of autophagy generally focuses on the examination of autophagosome formation and autophagic flux. Light chain 3B (LC3B) is considered as a marker of autophagy; it converts from cytosolic LC3B-I to autophagosomal membrane-bound LC3B-II through lipidation, and can be detected by Western blot analysis [156]. In addition, LC3B can be conjugated to green fluorescent protein (GFP) to form a fusion protein (GFP-LC3B), which enables detection of the subcellular location and migration of LC3B by immunohistochemistry or flow cytometry analysis. Also, GFP-LC3B has been applied to monitor the autophagic flux. Degradation of LC3B as an indicator of autophagic flux can be measured by quantification of free GFP fragments [155]. A HepG2-based cell line stably expressing GFP-LC3B has been established to facilitate the easy detection and quantification of autophagy [157]. Another characteristic of autophagic flux is the autophagy-induced degradation of p62, which can be examined using Western blot analysis [155]. Further exploration regarding the role of autophagy in DILI can be achieved by manipulation of autophagy through gene knockdown or application of inhibitors such as 3-methyladenine (3-MA) and chloroquine (CQ), followed by assessment of various cytotoxicity endpoints.

5 Challenges and Opportunities

Over decades, a variety of hepatic cell lines have been established. Their theoretically unlimited availability and friendly culture properties promote the intensive usage in the toxicological studies. Importantly, their applications in the high-content screening have greatly facilitated the early stage testing during drug development. In addition, the easy manipulation of these cell lines allow various genetic modifications and other approaches to be performed, which contributes markedly to our understanding of the mechanisms and related signaling pathways of DILI. Their long-term stability and proliferating properties enable research on the chronic drug effect, repeated dosing, and drug-induced changes in the cell cycle. Cell lines, including HepG2 and HepaRG, have shown promising predictive power in identifying the DILI risks, and advances in mechanistic studies could further facilitate the process.

However, as discussed above, most of the cell lines suffer from low capacity of drug metabolism, insufficient levels of transporters, and incomplete regulatory proteins such as nuclear receptors. Even HepaRG cells, the most promising surrogate of primary human hepatocytes in vitro, display reduced levels of certain CYP enzymes (e.g., CYP2D6) and other factors, such as BSEP [46, 58]. These deficiencies not only limit the basal levels but also the induction of the drug-metabolizing enzymes, and, hence, hinder the precise detection of metabolite-mediated toxic effects. Advance in the engineered cell lines, either expressing individual CYP enzymes, or expressing multiple factors simultaneously, partially overcome some of these drawbacks. These cell lines broaden the application of in vitro cell lines in metabolic studies, and have advantages in exploring the role of particular factors during drug processing. Nevertheless, the engineered cell lines still possess imbalanced metabolizing properties and cannot generate comprehensive drug-metabolism profiles. Therefore, they do not have the full capacity for detecting the DILI potential. Similar limitations are observed in mechanistic studies; some of the DILI mechanisms cannot be investigated using these cell lines due to the low expression of related factors, such as the reduced activity of BSEP. It can also obstruct our understanding of the connections between different mechanisms. This is of particular concern considering that DILI is a complex process resulting from the orchestration of multiple mechanisms. Due to these reasons, currently in vitro cell lines cannot fully replace primary human hepatocytes in toxicological testing and related studies, and caution should be exercised when extrapolating in vitro data to clinical outcomes.

Advances in technology have brought many new opportunities into this field. The establishment of new cell lines by immortalizing hepatocytes or other methods is expected to result in better in vitro models. The recent development of Upcyte® hepatocytes, which renders proliferation properties to human hepatocytes, is one example [158, 159]. Generating hepatocyte-like cells from induced pluripotent stem cells (iPSC) is another trend receiving considerable research interest (See stem cell chapter). Simultaneous transfection of multiple metabolizing enzymes into available cell lines, as discussed above, has introduced new capabilities to these cell models. Furthermore, the development of new platforms, such as 3D cultures, cocultures, liver-on-a-chip, and bioartificial livers, using in vitro cell lines alone or in combination with other cells/materials, has established microenvironments more similar to in vivo conditions [160] (See other chapters in the book). Manipulation of the oxygen levels in cell culture by external chambers or channels has also been shown to improve the metabolic activity of the cell lines [161, 162]. These new developments will make hepatic cell lines better in vitro tools in DILI studies in the future.

Disclaimer

This chapter is not an official guidance or policy statement of the US Food and Drug Administration (FDA). No official support or endorsement by the US FDA is intended or should be inferred.

References

1. Olson H, Betton G, Robinson D, Thomas K, Monro A, Kolaja G, Lilly P, Sanders J, Sipes G, Bracken W, Dorato M, Van Deun K, Smith P, Berger B, Heller A (2000) Concordance of the toxicity of pharmaceuticals in humans and in animals. Regul Toxicol Pharmacol 32(1):56–67. https://doi.org/10.1006/rtph.2000.1399

2. Gebhardt R, Hengstler JG, Muller D, Glockner R, Buenning P, Laube B, Schmelzer E, Ullrich M, Utesch D, Hewitt N, Ringel M, Hilz BR, Bader A, Langsch A, Koose T, Burger HJ, Maas J, Oesch F (2003) New hepatocyte in vitro systems for drug metabolism: metabolic capacity and recommendations for application in basic research and drug development, standard operation procedures. Drug Metab Rev 35(2–3):145–213. https://doi.org/10.1081/DMR-120023684

3. Guo L, Dial S, Shi L, Branham W, Liu J, Fang JL, Green B, Deng H, Kaput J, Ning B (2011) Similarities and differences in the expression of drug-metabolizing enzymes between human hepatic cell lines and primary human hepatocytes. Drug Metab Dispos 39(3):528–538. https://doi.org/10.1124/dmd.110.035873

4. den Braver-Sewradj SP, den Braver MW, Vermeulen NP, Commandeur JN, Richert L, Vos JC (2016) Inter-donor variability of phase I/phase II metabolism of three reference drugs in cryopreserved primary human hepatocytes in suspension and monolayer. Toxicol In Vitro 33:71–79. https://doi.org/10.1016/j.tiv.2016.02.013

5. Aden DP, Fogel A, Plotkin S, Damjanov I, Knowles BB (1979) Controlled synthesis of HBsAg in a differentiated human liver carcinoma-derived cell line. Nature 282(5739):615–616

6. Knowles BB, Howe CC, Aden DP (1980) Human hepatocellular carcinoma cell lines secrete the major plasma proteins and hepatitis B surface antigen. Science 209(4455):497–499

7. Berger E, Vega N, Weiss-Gayet M, Geloen A (2015) Gene network analysis of glucose linked signaling pathways and their role in human hepatocellular carcinoma cell growth and survival in HuH7 and HepG2 cell lines. Biomed Res Int 2015:821761. https://doi.org/10.1155/2015/821761

8. Costantini S, Di Bernardo G, Cammarota M, Castello G, Colonna G (2013) Gene expression signature of human HepG2 cell line. Gene 518(2):335–345. https://doi.org/10.1016/j.gene.2012.12.106

9. Wisniewski JR, Vildhede A, Noren A, Artursson P (2016) In-depth quantitative analysis and comparison of the human hepatocyte and hepatoma cell line HepG2 proteomes. J Proteomics 136:234–247. https://doi.org/10.1016/j.jprot.2016.01.016

10. Marroquin LD, Hynes J, Dykens JA, Jamieson JD, Will Y (2007) Circumventing the Crabtree effect: replacing media glucose with galactose increases susceptibility of HepG2 cells to mitochondrial toxicants. Toxicol Sci 97(2):539–547. https://doi.org/10.1093/toxsci/kfm052

11. O'Brien PJ, Irwin W, Diaz D, Howard-Cofield E, Krejsa CM, Slaughter MR, Gao B, Kaludercic N, Angeline A, Bernardi P, Brain P, Hougham C (2006) High concordance of drug-induced human hepatotoxicity with in vitro cytotoxicity measured in a novel cell-based model using high content screening. Arch Toxicol 80(9):580–604. https://doi.org/10.1007/s00204-006-0091-3

12. Noor F, Niklas J, Muller-Vieira U, Heinzle E (2009) An integrated approach to improved toxicity prediction for the safety assessment during preclinical drug development using Hep G2 cells. Toxicol Appl Pharmacol 237(2):221–231. https://doi.org/10.1016/j.taap.2009.03.011

13. O'Leary KA, Day AJ, Needs PW, Mellon FA, O'Brien NM, Williamson G (2003) Metabolism of quercetin-7- and quercetin-3-glucuronides by an in vitro hepatic model: the role of human beta-glucuronidase, sulfotransferase, catechol-O-methyltransferase and multi-resistant protein 2 (MRP2) in flavonoid metabolism. Biochem Pharmacol 65(3):479–491

14. Sassa S, Sugita O, Galbraith RA, Kappas A (1987) Drug metabolism by the human hepatoma cell, Hep G2. Biochem Biophys Res Commun 143(1):52–57

15. Hewitt NJ, Hewitt P (2004) Phase I and II enzyme characterization of two sources of HepG2 cell lines. Xenobiotica 34(3):243–256. https://doi.org/10.1080/004982503 10001657568

16. Brandon EF, Raap CD, Meijerman I, Beijnen JH, Schellens JH (2003) An update on in vitro test methods in human hepatic drug biotransformation research: pros and cons. Toxicol Appl Pharmacol 189(3):233–246

17. Wilkening S, Stahl F, Bader A (2003) Comparison of primary human hepatocytes and hepatoma cell line Hepg2 with regard to their biotransformation properties. Drug Metab Dispos 31(8):1035–1042. https://doi.org/10.1124/dmd.31.8.1035

18. Westerink WM, Schoonen WG (2007) Cytochrome P450 enzyme levels in HepG2 cells and cryopreserved primary human hepatocytes and their induction in HepG2 cells. Toxicol In Vitro 21(8):1581–1591. https://doi.org/10.1016/j.tiv.2007.05.014

19. Gerets HH, Tilmant K, Gerin B, Chanteux H, Depelchin BO, Dhalluin S, Atienzar FA (2012) Characterization of primary human hepatocytes, HepG2 cells, and HepaRG cells at the mRNA level and CYP activity in response to inducers and their predictivity for the detection of human hepatotoxins. Cell Biol Toxicol 28(2):69–87. https://doi.org/10.1007/s10565-011-9208-4

20. Ahlin G, Hilgendorf C, Karlsson J, Szigyarto CA, Uhlen M, Artursson P (2009) Endogenous gene and protein expression of drug-transporting proteins in cell lines routinely used in drug discovery programs. Drug Metab Dispos 37(12):2275–2283. https://doi.org/10.1124/dmd.109.028654

21. Sison-Young RL, Mitsa D, Jenkins RE, Mottram D, Alexandre E, Richert L, Aerts H, Weaver RJ, Jones RP, Johann E, Hewitt PG, Ingelman-Sundberg M, Goldring CE, Kitteringham NR, Park BK (2015) Comparative proteomic characterization of 4 human liver-derived single cell culture models reveals significant variation in the capacity for drug disposition, bioactivation, and detoxication. Toxicol Sci 147(2):412–424. https://doi.org/10.1093/toxsci/kfv136

22. Lin J, Schyschka L, Muhl-Benninghaus R, Neumann J, Hao L, Nussler N, Dooley S, Liu L, Stockle U, Nussler AK, Ehnert S (2012) Comparative analysis of phase I and II enzyme activities in 5 hepatic cell lines identifies Huh-7 and HCC-T cells with the highest potential to study drug metabolism. Arch Toxicol 86(1):87–95. https://doi.org/10.1007/s00204-011-0733-y

23. Doostdar H, Duthie SJ, Burke MD, Melvin WT, Grant MH (1988) The influence of culture medium composition on drug metabolising enzyme activities of the human liver derived Hep G2 cell line. FEBS Lett 241(1–2):15–18

24. Wilkening S, Bader A (2003) Influence of culture time on the expression of drug-metabolizing enzymes in primary human hepatocytes and hepatoma cell line HepG2. J Biochem Mol Toxicol 17(4):207–213. https://doi.org/10.1002/jbt.10085

25. Majer BJ, Mersch-Sundermann V, Darroudi F, Laky B, de Wit K, Knasmuller S (2004) Genotoxic effects of dietary and lifestyle related carcinogens in human derived hepatoma (HepG2, Hep3B) cells. Mutat Res 551(1–2):153–166. https://doi.org/10.1016/j.mrfmmm.2004.02.022

26. Tyakht AV, Ilina EN, Alexeev DG, Ischenko DS, Gorbachev AY, Semashko TA, Larin AK, Selezneva OV, Kostryukova ES, Karalkin PA, Vakhrushev IV, Kurbatov LK, Archakov AI, Govorun VM (2014) RNA-Seq gene expression profiling of HepG2 cells: the influence of experimental factors and comparison with liver tissue. BMC Genomics 15:1108. https://doi.org/10.1186/1471-2164-15-1108

27. Sison-Young RL, Lauschke VM, Johann E, Alexandre E, Antherieu S, Aerts H, Gerets HH, Labbe G, Hoet D, Dorau M, Schofield CA, Lovatt CA, Holder JC, Stahl SH, Richert L, Kitteringham NR, Jones RP, Elmasry M, Weaver RJ, Hewitt PG, Ingelman-Sundberg M, Goldring CE, Park BK (2016) A multicenter assessment of single-cell models aligned to standard measures of cell health for prediction of acute hepatotoxicity. Arch Toxicol. https://doi.org/10.1007/s00204-016-1745-4

28. Choi JM, Oh SJ, Lee SY, Im JH, Oh JM, Ryu CS, Kwak HC, Lee JY, Kang KW, Kim SK (2015) HepG2 cells as an in vitro model for evaluation of cytochrome P450 induction by xenobiotics. Arch Pharm Res 38(5):691–704. https://doi.org/10.1007/s12272-014-0502-6

29. Nakabayashi H, Taketa K, Miyano K, Yamane T, Sato J (1982) Growth of human hepatoma cells lines with differentiated functions in chemically defined medium. Cancer Res 42(9):3858–3863

30. Fang C, Yi Z, Liu F, Lan S, Wang J, Lu H, Yang P, Yuan Z (2006) Proteome analysis of human liver carcinoma Huh7 cells harboring hepatitis C virus subgenomic replicon. Proteomics 6(2):519–527. https://doi.org/10.1002/pmic.200500233

31. Jouan E, Le Vee M, Denizot C, Parmentier Y, Fardel O (2016) Drug transporter expression and activity in human hepatoma HuH-7 cells. Pharmaceutics 9(1). https://doi.org/10.3390/pharmaceutics9010003

32. Louisa M, Suyatna FD, Wanandi SI, Asih PB, Syafruddin D (2016) Differential expression of several drug transporter genes in HepG2 and Huh-7 cell lines. Adv Biomed Res 5:104. https://doi.org/10.4103/2277-9175.183664

33. Sainz B, Jr., Chisari FV (2006) Production of infectious hepatitis C virus by well-differentiated, growth-arrested human hepatoma-derived cells. J Virol 80 (20):10253–10257. https://doi.org/10.1128/JVI.01059-06.

34. Choi S, Sainz B, Jr., Corcoran P, Uprichard S, Jeong H (2009) Characterization of increased drug metabolism activity in dimethyl sulfoxide (DMSO)-treated Huh7 hepatoma cells. Xenobiotica 39 (3):205–217. doi:https://doi.org/10.1080/00498250802613620.

35. Liu Y, Flynn TJ, Xia M, Wiesenfeld PL, Ferguson MS (2015) Evaluation of CYP3A4 inhibition and hepatotoxicity using DMSO-treated human hepatoma HuH-7 cells. Cell Biol Toxicol 31(4–5):221–230. https://doi.org/10.1007/s10565-015-9306-9

36. Sivertsson L, Ek M, Darnell M, Edebert I, Ingelman-Sundberg M, Neve EP (2010) CYP3A4 catalytic activity is induced in confluent Huh7 hepatoma cells. Drug Metab Dispos 38(6):995–1002. https://doi.org/10.1124/dmd.110.032367

37. Sivertsson L, Edebert I, Palmertz MP, Ingelman-Sundberg M, Neve EP (2013) Induced CYP3A4 expression in confluent Huh7 hepatoma cells as a result of decreased cell proliferation and subsequent pregnane X receptor activation. Mol Pharmacol 83(3):659–670. https://doi.org/10.1124/mol.112.082305

38. Gripon P, Rumin S, Urban S, Le Seyec J, Glaise D, Cannie I, Guyomard C, Lucas J, Trepo C, Guguen-Guillouzo C (2002) Infection of a human hepatoma cell line by hepatitis B virus. Proc Natl Acad Sci U S A 99 (24):15655–15660. https://doi.org/10.1073/pnas.232137699.

39. Hart SN, Li Y, Nakamoto K, Subileau EA, Steen D, Zhong XB (2010) A comparison of whole genome gene expression profiles of HepaRG cells and HepG2 cells to primary human hepatocytes and human liver tissues. Drug Metab Dispos 38(6):988–994. https://doi.org/10.1124/dmd.109.031831

40. Antherieu S, Chesne C, Li R, Guguen-Guillouzo C, Guillouzo A (2012) Optimization of the HepaRG cell model for drug metabolism and toxicity studies. Toxicol In Vitro 26(8):1278–1285. https://doi.org/10.1016/j.tiv.2012.05.008

41. Parent R, Marion MJ, Furio L, Trepo C, Petit MA (2004) Origin and characterization of a human bipotent liver progenitor cell line. Gastroenterology 126(4):1147–1156

42. Cerec V, Glaise D, Garnier D, Morosan S, Turlin B, Drenou B, Gripon P, Kremsdorf D, Guguen-Guillouzo C, Corlu A (2007) Transdifferentiation of hepatocyte-like cells from the human hepatoma HepaRG cell line through bipotent progenitor. Hepatology 45(4):957–967. https://doi.org/10.1002/hep.21536

43. Jennen DG, Magkoufopoulou C, Ketelslegers HB, van Herwijnen MH, Kleinjans JC, van Delft JH (2010) Comparison of HepG2 and HepaRG by whole-genome gene expression analysis for the purpose of chemical hazard identification. Toxicol Sci 115 (1):66–79. doi:https://doi.org/10.1093/toxsci/kfq026.

44. Aninat C, Piton A, Glaise D, Le Charpentier T, Langouet S, Morel F, Guguen-Guillouzo C, Guillouzo A (2006) Expression of cytochromes P450, conjugating enzymes and nuclear receptors in human hepatoma HepaRG cells. Drug Metab Dispos 34 (1):75–83. doi:https://doi.org/10.1124/dmd.105.006759.

45. Josse R, Aninat C, Glaise D, Dumont J, Fessard V, Morel F, Poul JM, Guguen-Guillouzo C, Guillouzo A (2008) Long-term functional stability of human HepaRG hepatocytes and use for chronic toxicity and genotoxicity studies. Drug Metab Dispos 36(6):1111–1118. https://doi.org/10.1124/dmd.107.019901

46. Antherieu S, Chesne C, Li R, Camus S, Lahoz A, Picazo L, Turpeinen M, Tolonen A, Uusitalo J, Guguen-Guillouzo C, Guillouzo A (2010) Stable expression, activity, and inducibility of cytochromes P450 in differentiated HepaRG cells. Drug Metab Dispos 38(3):516–525. https://doi.org/10.1124/dmd.109.030197

47. Le Vee M, Jigorel E, Glaise D, Gripon P, Guguen-Guillouzo C, Fardel O (2006) Functional expression of sinusoidal and canalicular hepatic drug transporters in the differentiated human hepatoma HepaRG cell line. Eur J Pharm Sci 28(1–2):109–117. https://doi.org/10.1016/j.ejps.2006.01.004

48. Le Vee M, Noel G, Jouan E, Stieger B, Fardel O (2013) Polarized expression of drug transporters in differentiated human hepatoma HepaRG cells. Toxicol In Vitro 27(6):1979–1986. https://doi.org/10.1016/j.tiv.2013.07.003

49. Klein S, Mueller D, Schevchenko V, Noor F (2014) Long-term maintenance of HepaRG cells in serum-free conditions and application in a repeated dose study. J Appl Toxicol 34(10):1078–1086. https://doi.org/10.1002/jat.2929

50. Lubberstedt M, Muller-Vieira U, Mayer M, Biemel KM, Knospel F, Knobeloch D, Nussler AK, Gerlach JC, Zeilinger K (2011) HepaRG human hepatic cell line utility as a surrogate for primary human hepatocytes in drug

metabolism assessment in vitro. J Pharmacol Toxicol Methods 63(1):59–68. https://doi.org/10.1016/j.vascn.2010.04.013

51. Lambert CB, Spire C, Renaud MP, Claude N, Guillouzo A (2009) Reproducible chemical-induced changes in gene expression profiles in human hepatoma HepaRG cells under various experimental conditions. Toxicol In Vitro 23(3):466–475. https://doi.org/10.1016/j.tiv.2008.12.018

52. Tomida T, Okamura H, Satsukawa M, Yokoi T, Konno Y (2015) Multiparametric assay using HepaRG cells for predicting drug-induced liver injury. Toxicol Lett 236(1):16–24. https://doi.org/10.1016/j.toxlet.2015.04.014

53. Saito J, Okamura A, Takeuchi K, Hanioka K, Okada A, Ohata T (2016) High content analysis assay for prediction of human hepatotoxicity in HepaRG and HepG2 cells. Toxicol In Vitro 33:63–70. https://doi.org/10.1016/j.tiv.2016.02.019

54. Wu Y, Geng XC, Wang JF, Miao YF, Lu YL, Li B (2016) The HepaRG cell line, a superior in vitro model to L-02, HepG2 and hiHeps cell lines for assessing drug-induced liver injury. Cell Biol Toxicol 32(1):37–59. https://doi.org/10.1007/s10565-016-9316-2

55. Kanebratt KP, Andersson TB (2008) HepaRG cells as an in vitro model for evaluation of cytochrome P450 induction in humans. Drug Metab Dispos 36(1):137–145. https://doi.org/10.1124/dmd.107.017418

56. Kaneko A, Kato M, Sekiguchi N, Mitsui T, Takeda K, Aso Y (2009) In vitro model for the prediction of clinical CYP3A4 induction using HepaRG cells. Xenobiotica 39(11):803–810. https://doi.org/10.3109/00498250903184018

57. Ferreira A, Rodrigues M, Silvestre S, Falcao A, Alves G (2014) HepaRG cell line as an in vitro model for screening drug-drug interactions mediated by metabolic induction: amiodarone used as a model substance. Toxicol In Vitro 28(8):1531–1535. https://doi.org/10.1016/j.tiv.2014.08.004

58. Szabo M, Veres Z, Baranyai Z, Jakab F, Jemnitz K (2013) Comparison of human hepatoma HepaRG cells with human and rat hepatocytes in uptake transport assays in order to predict a risk of drug induced hepatotoxicity. PLoS One 8(3):e59432. https://doi.org/10.1371/journal.pone.0059432

59. Bachour-El Azzi P, Sharanek A, Burban A, Li R, Guevel RL, Abdel-Razzak Z, Stieger B, Guguen-Guillouzo C, Guillouzo A (2015) Comparative localization and functional activity of the main hepatobiliary transporters in HepaRG cells and primary human hepato-cytes. Toxicol Sci 145(1):157–168. https://doi.org/10.1093/toxsci/kfv041

60. Jackson JP, Li L, Chamberlain ED, Wang H, Ferguson SS (2016) Contextualizing hepatocyte functionality of cryopreserved HepaRG cell cultures. Drug Metab Dispos 44(9):1463–1479. https://doi.org/10.1124/dmd.116.069831

61. Glaise D, Ilyin GP, Loyer P, Cariou S, Bilodeau M, Lucas J, Puisieux A, Ozturk M, Guguen-Guillouzo C (1998) Cell cycle gene regulation in reversibly differentiated new human hepatoma cell lines. Cell Growth Differ 9(2):165–176

62. Gomez-Lechon MJ, Donato T, Jover R, Rodriguez C, Ponsoda X, Glaise D, Castell JV, Guguen-Guillouzo C (2001) Expression and induction of a large set of drug-metabolizing enzymes by the highly differentiated human hepatoma cell line BC2. Eur J Biochem 268(5):1448–1459

63. Donato MT, Lahoz A, Castell JV, Gomez-Lechon MJ (2008) Cell lines: a tool for in vitro drug metabolism studies. Curr Drug Metab 9(1):1–11

64. O'Connor JE, Martinez A, Castell JV, Gomez-Lechon MJ (2005) Multiparametric characterization by flow cytometry of flow-sorted subpopulations of a human hepatoma cell line useful for drug research. Cytometry A 63(1):48–58. https://doi.org/10.1002/cyto.a.20095

65. Fabre N, Arrivet E, Trancard J, Bichet N, Roome NO, Prenez A, Vericat JA (2003) A new hepatoma cell line for toxicity testing at repeated doses. Cell Biol Toxicol 19(2):71–82

66. Pfeifer AM, Cole KE, Smoot DT, Weston A, Groopman JD, Shields PG, Vignaud JM, Juillerat M, Lipsky MM, Trump BF et al (1993) Simian virus 40 large tumor antigen-immortalized normal human liver epithelial cells express hepatocyte characteristics and metabolize chemical carcinogens. Proc Natl Acad Sci U S A 90(11):5123–5127

67. Mace K, Aguilar F, Wang JS, Vautravers P, Gomez-Lechon M, Gonzalez FJ, Groopman J, Harris CC, Pfeifer AM (1997) Aflatoxin B1-induced DNA adduct formation and p53 mutations in CYP450-expressing human liver cell lines. Carcinogenesis 18(7):1291–1297

68. Bort R, Castell JV, Pfeifer A, Gomez-Lechon MJ, Mace K (1999) High expression of human CYP2C in immortalized human liver epithelial cells. Toxicol In Vitro 13(4–5):633–638

69. Soltanpour Y, Hilgendorf C, Ahlstrom MM, Foster AJ, Kenna JG, Petersen A, Ungell AL (2012) Characterization of THLE-cytochrome P450 (P450) cell lines: gene expression background and relationship to P450-enzyme activity. Drug Metab

Dispos 40(11):2054–2058. https://doi.org/10.1124/dmd.112.045815

70. Mills JB, Rose KA, Sadagopan N, Sahi J, de Morais SM (2004) Induction of drug metabolism enzymes and MDR1 using a novel human hepatocyte cell line. J Pharmacol Exp Ther 309(1):303–309. https://doi.org/10.1124/jpet.103.061713

71. Hariparsad N, Carr BA, Evers R, Chu X (2008) Comparison of immortalized Fa2N-4 cells and human hepatocytes as in vitro models for cytochrome P450 induction. Drug Metab Dispos 36(6):1046–1055. https://doi.org/10.1124/dmd.108.020677

72. Ripp SL, Mills JB, Fahmi OA, Trevena KA, Liras JL, Maurer TS, de Morais SM (2006) Use of immortalized human hepatocytes to predict the magnitude of clinical drug-drug interactions caused by CYP3A4 induction. Drug Metab Dispos 34(10):1742–1748. https://doi.org/10.1124/dmd.106.010132

73. Molden E, Asberg A, Christensen H (2000) CYP2D6 is involved in O-demethylation of diltiazem. An in vitro study with transfected human liver cells. Eur J Clin Pharmacol 56(8):575–579

74. Barcelo S, Mace K, Pfeifer AM, Chipman JK (1998) Production of DNA strand breaks by N-nitrosodimethylamine and 2-amino-3 methylimidazo[4,5-f]quinoline in THLE cells expressing human CYP isoenzymes and inhibition by sulforaphane. Mutat Res 402(1–2):111–120

75. Dambach DM, Andrews BA, Moulin F (2005) New technologies and screening strategies for hepatotoxicity: use of in vitro models. Toxicol Pathol 33(1):17–26. https://doi.org/10.1080/01926230590522284

76. Vignati L, Turlizzi E, Monaci S, Grossi P, Kanter R, Monshouwer M (2005) An in vitro approach to detect metabolite toxicity due to CYP3A4-dependent bioactivation of xenobiotics. Toxicology 216(2–3):154–167. https://doi.org/10.1016/j.tox.2005.08.003

77. Thompson RA, Isin EM, Li Y, Weidolf L, Page K, Wilson I, Swallow S, Middleton B, Stahl S, Foster AJ, Dolgos H, Weaver R, Kenna JG (2012) In vitro approach to assess the potential for risk of idiosyncratic adverse reactions caused by candidate drugs. Chem Res Toxicol 25(8):1616–1632. https://doi.org/10.1021/tx300091x

78. Gustafsson F, Foster AJ, Sarda S, Bridgland-Taylor MH, Kenna JG (2014) A correlation between the in vitro drug toxicity of drugs to cell lines that express human P450s and their propensity to cause liver injury in humans. Toxicol Sci 137(1):189–211. https://doi.org/10.1093/toxsci/kft223

79. Yoshitomi S, Ikemoto K, Takahashi J, Miki H, Namba M, Asahi S (2001) Establishment of the transformants expressing human cytochrome P450 subtypes in HepG2, and their applications on drug metabolism and toxicology. Toxicol In Vitro 15(3):245–256

80. Xuan J, Chen S, Ning B, Tolleson WH, Guo L (2015) Development of HepG2-derived cells expressing cytochrome P450s for assessing metabolism-associated drug-induced liver toxicity. Chem Biol Interact. https://doi.org/10.1016/j.cbi.2015.10.009

81. Wu Q, Ning B, Xuan J, Ren Z, Guo L, Bryant MS (2016) The role of CYP 3A4 and 1A1 in amiodarone-induced hepatocellular toxicity. Toxicol Lett 253:55–62. https://doi.org/10.1016/j.toxlet.2016.04.016

82. Gomez-Lechon MJ, Tolosa L, Donato MT (2017) Upgrading HepG2 cells with adenoviral vectors that encode drug-metabolizing enzymes: application for drug hepatotoxicity testing. Expert Opin Drug Metab Toxicol 13(2):137–148. https://doi.org/10.1080/17425255.2017.1238459

83. Hashizume T, Yoshitomi S, Asahi S, Uematsu R, Matsumura S, Chatani F, Oda H (2010) Advantages of human hepatocyte-derived transformants expressing a series of human cytochrome p450 isoforms for genotoxicity examination. Toxicol Sci 116(2):488–497. https://doi.org/10.1093/toxsci/kfq154

84. Wu Y, Chitranshi P, Loukotkova L, Gamboa da Costa G, Beland FA, Zhang J, Fang JL (2016) Cytochrome P450-mediated metabolism of triclosan attenuates its cytotoxicity in hepatic cells. Arch Toxicol. https://doi.org/10.1007/s00204-016-1893-6

85. Kublbeck J, Reinisalo M, Mustonen R, Honkakoski P (2010) Up-regulation of CYP expression in hepatoma cells stably transfected by chimeric nuclear receptors. Eur J Pharm Sci 40(4):263–272. https://doi.org/10.1016/j.ejps.2010.03.022

86. Naiki T, Nagaki M, Shidoji Y, Kojima H, Moriwaki H (2004) Functional activity of human hepatoma cells transfected with adenovirus-mediated hepatocyte nuclear factor (HNF)-4 gene. Cell Transplant 13(4):393–403

87. Tolosa L, Donato MT, Perez-Cataldo G, Castell JV, Gomez-Lechon MJ (2012) Upgrading cytochrome P450 activity in HepG2 cells co-transfected with adenoviral vectors for drug hepatotoxicity assessment. Toxicol In Vitro 26(8):1272–1277. https://doi.org/10.1016/j.tiv.2011.11.008

88. Tolosa L, Gomez-Lechon MJ, Perez-Cataldo G, Castell JV, Donato MT (2013) HepG2 cells simultaneously expressing five P450

enzymes for the screening of hepatotoxicity: identification of bioactivable drugs and the potential mechanism of toxicity involved. Arch Toxicol 87(6):1115–1127. https://doi.org/10.1007/s00204-013-1012-x

89. Sawada M, Kamataki T (1998) Genetically engineered cells stably expressing cytochrome P450 and their application to mutagen assays. Mutat Res 411(1):19–43

90. Goldring CE, Kitteringham NR, Jenkins R, Lovatt CA, Randle LE, Abdullah A, Owen A, Liu X, Butler PJ, Williams DP, Metcalfe P, Berens C, Hillen W, Foster B, Simpson A, McLellan L, Park BK (2006) Development of a transactivator in hepatoma cells that allows expression of phase I, phase II, and chemical defense genes. Am J Physiol Cell Physiol 290(1):C104–C115. https://doi.org/10.1152/ajpcell.00133.2005

91. van der Mark VA, Rudi de Waart D, Shevchenko V, Elferink RP, Chamuleau RA, Hoekstra R (2017) Stable overexpression of the constitutive androstane receptor reduces the requirement for culture with dimethyl sulfoxide for high drug metabolism in HepaRG cells. Drug Metab Dispos 45 (1):56–67. doi:https://doi.org/10.1124/dmd.116.072603.

92. Chu CC, Pan KL, Yao HT, Hsu JT (2011) Development of a whole-cell screening system for evaluation of the human CYP1A2-mediated metabolism. Biotechnol Bioeng 108(12):2932–2940. https://doi.org/10.1002/bit.23256

93. Sharanek A, Azzi PB, Al-Attrache H, Savary CC, Humbert L, Rainteau D, Guguen-Guillouzo C, Guillouzo A (2014) Different dose-dependent mechanisms are involved in early cyclosporine a-induced cholestatic effects in hepaRG cells. Toxicol Sci 141(1):244–253. https://doi.org/10.1093/toxsci/kfu122

94. Xu JJ, Henstock PV, Dunn MC, Smith AR, Chabot JR, de Graaf D (2008) Cellular imaging predictions of clinical drug-induced liver injury. Toxicol Sci 105 (1):97–105. doi:https://doi.org/10.1093/toxsci/kfn109.

95. Atienzar FA, Blomme EA, Chen M, Hewitt P, Kenna JG, Labbe G, Moulin F, Pognan F, Roth AB, Suter-Dick L, Ukairo O, Weaver RJ, Will Y, Dambach DM (2016) Key challenges and opportunities associated with the use of in vitro models to detect human DILI: integrated risk assessment and mitigation plans. Biomed Res Int 2016:9737920. https://doi.org/10.1155/2016/9737920

96. Nikoletopoulou V, Markaki M, Palikaras K, Tavernarakis N (2013) Crosstalk between apoptosis, necrosis and autophagy. Biochim Biophys Acta 1833(12):3448–3459. https://doi.org/10.1016/j.bbamcr.2013.06.001

97. Senft D, Ronai ZA (2015) UPR, autophagy, and mitochondria crosstalk underlies the ER stress response. Trends Biochem Sci 40(3):141–148. https://doi.org/10.1016/j.tibs.2015.01.002

98. Nagiah S, Phulukdaree A, Chuturgoon A (2015) Mitochondrial and oxidative stress response in HepG2 cells following acute and prolonged exposure to antiretroviral drugs. J Cell Biochem 116(9):1939–1946. https://doi.org/10.1002/jcb.25149

99. Li X, Wang Y, Wang H, Huang C, Huang Y, Li J (2015) Endoplasmic reticulum stress is the crossroads of autophagy, inflammation, and apoptosis signaling pathways and participates in liver fibrosis. Inflamm Res 64(1):1–7. https://doi.org/10.1007/s00011-014-0772-y

100. Vanden Berghe T, Linkermann A, Jouan-Lanhouet S, Walczak H, Vandenabeele P (2014) Regulated necrosis: the expanding network of non-apoptotic cell death pathways. Nat Rev Mol Cell Biol 15(2):135–147. https://doi.org/10.1038/nrm3737

101. Krysko DV, Vanden Berghe T, D'Herde K, Vandenabeele P (2008) Apoptosis and necrosis: detection, discrimination and phagocytosis. Methods 44(3):205–221. https://doi.org/10.1016/j.ymeth.2007.12.001

102. Hinson JA, Roberts DW, James LP (2010) Mechanisms of acetaminophen-induced liver necrosis. Handb Exp Pharmacol 196:369–405. https://doi.org/10.1007/978-3-642-00663-0_12

103. Jaeschke H, McGill MR, Ramachandran A (2012) Oxidant stress, mitochondria, and cell death mechanisms in drug-induced liver injury: lessons learned from acetaminophen hepatotoxicity. Drug Metab Rev 44(1):88–106. https://doi.org/10.3109/03602532.2011.602688

104. Lin T, Yang MS (2008) Benzo[a]pyrene-induced necrosis in the HepG(2) cells via PARP-1 activation and NAD(+) depletion. Toxicology 245(1–2):147–153. https://doi.org/10.1016/j.tox.2007.12.020

105. Golstein P, Kroemer G (2007) Cell death by necrosis: towards a molecular definition. Trends Biochem Sci 32(1):37–43. https://doi.org/10.1016/j.tibs.2006.11.001

106. Danial NN, Korsmeyer SJ (2004) Cell death: critical control points. Cell 116(2):205–219

107. Taylor RC, Cullen SP, Martin SJ (2008) Apoptosis: controlled demolition at the cellular level. Nat Rev Mol Cell Biol 9(3):231–241. https://doi.org/10.1038/nrm2312

108. Kroemer G, Galluzzi L, Brenner C (2007) Mitochondrial membrane permeabilization in cell death. Physiol Rev 87(1):99–163. https://doi.org/10.1152/physrev.00013.2006

109. Chao DT, Korsmeyer SJ (1998) BCL-2 family: regulators of cell death. Annu Rev Immunol 16:395–419. https://doi.org/10.1146/annurev.immunol.16.1.395

110. Zimmermann KC, Green DR (2001) How cells die: apoptosis pathways. J Allergy Clin Immunol 108(4 Suppl):S99–103

111. Degterev A, Boyce M, Yuan J (2003) A decade of caspases. Oncogene 22(53):8543–8567. https://doi.org/10.1038/sj.onc.1207107

112. Dykens JA, Jamieson JD, Marroquin LD, Nadanaciva S, Xu JJ, Dunn MC, Smith AR, Will Y (2008) In vitro assessment of mitochondrial dysfunction and cytotoxicity of nefazodone, trazodone, and buspirone. Toxicol Sci 103(2):335–345. https://doi.org/10.1093/toxsci/kfn056

113. Labbe G, Pessayre D, Fromenty B (2008) Drug-induced liver injury through mitochondrial dysfunction: mechanisms and detection during preclinical safety studies. Fundam Clin Pharmacol 22(4):335–353. https://doi.org/10.1111/j.1472-8206.2008.00608.x

114. Will Y, Dykens J (2014) Mitochondrial toxicity assessment in industry—a decade of technology development and insight. Expert Opin Drug Metab Toxicol 10(8):1061–1067. https://doi.org/10.1517/17425255.2014.939628

115. Brand MD, Nicholls DG (2011) Assessing mitochondrial dysfunction in cells. Biochem J 435(2):297–312. https://doi.org/10.1042/BJ20110162

116. Li Y, Couch L, Higuchi M, Fang JL, Guo L (2012) Mitochondrial dysfunction induced by sertraline, an antidepressant agent. Toxicol Sci 127(2):582–591. https://doi.org/10.1093/toxsci/kfs100

117. Tirmenstein MA, Hu CX, Gales TL, Maleeff BE, Narayanan PK, Kurali E, Hart TK, Thomas HC, Schwartz LW (2002) Effects of troglitazone on HepG2 viability and mitochondrial function. Toxicol Sci 69(1):131–138

118. Kamalian L, Chadwick AE, Bayliss M, French NS, Monshouwer M, Snoeys J, Park BK (2015) The utility of HepG2 cells to identify direct mitochondrial dysfunction in the absence of cell death. Toxicol In Vitro 29(4):732–740. https://doi.org/10.1016/j.tiv.2015.02.011

119. Wang C, Youle RJ (2009) The role of mitochondria in apoptosis. Annu Rev Genet 43:95–118. https://doi.org/10.1146/annurev-genet-102108-134850

120. Hatok J, Racay P (2016) Bcl-2 family proteins: master regulators of cell survival. Biomol Concepts 7(4):259–270. https://doi.org/10.1515/bmc-2016-0015

121. Videla LA (2009) Oxidative stress signaling underlying liver disease and hepatoprotective mechanisms. World J Hepatol 1(1):72–78. https://doi.org/10.4254/wjh.v1.i1.72

122. Pereira CV, Nadanaciva S, Oliveira PJ, Will Y (2012) The contribution of oxidative stress to drug-induced organ toxicity and its detection in vitro and in vivo. Expert Opin Drug Metab Toxicol 8(2):219–237. https://doi.org/10.1517/17425255.2012.645536

123. Wang X, Fang H, Huang Z, Shang W, Hou T, Cheng A, Cheng H (2013) Imaging ROS signaling in cells and animals. J Mol Med (Berl) 91(8):917–927. https://doi.org/10.1007/s00109-013-1067-4

124. Chen S, Zhang Z, Qing T, Ren Z, Yu D, Couch L, Ning B, Mei N, Shi L, Tolleson WH, Guo L (2016) Activation of the Nrf2 signaling pathway in usnic acid-induced toxicity in HepG2 cells. Arch Toxicol. https://doi.org/10.1007/s00204-016-1775-y

125. Raza H, John A (2012) Streptozotocin-induced cytotoxicity, oxidative stress and mitochondrial dysfunction in human hepatoma HepG2 cells. Int J Mol Sci 13(5):5751–5767. https://doi.org/10.3390/ijms13055751

126. Gao Y, Chu S, Zhang Z, Zuo W, Xia C, Ai Q, Luo P, Cao P, Chen N (2016) Early stage functions of mitochondrial autophagy and oxidative stress in acetaminophen-induced liver injury. J Cell Biochem. https://doi.org/10.1002/jcb.25788

127. Anthérieu S, Bachour-El Azzi P, Dumont J, Abdel-Razzak Z, Guguen-Guillouzo C, Fromenty B, Robin MA, Guillouzo A (2013) Oxidative stress plays a major role in chlorpromazine-induced cholestasis in human HepaRG cells. Hepatology 57(4):1518–1529. https://doi.org/10.1002/hep.26160

128. Nguyen T, Nioi P, Pickett CB (2009) The Nrf2-antioxidant response element signaling pathway and its activation by oxidative stress. J Biol Chem 284(20):13291–13295. https://doi.org/10.1074/jbc.R900010200

129. Kobayashi A, Kang MI, Okawa H, Ohtsuji M, Zenke Y, Chiba T, Igarashi K, Yamamoto M (2004) Oxidative stress sensor Keap1 functions as an adaptor for Cul3-based E3 ligase to regulate proteasomal degradation of Nrf2. Mol Cell Biol 24(16):7130–7139. https://doi.org/10.1128/MCB.24.16.7130-7139.2004

130. Chen S, Melchior WB, Jr., Guo L (2014) Endoplasmic reticulum stress in drug- and environmental toxicant-induced liver toxicity. J Environ Sci Health C Environ Carcinog Ecotoxicol Rev 32 (1):83–104. doi:https://doi.org/10.1080/10590501.2014.881648.

131. Iurlaro R, Munoz-Pinedo C (2016) Cell death induced by endoplasmic reticulum stress. FEBS J 283(14):2640–2652. https://doi.org/10.1111/febs.13598

132. Samali A, Fitzgerald U, Deegan S, Gupta S (2010) Methods for monitoring endoplasmic reticulum stress and the unfolded protein response. Int J Cell Biol 2010:830307. https://doi.org/10.1155/2010/830307

133. Oslowski C, Urano F (2011) Measuring ER stress and the unfolded protein response using mammalian tissue culture system. Methods Enzymol 490:71–92. https://doi.org/10.1016/B978-0-12-385114-7.00004-0

134. Chen S, Xuan J, Couch L, Iyer A, Wu Y, Li QZ, Guo L (2014) Sertraline induces endoplasmic reticulum stress in hepatic cells. Toxicology 322:78–88. https://doi.org/10.1016/j.tox.2014.05.007

135. Ren Z, Chen S, Zhang J, Doshi U, Li AP, Guo L (2016) Endoplasmic reticulum stress induction and ERK1/2 activation contribute to nefazodone-induced toxicity in hepatic cells. Toxicol Sci. https://doi.org/10.1093/toxsci/kfw173

136. Chen S, Zhang Z, Wu Y, Shi Q, Yan H, Mei N, Tolleson WH, Guo L (2015) Endoplasmic reticulum stress and store-operated calcium entry contribute to usnic acid-induced toxicity in hepatic cells. Toxicol Sci 146(1):116–126. https://doi.org/10.1093/toxsci/kfv075

137. Uzi D, Barda L, Scaiewicz V, Mills M, Mueller T, Gonzalez-Rodriguez A, Valverde AM, Iwawaki T, Nahmias Y, Xavier R, Chung RT, Tirosh B, Shibolet O (2013) CHOP is a critical regulator of acetaminophen-induced hepatotoxicity. J Hepatol 59(3):495–503. https://doi.org/10.1016/j.jhep.2013.04.024

138. Park IJ, Kim MJ, Park OJ, Choe W, Kang I, Kim SS, Ha J (2012) Cryptotanshinone induces ER stress-mediated apoptosis in HepG2 and MCF7 cells. Apoptosis 17(3):248–257. https://doi.org/10.1007/s10495-011-0680-3

139. Boyce M, Bryant KF, Jousse C, Long K, Harding HP, Scheuner D, Kaufman RJ, Ma D, Coen DM, Ron D, Yuan J (2005) A selective inhibitor of eIF2alpha dephosphorylation protects cells from ER stress. Science 307(5711):935–939. https://doi.org/10.1126/science.1101902

140. Maiuri AR, Breier AB, Turkus JD, Ganey PE, Roth RA (2016) Calcium contributes to the cytotoxic interaction between diclofenac and cytokines. Toxicol Sci 149(2):372–384. https://doi.org/10.1093/toxsci/kfv249

141. Yusuf AT, Vian L, Sabatier R, Cano JP (2000) In vitro detection of indirect-acting genotoxins in the comet assay using Hep G2 cells. Mutat Res 468(2):227–234

142. Huang X, Halicka HD, Traganos F, Tanaka T, Kurose A, Darzynkiewicz Z (2005) Cytometric assessment of DNA damage in relation to cell cycle phase and apoptosis. Cell Prolif 38(4):223–243. https://doi.org/10.1111/j.1365-2184.2005.00344.x

143. Darzynkiewicz Z, Halicka DH, Tanaka T (2009) Cytometric assessment of DNA damage induced by DNA topoisomerase inhibitors. Methods Mol Biol 582:145–153. https://doi.org/10.1007/978-1-60761-340-4_12

144. Sharma A, Singh K, Almasan A (2012) Histone H2AX phosphorylation: a marker for DNA damage. Methods Mol Biol 920:613–626. https://doi.org/10.1007/978-1-61779-998-3_40

145. Chen S, Wan L, Couch L, Lin H, Li Y, Dobrovolsky VN, Mei N, Guo L (2013) Mechanism study of goldenseal-associated DNA damage. Toxicol Lett 221(1):64–72. https://doi.org/10.1016/j.toxlet.2013.05.641

146. Cover C, Mansouri A, Knight TR, Bajt ML, Lemasters JJ, Pessayre D, Jaeschke H (2005) Peroxynitrite-induced mitochondrial and endonuclease-mediated nuclear DNA damage in acetaminophen hepatotoxicity. J Pharmacol Exp Ther 315(2):879–887. https://doi.org/10.1124/jpet.105.088898

147. Poulsen KL, Olivero-Verbel J, Beggs KM, Ganey PE, Roth RA (2014) Trovafloxacin enhances lipopolysaccharide-stimulated production of tumor necrosis factor-alpha by macrophages: role of the DNA damage response. J Pharmacol Exp Ther 350(1):164–170. https://doi.org/10.1124/jpet.114.214189

148. Williams AB, Schumacher B (2016) p53 in the DNA-damage-repair process. Cold Spring Harb Perspect Med 6(5). https://doi.org/10.1101/cshperspect.a026070

149. Hsu IC, Tokiwa T, Bennett W, Metcalf RA, Welsh JA, Sun T, Harris CC (1993) p53 gene mutation and integrated hepatitis B viral DNA sequences in human liver cancer cell lines. Carcinogenesis 14(5):987–992

150. Lehman TA, Modali R, Boukamp P, Stanek J, Bennett WP, Welsh JA, Metcalf RA, Stampfer MR, Fusenig N, Rogan EM et al (1993) p53 mutations in human immortalized epithelial cell lines. Carcinogenesis 14(5):833–839

151. Stahler F, Roemer K (1998) Mutant p53 can provoke apoptosis in p53-deficient Hep3B cells with delayed kinetics relative to wild-type p53. Oncogene 17(26):3507–3512. https://doi.org/10.1038/sj.onc.1202245

152. Huang X, Darzynkiewicz Z (2006) Cytometric assessment of histone H2AX phosphorylation: a reporter of DNA damage. Methods Mol Biol 314:73–80. https://doi.org/10.1385/1-59259-973-7:073

153. Tanaka T, Halicka D, Traganos F, Darzynkiewicz Z (2009) Cytometric analysis of DNA damage: phosphoryla-

tion of histone H2AX as a marker of DNA double-strand breaks (DSBs). Methods Mol Biol 523:161–168. https://doi.org/10.1007/978-1-59745-190-1_11

154. Barth S, Glick D, Macleod KF (2010) Autophagy: assays and artifacts. J Pathol 221(2):117–124. https://doi.org/10.1002/path.2694

155. Mizushima N, Yoshimori T, Levine B (2010) Methods in mammalian autophagy research. Cell 140(3):313–326. https://doi.org/10.1016/j.cell.2010.01.028

156. Klionsky DJ et al (2016) Guidelines for the use and interpretation of assays for monitoring autophagy (3rd edition). Autophagy 12(1):1–222. https://doi.org/10.1080/15548627.2015.1100356

157. Chen S, Dobrovolsky VN, Liu F, Wu Y, Zhang Z, Mei N, Guo L (2014) The role of autophagy in usnic acid-induced toxicity in hepatic cells. Toxicol Sci 142(1):33–44. https://doi.org/10.1093/toxsci/kfu154

158. Burkard A, Dahn C, Heinz S, Zutavern A, Sonntag-Buck V, Maltman D, Przyborski S, Hewitt NJ, Braspenning J (2012) Generation of proliferating human hepatocytes using Upcyte(R) technology: characterisation and applications in induction and cytotoxicity assays. Xenobiotica 42(10):939–956. https://doi.org/10.3109/00498254.2012.675093

159. Tolosa L, Gomez-Lechon MJ, Lopez S, Guzman C, Castell JV, Donato MT, Jover R (2016) Human Upcyte hepatocytes: characterization of the hepatic phenotype and evaluation for acute and long-term hepatotoxicity routine testing. Toxicol Sci 152(1):214–229. https://doi.org/10.1093/toxsci/kfw078

160. Ware BR, Khetani SR (2016) Engineered liver platforms for different phases of drug development. Trends Biotechnol. https://doi.org/10.1016/j.tibtech.2016.08.001

161. Peng CC, Liao WH, Chen YH, Wu CY, Tung YC (2013) A microfluidic cell culture array with various oxygen tensions. Lab Chip 13(16):3239–3245. https://doi.org/10.1039/c3lc50388g

162. Oshikata-Miyazaki A, Takezawa T (2016) Development of an oxygenation culture method for activating the liver-specific functions of HepG2 cells utilizing a collagen vitrigel membrane chamber. Cytotechnology 68(5):1801–1811. https://doi.org/10.1007/s10616-015-9934-1

Chapter 9

Evaluation of Drug-Induced Liver Injuries (DILI) with Human Hepatocytes: Scientific Rationale and Experimental Approaches

Albert P. Li

Abstract

Preclinical safety evaluation with laboratory animals may not accurately predict human drug safety due to species differences in response to toxicants. Here the Human Cell Paradigm, namely, that human-specific drug properties can be obtained with in vitro human-based experimental systems is proposed. The success of the Human Cell Paradigm depends on the physiological relevance of the in vitro system, namely, the retention of human-specific and organ-specific properties. Human hepatocytes, with complete hepatic metabolizing enzymes, transporters and cofactors, represent a practical and useful experimental system to assess human-specific hepatic drug properties. In this chapter, the scientific rationale and experimental approaches for the application of primary cultured human hepatocytes to evaluate drug-induced liver injuries (DILI) is reviewed. This review focuses on experimental approaches based on the *Key Idiosyncratic Determinant* (KID) hypothesis—that drugs with KID are likely to cause idiosyncratic drug toxicity. We have identified that metabolism-dependent toxicity and induction of reactive oxygen species as two important KIDs. In vitro experimental approaches with primary cultured human hepatocytes that can be applied in drug development for optimization and prioritization of chemical structures based on human hepatotoxic potential are described.

Key words Drug-induced liver injury, Human hepatocytes, Preclinical safety, Key idiosyncratic determinant hypothesis, Metabolism-dependent toxicity, Induction of reactive oxygen species

1 Introduction

Drug-induced liver injury (DILI) continues to be a major challenge in drug development [1–4]. The routine safety evaluation approaches of preclinical evaluation in laboratory animals followed by phase I, II and III clinical trials, are inadequate in the identification of DILI drugs, as demonstrated by the occurrence of drug-induced liver failures for an alarming number of newly marketed drugs. Species-differences in drug toxicity, namely, that human-specific toxicity is not readily detected in nonhuman animals, is one plausible explanation for the ineffectiveness of preclinical safety trials.

Minjun Chen and Yvonne Will (eds.), *Drug-Induced Liver Toxicity*, Methods in Pharmacology and Toxicology,
https://doi.org/10.1007/978-1-4939-7677-5_9, © Springer Science+Business Media, LLC, part of Springer Nature 2018

This is further supported by the many cases of clinical trial failures due to unexpected liver toxicity for drug candidates that had no significant findings in preclinical safety evaluations. The rare incidence rate of DILI, namely, approximately 19 per 100,000 treated patients [5], cannot be readily detected in phase I, II, and III clinical trials due to the limited number of subjects.

It is clear that the current drug safety evaluation paradigm is not adequate in the elimination of drugs with human-specific drug toxicity that is detectable only after exposure to a relatively large human population due to the rare incidence of occurrence. In this chapter, I will present a proposal that evaluation of human-specific drug properties using physiologically relevant in vitro human cell-based experimental systems should be a critical part of the safety evaluation regimen. Specifically, I will review the scientific rationale and experimental approaches with human hepatocytes for the evaluation of drug-induced liver injuries that apparently are not detected in preclinical animal safety studies and clinical human safety trials.

2   Roles of the Liver in Drug Toxicity

The liver is the major organ for xenobiotic metabolism (biotransformation), with the parenchymal cells (hepatocytes) responsible for virtually all biotransformation activities [6]. Hepatocyte-mediated biotransformation is a key determinant of the following key drug properties:

1. Metabolic stability [7]: The rate of metabolism of the parent drug by hepatocytes is responsible for the plasma half-life, and therefore organ exposure to the parent.

2. Metabolite generation [8]: The parent drug is metabolized by the hepatocytes to various metabolites which may have biological properties different from that of the parent. Hepatic metabolism of a parent drug to toxic/reactive metabolites is a key mechanism for DILI.

3. Drug-drug interactions [9]: An average patient routinely takes several drugs simultaneously, usually for the treatment of multiple ailments. Some diseases like HIV infection and cancer require treatment by multiple drugs. DILI may be exacerbated in patients with enhanced metabolic activation via inductive drug-drug interactions: induction of drug-metabolizing enzyme activity (e.g., CYP3A4) by environmental agents (e.g., pollutants; foods) or coadministered drugs (e.g., rifampin). Hepatotoxicity potential of a drug may also be amplified via diminished detoxification pathways.

4. Hepatotoxicity [9]: While multiple cell types, including Kupffer cells and endothelial cells, are involved in the development of hepatotoxicity, the hepatocytes represent the key

target cells. Liver failure occurs when the majority of the hepatocytes in the liver are severely damaged, leading directly or indirectly to liver failure.

In summary, hepatocyte-associated liver functions are key determinants of drug toxicity. Metabolic stability determines the duration of drug exposure. Metabolite formation affects overall toxic potential via metabolic activation and detoxification. Drug-drug interaction leads to alterations in parent drug and metabolite exposure. Further, hepatocytes are the major in vivo target cells for initiation of hepatotoxicity, leading ultimately to hepatic failure. Primary human hepatocytes therefore represent a physiologically relevant experimental system for the evaluation of DILI [10, 11].

3   Species Difference in Drug Toxicity as a Result of Species Difference in Drug Metabolism

A major reason that human hepatocytes represent an important in vitro experimental system for the evaluation of human drug properties is that they retain human-specific biology. Evidence is accumulating that the effectiveness of the classical approach of safety evaluation in laboratory animals is limited by species-differences in drug properties, especially ADMET drug properties: absorption, disposition, metabolism, elimination and toxicity [9, 12, 13]. Species differences in drug metabolism is a well-established phenomenon. The most important drug-metabolizing enzymes belong to the cytochromes P450 which are localized mainly in the parenchymal cells (hepatocytes) of the liver and are found in other organ such as intestinal epithelium [14, 15], lung [16], and kidney [17]. Of the major isoforms involved in drug metabolism, namely, CYP isoforms 1A, 2B, 2C, 2D, 2E, and 3A, the human isoforms are substantially different from those found in rat, dog, and monkey (Table 1).

Drug metabolism is a key determinant in drug toxicity: a toxicant can be rendered more toxic (metabolic activation) or less toxic (detoxification) by biotransformation. Species differences in drug-metabolizing enzymes such as cytochromes P450 can lead to species differences in xenobiotic toxicity due to differences in rate of metabolic activation and detoxification, as well as differences in metabolite formation. A clear example is the finding of Easterbrook et al. [18] that coumarin to 7-hydroxycoumarin was observed in human but not in rat liver microsomes. The report of Lee et al. [19] is a pioneering study using animal and human hepatocytes to evaluate species-differences in metabolite formation to aid the selection of an appropriate animal model for drug development. The finding that metabolites formed by rat hepatocytes were different from those formed by human hepatocytes suggest that, for the drug candidate evaluated, the rat may not be an appropriate

Table 1
A comparison of hepatic P450 isoforms in human to the four commonly used laboratory animal species for safety evaluation (mouse, rat, dog, and monkey)

P450 isoform subfamily	Human	Mouse	Rat	Dog	Monkey
2A	**2A6**, **2A7**, **2A13**	2A4, 2A5, 2A12, 2A22	2A1, 2A2, 2A3	2A13, 2A25	2A23, 2A24
2B	**2B6**, **2B7**	2B9, 2B10	2B1, 2B2, 2B3	2B11	2B17
2C	**2C8**, **2C9**, **2C18**, **2C19**	2C29, 2C37, 2C38, 2C39, 2C40, 2C44, 2C50, 2C54, 2C55	2C6, 2C7, 2C11, 2C12, 2C13, 2C22, 2C23	2C21, 2C41	2C20, 2C43
2D	**2D6**, **2D7**, **2D8**	2D9, 2D10, 2D11, 2D12, 2D13, 2D22, 2D26, 2D34, 2D40	2D1, 2D2, 2D3, 2D4, 2D5, 2D18	2D15	2D17, 2D19, 2D29, 2D30, 2D42
2E	**2E1**	2E1	2E1	2E1	2E1
3A	**3A4**, **3A5**, **3A7**, **3A43**	3A11, 3A13, 3A16, 3A25, 3A41, 3A44	3A1, 3A2, 3A9, 3A18, 3A62	3A12, 3A26	3A8

Extensive species difference has been established, with P450 1A and 2E found to be the only isoforms that are conserved among the multiple animal species. Species difference in P450 isoforms has led to differences in metabolic stability, metabolite profiles, as well as drug toxicity and efficacy. The human isoforms commonly investigated are in bold

experimental model for the assessment of human drug properties. Species difference in metabolite formation is now a frequently observed phenomenon in drug development.

4   Human Cell Paradigm (HCP) for the Prediction of Human Drug Properties

Because of the known species differences in drug properties, I have proposed a new paradigm, the human cell paradigm (HCP) for drug development, namely, the application of physiologically relevant human-based in vitro experimental systems to evaluate human-specific drug properties, followed by extrapolation of the data to humans in vivo [20, 21]. Early assessment of human-drug properties will allow optimization of human drug properties as well as the selection of the most appropriate animal species for preclinical animal trials, thereby enhancing the probability of clinical success. A physiologically relevant in vitro human cell system is defined as one that retains both organ-specific and human-specific properties, as represented by primary human hepatocytes for the evaluation of human hepatic drug properties.

With the HCP paradigm, human-specific adverse drug properties are obtained using physiologically relevant human cell based in vitro experimental systems, followed by prediction of human in vivo effects using two methods: (1) Direct extrapolation of in vitro results to human in vivo using known human in vivo parameters (e.g., physiologically based pharmacokinetics data; genetic polymorphism; environment factors). This approach has been applied successful in the estimation of hepatic metabolic clearance and drug-drug interactions. (2) Develop in vitro animal results using similar cell systems from multiple species for the selection of the most relevant animal species for in vivo evaluation and extrapolation of results to humans in vivo. This approach is recommended for toxicological endpoints which can be adequately evaluated with in vitro approaches such as hepatotoxicity. The key emphasis is that human-specific drug properties obtained using in vitro human-based experimental systems are critical to the evaluation of human in vivo drug properties (Fig. 1).

5   Human Hepatocyte Cryopreservation as an Enabling Technology

Human hepatocytes can be isolated from human liver biopsies or whole livers which have been donated for but not used for transplantation. The application of human hepatocytes in research was limited by the general unavailability of human livers for research and the lack of hepatocyte isolation expertise in most laboratories. We dedicated extensive effort in our laboratory toward the optimization of hepatocyte isolation, cryopreservation, and recovery of hepatocytes from cryopreservation [9, 22–24]. A major advancement is the development of a specialized medium (Cryopreserved Hepatocyte Recovery Medium (CHRM™)) which greatly enhanced the viability of hepatocytes thawed from cryopreservation. Upon recovery in CHRM, the viability (based on dye exclusion) is routinely >85%, with drug-metabolizing enzyme activities similar to that in vivo [21]. Furthermore, approximately 50% of the human

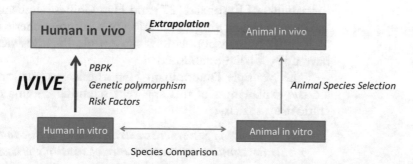

Fig. 1 Human cell paradigm (HCP) for the prediction of human drug properties. With the HCP paradigm, emphasis is placed on human-specific drug properties obtained with physiologically relevant human-based in vitro experimental systems. In vitro results are then extrapolated to in vivo based on known human in vivo parameters and/or via the selection of the most appropriate animal species using similar in vitro systems, followed by in vivo evaluation in the chosen animal species using a parallelogram approach as illustrated here

hepatocyte isolations resulted in cryopreserved hepatocytes that formed monolayer cultures with >80% confluency (plateable cryopreserved human hepatocytes) [21]. We now have extended human hepatocyte cryopreservation to the preparation of cryopreserved human hepatocytes pooled from multiple donors: cryopreserved hepatocytes from individual donors are thawed, cells from multiple donors are pooled, and the cells recryopreserved. While individual donors can be used to illustrate individual differences, the pooled cryopreserved hepatocytes can be used for the investigation of drug properties toward a "normalized" human population.

We are also successful in the cryopreservation of nonhuman animal hepatocytes. Cryopreserved hepatocytes from multiple animal species and human can be used in the same experiment for the selection of the animal species most resembling human in the drug property of interest based on the parallelogram approach as discussed earlier.

Drug-metabolizing enzyme activities of multiple lots of cryopreserved human hepatocytes are shown in Table 2. The morphology of cultured cryopreserved human and animal hepatocytes is shown in Fig. 2.

5.1 The "Multiple Determinant Hypothesis" for the Manifestation of Idiosyncratic Drug Toxicity

Idiosyncratic drug toxicity continues to be a challenge for drug developers and regulatory agencies. The low incidence of occurrence apparently explains the inability of its detection only after post-marketing when a large patient population has been exposed, but not in the routinely performed phase I, II and III clinical trials with limited patient populations. The Genome Wide Association Studies (GWAS) attempting to identify at risk populations identified apparent links between HLA genotype and susceptibility for DILI: HLA-DRB1*16: 01-DQB1*05: 02 genotype for flupirtine [25], HLA-B*5701 genotype for flucloxacillin [26], HLA-A*33:01 genotype for terbinafine, fenofibrate, and ticlopidine [27]. Some non-drug-specific risk factors have also been reported for patients of European [27] and Han Chinese descends [28]. At the time of this writing, application of common genetic risk factors to identify human populations susceptible for idiosyncratic DILI have not yet been established.

The Multiple Determinant Hypothesis was put forth [29] to aid the explanation of this apparent scientific enigma of idiosyncratic drug toxicity:

The low frequency of idiosyncratic drug toxicity is due to the requirements for simultaneous occurrence of multiple critical and discrete events, with the probability for the occurrence of idiosyncratic toxicity as a product of the probabilities of each event [29].

These critical and discrete events are considered "risk factors" which can be a combination of discrete environmental, genetic, and physiological (e.g., metabolic) factors. The hypothesis can

Table 2
Donor demographics, post-thawed viability, yield, and P450 isoform-selective substrate metabolism activities of cryopreserved human hepatocytes from 11 donors

Lot number	Gender	Ethnicity	Age	Viability	Yield (million cells per vial)	1A2	2A6	2B6	2C8	2C9	2C19	2D6	CYP2E1	3A4-MDZ	3A4-TEST
HH1016	F	H	64	88	5.7	154.0	81.4	10.1	1.7	44.2	20.9	4.4	41.3	67.1	454.7
HH1028	M	H	43	94	5.3	54.3	39.3	6.2	4.8	27.7	55.9	6.3	22.7	33.5	300.7
HH1030	M	C	31	35	5.2	68.9	8.6	4.1	3.7	29.6	14.0	4.6	51.7	19.1	106.7
HH1031	M	H	42	92	7.2	12.7	8.4	81	2.3	59.8	0.9	18	38	14.8	179.2
HH1032	F	C	68	95	7.8	7.0	20.0	8.1	0.7	21.4	4.9	7.3	29.8	16.3	102.7
HH1033	F	C	40	92	5.7	31.1	1.5	18.3	1.3	66	7.0	19.4	35.9	4.8	73.9
HH1037	M	C	45	88	3.3	83.7	45.2	6.8	8.2	20.6	9.7	5.2	9.4	23.4	256.7
HH1044	M	C	67	86	5.0	115	5.6	52.9	1.5	55.8	0.5	46.2	41.1	21.3	477.7
HH1041	M	C	53	87	7.8	21.7	41.4	15.7	6.4	34.7	0.3	7.3	27.8	3.4	33.1
HH1042	M	C	57	95	3.7	18.9	11.1	5.4	1.6	7.2	0.5	2.3	6.3	10.2	234.7

The consistently high (86–95% viability) is a function of the optimized procedures used in the isolation, cryopreservation, and thawing of the cryopreserved cells. Viability was determined by trypan blue exclusion. The metabolic pathways evaluated were: phenacetin 1-hydroxylation (CYP1A2), bupropion hydroxylation (CYP2B6), paclitaxel 6α-hydroxylation (CYP2C8), diclofenac hydroxylation (CYP2C9), dextromethorphan hydroxylation (CYP2D6), chlorzoxazone 6-hydroxylation (CYP2E1), midazolam and testosterone 6b-hydroxylation (CYP3A4-MDZ and CYP3A4-TEST, respectively), with activity expressed as pmol/million hepatocytes/min. (*F* female, *M* male, *C* Caucasian, *H* Hispanic, *C* Caucasian)

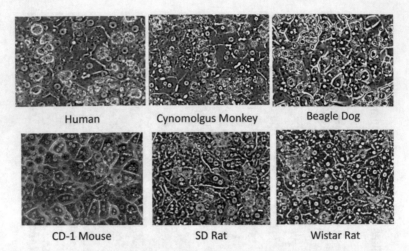

Fig. 2 Morphology of cultured cryopreserved human and animal hepatocytes. The cryopreserved hepatocytes formed highly confluent (near 100%) cultures and exhibited the cobble-stone cell shape typical of freshly isolated hepatocytes. The successful cryopreservation allows simultaneous experimentation of hepatocytes from human and multiple animal species for the selection of the most appropriate animal species for in vivo assessment of human drug properties as described for HCP. [Phase-contrast microphotograph (200× magnification)]

explain the low incidence rate (product of the incidence rate of each discrete risk factor). As nongenetic risk factors can be transient in nature, identification of the at-risk population is virtually impossible. A new paradigm for identification of drugs with idiosyncratic toxicity is therefore needed.

6 Identification of Drugs with Idiosyncratic Toxicity Based on Common Properties

I have previously proposed that drugs with idiosyncratic toxicity may have common properties which can be used for their early detection and therefore removed from drug development. The key to success of this approach is to apply experimental systems with human-specific and organ-specific properties, and that the common properties have mechanistic links to drug toxicity. I would like to propose here the following key common drug properties which have been modified based on my previous publication [29]:

1. Toxicity is related to metabolic activation of the parent drug to toxic metabolites (metabolically activated), including reactive oxygen species (ROS).

2. Metabolic activation is performed via pathways that can be enhanced by environmental and genetic factors (e.g., inducible P450).

3. The toxic metabolites can be detoxified by drug-metabolizing enzymes or cofactors (detoxification).

An individual who, due to environmental factors including exposure to foods, pollutants, and physiological factors such as stress, or genetic factors such as drug-metabolizing enzyme polymorphism, may be at risk if there is a confluence of risk factors such as the following:

1. Enhanced drug absorption due to decreased enteric drug metabolism and/or inhibition of transporter-mediated enteric efflux, thereby increasing systemic drug burden.

2. Enhanced drug-metabolizing enzyme activities for metabolic activation, leading to increased toxic/reactive metabolite formation in the target organ (e.g., liver).

3. Diminished drug-metabolizing enzyme for metabolic detoxification and/or detoxifying cofactors (e.g., reduced L-glutathione), thereby extending the half-life of toxic/reactive metabolites.

4. Enhanced/presensitized physiological response leading to exacerbated cellular damages (e.g., preactivated immune-toxicological responses due to exposure of environmental toxicants and/or pathological organisms).

5. Diminished capacity of the patients to repair and to reverse the cascade of events leading ultimately to organ failure.

Based on the above, I would like to discuss key drug properties that would define drugs with idiosyncratic drug toxicity—the "Key Idiosyncratic Determinants (KID)." I propose here that elucidation of KID may allow early identification of drugs with idiosyncratic toxicity.

7   Metabolism-Dependent Drug Toxicity as a Key Idiosyncratic Determinant (KID)

Individual variations in drug metabolism are a well-established phenomenon. A drug where metabolism plays a key role in its observed toxicity is likely to elicit individual differences in drug toxicity. I hereby propose that drugs that are metabolically activated to highly toxic metabolites are likely to be associated with idiosyncratic drug toxicity. As described earlier, the toxicity of these drugs may be significantly enhanced in individuals with a confluence of risk factors related to drug metabolism: increased exposure to parent drug plus increased formation of toxic metabolites due to enhanced bioactivating metabolic enzyme activity plus compromised detoxification mechanisms.

A corollary of metabolism-dependent drug toxicity as a KID is that an individual with a substantially high level drug-metabolizing enzyme activity would be more sensitive to the toxicity of a drug with metabolism-dependent toxicity. Drug-metabolizing enzyme activity is known to vary among individuals due to genetic

(genetic polymorphism) and environmental factors (environmental pollutants, foods, and medications that are inhibitors or inducers of drug-metabolizing enzymes). The most important drug-metabolizing enzymes are cytochrome P450 isoforms (CYP), especially CYP3A4, which is known to be responsible for the metabolism of over 50% of existing drugs. Large individual variation in CYP3A4 activity are known to occur in the human population. Cryopreserved human hepatocytes from different donors in our laboratory have an approximately 100-fold difference between lots with the lowest and highest activities (Fig. 3), consistent with clinical findings.

We evaluated in our laboratory the hypothesis that hepatic cytochrome P450-dependent monooxygenase (CYP) activity is one of the key risk factors for drug-induced liver injuries (DILI) in the human population, especially for drugs that are metabolically activated to cytotoxic/reactive metabolites. As CYP3A4 is known to be one of the most important P450 isoforms for drug metabolism, studies were performed to evaluate the relationship between the in vitro cytotoxicity of hepatotoxic drugs and CYP3A4 activity for four drugs known to be associated with acute liver failure: acetaminophen, cyclophosphamide, ketoconazole, and tamoxifen. Using hepatocytes from 19 donors, we observed that the human hepatocyte lots with the highest CYP3A4 activity were consistently more susceptible to the in vitro cytotoxicity of the hepatotoxic drugs, thereby supporting the hypothesis that elevated P450 activity may be a risk factor for drug-induced liver injuries (Fig. 3).

8   Concurrent Induction of Oxidative Stress and Cytotoxicity as KID

I have earlier proposed that DILI drugs can be identified based on the "common properties" hypothesis: drugs that cause idiosyncratic hepatotoxicity may have common chemical and biological properties which can be used for their identification [29].

Based on this hypothesis, our laboratory, via a collaboration with the National Center for Toxicological Research (NCTR) of the US Food and Drug Administration (FDA), embarked upon a vigorous research program to evaluate the possibility that toxicological responses of human hepatocytes in vitro could be used for the identification of DILI drugs [30]. We hypothesize that a vigorous, nonbiased, quantitative analysis of the dose-response relationship of cellular toxicological response in human hepatocytes may allow the identification of endpoints or combination of endpoints for accurate identification of drugs associated with severe DILI events. The study was performed with strict adherence to the following five requirements:

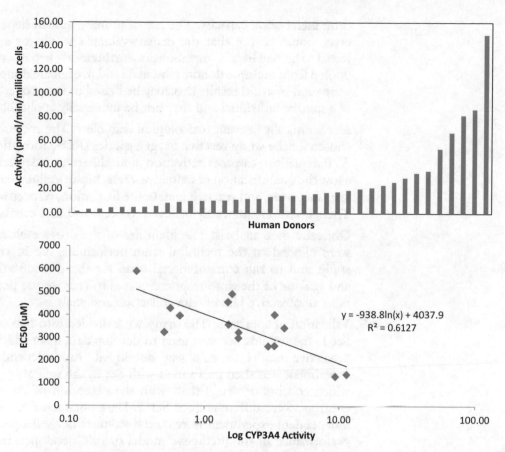

Fig. 3 Individual variation of CYP3A4 activity (top) and the inverse correlation of CYP3A4 activity with EC50 value for the hepatotoxicant, acetaminophen (bottom). Our results suggest that individual differences in drug-metabolizing enzyme activity may lead to differences in sensitivity to drug-induced liver injuries by drugs that are metabolically activated. The results suggest that metabolism-dependent drug toxicity may be a key idiosyncratic determinant

1. Accurate drug annotation: The drugs evaluated in the study were annotated as DILI and non-DILI drugs based on comprehensive review of the literature, with emphasis placed on a list of drugs associated with hepatotoxicity created by an international collaboration of multiple study groups/registries, which provided comprehensive information on hepatotoxicity (i.e., causality level, severity, reporting frequency, and regional difference) based on post-marketing safety experience in different countries [3], and three USA databases for drug-induced acute liver failure [31–33] were used for the annotation of the DILI status of the drugs.

2. Metabolic competent experimental system: Primary human hepatocytes, the generally accepted gold standard for in vitro human drug metabolism studies, were used in the study rather than hepatic cell lines which are known to have attenuated

drug metabolism capacity. The use of primary human hepatocytes would ensure that the drugs evaluated would be subjected to human hepatic metabolism. Furthermore, hepatocytes pooled from multiple donors (five male and five female donors) were used to avoid results that may be biased to the properties of a specific individual and may not be universally applicable.

3. Mechanistically relevant toxicological endpoints: The endpoints chosen for the study-reactive oxygen species (ROS) formation, ATP depletion, caspases activation, and glutathione depletion allow the quantification of oxidative stress, hepatocellular damage, apoptosis, and reactive metabolite formation, respectively. These events are generally believed to occur in DILI events.

4. Objective data analysis: The identities of the drugs evaluated were blinded to the technical team performing the in vitro study, and to the computational team for the quantification and analysis of the dose-response curves to remove the possibility of objective bias in data collection and analysis.

5. Validation of approach: The drugs were divided into two sets. Set 1, the training set, was used to develop data from which a predictive model or rule was developed. An independent experiment was then performed with Set 2, the validation set which consists of drugs that, with the exception of internal controls, were different from Set 1. Data obtained from this independent experiment were used to confirm or challenge the performance of the predictive model or rule developed from the data of the training set.

Our investigation led to a novel finding that the ratio of drug-induced reactive oxygen species to cellular ATP depletion (ROS/ATP ratio) quantitatively measured using human primary hepatocyte in response to drug treatment can accurately distinguish drugs that were associated with severe (sDILI) in a post-marketing setting from the nonsevere DILI (nsDILI) drugs (Fig. 4).

There are clinical data supporting the validity of the success of this assay. Watkins [4] made an interesting finding that hepatocellular injury was the major mechanism of toxicity for 16 drugs that have been withdrawn from the market or have received boxed warning labels due to their association with acute liver failure (ALF). This finding was supported by a survey of ALF cases in US for a 10.5-year period [33] which showed that 77.8% of all ALF reported were due to hepatocellular injury. These clinical findings support the use of human hepatocytes as an in vitro system to evaluate drug-induced hepatic injury [9, 34]. Results of our study support the hypothesis that the ALF dominated mainly by hepatocellular injury is most likely predicted by a hepatocyte-based in vitro system with well-defined biological endpoint(s). Future research will include the development of assays for DILI events not related to direct hepatocellular injury such as steatosis, cholestasis, and immune-mediated hepatotoxicity.

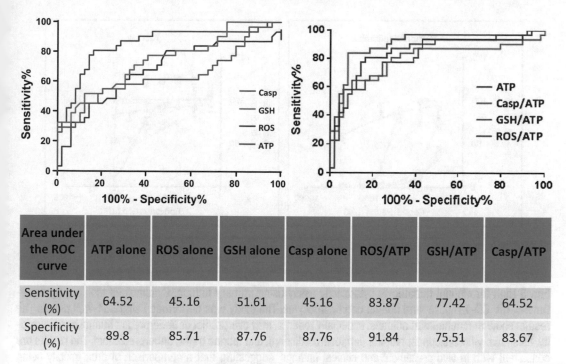

Area under the ROC curve	ATP alone	ROS alone	GSH alone	Casp alone	ROS/ATP	GSH/ATP	Casp/ATP
Sensitivity (%)	64.52	45.16	51.61	45.16	83.87	77.42	64.52
Specificity (%)	89.8	85.71	87.76	87.76	91.84	75.51	83.67

Fig. 4 Specificity and sensitivity in the identification of drugs with severe DILI properties using the Human Hepatocyte ROC/ATP assay. ROS/ATP ratio was found to yield the highest sensitivity (84%) and specificity (92%). The assay was developed as a collaboration with the National Center for Toxicology Research of US Food and Drug Administration using over 100 clinically hepatotoxic and nonhepatotoxic drugs

9   Human Hepatocyte Assays for Hepatotoxicity Potential in Drug Development

The following are assays developed with human hepatocytes in our laboratory for applications in early drug development to minimize hepatotoxic potential.

1. High throughput screening for in vitro hepatotoxicity:

    In this assay, plateable cryopreserved human hepatocytes are cultured for 4 h, followed by treatment with the test articles for a designated time-period (e.g., 24 h), followed by quantification of viability. This assay can be performed in 96-, 384-, and 1536-well plates. In our laboratory, quantification of cellular ATP contents is a preferred viability endpoint for its robust signal, high sensitivity and low background values (Fig. 5).

2. Evaluation of metabolism-dependent cytotoxicity:

    As described earlier, drugs with metabolism-dependent toxicity are likely to cause idiosyncratic drug toxicity due to individual differences in drug metabolism as well as fluctuations in drug metabolism capacity in an individual due to environmental factors. Further, these drugs may exhibit species difference in toxicity due to species difference in drug metabolism.

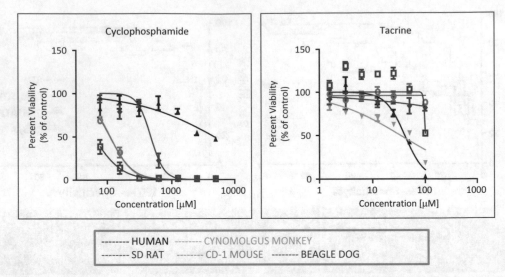

Fig. 5 High throughput hepatocyte cytotoxicity assay using primary human, Cynomolgus monkey, Sprague-Dawley rat, CD-1 mouse, and beagle dog hepatocytes. The study was performed using 384-well plates. The results show that nonhuman animals, especially rodents, may overpredict or underpredict human hepatotoxicity, as shown with cyclophosphamide (left; overprediction), and tacrine (right; underprediction). The results are consistent with in vivo preclinical and clinical findings, suggesting that a comparison of drug toxicity using animal and human hepatocytes may allow early determination of species differences and the selection of the most appropriate animal species for safety evaluation

Metabolism-dependent drug toxicity can be evaluated using two approaches [35]: (1) Metabolic comparative cytotoxicity assay (MCCA): Comparison of cytotoxicity in a metabolically competent cell system (e.g., primary hepatocytes) versus that in a metabolically incompetent cell system (e.g., Chinese hamster ovary cells); (2) Cytotoxic metabolic pathway identification assay: Evaluation of cytotoxicity in primary hepatocytes in the presence and absence of a P450 inhibitor (e.g., 1-aminobenzotriazole). A decrease in cytotoxicity with absent or diminished drug metabolism would suggest that the drug evaluated exhibits metabolism-dependent toxicity (Fig. 6).

3. ROS/ATP assay for sDILI

As described earlier, this assay was codeveloped between our laboratory and FDA National Center for Toxicological Research [30]. The assay identifies drugs with severe DILI properties (drugs known to cause liver failure) with >85% specificity and sensitivity. In this assay, primary cultured human hepatocytes are treated with seven concentrations of the test articles for 48 h, followed by evaluation of both reactive oxygen species (ROS) formation and viability based on cellular ATP contents. The area-under-the curve of a plot of the ROS/ATP ratio vs drug concentration is used to delineate sDILI and non-sDILI drugs (Fig. 4).

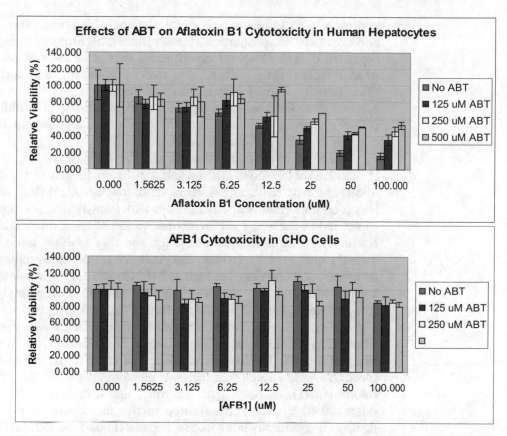

Fig. 6 Human hepatocyte assays for the identification of metabolism-dependent cytotoxicity. Results with a model metabolically activated hepatotoxicant, aflatoxin B1, is shown. That metabolism is critical to aflatoxin B1 hepatotoxicity is demonstrated by the attenuation of its cytotoxicity by a nonselective P450 inhibitor, 1-aminobenzotrizole, in human hepatocytes (top), as well as the lack of cytotoxicity in the metabolically incompetent CHO cell line (bottom)

10   Conclusion

Drugs with idiosyncratic drug toxicity cannot be readily identified using routine preclinical and clinical safety regiments due to its human specificity (thereby cannot be detected in laboratory animals during preclinical trials), and/or its low incidence (thereby cannot be readily detected in clinical trials due to the limited number of subjects). I have previously proposed the Multiple Determinant Hypothesis to explain the idiosyncratic phenomenon, namely, that the low incidence of idiosyncratic drug toxicity is due to the rare, concurrent existence of multiple discrete risk factors in the affected individuals. The hypothesis led to my proposal that definition of the risk factors may allow the establishment of an effective approach to identify drugs with idiosyncratic toxicity.

I also proposed the Human Cell Paradigm which states that human drug properties can be evaluated with human-cell based experimental approaches. The prerequisite for the success of the approach is to utilize experimental systems with human-specific and organ-specific properties. Primary human hepatocytes thereby represent the most relevant experimental system for the evaluation of idiosyncratic drug-induced liver toxicity in the human population. Primary human hepatocytes are known to retain human-specific drug-metabolizing enzymes and cofactors, and unlike cell-free systems such as liver microsomes, can be used for the evaluation of toxicological responses.

I have identified metabolism-dependent drug toxicity and the co-occurrence of oxidative stress and hepatocyte toxicity as the key idiosyncratic determinants. That metabolism-dependent drug toxicity is an important property of drugs with idiosyncratic toxicity is supported by the well-established observation of vast individual differences in drug metabolism capacity, and that multiple environmental and genetic factors can upregulate or downregulate drug-metabolizing enzymes such as P450 isoforms. Further, similar environmental factors can downregulate detoxification pathways. Another strong support for metabolism-dependent drug toxicity as a key determinant of idiosyncratic drug toxicity is that a vast majority of drugs with idiosyncratic drug toxicity are known to form reactive metabolites. Reactive metabolites can exert initial cell stress through a wide range of mechanisms including depletion of glutathione (GSH), or binding to enzymes, lipids, nucleic acids and other cell structures. Furthermore, reactive metabolites or parent drugs may specifically inhibit other hepatocellular functions such as the apical (canalicular) bile salt efflux pump (BSEP), in which case the subsequent intracellular accumulation of its substrates may cause secondary toxic hepatocyte damage [36, 37]. Covalent interaction of reactive metabolites with cellular and mitochondrial macromolecules which, in conjunction with ROS induction may initiate cytotoxic events critical to the onset and propagation of liver injuries, leading ultimately to total liver failure. Elimination of drug candidates in drug development based purely on reactive metabolite formation using human liver microsomes has not been productive due to apparent false positive results. I propose here to identify drugs with metabolism-dependent toxicity based on in vitro hepatotoxicity in primary culture human hepatocytes to minimize artifacts of cell free experimental systems.

Our empirical finding that the ROS/ATP ratio accurately identifies drugs with severe DILI properties suggests that co-occurrence of reactive oxygen species and cytotoxicity is a key idiosyncratic determinant. Our observation is consistent with a current hypothesis suggesting that causative events of liver injuries involve impairment of ATP synthesis, opening of mitochondrial permeability transition pore, specific changes in mitochondrial morphology, impaired Ca^{2+} uptake, generation of mitochondrial reactive oxygen species (mtROS) which initiate inflammatory events critical to the ultimate onset of liver injuries [38]. ROS production and reduction of cellular ATP may not be the ultimate mechanism of liver failure, but could be key initiating events.

Lastly, I would like to emphasize the following: We need to accept the inadequacy of current safety testing regimes in the identification of drugs with idiosyncratic hepatotoxicity. Toxicology as a discipline in the past relies on the generalized doctrine that in vivo animal experimentation represents the most accurate preclinical approach to predict human drug toxicity. This approach of course is valuable in the elimination of drugs with toxicity both in animals and humans, but not for drugs with human-specific toxicity. I propose that drugs with human-specific toxicity need to be evaluated with mechanistic approaches in experimental systems with human-specific biology relevant to the toxic events. Primary human hepatocytes accompanied with toxicologically relevant experimental approaches as described in this review represent a logical and hopefully useful approach to overcome the challenge of drug-induced idiosyncratic hepatotoxicity.

References

1. Li AP, Zhang J (2016) Editorial: promising approaches to identify DILI drugs. Chem Biol Interact 255.1–2

2. Lo Re V 3rd, Haynes K, Forde KA, Goldberg DS, Lewis JD, Carbonari DM, Leidl KB, Reddy KR, Nezamzadeh MS, Roy J, Sha D, Marks AR, De Boer J, Schneider JL, Strom BL, Corley DA (2015) Risk of acute liver failure in patients with drug-induced liver injury: evaluation of Hy's law and a new prognostic model. Clin Gastroenterol Hepatol 13:2360–2368

3. Suzuki A, Andrade RJ, Bjornsson E, Lucena MI, Lee WM, Yuen NA, Hunt CM, Freston JW (2010) Drugs associated with hepatotoxicity and their reporting frequency of liver adverse events in VigiBase: unified list based on international collaborative work. Drug Saf 33:503–522

4. Watkins PB (2005) Idiosyncratic liver injury: challenges and approaches. Toxicol Pathol 33:1–5

5. Hussaini SH, Farrington EA (2014) Idiosyncratic drug-induced liver injury: an update on the 2007 overview. Expert Opin Drug Saf 13:67–81

6. Li AP (2004) In vitro approaches to evaluate ADMET drug properties. Curr Top Med Chem 4:701–706

7. Di L, Atkinson K, Orozco CC, Funk C, Zhang H, McDonald TS, Tan B, Lin J, Chang C, Obach RS (2013) In vitro-in vivo correlation for low-clearance compounds using hepatocyte relay method. Drug Metab Dispos 41:2018–2023

8. Wohlfarth A, Scheidweiler KB, Pang S, Zhu M, Castaneto M, Kronstrand R, Huestis MA (2016) Metabolic characterization of AH-7921, a synthetic opioid designer drug: in vitro metabolic stability assessment and metabolite identification, evaluation of in silico prediction, and in vivo confirmation. Drug Test Anal 8:779–791

9. Li AP (2010) Evaluation of drug metabolism, drug-drug interactions, and in vitro hepatotoxicity with cryopreserved human hepatocytes. Methods Mol Biol 640:281–294

10. Li AP (2014) In vitro human hepatocyte-based experimental systems for the evaluation of human drug metabolism, drug-drug interactions, and drug toxicity in drug development. Curr Top Med Chem 14:1325–1338

11. Funk C, Roth A (2017) Current limitations and future opportunities for prediction of DILI from in vitro. Arch Toxicol 91:131–142

12. Li AP (2004) Accurate prediction of human drug toxicity: a major challenge in drug development. Chem Biol Interact 150:3–7

13. Baillie TA, Rettie AE (2011) Role of biotransformation in drug-induced toxicity: influence of intra- and inter-species differences in drug metabolism. Drug Metab Pharmacokinet 26:15–29

14. Ho MD, Ring N, Amaral K, Doshi U, Li AP (2017) Human enterocytes as an in vitro model for the evaluation of intestinal drug metabolism: characterization of drug-metabolizing enzyme activities of cryopreserved human enterocytes from twenty-four donors. Drug Metab Dispos 45:686–691

15. von Richter O, Burk O, Fromm MF, Thon KP, Eichelbaum M, Kivisto KT (2004) Cytochrome P450 3A4 and P-glycoprotein expression in human small intestinal enterocytes and hepatocytes: a comparative analysis in paired tissue specimens. Clin Pharmacol Ther 75:172–183

16. Somers GI, Lindsay N, Lowdon BM, Jones AE, Freathy C, Ho S, Woodrooffe AJ, Bayliss MK, Manchee GR (2007) A comparison of the expression and metabolizing activities of phase I and II enzymes in freshly isolated human lung parenchymal cells and cryopreserved human hepatocytes. Drug Metab Dispos 35:1797–1805

17. Dixon J, Lane K, Macphee I, Philips B (2014) Xenobiotic metabolism: the effect of acute kidney injury on non-renal drug clearance and hepatic drug metabolism. Int J Mol Sci 15:2538–2553

18. Easterbrook J, Fackett D, Li AP (2001) A comparison of aroclor 1254-induced and uninduced rat liver microsomes to human liver microsomes in phenytoin O-deethylation, coumarin 7-hydroxylation, tolbutamide 4-hydroxylation, S-mephenytoin 4'-hydroxylation, chloroxazone 6-hydroxylation and testosterone 6beta-hydroxylation. Chem Biol Interact 134:243–249

19. Lee K, Vandenberghe Y, Herin M, Cavalier R, Beck D, Li A, Verbeke N, Lesne M, Roba J (1994) Comparative metabolism of SC-42867 and SC-51089, two PGE2 antagonists, in rat and human hepatocyte cultures. Xenobiotica 24:25–36

20. Li AP (2007) Human-based in vitro experimental systems for the evaluation of human drug safety. Curr Drug Saf 2:193–199

21. Li AP (2015) Evaluation of adverse drug properties with cryopreserved human hepatocytes and the integrated discrete multiple organ co-culture (IdMOC(TM)) system. Toxicol Res 31:137–149

22. Loretz LJ, Li AP, Flye MW, Wilson AG (1989) Optimization of cryopreservation procedures for rat and human hepatocytes. Xenobiotica 19:489–498

23. Li AP, Lu C, Brent JA, Pham C, Fackett A, Ruegg CE, Silber PM (1999) Cryopreserved human hepatocytes: characterization of drug-metabolizing enzyme activities and applications in higher throughput screening assays for hepatotoxicity, metabolic stability, and drug-drug interaction potential. Chem Biol Interact 121:17–35

24. Li AP (2007) Human hepatocytes: isolation, cryopreservation and applications in drug development. Chem Biol Interact 168:16–29

25. Nicoletti P, Werk AN, Sawle A, Shen Y, Urban TJ, Coulthard SA, Bjornsson ES, Cascorbi I, Floratos A, Stammschulte T, Gundert-Remy U, Nelson MR, Aithal GP, Daly AK (2016) HLA-DRB1*16: 01-DQB1*05: 02 is a novel genetic risk factor for flupirtine-induced liver injury. Pharmacogenet Genomics 26:218–224

26. Daly AK, Donaldson PT, Bhatnagar P, Shen Y, Pe'er I, Floratos A, Daly MJ, Goldstein DB, John S, Nelson MR, Graham J, Park BK, Dillon JF, Bernal W, Cordell HJ, Pirmohamed M, Aithal GP, Day CP (2009) HLA-B*5701 genotype is a major determinant of drug-induced liver injury due to flucloxacillin. Nat Genet 41:816–819

27. Nicoletti P, Aithal GP, Bjornsson ES, Andrade RJ, Sawle A, Arrese M, Barnhart HX, Bondon-Guitton E, Hayashi PH, Bessone F, Carvajal A, Cascorbi I, Cirulli ET, Chalasani N, Conforti A, Coulthard SA, Daly MJ, Day CP, Dillon JF, Fontana RJ, Grove JI, Hallberg P, Hernandez N, Ibanez L, Kullak-Ublick GA, Laitinen T, Larrey D, Lucena MI, Maitland-van der Zee AH, Martin JH, Molokhia M, Pirmohamed M, Powell EE, Qin S, Serrano J, Stephens C, Stolz A, Wadelius M, Watkins PB, Floratos A, Shen Y, Nelson MR, Urban TJ, Daly AK (2017) Association of liver injury from specific drugs, or groups of drugs, with polymorphisms in HLA and other genes in a genome-wide association study. Gastroenterology 152:1078–1089

28. Jiang J, Zhang X, Huo R, Li X, Yang Y, Gai Z, Xu M, Shen L, Cai L, Wan C, Li B, He L, Qin S (2015) Association study of UGT1A9 promoter polymorphisms with DILI based on systematically regional variation screen in Chinese population. Pharmacogenomics J 15:326–331

29. Li AP (2002) A review of the common properties of drugs with idiosyncratic hepatotoxicity and the "multiple determinant hypothesis" for the manifestation of idiosyncratic drug toxicity. Chem Biol Interact 142:7–23

30. Zhang J, Doshi U, Suzuki A, Chang CW, Borlak J, Li AP, Tong W (2016) Evaluation of multiple mechanism-based toxicity endpoints in primary cultured human hepatocytes for the identification of drugs with clinical hepatotoxicity: results from 152 marketed drugs with known liver injury profiles. Chem Biol Interact 255:3–11

31. Chalasani N, Fontana RJ, Bonkovsky HL, Watkins PB, Davern T, Serrano J, Yang H, Rochon J (2008) Causes, clinical features, and outcomes from a prospective study of drug-induced liver injury in the United States. Gastroenterology 135:1924–1934.e4

32. Mindikoglu AL, Magder LS, Regev A (2009) Outcome of liver transplantation for drug-induced acute liver failure in the United States: analysis of the united network for organ sharing database. Liver Transpl 15: 719–729

33. Reuben A, Koch DG, Lee WM (2010) Drug-induced acute liver failure: results of a U.S. multicenter, prospective study. Hepatology 52:2065–2076

34. Gomez-Lechon MJ, Donato MT, Castell JV, Jover R (2003) Human hepatocytes as a tool for studying toxicity and drug metabolism. Curr Drug Metab 4:292–312

35. Li AP (2009) Metabolism comparative cytotoxicity assay (MCCA) and cytotoxic metabolic pathway identification assay (CMPIA) with cryopreserved human hepatocytes for the evaluation of metabolism-based cytotoxicity in vitro: proof-of-concept study with aflatoxin B1. Chem Biol Interact 179:4–8

36. Yucha RW, He K, Shi Q, Cai L, Nakashita Y, Xia CQ, Liao M (2017) In vitro drug-induced liver injury prediction: criteria optimization of efflux transporter IC50 and physicochemical properties. Toxicol Sci 157:487–499

37. Guo YX, Xu XF, Zhang QZ, Li C, Deng Y, Jiang P, He LY, Peng WX (2015) The inhibition of hepatic bile acids transporters Ntcp and Bsep is involved in the pathogenesis of isoniazid/rifampicin-induced hepatotoxicity. Toxicol Mech Methods 25:382–387

38. Kozlov AV, Lancaster JR Jr, Meszaros AT, Weidinger A (2017) Mitochondria-meditated pathways of organ failure upon inflammation. Redox Biol 13:170–181

Chapter 10

Status and Use of Induced Pluripotent Stem Cells (iPSCs) in Toxicity Testing

Min Wei Wong, Chris S. Pridgeon, Constanze Schlott,
B. Kevin Park, and Christopher E.P. Goldring

Abstract

Adverse drug reactions (ADRs) are a major cause of drug attrition during development and withdrawal from market. Hepatotoxicity is among the most common reasons given for drug attrition or withdrawal; this occurs for a multitude of reasons among which is certainly the lack of adequate models able to recapitulate hepatotoxicity in vitro. The loss of compounds in late-stage testing or after marketing is a major financial burden for the pharmaceutical industry and improved models capable of predicting human toxicity of novel compounds at the early stages of testing are highly sought-after. An ideal novel hepatotoxicity model of should be amenable to high-throughput screening and able to recapitulate the hepatic phenotype over an extended period and also model idiosyncratic drug-induced liver injury (DILI). There are no currently models able to fulfill these requirements.

Pluripotent stem cell-derived hepatocyte-like cells (PSC-HLCs) are a developing model which show promise for hepatotoxicity testing. However, the current phenotype of PSC-HLCs is closer to a fetal hepatocyte than an adult hepatocyte. The methodologies for generating mature PSC-HLCs close to an idealized hepatotoxicity model remain to be developed, though incremental improvements to the state-of-the-art are frequently made. Novel PSC-HLC technologies are being developed independently in many research groups; as such there is a need for standardization in benchmarking of these cells and for evaluating the performance and functionality of newly developed HLC models.

Key words iPSC, ADR, DILI, Hepatotoxicity, HLCs, Drug safety

1 Introduction

Adverse drug reactions (ADR) are a major problem for clinicians and pharmaceutical industry. Of all the different targets of ADRs, the liver is the most susceptible organ; drug-induced liver injury (DILI) is the second highest cause of drug attrition [1] and accounts for more than 50% of cases of acute liver failure [2, 3] and therefore is related to a high morbidity and mortality [4]. DILI is a major financial burden for healthcare providers and the

---

Min Wei Wong and Chris S. Pridgeon contributed equally to this work.

Minjun Chen and Yvonne Will (eds.), *Drug-Induced Liver Toxicity*, Methods in Pharmacology and Toxicology,
https://doi.org/10.1007/978-1-4939-7677-5_10, © Springer Science+Business Media, LLC, part of Springer Nature 2018

pharmaceutical industry and therefore, early detection of DILI during the drug discovery process would be beneficial to minimize costs, improve patient safety and save resources. A reliable in vitro model for predicting DILI in humans should resemble the in vivo liver phenotype and be able to support long term studies and high throughput screening (HTS) for toxicity assessment.

Currently several in vitro models are used to predict the hepatotoxicity of new chemical entities (NCEs), including HepG2 and HepaRG cells, which are widely used in the pharmaceutical and chemical industries for initially screening of NCEs. These models have high proliferative capacity and their ease of culture, economical and ready availability and amenability for HTS in the industry make them convenient for generating reproducible data [5, 6]. HepG2 cells are an immortalized cell line derived from a hepatocellular carcinoma of a 15-year-old Caucasian male and are the most widely used line. These cells are highly differentiated and exhibit several genotypic features of normal human liver cells and therefore can be used in the screening of cytotoxicity at the lead generation phase of NCEs [7, 8]. The main disadvantage of HepG2 cells is their negligible phase I metabolism when compared with human primary hepatocytes (hPH) [9, 10]. Consequently, HepG2 cells are suitable for testing parent drug-toxicity but inappropriate for metabolite toxicity testing.

The HepaRG cell line shows better metabolic activity than HepG2 cells though still less than hPH [10, 11]. Gerets et al. showed that 21 out of 45 investigated drug metabolism related genes were significantly more highly expressed in HepaRG compared to HepG2, including CYP3A4, one of the most important xenobiotic metabolism enzymes [5]. Furthermore, they found that HepaRGs are the most inducible model in comparison to HepG2 and hPH and showed a comparable level of liver-specific gene expression to hPH, making them preferable in toxicity testing [12]. In spite of this, immortalized cell lines in general are not an ideal option for modeling DILI due to their limited metabolic capacities [13]. It also should be remembered that they are derived from hepatocellular carcinoma and may exhibit abnormal karyotypes and expression patterns, which do not mimic normal in vivo hPH [14].

HPHs are probably the cells that are the nearest model we have to a gold standard to provide human predictive DILI data. They can retain much of the liver specific phenotype for a short period under simple culture conditions [15], and are at present the closest in vitro cell model to human liver. However, the scarcity of suitable donor tissues and the nonproliferative nature of hPH results in a limited availability and life span of hPHs [16–18]. In vitro, they also rapidly undergo a progressive dedifferentiation process culminating in dramatic loss of the liver-specific phenotype [19, 20]. These drawbacks associated with the use of hPH means that despite their close resemblance to human liver, they are a suboptimal model for toxicological studies. Moreover, their use is confounded by interindividual variability between hPH donors where repeat studies on a single genetic background are not possible, which may complicate the interpretation and analysis for studies involving NCEs. In addition, these disadvantages make hPH challenging to apply to HTS. However, since hPH are the only cell type to faithfully recapitulate the key metabolic enzymes in the liver, they remain a standard model against which other cell models should be compared [21].

In recent years, numerous attempts have been made to improve the longevity of hPH in vitro. Media supplements including nicotinamide [22, 23] and DMSO together with several growth factors [24] improved the phenotypic stability and lifespan of the hPH. Other efforts to overcome the short lifespan include the development of 2D-coculture systems [25], 3D-culture systems [26–28] and 3D-bioreactor technology [29]. These systems enable better cell–cell and cell–ECM interactions, which have been reported to be crucial for maintaining liver specific pathways and functions [30, 31].

Despite promising developments in hPH culture, they have never been shown to exactly duplicate cells as they exist in an intact liver in vivo, and interdonor variability also remains an issue, causing differences in the expression of drug-metabolizing enzymes and transporters leading to varying detoxification potentials and hindering reproducibility [32]. Rodent primary hepatocytes and cell lines are commonly used as an alternative to hPH for toxicological screening purposes but interspecies differences for these cell lines compared to hPH may negatively impact the predictivity of human DILI [33].

An attractive alternative for modeling DILI is the use of hepatocyte-like cells (HLCs) derived from human induced pluripotent stem cells (hiPSCs). Their proliferative ability and the potential to mimic disease-susceptible phenotypes are major assets. These cells will be the focus of the remainder of this chapter.

2   Production of Pluripotent Stem Cells

Induced pluripotent stem cells (iPSCs) may be reprogrammed from theoretically any cell type by inducing ectopic expression of the so-called "Yamanaka Factors." The efficacy of these factors in iPSCs was first observed in mice in 2006 and was subsequently developed in human cells [34, 35]. Typically the factors used in the induction of pluripotency are OSKM (OCT4, SOX2, KLF4, and MYC), although MYC is sometimes not used due to its role at a potent oncogene [36, 37]. In addition, OSNL, instead of OSKM, has been used to generate PSCs where KLF4 and MYC are replaced with NANOG and Lin-28 [38].

The method of delivery of these factors can determine what downstream purposes the resultant iPSCs are suitable for. Integrative methods rely upon integrating new copies of the genes into the host genome where they can be highly expressed. These methods tend to be the most efficient but the transgenes cannot easily be removed once pluripotency has been achieved; this is not ideal as the transgenes may pose an oncogenic risk if used therapeutically [39]. Integrative methods, such as those used to generate the first iPSCs, require the use of retroviruses, lentiviruses or the use of an integrating plasmid [34, 35, 38].

In contrast, non-integrative methods tend to be less efficient than integrative methods but do not continue ectopic expression of the chosen factors after pluripotency has been achieved. Pluripotency can be maintained without constant, high levels of expression of the pluripotency factors. These methods typically include the use of integration incompetent or deficient viruses, such as Sendai virus or adenovirus; nonintegrating plasmids, or through the delivery of RNA or proteins of the pluripotency factors. iPSCs generated by non-integrative methods may be deemed suitable for therapeutic use. However, when using DNA-based methods the possibility of integration, however slight, remains. RNA- or protein-based reprogramming methods have no possibility of integrating into the host genome, although these methods are labor-intensive and in the case of protein delivery, relatively inefficient [40–42].

3   Developing iPSC-Derived Models for Toxicological Studies

Sison-Young et al. recently investigated protein expression in cryopreserved hPH and several cell lines (HepG2, Upcyte, and HepaRG) and concluded that none of the cell lines display cytochromes P450 expression comparable to those found in hPH with the exception of satisfactory CYP3A4 expression in HepaRG cells [10]. Therefore, the authors proposed that since these cell lines do not express the relevant metabolic enzymes at satisfactory levels, they are poor sources for the acquisition of relevant toxicological data which relies on metabolite formation or drug bioactivation (Fig. 1).

The expression profile of phase II enzymes was also examined and was shown to be more promising; HepG2 cells and Upcytes have GSTM3 (a major glutathione transferase) expression comparable to hPH, indicating their applicability in GSH conjugation studies. The authors also reported that the phase II expression profile of HepaRG cells shows multiple glutathione S-transferases equivalent to cryopreserved hPH. These cell lines were shown to

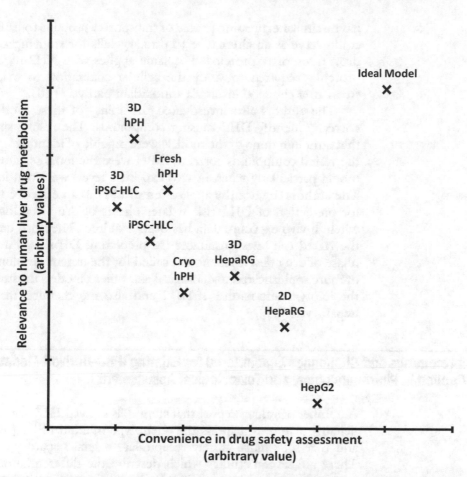

Fig. 1 Postulated convenience in drug safety assessment of different human cell culture models relative to physiological (metabolic) relevance of different current human liver models: a viewpoint. Currently, no ideal in vitro model of hepatotoxicity exists. An ideal model would fully recapitulate toxicity observed in human liver and also be cheap, easy to culture long-term and amenable to HTS (high throughput screening). This figure shows the metabolic relevance of current in vitro human liver models (*y*-axis) against their convenience for drug safety testing (*x*-axis). This encompasses factors such as ease of culture, availability, cost, amenability to HTS and similar factors. It is not implied that convenience necessarily has any impact on the value of the data or that it is inherently more or less useful than a less convenient model. A hypothetical 'ideal model' is shown for comparison. 3D culture typically improved metabolic relevance but makes routine culture and implementation of HTS more challenging. None of these models encompass any aspects of the immune system that may be implicated in relatively simple DILI and is certainly involved in the difficult-to-predict idiosyncratic DILI. *hPH*—Highly relevant to human liver when fresh, extremely difficult to culture long-term without loss of phenotype. Difficult to effectively cryopreserve [98], confounded by scarcity and interdonor variability. *iPSC-HLCs*—Non-static model with constantly improving protocols, overcomes hPH issues of scarcity and interdonor variability while retaining advantages of multiple genetic backgrounds, currently difficult to culture large-scale and confounded by low metabolic relevance. *Advanced cell lines*—e.g., HepaRG. Static model from a single genetic background showing improvement over traditional cancer cell lines. Expensive and more laborious to culture than traditional cell lines. *Traditional cell lines*—e.g., HepG2. Static model from a single genetic background with minimal expression of hepatic-specific genes, inexpensive and readily available, simple to culture and highly amenable to HTS. Lack of phase I metabolism makes them unsuitable for testing compounds requiring metabolism for toxicological events

have a similar expression profile of transporter proteins to hPH and could serve as an alternative to primary cells for studying certain drug transporter proteins. The same applies with Nrf2-regulated proteins, required to study the cellular adaptation to oxidative stress after chemical insult via antioxidant pathway [10].

The authors also investigated the ability of these models to correctly identify DILI-causing compounds. The results showed that although none of the models were capable of identifying all of the tested compounds correctly, hPH were the most sensitive cell model particularly when in vivo exposure levels were considered. The authors suggest the application of hPH as an effective model for prediction of DILI risk at later phases of drug development when in vivo exposure data has been acquired. They also deemed the tested cell lines unsuitable for predicting DILI risks in early phase of drug development and called for the urgent development of more sophisticated toxicological assessment models for studying the idiosyncratic nature of DILI and also the chemical insult in hepatocytes [21].

4   Shortcomings and Challenges Encountered for Existing iPSC-Derived Models to be Applied in Pharmacological and Toxicological Assessment

A number of studies report that stem cells derived HLCs are insufficiently mature to express the phenotype of adult hPHs [43–76] and that they more closely recapitulate a fetal hepatocyte [77]. There are several studies which describe the differentiation of a mature hepatic phenotype in HLCs, however these studies are often set backed by poor handling of controls cells (for example, the use of dedifferentiated rather than freshly isolated hPHs) or non-physiologically relevant controls (e.g., HepG2). Furthermore, the phenotyping of these models is often inadequate and fails to implement quantitatively relevant assays such as mass spectrometry. This lack of benchmarking in assessing HLCs has hindered the development of the model [78] (Fig. 2).

More positively, it has recently been demonstrated that the phenotype of HLCs retains some of the phenotype of the donor cells. For example, Yusa et al. demonstrated that α1-antitrypsin deficiency could be modeled and reversed in HLCs [79]. Another study showed that the expression profile of CYP2C9 and CYP2D6 were retained from the donor cell, which is particularly useful for toxicity elicited by drugs where these metabolic enzymes are required, such as benzbromarone and tamoxifen [80, 81]. CYPs are phase I xenobiotic metabolism enzymes that are fundamental for chemical functionality and drug elimination of the liver. However, xenobiotic metabolism can lead to the production of chemically reactive metabolites which damage cellular macromolecules and, at sufficient abundance, lead to DILI [82]. For this reason, the ability to reproducibly model rarer phenotypes which

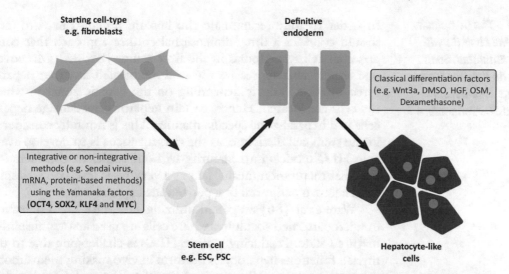

Fig. 2 Simple illustration of how HLCs may be generated from somatic cells. The starting cell type, which could be any cell type in the body, is reprogrammed to yield induced iPSCs via integrative or non-integrative methods [39, 40]. The iPSCs are then typically subjected to a series of differentiation processes via classical differentiation factors (e.g., Wnt3a, DMSO, HGF, OSM, Dexamethasone, and also using other novel methods including small molecule differentiation, e.g., dihexa) to generate hepatocyte-like cells (HLCs)

may be more prone to DILI is likely to be a major advantage for HLCs and is something that cannot easily be achieved with other current models.

The possibility of using HLCs as a hepatic model to study DILI, which is able to combine the most sought-after aspects of hPH metabolic capability and cancer cell line longevity and reproducibility has long been suggested. However, there are several key challenges which must be overcome before this goal can be fully realized:

4.1 HLC Differentiation Protocols must Mimic Several Months of Embryonic Development and Beyond

Current HLC differentiation protocols condense the entirety of *in utero* development to just a few weeks [43, 44, 83]. This may explain the lack of maturity found in current HLC models. Moreover, it is well known that cytochromes P450 maturation in the liver continues postpartum in the first months of life [78]. As such, it is necessary to improve the methodologies of the model development using in vivo liver development as a guide. Some recent published works using vitamin K and lithocholic acid to model environmental exposure postpartum showed improvements in the hepatic phenotype [75]. Other similar developments should also be investigated.

4.2 Currently HLCs in Culture Are Unstable, Similar to hPH—An Ideal Model Should Exhibit Stability In Vitro

A recent study showed that HLCs should maintain their hepatic phenotypes (assessed by rate of albumin and urea secretion) for a longer term when co-cultured with a supportive cell type, e.g., fibroblasts. Similar to hPH, HLCs undergo dedifferentiation when cultured in isolation [84]. An ideal model should be stable and long-term for the study of chronic toxicity.

4.3 The Complexity of the Liver Should Be Emulated, Such As Its Role for First-Pass Metabolism and 3D Architecture

In order to fully recapitulate the hepatic function in vitro, one should consider a three-dimensional culture approach that comprises all cell types found in the liver acinus [84, 85]. Moreover, one should also appreciate the well-established fact that hepatocytes function variably depending on the hepatic zones in which the cells are located. Hence, certain hepatotoxins damage hepatic cells in a hepatic-zone specific manner. This is not fully considered in the stem cell discipline, as the current focus is to develop available HLC models into maturity without sufficient consideration for what maturation means, i.e., at a very basic level, do we aspire to generate a periportal or a perivenous hepatocyte?

Ware et al. [86] suggested utilizing HLCs for DILI detection in micropatterned cocultures where cells are used at a "sufficiently" matured state. Producing mature HLCs is challenging due to the myriad functions hepatocytes perform in vivo making them among the most complex cell types, and therefore it may be beneficial to use HLCs in an "as is" state rather than wait until "perfect" hepatocytes are generated.

5 Suggested Culture Methods to Improve the Phenotype of Hepatocyte-like Cells

It is understood that 2D single-cell models are insufficient for the recapitulation of the full complexity of DILI development, and current research efforts are focused on developing complex models to study it and enhance HLCs [10]. Other DILI models are also under development, including co-culture models, spheroids, and microfluidics systems [28, 87, 88]. It is suggested that the methodologies used in developing the models could be modified and used in maturing the phenotype of HLC models.

Multiple studies have investigated hepatic spheroids; For example InSphero have utilized a hanging drop system to produce microtissues using both single cell and multi-cell type formats with both primary cells or cancer cell lines [89]. It has been shown that culturing HepG2 and HepaRG cells in a hanging drop system enhances their expression and inducibility of CYP mRNAs compared with 2D culture [90]. 3D culture may also prove beneficial if applied to HLCs. Recently, proteomic experiments have shown that paracetamol treatment of hPH spheroids in hanging drop produced novel mitochondrial protein adducts indicating the ability of these cells to bioactivate paracetamol to NAPQI [91].

Micropatterned plates have been reported to improve the phenotype of hPH in culture. Micropatterned co-culture of hPH with fibroblasts showed improved predictive capacity with a panel of at least 17 test compounds [92]. In addition, when elements of the innate immune system such as the Kupffer cells are included, the system may be able to model some of the mechanisms underlying idiosyncratic DILI [93]. Other innovative liver models may also be considered for improvement of the HLC phenotype including 3D bioprinted systems and perfused microtiter plate cultures [94].

6 Phenotyping iPSC Models Is Essential for Standardization

Many research groups are producing HLCs using their own methodologies for toxicological assessment. These assessments often lack intergroup standardization, which presents a challenge when comparing results from different labs [43–76]. Therefore, a benchmark requirement for evaluating HLCs' drug-metabolizing phenotype should be established, especially in comparison to common cell types used in industry (e.g., hPH, HepG2, and HepaRG cells). Standardization of phenotyping for all HLC lines would enable direct comparison between lines and protocols to simplify the identification of true advancement in the field without interference from methodological, clonal, or donor variation.

There are several other criteria for standardizing HLCs: their generation and application should be reproducible and the pharmacological phenotype should be characterized using a defined panel of training compounds and compared with a fixed reference to determine true progress. Mass spectrometry is essential as part of this benchmarking and should be integrated as part of the assays. The ideal technique for toxicological assessment is global proteomic assessment, as this approach provides an overarching visualization of the model's physiological phenotype. Due to recent advancement in mass spectrometry technique [95], it can now provide a platform for readily comparing HLCs with other cell models.

Finally, the phenotypic characterization of hepatic models could be enhanced by better understanding of the mechanisms underlying the dedifferentiation in hPH. Considering that hPH start to lose phenotype once removed from the body and original neighboring non-parenchymal cells [96, 97], this presents a challenge in maintenance and culture. Improved understanding of dedifferentiation may inform novel approaches for differentiation of HLCs [20].

7 Conclusions and Future Requirements

The complex and often idiosyncratic nature of DILI is probably due to interindividual variability as well as the multidimensional nature of the pathology of DILI—this presents a challenge for researchers to generate in vitro models that can begin to recapitulate the liver biology and the DILI phenotypes [82]. For example, Sison-Young et al. recently showed that there are currently no ideal in vitro models that can replicate the toxicological data generated by hPH which is also an imperfect model [10]. hPH quickly dedifferentiate and lose most of their xenobiotic metabolism capabilities, hindering the collection of reproducible data [20]. We still do not fully understand the physiological relevance of data generated from immortalized cell lines, which often lack the xenobiotic enzymes required for bioactivation, therefore there is an urgent demand for new in vitro models [10]. The next generation of in vitro models must have a pharmacological phenotype relevant to human liver so that the generated data are reliable for investigating xenobiotic bioactivation and/or bioaccumulation [10]. Multicellular models incorporating HLCs with non-parenchymal liver cells or immune cells have the potential to become a platform for studying DILI and as an alternative to hPH for generating reproducible data to study the interaction of NCEs with human liver—but these multicell models have to depend on the "quality" or maturity, of the cells, including iPSC-derived cells, that will be used to build them.

References

1. Laverty H et al (2011) How can we improve our understanding of cardiovascular safety liabilities to develop safer medicines? Br J Pharmacol 163(4):675–693

2. Ostapowicz G et al (2002) Results of a prospective study of acute liver failure at 17 tertiary care centers in the United States. Ann Intern Med 137(12):947–954

3. Mindikoglu AL, Magder LS, Regev A (2009) Outcome of liver transplantation for drug-induced acute liver failure in the United States: analysis of the United Network for Organ Sharing database. Liver Transpl 15(7):719–729

4. Pirmohamed M et al (2004) Adverse drug reactions as cause of admission to hospital: prospective analysis of 18 820 patients. BMJ 329(7456):15–19

5. Gerets HH et al (2012) Characterization of primary human hepatocytes, HepG2 cells, and HepaRG cells at the mRNA level and CYP activity in response to inducers and their predictivity for the detection of human hepatotoxins. Cell Biol Toxicol 28(2):69–87

6. O'Brien PJ et al (2006) High concordance of drug-induced human hepatotoxicity with in vitro cytotoxicity measured in a novel cell-based model using high content screening. Arch Toxicol 80(9):580–604

7. Gerets HH et al (2009) Selection of cytotoxicity markers for the screening of new chemical entities in a pharmaceutical context: a preliminary study using a multiplexing approach. Toxicol In Vitro 23(2):319–332

8. Sassa S et al (1987) Drug metabolism by the human hepatoma cell, Hep G2. Biochem Biophys Res Commun 143(1):52–57

9. Xu JJ, Diaz D, O'Brien PJ (2004) Applications of cytotoxicity assays and pre-lethal mechanistic assays for assessment of human hepatotoxicity potential. Chem Biol Interact 150(1):115–128

10. Sison-Young RL et al (2015) Comparative proteomic characterization of 4 human liver-derived single cell culture models reveals significant variation in the capacity for drug disposition, bioactivation, and detoxication. Toxicol Sci 147(2):412–424

11. Nelson LJ et al (2017) Human hepatic HepaRG cells maintain an organotypic phenotype with high intrinsic CYP450 activity/metabolism and significantly outperform standard HepG2/C3A cells for pharmaceutical and therapeutic applications. Basic Clin Pharmacol Toxicol 120(1):30–37

12. Wu Y et al (2016) The HepaRG cell line, a superior in vitro model to L-02, HepG2 and hiHeps cell lines for assessing drug-induced liver injury. Cell Biol Toxicol 32(1):37–59

13. Guo L et al (2011) Similarities and differences in the expression of drug-metabolizing enzymes between human hepatic cell lines and primary human hepatocytes. Drug Metab Dispos 39(3):528–538

14. Wong N et al (2000) A comprehensive karyotypic study on human hepatocellular carcinoma by spectral karyotyping. Hepatology 32(5):1060–1068

15. Smith CM et al (2012) A comprehensive evaluation of metabolic activity and intrinsic clearance in suspensions and monolayer cultures of cryopreserved primary human hepatocytes. J Pharm Sci 101(10):3989–4002

16. Guillouzo A et al (2007) The human hepatoma HepaRG cells: a highly differentiated model for studies of liver metabolism and toxicity of xenobiotics. Chem Biol Interact 168(1):66–73

17. Madan A et al (2003) Effects of prototypical microsomal enzyme inducers on cytochrome P450 expression in cultured human hepatocytes. Drug Metab Dispos 31(4):421–431

18. Richert L et al (2006) Gene expression in human hepatocytes in suspension after isolation is similar to the liver of origin, is not affected by hepatocyte cold storage and cryopreservation, but is strongly changed after hepatocyte plating. Drug Metab Dispos 34(5):870

19. Sjogren AK et al (2014) Critical differences in toxicity mechanisms in induced pluripotent stem cell-derived hepatocytes, hepatic cell lines and primary hepatocytes. Arch Toxicol 88(7):1427–1437

20. Heslop JA et al (2017) Mechanistic evaluation of primary human hepatocyte culture using global proteomic analysis reveals a selective dedifferentiation profile. Arch Toxicol 91(1):439–452

21. Sison-Young RL et al (2017) A multicenter assessment of single-cell models aligned to standard measures of cell health for prediction of acute hepatotoxicity. Arch Toxicol 91(3):1385–1400

22. Inoue C et al (1989) Nicotinamide prolongs survival of primary cultured hepatocytes without involving loss of hepatocyte specific functions. J Biol Chem 264(9):4747–4750

23. Katsura N et al (2002) Long-term culture of primary human hepatocytes with preservation of proliferative capacity and differentiated functions. J Surg Res 106(1):115–123

24. Kost DP, Michalopoulos GK (1991) Effect of 2% dimethyl sulfoxide on the mitogenic properties of epidermal growth factor and hepatocyte growth factor in primary hepatocyte culture. J Cell Physiol 147(2):274–280

25. Bale SS et al (2015) Long-term coculture strategies for primary hepatocytes and liver sinusoidal endothelial cells. Tissue Eng Part C Methods 21(4):413–422

26. Gomez-Lechon MJ et al (1998) Long-term expression of differentiated functions in hepatocytes cultured in three-dimensional collagen matrix. J Cell Physiol 177(4):553–562

27. Bachmann A et al (2015) 3D cultivation techniques for primary human hepatocytes. Microarrays 4(1):64–83

28. Bell CC et al (2016) Characterization of primary human hepatocyte spheroids as a model system for drug-induced liver injury, liver function and disease. Sci Rep 6:25187

29. Knospel F et al (2016) In vitro model for hepatotoxicity studies based on primary human hepatocyte cultivation in a perfused 3D bioreactor system. Int J Mol Sci 17(4):584

30. LeCluyse EL, Audus KL, Hochman JH (1994) Formation of extensive canalicular networks by rat hepatocytes cultured in collagen-sandwich configuration. Am J Phys 266(6 Pt 1):C1764–C1774

31. Bedossa P, Paradis V (2003) Liver extracellular matrix in health and disease. J Pathol 200(4):504–515

32. den Braver-Sewradj SP et al (2016) Inter-donor variability of phase I/phase II metabolism of three reference drugs in cryopreserved primary human hepatocytes in suspension and monolayer. Toxicol In Vitro 33:71–79

33. Olson H et al (2000) Concordance of the toxicity of pharmaceuticals in humans and in animals. Regul Toxicol Pharmacol 32(1):56–67

34. Takahashi K, Yamanaka S (2006) Induction of pluripotent stem cells from mouse embryonic and adult fibroblast cultures by defined factors. Cell 126(4):663–676

35. Takahashi K et al (2007) Induction of pluripotent stem cells from adult human fibroblasts by defined factors. Cell 131(5):861–872

36. Nakagawa M et al (2008) Generation of induced pluripotent stem cells without Myc from mouse and human fibroblasts. Nat Biotechnol 26(1):101–106

37. Okita K, Ichisaka T, Yamanaka S (2007) Generation of germline-competent induced pluripotent stem cells. Nature 448(7151):313–317

38. Yu J et al (2007) Induced pluripotent stem cell lines derived from human somatic cells. Science 318(5858):1917–1920

39. Gonzalez F, Boue S, Izpisua Belmonte JC (2011) Methods for making induced pluripotent stem cells: reprogramming a la carte. Nat Rev Genet 12(4):231–242

40. Warren L et al (2010) Highly efficient reprogramming to pluripotency and directed differentiation of human cells with synthetic modified mRNA. Cell Stem Cell 7(5):618–630

41. Zhou H et al (2009) Generation of induced pluripotent stem cells using recombinant proteins. Cell Stem Cell 4(5):381–384

42. Kim D et al (2009) Generation of human induced pluripotent stem cells by direct delivery of reprogramming proteins. Cell Stem Cell 4(6):472–476

43. Cameron K et al (2015) Recombinant laminins drive the differentiation and self-organization of hESC-derived hepatocytes. Stem Cell Reports 5(6):1250–1262

44. Godoy P et al (2015) Gene networks and transcription factor motifs defining the differentiation of stem cells into hepatocyte-like cells. J Hepatol 63(4):934–942

45. Kia R et al (2013) Stem cell-derived hepatocytes as a predictive model for drug-induced liver injury: are we there yet? Br J Clin Pharmacol 75(4):885–896

46. Cai J et al (2007) Directed differentiation of human embryonic stem cells into functional hepatic cells. Hepatology 45(5):1229–1239

47. Ek M et al (2007) Expression of drug metabolizing enzymes in hepatocyte-like cells derived from human embryonic stem cells. Biochem Pharmacol 74(3):496–503

48. Söderdahl T et al (2007) Glutathione transferases in hepatocyte-like cells derived from human embryonic stem cells. Toxicol In Vitro 21(5):929–937

49. Hay DC et al (2008) Highly efficient differentiation of hESCs to functional hepatic endoderm requires ActivinA and Wnt3a signaling. Proc Natl Acad Sci U S A 105(34):12301–12306

50. Shiraki N et al (2008) Differentiation of mouse and human embryonic stem cells into hepatic lineages. Genes Cells 13(7):731–746

51. Agarwal S, Holton KL, Lanza R (2008) Efficient differentiation of functional hepatocytes from human embryonic stem cells. Stem Cells 26(5):1117–1127

52. Moore RN, Moghe PV (2009) Expedited growth factor-mediated specification of human embryonic stem cells toward the hepatic lineage. Stem Cell Res 3(1):51–62

53. Basma H et al (2009) Differentiation and transplantation of human embryonic stem cell-derived hepatocytes. Gastroenterology 136(3):990–999

54. Song Z et al (2009) Efficient generation of hepatocyte-like cells from human induced pluripotent stem cells. Cell Res 19(11):1233–1242

55. Duan Y et al (2010) Differentiation and characterization of metabolically functioning hepatocytes from human embryonic stem cells. Stem Cells 28(4):674–686

56. Synnergren J et al (2010) Transcriptional profiling of human embryonic stem cells differentiating to definitive and primitive endoderm and further toward the hepatic lineage. Stem Cells Dev 19(7):961–978

57. Touboul T et al (2010) Generation of functional hepatocytes from human embryonic stem cells under chemically defined conditions that recapitulate liver development. Hepatology 51(5):1754–1765

58. Brolen G et al (2010) Hepatocyte-like cells derived from human embryonic stem cells specifically via definitive endoderm and a progenitor stage. J Biotechnol 145(3):284–294

59. Ghodsizadeh A et al (2010) Generation of liver disease-specific induced pluripotent stem cells along with efficient differentiation to functional hepatocyte-like cells. Stem Cell Rev 6(4):622–632

60. Liu H et al (2010) Generation of endoderm-derived human induced pluripotent stem cells from primary hepatocytes. Hepatology 51(5):1810–1819

61. Si-Tayeb K et al (2010) Highly efficient generation of human hepatocyte-like cells from induced pluripotent stem cells. Hepatology 51(1):297–305

62. Sullivan GJ et al (2010) Generation of functional human hepatic endoderm from human induced pluripotent stem cells. Hepatology 51(1):329–335

63. Rashid ST et al (2010) Modeling inherited metabolic disorders of the liver using human induced pluripotent stem cells. J Clin Invest 120(9):3127–3136

64. Zhang S et al (2011) Rescue of ATP7B function in hepatocyte-like cells from Wilson's disease induced pluripotent stem cells using gene therapy or the chaperone drug curcumin. Hum Mol Genet 20(16):3176–3187

65. Bone HK et al (2011) A novel chemically directed route for the generation of definitive endoderm from human embryonic stem cells based on inhibition of GSK-3. J Cell Sci 124(Pt 12):1992–2000

66. Yildirimman R et al (2011) Human embryonic stem cell derived hepatocyte-like cells as a tool for in vitro hazard assessment of chemical carcinogenicity. Toxicol Sci 124(2):278–290

67. Chen YF et al (2012) Rapid generation of mature hepatocyte-like cells from human induced pluripotent stem cells by an efficient three-step protocol. Hepatology 55(4):1193–1203

68. Cayo MA et al (2012) JD induced pluripotent stem cell-derived hepatocytes faithfully recapitulate the pathophysiology of familial hypercholesterolemia. Hepatology 56(6):2163–2171

69. Schwartz RE et al (2012) Modeling hepatitis C virus infection using human induced pluripotent stem cells. Proc Natl Acad Sci U S A 109(7):2544–2548

70. Takayama K et al (2012) Efficient generation of functional hepatocytes from human embryonic stem cells and induced pluripotent stem cells by HNF4alpha transduction. Mol Ther 20(1):127–137

71. Choi SM et al (2013) Efficient drug screening and gene correction for treating liver disease using patient-specific stem cells. Hepatology 57(6):2458–2468

72. Ramasamy TS et al (2013) Application of three-dimensional culture conditions to human embryonic stem cell-derived definitive endoderm cells enhances hepatocyte differentiation and functionality. Tissue Eng Part A 19(3–4):360–367

73. Gieseck Iii RL et al (2014) Maturation of induced pluripotent stem cell derived hepatocytes by 3D-culture. PLoS One 9(1):e86372

74. Jia B et al (2014) Modeling of hemophilia A using patient-specific induced pluripotent stem cells derived from urine cells. Life Sci 108(1):22–29

75. Avior Y et al (2015) Microbial-derived lithocholic acid and vitamin K2 drive the metabolic maturation of pluripotent stem cells-derived and fetal hepatocytes. Hepatology 62(1):265–278

76. Chien Y et al (2015) Synergistic effects of carboxymethyl-hexanoyl chitosan, cationic polyurethane-short branch PEI in miR122 gene delivery: accelerated differentiation of iPSCs into mature hepatocyte-like cells and improved stem cell therapy in a hepatic failure model. Acta Biomater 13:228–244

77. Baxter M et al (2015) Phenotypic and functional analyses show stem cell-derived hepatocyte-like cells better mimic fetal rather than adult hepatocytes. J Hepatol 62(3):581–589

78. Goldring C et al (2017) Stem cell-derived models to improve mechanistic understanding and prediction of human drug-induced liver injury. Hepatology 65(2):710–721

79. Yusa K et al (2011) Targeted gene correction of alpha1-antitrypsin deficiency in induced pluripotent stem cells. Nature 478(7369):391–394

80. Ulvestad M et al (2013) Drug metabolizing enzyme and transporter protein profiles of hepatocytes derived from human embryonic and induced pluripotent stem cells. Biochem Pharmacol 86(5):691–702

81. Takayama K et al (2014) Prediction of interindividual differences in hepatic functions and drug sensitivity by using human iPS-derived hepatocytes. Proc Natl Acad Sci U S A 111(47):16772–16777

82. Park BK et al (2011) Managing the challenge of chemically reactive metabolites in drug development. Nat Rev Drug Discov 10(4):292–306

83. Liu J et al (2015) Efficient episomal reprogramming of blood mononuclear cells and differentiation to hepatocytes with functional drug metabolism. Exp Cell Res 338(2):203–213

84. Berger DR et al (2015) Enhancing the functional maturity of induced pluripotent stem cell-derived human hepatocytes by controlled presentation of cell-cell interactions in vitro. Hepatology 61(4):1370–1381

85. Davidson MD, Ware BR, Khetani SR (2015) Stem cell-derived liver cells for drug testing and disease modeling. Discov Med 19(106):349–358

86. Ware BR, Berger DR, Khetani SR (2015) Prediction of drug-induced liver injury in micropatterned co-cultures containing iPSC-derived human hepatocytes. Toxicol Sci 145(2):252–262

87. Bhushan A et al (2013) Towards a three-dimensional microfluidic liver platform for predicting drug efficacy and toxicity in humans. Stem Cell Res Ther 4(Suppl 1):S16

88. Goers L, Freemont P, Polizzi KM (2014) Co-culture systems and technologies: taking synthetic biology to the next level. J R Soc Interface 11(96):20140065

89. Marx V (2013) Cell culture: a better brew. Nature 496(7444):253–258

90. Takahashi Y et al (2015) 3D spheroid cultures improve the metabolic gene expression profiles of HepaRG cells. Biosci Rep 35(3):e00208

91. Bruderer R et al (2015) Extending the limits of quantitative proteome profiling with data-independent acquisition and application to acetaminophen-treated three-dimensional liver microtissues. Mol Cell Proteomics 14(5):1400–1410

92. Chan TS et al (2013) Meeting the challenge of predicting hepatic clearance of compounds slowly metabolized by cytochrome P450 using a novel hepatocyte model, HepatoPac. Drug Metab Dispos 41(12):2024–2032

93. Nguyen TV et al (2015) Establishment of a hepatocyte-kupffer cell coculture model for

assessment of proinflammatory cytokine effects on metabolizing enzymes and drug transporters. Drug Metab Dispos 43(5): 774–785

94. Domansky K et al (2010) Perfused multiwell plate for 3D liver tissue engineering. Lab Chip 10(1):51–58

95. Kitteringham NR et al (2009) Multiple reaction monitoring for quantitative biomarker analysis in proteomics and metabolomics. J Chromatogr B Analyt Technol Biomed Life Sci 877(13):1229–1239

96. Bhatia SN et al (1998) Probing heterotypic cell interactions: hepatocyte function in microfabricated co-cultures. J Biomater Sci Polym Ed 9(11):1137–1160

97. Zinchenko YS et al (2006) Hepatocyte and kupffer cells co-cultured on micropatterned surfaces to optimize hepatocyte function. Tissue Eng 12(4):751–761

98. Terry C et al (2010) Optimization of the cryopreservation and thawing protocol for human hepatocytes for use in cell transplantation. Liver Transpl 16(2):229–237

Chapter 11

Engineered Human Liver Cocultures for Investigating Drug-Induced Liver Injury

Chase P. Monckton and Salman R. Khetani

Abstract

Drug-induced liver injury (DILI) remains a major cause of drug attrition, black-box warnings on marketed drugs, and acute liver failures. It is clear with several high-profile drug failures that animal models do not suffice for predicting human DILI largely due to species-specific differences in drug metabolism pathways. Thus, in vitro models of the human liver are playing an ever-important role in mitigating DILI risk during preclinical testing. Methods to isolate and culture hepatocytes on collagen-coated plastic in the presence of supportive liver- and non-liver-derived nonparenchymal cell types (NPCs) were developed several decades ago; however, improvements were needed to stabilize diverse hepatic functions for several weeks to enable chronic drug treatment as in the clinic. Today, engineering tools such as protein micropatterning, microfluidics, specialized plates, biomaterial scaffolds, and bioprinting enable precise control over the cellular microenvironment for enhancing and stabilizing hepatic functions in the presence of NPC types, including those derived from the liver towards determining their impact on DILI progression. The introduction of induced pluripotent stem cell-derived human hepatocyte-like cells can potentially allow a better understanding of inter-individual differences in idiosyncratic DILI. Here, we review the abovementioned advances in the engineering of human liver cocultures and their utilization for predicting clinical DILI with high sensitivity/specificity and elucidating underlying mechanisms. Key platforms and associated validation data sets are presented to highlight major trends and pending issues to be addressed moving forward. In the future, engineered human liver cocultures will reduce drug attrition, animal usage, and cases of DILI in humans.

Key words Microfabrication, Soft lithography, Microfluidics, Micropatterned cocultures, Liver-on-a-chip, Hepatocytes, Nonparenchymal cells, 3D liver spheroids

1 Introduction

Drug-induced liver injury (DILI) remains a leading cause of pre-clinical and clinical drug attrition, black-box warnings on marketed drugs, and acute liver failures in the USA alone [1]. Numerous marketed drugs can cause DILI that can manifest itself as cellular necrosis, hepatitis, cholestasis, fibrosis, or a mixture of injury types [2]. DILI phenomena can occur through intrinsic or idiosyncratic pathways, the latter being the greater concern for drug development because its mechanism of action is variable in the clinic and not

Minjun Chen and Yvonne Will (eds.), *Drug-Induced Liver Toxicity*, Methods in Pharmacology and Toxicology, https://doi.org/10.1007/978-1-4939-7677-5_11, © Springer Science+Business Media, LLC, part of Springer Nature 2018

well characterized. The severity of idiosyncratic DILI can be exacerbated by states of stress (i.e., inflammation), patient-specific risk factors (i.e., genetics, age, gender, diet), and underlying disease states (i.e., hepatitis, cholestasis, and fibrosis). Unfortunately, the live animal testing required by the Food and Drug Administration (FDA) during preclinical drug development is only capable of identifying <50% of human DILI, largely due to differences in species-specific drug metabolism pathways [3]. Additionally, traditional animal testing is time-consuming, requires a large capital investment, and does not capture human patient risk factors for DILI such as genetics and disease.

Given the abovementioned challenges with screening drugs in animals, regulatory agencies and the pharmaceutical/biotech industry are under increased pressures to develop and adopt human-relevant methods to mitigate DILI risk prior to human clinical trials. With such an urgent need, the field of human liver culture platforms has grown rapidly over the last 5–10 years [4]. The utilization of engineering tools such as protein micropatterning, microfluidics, specialized plates, biomaterial scaffolds, and bioprinting has enabled greater control over the cellular microenvironment which has increased the longevity and reproducibility of cellular responses. Regardless of the specific technology utilized to build in vitro liver models, coculture with nonparenchymal cell (NPC) types has been shown to enhance and stabilize the phenotype of primary hepatocytes from several species for several weeks. In this chapter, we will discuss the use of the abovementioned engineering tools to create liver cocultures that have shown utility in detecting DILI. We begin with a brief description of conventional/traditional coculture models and then discuss engineered liver models starting with static micropatterned cocultures, followed by static spheroidal and bioprinted liver cocultures, and finally perfused platforms that can be adapted to different types of cocultures. Where appropriate, we discuss the initial development of engineered cocultures using animal hepatocytes or cancerous cell lines as is common practice in this field. We then discuss best practices in appraising the phenotype of liver cocultures before and after drug treatment, followed by the more recent use of liver cocultures for modeling diseases that can affect DILI outcomes and enable the simultaneous assessment of drug efficacy and toxicity. Finally, we summarize the key trends and the pending issues that we believe will need to be addressed moving forward. We highlight representative platforms, some in commercial practice, to demonstrate major points instead of being exhaustive in discussing every liver coculture model developed in the field.

2   Conventional Cocultures of Hepatocytes and Nonparenchymal Cell Types

Heterotypic interactions between parenchymal cells and NPCs are important in many organ systems and the liver is no exception. The formation of the liver in the embryo from the endodermal foregut and mesenchymal vascular structures is thought to be mediated by heterotypic interactions [5]. Indeed, without the interaction with the mesenchyme, the endoderm does not fully undergo hepatic differentiation [6, 7]. Heterotypic cell–cell interactions also play critical roles in the adult liver [8]. In the liver sinusoid, hepatocytes are separated from the fenestrated liver sinusoidal endothelial cells (LSECs) by a thin extracellular matrix (ECM) protein region called the Space of Disse. Hepatic stellate cells (HSCs), which normally store vitamin A droplets, have elaborate, extensive processes that contact the hepatocytes within the sinusoid. The Kupffer cells (KCs), the resident macrophages of the liver, are free to roam through the blood and liver tissue compartments. Lastly, cholangiocytes (biliary ductal cells) line the bile ducts that drain the contents of the hepatic bile canaliculi into the gall bladder.

In vitro, coculture with both liver- and non-liver-derived NPC types can transiently induce functions in primary hepatocytes from multiple species, including humans [5, 9]. Langenbach et al. reported in 1979 the first coculture to our knowledge of adult rat hepatocytes on a layer of irradiated C3H/10T1/2 mouse embryo cells [10]. The cocultured hepatocytes maintained in vivo-like morphological characteristics and were capable of metabolizing N-2-acetylaminofluorene to water-soluble products at 14 days in culture at ~70% of the levels observed on the day of seeding. In contrast, hepatocytes cultured on their own lost metabolic activity after 5 days. Michalopoulus et al. also showed in 1979 that adult rat hepatocytes cultured on confluent human fibroblasts maintained characteristic morphology, basal cytochrome P450 (CYP450) activity, and inducibility of CYP450 enzymes via phenobarbital and methylcholanthrene for 10 days [11]. Subsequently, the Guillouzo group in 1983–1984 demonstrated long-term (40+ days) retention of albumin secretion from adult rat and human hepatocytes upon cocultivation with rat liver epithelial cells [12, 13].

Since the abovementioned pioneering studies, liver-derived NPC types that have been shown to induce phenotypic changes in hepatocytes include HSCs [14], LSECs [15], KCs [16], and the entire NPC fraction of the liver [17]. Interestingly, functions in hepatocytes can also be modulated via cocultivation with NPC types from other organ systems and species, such as murine embryonic 3T3 fibroblasts [18], rat dermal fibroblasts [19], Chinese hamster ovary cells [20], canine kidney epithelial cells [21], bovine aortic epithelial cells [19, 22], and lung epithelial cells [23]. Furthermore, hepatocytes isolated from adult and fetal human [13, 24], rat [12, 25], chick [26], and porcine [27] liver have been shown to benefit functionally upon coculture with NPCs. In addition to viable NPCs, hepatocyte functions can be induced on NPC feeder layers that are desiccated and heated [17], glutaraldehyde-fixed [15], or growth-arrested via mitomycin C treatment [28]. In some instances, the functions of select NPCs are also modulated when cocultured with hepatocytes [29].

There have been several studies which have elucidated the role of potential molecular mediators (i.e., receptors, gap junctions, cytokines, cadherins, and ECM proteins) of the so-called "coculture effect" between hepatocytes and NPC types. To date, the data suggest that both matrix deposition and direct cell–cell contact play roles in the coculture effect [5, 19, 20, 30–33], whereas soluble factors alone (i.e., NPC conditioned medium) have proven largely ineffective [17, 28, 34]. However, the complete molecular mechanism underlying the coculture effect remains undefined. Given the plethora of different NPC types that can induce hepatospecific functions with varying kinetics, it is likely that many distinct mechanisms may operate in concert, each modulating a subset of liver functions.

Conventional (randomly distributed) hepatocyte–NPC cocultures described above have proven useful to investigate physiological and pathophysiological processes such as host response to sepsis [35], mutagenesis [36], xenobiotic metabolism and toxicity [37], response to oxidative stress [38], lipid metabolism [39], and induction of the acute phase response [40]. Such cocultures have also been explored for their potential use in clinical bioartificial liver devices [41]. However, randomly distributed cocultures inherently contain areas of the monolayer with suboptimal homotypic and heterotypic cell–cell interactions due to a lack of control over the cellular architecture. Such suboptimal cell–cell interactions can lead to an instability and low levels of liver functions over long-term culture [42]. For example, randomly distributed cocultures of primary human hepatocytes (PHHs) and 3T3-J2 murine embryonic fibroblasts are not able to sustain infection with hepatitis B/C viruses [43, 44] and malaria [45], which is likely due to the incomplete polarization and functions of the hepatocytes. Lastly, randomly distributed cocultures do not allow investigations into how homotypic and heterotypic cell–cell interactions between hepatocytes and their NPC neighbors affects liver functions without the confounding effects of cell density variations on cell numbers/ratios and nutrient depletion rates.

3 Micropatterned Cocultures

In contrast to a random seeding of two cell types on a surface as in the abovementioned conventional hepatocyte-NPC cocultures, microfabrication tools adapted from the semiconductor industry allow for the creation of heterogeneous surfaces with precise features that can range in sizes from a few nanometers to micrometers [46]. In the case of the liver, Singhvi et al. in 1994 first micropatterned rat hepatocytes on laminin-coated monolayers of self-assembled alkanethiols that were surrounded by nonadhesive polyethylene glycol (PEG) to keep the cells from migrating off the laminin-coated domains [47]. Such micropatterned hepatocytes secreted higher levels of albumin and exhibited reduced DNA synthesis on adhesive domains of a smaller surface area that restricted cell spreading as opposed to surfaces uniformly coated with laminin that allowed complete cell spreading. However, modulating cell spreading alone was not sufficient to stabilize the hepatocyte phenotype beyond 3 days in culture.

Bhatia et al. subsequently employed photolithographic tools to first micropattern rat hepatocytes on collagen-coated circular domains and then surround these domains with 3T3-J2 murine embryonic fibroblasts [18, 48], an NPC type that is also used to support keratinocytes in coculture [49]. Such micropatterned cocultures (MPCCs) allowed tuning of homotypic interactions between hepatocytes and the heterotypic interface between hepatocytes and the fibroblasts while keeping cell numbers/ratios constant across the various patterned configurations. Overall, several key findings emerged from these pioneering studies: (a) circular domains, as opposed to patterns with sharp corners (i.e., rectangles, squares, and triangles), led to better retention of patterning fidelity over several weeks in culture; (b) controlling homotypic interactions between hepatocytes alone was not sufficient to rescue liver-specific functions in the absence of coculture with the fibroblasts; (c) increasing the heterotypic interface between fibroblasts and hepatocytes via a reduction in the diameter of the collagen-coated domains led to higher hepatospecific functions (albumin and urea secretion) than when the domain diameter was larger; and, (d) contact with fibroblasts was necessary since both fibroblast- and coculture-conditioned media were not able to rescue the phenotype of hepatocyte-only cultures. Khetani et al. subsequently showed that the J2 sub-clone of the 3T3 fibroblasts induced optimal functions in hepatocytes than other 3T3 subclones such as NIH/3T3, 3T3-Swiss, and 3T3-L1 [31].

Creation of MPCCs using PHHs, both freshly isolated and cryopreserved, and 3T3-J2 fibroblasts showed a similar induction of liver-specific functions relative to pure hepatocyte cultures as observed with rat hepatocytes [42]. However, in contrast to studies using rat hepatocytes, PHHs displayed highest functions on collagen-coated domains of intermediate diameters (~500 μm domain diameter with 1200 μm center-to-center spacing between domains), suggesting a species-specific balance in homotypic interactions between hepatocytes and their heterotypic interactions with the fibroblasts. This example illustrates the need to empirically determine the effects of an engineering technique on the functions of animal versus human liver cells. More importantly, exercising precise control over homotypic and heterotypic cell–cell interactions via the MPCC technique led to high and stable PHH functions, including activities of drug metabolism enzymes and transporters, for 4–6 weeks as compared to an unstable phenotype observed in randomly distributed cocultures of the same two cell types with similar ratios.

The abovementioned photolithographic micropatterning process is time-consuming, requires a clean room and several specialized pieces of equipment, and is compatible only with one culture dish at a time (i.e., serial). Therefore, Khetani and Bhatia developed stencils using polydimethylsiloxane (PDMS) to enable the rapid creation of MPCCs in a 24-well plate format for medium-throughput drug screening [42]. However, since PDMS is a porous and hydrophobic material, drugs and proteins in the culture medium tended to get wicked up in the material, thereby reducing the molecule concentration available to the cells. Furthermore, the stencil process was not adaptable to 96-well plates for higher-throughput screening. Thus, a new process utilizing a PDMS mask to protect desired regions of an ECM protein coat on a surface was developed to create MPCCs in industry-standard polystyrene 24- and 96-well plates (Fig. 1a–c); this process has been described in precise detail [50, 51]. The Bhatia group at MIT has recently used a similar process to further miniaturize MPCCs into 384-well plates. Miniaturized human MPCCs in a multiwell format have been extensively validated for several applications in drug development, such as drug clearance predictions [52–54], drug–drug interactions [42, 53, 55, 56], drug metabolite profiling [57–59], drug–transporter interactions [56, 60], DILI prediction [61, 62], and infection with hepatitis B/C viruses [43, 44] and malaria [45, 63]. More recently, MPCCs allowed investigations into the effects of chronic hyperglycemia as in type 2 diabetes mellitus on PHH functions [64, 65]. Below, we focus on data sets that pertain to DILI prediction.

MPCCs created with PHHs or primary rat hepatocytes were treated for up to 9 days with 45 drugs of which 35 have known DILI liabilities in the clinic while ten are generally considered not toxic to the liver [62] (Fig. 1d). Given inter-individual differences in drug concentrations in plasma and within the liver, MPCCs were treated with drug concentrations up to 100-fold of the reported C_{max} (maximum drug concentration in human plasma) for each drug, which is also common with other platforms and does not increase the false positive rate for DILI detection [66]. Overall, several key findings emerged from this pioneering study using MPCCs: (a) repeat drug treatment for at least 9 days improved the sensitivity for DILI detection without a reduction in specificity; (b) secreted albumin and urea as liver function biomarkers were as sensitive for DILI prediction as the classic hepatotoxicity marker, ATP, which allows monitoring of the same culture wells for drug effects over many time-points while conserving the use of limited PHHs; (c) human MPCCs showed a 2.3-fold improvement in sensitivity without compromising specificity for

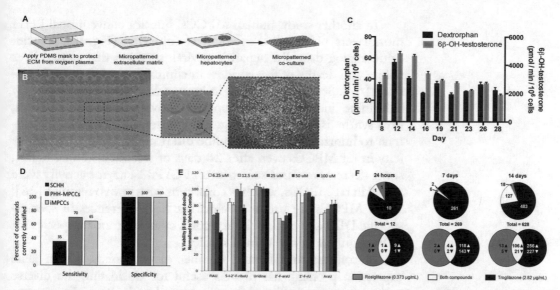

Fig. 1 The micropatterned coculture platform. (**a**) Tissue culture polystyrene (or glass) can be uniformly coated with extracellular matrix protein (ECM) such as collagen and protected with a polydimethylsiloxane (PDMS) stamp [70]. Exposed areas of ECM are ablated under oxygen plasma, leaving micropatterned ECM islands that match the geometry of the PDMS stamp. Hepatocytes, either primary or induced pluripotent stem cell-derived, selectively attach to ECM islands, and nonparenchymal cells (NPCs) fill in the surrounding area. (**b**) An industry standard 96-well plate showing uniform hepatocyte islands micropatterned using the process in panel (**a**). The NPCs used in this example are 3T3-J2 murine embryonic fibroblasts surrounding the primary human hepatocyte (PHH) colonies. (**c**) MPCCs created using PHHs maintain high levels of CYP450 activities for several weeks. Reprinted with permission from [53]. CYP3A4 activity was assessed via metabolism of testosterone into 6β-OH-testosterone, while CYP2D6 activity was assessed via metabolism of dextromethorphan into dextrorphan. (**d**) Sensitivity and specificity for DILI prediction in sandwich cultured PHHs (SCHH), MPCCs created using PHHs (PHH-MPCCs), and MPCCs created using iPSC-derived human hepatocyte-like cells (iMPCCs). All culture models were treated with 37 hepatotoxic drugs and ten non-liver-toxic drugs (24-h treatment for SCHH, 9-day treatment for PHH-MPCCs, and 6-day treatment for iMPCCs) to calculate the sensitivity and specificity. Reprinted with permission from [62, 72]. (**e**) MPCCs containing PHHs that were dosed for 8 days with 0, 6.25, or 50 μM fialuridine and five other analog compounds [68]. Culture viability was assessed using the MTT assay and normalized to vehicle-only controls. Only fialuridine caused a dose-dependent toxicity in the MPCCs. On the other hand, no dose-dependent toxicity was observed in MPCCs created using primary rat hepatocytes and dosed with the same compounds at the same doses for 8 days (data not shown). (**f**) Time-dependent global gene expression changes in MPCCs treated with troglitazone or rosiglitazone at their respective C_{max} levels for up to 14 days. Reprinted with permission from [69]. Number of genes upregulated or downregulated (|fold change| > 2.0 and |difference in expression| > 100 using Affymetrix whole genome human microarrays) in MPCCs by troglitazone (2.82 μg/mL) or rosiglitazone (0.373 μg/mL) or both drugs relative to vehicle (DMSO) control after treatment for 24 h (*left*), 7 days (*middle*), and 14 days (*right*)

DILI detection as compared to a 24-h treatment of ECM-sandwiched PHH monolayers with the same drugs; (d) human MPCCs were more sensitive (65.7%) than their rat counterparts (48.6%) for detecting human DILI across a wide range of drugs; (e) human MPCCs displayed a 100% sensitivity for drugs with the highest DILI concern (i.e., black-box warnings or withdrawn from the marketplace) when at least two PHH donors were utilized.

In another study, human MPCCs, but not conventional PHH monolayers, picked up the toxicity of fialuridine (Fig. 1e), a nucleoside analog drug for hepatitis B viral infection that caused liver failure and deaths of five patients in clinical trials due to lactic acidosis [67]. Several end-points in human MPCCs were affected by fialuridine including mitochondrial activity, albumin secretion, urea synthesis, and morphological integrity of the PHHs. In contrast to human MPCCs, fialuridine did not cause overt hepatotoxicity in rat MPCCs even after 28 days of treatment. Nonetheless, some decreases in urea secretion and CYP3A enzyme activity were noted in rat MPCCs, which is consistent with in vivo findings [68]. Thus, MPCCs are useful to elucidate key differences in species-specific DILI and enable the selection of an appropriate species for FDA-required in vivo animal studies.

In contrast to a limited number of end-points, global gene expression profiling has proven useful for elucidating the diverse pathways that are affected in cells treated with drugs. In a recent study [69], Ware et al. found that human MPCCs treated for up to 14 days with troglitazone (clinical hepatotoxin) or rosiglitazone (non-liver-toxic structural analog of troglitazone) at each drug's respective C_{max} did not cause overt hepatotoxicity, as is the case in the majority of patients who were administered these drugs safely without experiencing severe DILI. However, when analyzing MPCCs at the gene expression level using Affymetrix whole-genome human microarrays, 12, 269, and 628 genes were differentially expressed after 1, 7, and 14 days of drug treatment, respectively, relative to the vehicle control (Fig. 1f). Troglitazone modulated >75% of these differentially expressed genes across pathways such as fatty acid and drug metabolism, oxidative stress, inflammatory response, and complement/coagulation cascades. Escalating rosiglitazone's dose to that of troglitazone's C_{max} increased rosiglitazone-modulated transcripts relative to the lower dose; however, over half the identified transcripts were still exclusively modulated by troglitazone, thereby suggesting that troglitazone's effects on PHHs are partly due to troglitazone's intrinsic properties as opposed to its higher C_{max} than rosiglitazone. More generally, other hepatotoxins including nefazodone, ibufenac, and tolcapone also induced a greater number of differentially expressed genes in MPCCs than their non-liver-toxic analogs, buspirone, ibuprofen, and entacapone, after 7 days of treatment. This study showed for the first time that extraction of global gene expression profiles from PHHs repeatedly treated with drugs for up to 2 weeks can be highly useful to distinguish hepatotoxic drugs from their nontoxic analogs and understand mechanism of action at drug doses that are pharmacologically relevant and may not necessarily lead to overt hepatotoxicity in a majority of the patients.

The MPCC technology has also been adapted to induced pluripotent stem cell-derived human hepatocyte-like cells (iHeps) [70], which afford the opportunity to sustainably evaluate drug toxicity across diverse genetic backgrounds [71]. Berger et al. found that as compared to a severely immature and declining iHep phenotype in conventional monolayers, both micropatterning and cocultivation with 3T3-J2 fibroblasts were beneficial to functionally mature iHeps towards the adult PHH phenotype and stabilize iHep phenotype for at least 4 weeks in vitro at previously unprecedented levels [70]. More importantly, when MPCCs containing iHeps were dosed with a set of 47 drugs for 6 days and assessed for hepatotoxicity (ATP) and liver functions (albumin and urea), the sensitivity (65%) and specificity (100%) for DILI detection were remarkably similar to the values obtained with MPCCs containing PHHs treated with the same drugs (70% sensitivity and 100% specificity) (Fig. 1d) [72]. These results suggest that MPCCs containing iHeps may be useful for an initial drug toxicity screen during drug development; however, mechanistic inquiries into DILI outcomes will require further probing of active pathways within stabilized iHeps relative to PHHs.

The MPCC platform was designed to be modular in that the NPC type/population can be modified without significantly affecting the hepatocyte homotypic interactions on the micropatterned domains, which are important for maintaining cell polarity. Nguyen et al. augmented preestablished MPCCs with primary human KCs once the hepatic phenotype was stable after 5–7 days [73]. Stimulating the KCs in MPCCs with bacterial derived endotoxin, lipopolysaccharide (LPS), led to cytokine-mediated downregulation of CYP450s in PHHs, which can affect DILI outcomes. Davidson et al. have recently augmented MPCCs with primary human HSCs at physiological ratios with PHHs and demonstrated effects on hepatic functions that are reminiscent of a nonalcoholic steatohepatitis/early fibrosis phenotype [74] as discussed further below in the "Modeling Diseases Using Cocultures" section. We are now augmenting MPCCs with LSECs and all of the liver NPCs combined to enable the crosstalk between liver cell types in modeling different types of DILI. Ultimately, different configurations of MPCCs with respect to the source/species of hepatocytes as well as the type of NPC population may be useful for elucidating the role of cell–cell interactions in DILI.

4   Spheroidal and Bioprinted Cocultures

In addition to cocultivation with NPC types, another strategy to stabilize hepatocyte functions is to culture them in spheroidal configurations, which leads to the establishment of homotypic cell–cell interactions and the presence of ECM proteins within and around the spheroids [75]. While coculture with NPC types is not entirely necessary in spheroidal configurations, functions can be further enhanced and the role of heterotypic cell–cell interactions on drug outcomes can be properly studied. Thus, most of the commercially available liver spheroidal platforms contain cocultures of hepato-cytes with one or more NPC types. Hepatic spheroids can sponta-neously form on nontreated culture plates or those coated with polymers such as poly (2-hydroxymethyl methacrylate) (HEMA) [76] or proprietary coatings (i.e., Corning's ultralow attachment surface [77]). Such spheroids have been shown to display high viability, albumin secretion, and activities of major CYP450 enzymes for 5 weeks [77]. Chronic treatment with hepatotoxins, including fialuridine, for up to 28 days showed time- and dose-dependent hepatotoxicity (Fig. 2a–c).

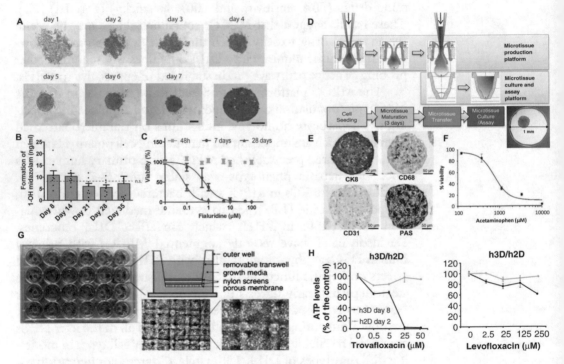

Fig. 2 Spheroidal liver cocultures. (**a**) Time series showing progressing spheroid aggregation over time on ultra-low attachment 96-well plates from Corning [77]. Scale bar is 100 μm. (**b**) CYP3A4 activity over 35 days in the spheroids of panel (**a**) treated with midazolam. No change in the rate of midazolam hydroxylation was detected over 5 weeks (n.s. corresponds to $p > 0.05$, F-test). (**c**) Viability of the spheroids of panel (**a**) treated with fialuridine over 28 days. (**d**) The InSphero strategy to create multicellular spheroids. The GravityPLUS 96-well plate allows a single microtissue to form in each drop [78]. Once the microtissues are formed, they are transferred to a GravityTRAP plate that has a proprietary nonadhesive coating to enable the long-term culture of the microtissues without attachment. Brightfield image of a single microtissue is shown. (**e**) Immunohistochemistry staining for markers in microtissue of panel (**d**). CK8 is an epithelial (hepatocyte) marker; CD68 is a macrophage marker; CD31 is an endothelial marker; and, PAS (periodic acid Schiff stain) is a glycogen stain, typically found in hepatocytes in the liver. (**f**) Dose-dependent toxicity of acetaminophen in microtissues of panel (**d**) that were treated with drug for 14 days and assessed for ATP content. (**g**) 24-well insert plate system for growth of liver cocultures on nylon scaffolds. Reprinted with permission from [80]. Phase-contrast micrographs of the morphology of 30-day-old human liver coculture. Scale bars are 100 μm. (**h**) Dose-dependent toxicity of hepatotoxic drug, trovafloxacin (*left*), and its non-liver-toxic analog, levofloxacin (*right*), in human cocultures of panel (**g**) (h3D) in comparison with hepatocyte monolayers (h2D)

With the abovementioned strategy of forming spheroids on uniformly coated nonadhesive surfaces, it is difficult to control the spheroid size and smaller spheroids can merge to form larger spheroids that can have necrotic cores due to limitations in oxygen/nutrient diffusion. To mitigate such a challenge, specialized plates and scaffolds have been developed to direct the assembly of uniformly sized spheroids that remain separated for interrogation following drug treatment. For instance, InSphero Inc. developed a specialized plate for creating hanging liquid drops that allow the formation of hepatic spheroids (one per well) of controlled diameters, which remain viable and secrete albumin for ~1 month (Fig. 2d–f) [78]. The introduction of KCs into the hepatic spheroids allows investigation into the effects of LPS-activated KCs on drug-induced hepatotoxicity. Proctor et al. recently carried out a relatively comprehensive validation of the InSphero platform-generated PHH/KC spheroids for hepatotoxicity detection by measuring ATP levels in the lysates of spheroids that were treated for up to 14 days with a panel of 110 drugs with and without reported cases of clinical DILI [79]. Irrespective of comparing IC_{50} values or exposure-corrected margin of safety values (IC_{50}/C_{max}), the spheroids demonstrated increased sensitivity in identifying known hepatotoxicants than short-term PHH monolayers (~60% versus ~40%), while specificity was similar across both assays (~80–85%). Using another commercial platform by Regenemed Inc., Kostadinova et al. seeded a mixture of liver NPCs onto a porous nylon scaffold placed within a removable transwell followed by seeding of PHHs onto the preestablished liver NPC/nylon culture [80]. PHHs in this platform secreted liver proteins (albumin, transferrin, and fibrinogen) and displayed CYP450 activities for 77–90 days, and were more sensitive to hepatotoxic drugs than monolayer controls (Fig. 2g and h).

Academic groups have also developed devices to create controlled sized spheroidal cultures. For instance, Miyamoto et al. utilized a "Tapered Stencil for Cluster Culture" device to form HepG2 spheroids [81]. Tong et al. immobilized hepatocyte spheroids between a glass coverslip and a porous Parylene C membrane that were modified with PEG and galactose for enhanced spheroid formation and retention during medium changes [82]. In another study, coculturing PHHs with human adipose-derived stem cells in concave microwells increased the rate of formation and stability of liver functions over monocultured spheroids [83]. Similarly, PHHs cocultured with bone marrow-mesenchymal stem cells into spheroidal structures through automated, stir-tank bioreactors showed increased viability and expression of drug metabolism enzymes, which is useful for long-term drug treatment [84]. Takayama et al. utilized a nanopillar plate to create spheroidal cultures of iHeps or HepG2 cells and assessed the toxicity of 24 hepatotoxic drugs [85]. The iHep spheroids were more sensitive to the drugs as compared to the HepG2 spheroids, though iHep spheroids displayed lower sensitivity than conventional PHH monolayers, which could be due to the immature phenotype of the iHeps. Liu et al. loaded primary rat hepatocytes, NIH/3T3 fibroblasts, and human umbilical vein endothelial cells (HUVECs) onto micropatterned electrospun fibrous mats to form spatially controlled spheroidal structures [86]. Such structures secreted albumin and urea and displayed CYP450 activities for 15 days.

The abovementioned spheroidal cultures rely on cell secreted ECM; however, such an approach does not allow precise and reproducible tuning of the biochemical and biomechanical microenvironment around cells. In contrast, naturally derived (i.e., alginate, chitosan, and cellulose) and synthetic biomaterials (i.e., PEG) can be used to mitigate such a limitation by presenting an engineered polymer matrix to cells [75, 87]. For instance, biocompatible PEG hydrogels provide control over mechanical properties via customization of chain length and control over biochemical properties by the tethering of ligands such as cell adhesion peptides and growth factors [87]. Chen et al. cocultivated PHHs, 3T3-J2 fibroblasts, and immortalized LSECs in RGDS-modified PEG to enable cell attachment and observed relatively stable albumin and urea secretion for at least 8 days in vitro [88]. A microfluidic droplet generator was subsequently used to generate PEG-based hepatic microtissues [89], which are more amenable to high-throughput drug studies than bulk gels. In a study utilizing a naturally derived biomaterial, Tasnim et al. encapsulated human pluripotent stem cell-derived hepatocyte-like cells (hPSC-HLC) in galactosylated cellulosic sponges, which promoted the formation and retention of spheroids [90]. The hPSC-HLC spheroids were more sensitive to the toxicity of hepatotoxins (acetaminophen, troglitazone, and methotrexate) as compared to conventional hPSC-HLC monolayers, and responses in hPSC-HLC spheroids were similar to those observed in PHHs. Larkin et al. designed a detachable, nanoscale, and mechanically tunable Space of Disse (i.e., overlay) to separate rat hepatocyte cultures from a mixture of LSECs and KCs using self-assembled polyelectrolyte multilayers of chitosan and hyaluronic acid (HA) [91]. When tuned to exhibit liver-like stiffness, the polymeric space of Disse enabled higher albumin secretion and CYP1A activity in the hepatocytes, while hepatocytes and KCs showed some proliferation as compared to the nonpolymeric controls. More recently, the same group has created a detachable Space of Disse using a mixture of collagen and HA, and demonstrated acetaminophen-mediated toxicity to rat LSECs and hepatocytes, as well as higher cytokine secretion by the KCs [92]. The cocultures exhibited increased aspartate aminotransferase (AST):alanine aminotransferase (ALT) ratios of 2.1–2.5, which were similar to values obtained in vivo in rats dosed with acetaminophen.

While spheroidal cocultures containing PHHs and NPCs have shown the robust longevity of functions and utility for DILI detection, it is difficult to precisely control the spatial arrangement of different cell types (as in vivo) except for that which is induced by the spontaneous sorting of specific cell types. On the other hand, bioprinting has emerged as a method to position different cell populations in relatively large constructs that can have utility in both drug screening and ultimately regenerative medicine. Organovo Inc. has

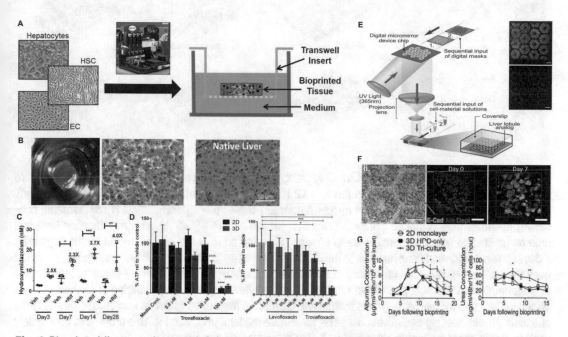

Fig. 3 Bioprinted liver cocultures. (**a**) Schematic of transverse cross section of bioprinted liver tissue from Organovo Inc. containing hepatocytes, endothelial cells (ECs) and hepatic stellate cells (HSCs). Reprinted with permission from [93]. (**b**) Gross image of bioprinted human liver tissue created using the process of panel (**a**) with 2.5 mm diameter and 0.5 mm thickness (*left*). Comparison of H&E stained bioprinted liver (*center*) and native human liver (*right*). (**c**) Basal and rifampicin-induced CYP3A4 activity in bioprinted human liver tissues of panel (**b**), measured by the formation of 4-hydroxymidazolam from midazolam. (**d**) Dose-dependent toxicity of trovafloxacin to 2D hepatocyte monolayers and 3D bioprinted human liver tissues of panel (**b**) following 7 days of treatment (*left*). Dose-dependent toxicity of hepatotoxin, trovafloxacin, and its non-liver-toxic structural analog, levofloxacin, to bioprinted human liver tissues following 7 days of treatment (*right*). (**e**) Schematic of a two-step 3D bioprinting approach in which first cell type is patterned by the first digital mask followed by the patterning of supporting cells using a second digital mask. Reprinted with permission from [95]. Images show bioprinted fluorescently labeled human induced pluripotent stem cell-derived hepatic progenitor cells or hiPSC-HPCs (*green*) in 5% (wt/vol) gelatin methacrylate and supporting cells containing a mixture of human umbilical endothelial vein cells and adipose-derived stem cells (*red*) in 2.5% (wt/vol) GelMA with 1% glycidal methacrylate. Scale bars are 500 μm. (**f**) Phase contrast and confocal immunofluorescence images showing albumin (Alb), E-cadherin (E-Cad), and nucleus (DAPI) staining of hiPSC-HPCs in bioprinted cocultures of panel (**e**) on the day of seeding (day 0) and 7 days later. Scale bars are 500 μm in brightfield and 100 μm in fluorescent images. (**g**) Albumin (*left*) and urea (*right*) secretions from 3D bioprinted cultures of panel (**e**) containing hiPSC-HPCs with (3D-triculture) or without (3D HPC-only) supportive cells as compared to 2D hiPSC-HPC monolayers

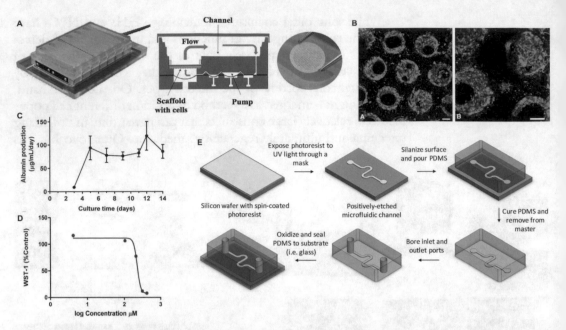

Fig. 4 Perfused liver cocultures. (**a**) The LiverChip platform. Reprinted with permission from [104]. A cell culture plate is attached to a pneumatic plate forming 12 fluidically isolated bioreactors per plate footprint (*left*). Bioreactor cross section is shown in the middle. A collagen-coated polystyrene scaffold (1 cm diameter) containing microchannels is placed into each bioreactor for cell culture (*right*). (**b**) Low-magnification (*left*) and high magnification (*right*) immunofluorescent images showing primary human hepatocyte morphology after 7 days (*green*: f-actin and *blue*: Hoescht) in the platform of panel (**a**). Scale bar is 100 μm. (**c**) Albumin secretion from the platform of panel (**a**). (**d**) Toxicity of hepatotoxin, diclofenac, to the platform of panel (**a**) after 6 days of treatment. Reprinted with permission from [105]. (**e**) Soft-lithographic process utilizing photoresist-coated silicon wafers and molding of polydimethylsiloxane (PDMS) on the wafers to create microfluidic devices with channels for cell seeding and inlet/outlet ports for culture medium perfusion [4]. This process is now widely used to create organ-on-a-chip platforms, including those for liver cocultures

developed a bioprinted human liver tissue containing a compartment of PHHs next to an NPC compartment containing HSCs and HUVECs housed in a 24-well transwell format [93]. These bioprinted liver tissues displayed high viability, albumin secretion, and CYP3A4 activity for 28 days, and were more sensitive to the toxicity of trovafloxacin after 7 days of treatment than conventional monolayers (Fig. 3a–d). Academic groups have also created bioprinted liver tissues. Jeon et al. used a 3D bioprinting system to create structures containing HepG2 cells in alginate and found better growth and expression of liver-specific genes in the bioprinted structures as compared to the monolayer controls [94]. Ma et al. utilized 3D bioprinting to create liver lobule-like hexagonal structures of iHeps, endothelial cells, and adipose-derived stem cells embedded in a hydrogel (Fig. 3e–g) [95]. Albumin secretion from the iHeps in such bioprinted tissues was detected for 32 days, urea secretion was detected for 15 days, while CYP450 mRNA transcripts were detected for 7 days. Furthermore, the levels of these markers were higher in the cocultured bioprinted tissues than bioprinted iHeps alone or conventional monolayers.

5   Perfused Cocultures

In contrast to static platforms, perfusion systems or bioreactors can allow automated control over culture medium pH, temperature, fluid pressures, cell shear stress, nutrient supply, and waste removal. The Griffith group at MIT pioneered one of the first perfused liver platforms for drug screening (Fig. 4a–d). In an earlier version of this so-called "LiverChip," Powers et al. cultured primary rat hepatocytes within an array of collagen-coated microchannels created via deep reaction ion etching of silicon wafers [96, 97]. Reactor dimensions were such that the perfusate flow rates met both the oxygen demands of the hepatocytes and subjected the cells to low shear stress as in vivo. Over 2 weeks, the hepatocytes rearranged extensively to form tissue-like structures and preaggregating the cells for 2–3 days prior to introduction into the bioreactor further aided the reorganization process. Additionally, the hepatocyte aggregates maintained near constant rates of albumin secretion and urea synthesis under perfusion that were an order of magnitude higher than in static controls. CYP450 activities were up to 33-fold higher in the perfused microreactors as compared to hepatocytes in a collagen gel sandwich after 7 days of culture [98]. Coculture of rat LSECs with rat hepatocytes in the LiverChip showed that the LSECs demonstrated moderate proliferation and were positive for the prototypical marker, SE-1, whereas LSECs entirely disappeared from conventional monolayers after 13 days in culture [99]. Domansky et al. subsequently miniaturized the LiverChip into 12 polycarbonate microreactors in a multiwell plate footprint such that each microreactor had its own fluid reservoir and an integrated micropump for continuous perfusion [100]. When rat hepatocytes were cocultured with a mixture of liver NPCs in this multiwell LiverChip and subsequently stimulated with LPS for 48 h, elevated levels of proinflammatory and anti-inflammatory cytokines were observed [101]. When LPS was administered to these cocultures with known idiosyncratic toxin, ranitidine, lactate dehydrogenase (LDH) release into the culture medium was markedly increased as compared to control cocultures and when the cocultures were treated with the nontoxic analog, famotidine [101].

The abovementioned LiverChip multiwell platform is now commercially available through CN Bio Innovations Limited and it has been adapted to human hepatocyte-KC cocultures that display stable albumin secretion for 2 weeks and respond to LPS stimulation by increasing the secretion of 11 different pro-inflammatory cytokines (i.e., IL-6, TNFα, and RANTES) [102, 103]. Stimulating these cocultures with IL-6 caused a dose-dependent decrease in CYP3A4 activity, an increase in C-reactive protein (CRP) secretion, and a decrease in shed soluble IL-6-receptor levels, which demonstrates an in vivo-like response of PHHs to IL-6 [104]. Treating the IL-6-stimulated cocultures with tocilizumab, an anti-IL-6R monoclonal antibody, led to the recovery of CYP3A4 activity and reduction in CRP levels following 72 h of treatment. More recently, major phase I and II metabolites of diclofenac produced from the cocultures were similar to those observed in humans [105]. Furthermore, a glycine-conjugated bile acid was found to be a sensitive marker of dose-dependent diclofenac toxicity in the perfused cocultures.

Other groups have used PDMS-based microfluidic devices (Fig. 4e) to perfuse liver cocultures for drug screening. For instance, Kane et al. developed an 8 × 8 element nonaddressable array of microfluidic wells containing MPCCs of rat hepatocytes and 3T3-J2 fibroblasts that were independently perfused with culture medium and oxygen [106]. While perfused cocultures displayed stable albumin and urea secretions for 32 days, the static controls surprisingly secreted higher amounts of these biomarkers. However, in another platform containing randomly distributed cocultures of PHHs and endothelial cells, production of drug metabolites was observed at a greater rate in perfused cocultures relative to static controls [107]. Similarly, Esch et al. found higher albumin and urea secretions in perfused cocultures of PHHs and a liver NPC mixture (fibroblasts, HSCs, and KCs) as compared to static controls [108].

Multichamber and/or multilayered microfluidic devices are now being used for liver cocultures to mimic the architecture of the liver sinusoid in vivo. For instance, Kang et al. found that primary rat hepatocytes maintained normal morphology and produced urea for 30 days when they were cultured on one side of a transwell membrane while immortalized bovine aortic endothelial cells were cultured on the other side of the membrane that was subjected to dual-channel microfluidic perfusion [109]. In another example, Rennert et al. cultured a mixture of HUVECs and monocyte-derived macrophages on one side of a polyethylene terephthalate (PET) membrane and a mixture of HepaRG cancerous cell line and LX-2 immortalized stellate cell line on the other side of the membrane [110]; the layered cocultures on the membrane were then perfused in a biochip that had integrated luminescent-based sensors for real-time measurement of oxygen consumption levels. Albumin and urea secretions were detected for 4 days at higher levels in perfused biochips as compared to static controls. Prodanov et al. also utilized a PET membrane to separate two cell culture chambers in a microfluidic device [111]. PHHs were seeded in the bottom chamber and overlaid with a collagen gel containing LX-2 cells, while a mixture of EA.hy926 endothelial cell line and U937 monocyte cell line was seeded in the top chamber. The perfused cocultures displayed higher albumin and urea secretions for ~4 weeks than static cocultures; however, CYP3A4 activity was statistically similar across both perfused and static cocultures.

Using a similar cellular makeup as that by Prodanov mentioned above [111], Vernetti et al. created layered liver cocultures in a single chamber commercially available microfluidic device;

PHHs were allowed to first attach overnight, followed by seeding of a mixture of EA.hy926 cells and U937 cells on top of the attached PHHs, and then the coculture was covered with LX-2 cells embedded in a collagen gel [112]. In this so-called "SQL-SAL" (sequentially layered self-assembled liver), about 20% of the PHHs were transduced with lentivirus carrying biosensors for apoptosis (cytochrome C) and reactive oxygen species or ROS (hydrogen peroxide). In contrast to static controls, perfused cocultures displayed higher albumin and urea secretions for 25 days; the perfused cocultures also produced CYP450 and glucuronidated metabolites of prototypical substrates. Hepatotoxicity of troglitazone in the perfused cocultures was observed via LDH release, albumin secretion, urea synthesis, a decrease in cytochrome C biosensor intensity inside the transduced PHHs, and an increase in ROS biosensor intensity. Caffeine, on the other hand, did not cause hepatotoxicity to the perfused cocultures. When the perfused cocultures were treated with LPS, a dose-dependent increase in TNFα secretion was measured. Coincubating LPS with trovafloxacin led to an expected and marked increase in toxicity as assessed via LDH release, whereas such did not occur to the same extent with LPS + levofloxacin. This same group has recently published a second generation version of their platform called "LAMPS" (liver acinus microphysiological system) that uses a gel composed of porcine-derived whole liver extracellular matrix (P-LECM) instead of rat tail collagen, primary human microvascular endothelial cells instead of the EA.hy926 cell line, THP-1 monocyte cell line instead of the U-937 cell line, and culture medium with reduced serum as well as soluble P-LECM, which better supports NPC functions [113].

In addition to any potential benefits of perfusion on the functions of liver cocultures, perfusion can also subject the cells to gradients of oxygen, nutrients, and hormones, which have been shown to lead to zonation or differential functions in hepatocytes across the length of the sinusoid in vivo [114, 115]. DILI can also manifest itself with a zonal pattern dependent on the mechanism of action of the drug and its metabolism by specific isoenzymes in the hepatocytes [116, 117]. Allen et al. described the first parallel-plate bioreactor with oxygen gradients that was used to induce a zonal pattern of CYP450s in rat hepatocyte cultures (Fig. 5a–d) [118]. Cells were cultured on a glass slide which was then placed inside a gas impermeable polycarbonate block with inlet and outlet for culture medium perfusion. After assembly, the chamber was inserted into the flow circuit containing a culture medium reservoir, gas exchanger, Clark-type oxygen probe, and syringe pump. A model of oxygen transport in the bioreactor was developed to estimate oxygen distribution at the cell surface, and then experimental measurements of outlet oxygen concentrations across various flow conditions were used to validate model predictions. Hepatic viability was maintained across the entire chamber length for at least 24 h while the cells were subjected to a physiologic oxygen gradient at the cell surface from 76 mmHg at the bioreactor inlet to 5 mmHg at the outlet. Such an oxygen gradient led to higher levels of phosphoenolpyruvate carboxykinase protein at the upstream (high oxygen) regions, while higher levels of CYP2B protein were localized at the downstream (low oxygen) regions as expected from in vivo data. The same group then extended the bioreactor design to higher functioning cocultures of rat hepatocytes and 3T3-J2 fibroblasts and showed greater cell toxicity at the downstream (low oxygen) regions following acetaminophen treatment, presumably due to the higher CYP450 activities in the downstream regions as compared to the upstream regions [119].

Two other groups have adapted microfluidic systems to models of liver zonation. The abovementioned LAMPS was used to subject perfused human liver cocultures to zone 1 oxygen (10–12%) or

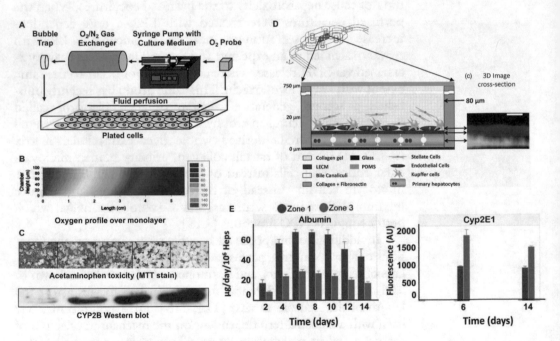

Fig. 5 Zonated liver cocultures. (**a**) Parallel-plate bioreactor schematic to expose cells to an oxygen gradient. Reprinted with permission from [118, 119]. (**b**) Two-dimensional contour plot of predicted oxygen concentration profile in cross section of bioreactor of panel (**a**). Cells at the bioreactor outlet are exposed to a lower oxygen tension than cells at the bioreactor inlet. (**c**) Rat hepatocyte bioreactor of panel (**a**) treated with acetaminophen showed greater (zonal) toxicity near the bioreactor outlet as assessed by the MTT stain (*top*). Higher (zonal) expression of CYP2B enzyme at the outlet of the bioreactor (*bottom*). (**d**) Structure of a multilayered liver coculture housed in a commercially available microfluidic device from Nortis Bio [113]. An *X–Z* projection is shown that demonstrates the layering of the cells with the reconstructed liver acinus from confocal images of labeled hepatocytes, the porcine liver ECM (LECM), and endothelial cells. The white scale bar is 10 μm. (**e**) The device of panel (**e**) was operated with different perfusion rates (5 μL/h for zone 1, periportal, and 15 μL/h for zone 3, perivenous) to subject the liver cocultures to different oxygen tensions as in liver zonation in vivo. Albumin level was measured in the efflux at the device outlet (*left*), while CYP2E1 protein expression level was measured via imaging of a fluorescently labeled antibody (*right*)

zone 3 oxygen (3–5%) levels in separate devices (Fig. 5e–g) [113]. The oxygen tension in each configuration was computationally modeled using the microfluidic device dimensions, culture medium flow rate, cell numbers, oxygen consumption rate of hepatocytes, and the diffusion coefficients of oxygen in different materials. The computational model of oxygen tensions was validated using oxygen sensitive and insensitive dyes. At the functional level, zone 1 cocultures exhibited greater levels of oxidative phosphorylation, albumin secretion, and urea synthesis as compared to zone 3 cocultures, which is consistent with zonal functions in vivo. On the other hand, zone 3 cocultures exhibited greater levels of alpha-1-antitrypsin activity, glycolysis, steatosis, CYP2E1 activity, and acetaminophen toxicity as compared to zone 1 cocultures. In contrast to an oxygen gradient, McCarty et al. generated a gradient of soluble factors (i.e., hormones and drugs) onto a rat hepatocyte monolayer using a microfluidic device [120]. Subjecting the cells to glucagon and insulin gradients, but in opposite directions (i.e., high glucagon with low insulin, and low glucagon with high insulin), led to an expected staining pattern for glycogen, such that cells contained less cytoplasmic glycogen in the presence of high levels of glucagon and more glycogen in the presence of high levels of insulin. For carbomyl phosphate synthetase 1 (CPS1, a urea cycle enzyme) staining, the opposite trends than glycogen were observed. Finally, cultures that were subjected to a gradient of 3-methylcholanthrene (3-MC), an inducer of glutathione S-transferase and CYP450 enzymes, displayed greater hepatotoxicity of allyl alcohol in the low 3-MC region and greater hepatotoxicity of acetaminophen in the high 3-MC region. Such a trend could be due to a greater level of protective glutathione conjugation of the reactive (toxic) metabolite of allyl alcohol in the high 3-MC region, and a greater level of CYP450-mediated generation of the toxic metabolite of acetaminophen in the high 3-MC region.

6   Appraising Coculture Phenotype Before and After Drug Treatment

It is important that prior to treatment with any drugs, the phenotypes of the various cell types in the liver cocultures are appraised using well-accepted markers towards providing the highest probability of obtaining a robust in vitro-to-in vivo correlation in the measured DILI endpoints. The phenotypic stability of hepatocytes can be assessed over time without having to lyse the cells by measuring albumin and urea secretions in the cell culture supernatants, and probing the activities of major CYP450 (i.e., CYP1A2, 2A6, 2B6, 2C8, 2C9, 2C19, 2D6, and 3A4) and phase II (i.e., UGTs) enzymes using prototypical substrates, in some cases with fluorescent or luminescent readouts. We refer the reader to a previous article that details methods for these phenotypic markers [51]. While the stability of the abovementioned phenotypic markers typically indicates a healthy hepatocyte, other proteins that are pertinent to the line of inquiry may need to be measured in supernatants and/or cell lysates. For liver NPC types, there is less consensus on which are the most appropriate markers to measure in vitro relative to in vivo biology. Nonetheless, we refer the reader to another review article that summarizes markers which have been most commonly used for different liver NPC types [121]. In some cases, global gene expression profiles extracted from the liver cocultures followed by RT-qPCR validation can also be useful to analyze diverse pathways expressed over time in culture; however, with mixed cocultures, it is not always trivial to discern which cell type is contributing to a given gene expression signal. Finally, it is important to compare the phenotype of cells in cocultures over time to freshly isolated cell counterparts (prior to any plating) from the same donor(s) to determine the extent to which cultured cells are like a phenotype that is closest to the in vivo liver. With the increased use of commercially available cryopreserved cells for on-demand drug screening, fresh tissues/cells are not always available and/or desired. In that case, the phenotype of cultured cells over time should be compared to cells immediately after thawing.

After treatment with drugs, the phenotype and viability of liver cocultures can be evaluated as a function of the dose and time of drug incubation. However, for general/nonspecific cytotoxicity markers like ATP or LDH, control cultures of the NPC types may need to be carried out if the objective is to determine hepatotoxicity versus cytotoxicity to the entire liver tissue. Regardless, it is important to evaluate cell type-specific markers (i.e., albumin secretion, urea synthesis, and ALT leakage for hepatocytes) alongside the cytotoxicity markers to provide a complete picture of how different cell types are affected by the drug of interest. High content screening (HCS) of multiplexed fluorescent readouts can also be used to obtain an understanding of cell-specific and organelle-specific mechanisms underlying DILI. Several commercial HCS systems (e.g., Thermo Fisher ArrayScan, Molecular Devices ImageXpress, GE Healthcare IN Cell Analyzer, and PerkinElmer Opera Phenix) couple automated and multispectral epifluorescent microscopy with software for real-time analysis of fluorescent intensities within individual cells. HCS for DILI detection was initially implemented by O'Brien et al. using HepG2 cells [122], extended by Xu et al. to short-term ECM-sandwich cultures of PHHs [66], and more recently applied to MPCCs containing PHHs and 3T3-J2 fibroblasts [61]. Several parameters can be assessed using HCS such as cell number via nuclei count, reactive oxygen species, mitochondrial membrane potential, apoptosis, cell cycle arrest, cell stress response, phospholipidosis, and neutral lipid accumulation [123, 124].

7 Modeling Diseases Using Cocultures

Liver diseases can also potentially affect the severity of DILI in patients [125], and therefore drugs that are being developed for treating diseases of the liver, such as chronic inflammation, hepatitis B/C viral infections, malaria, nonalcoholic fatty liver disease, and fibrosis, need special attention for testing both efficacy and toxicity. While still a relatively new direction, engineered human liver cocultures have the potential to be used for such a dual-purpose scenario by first mimicking aspects of the disease in an in vitro setting. For instance, to model "resident" liver inflammation, a few groups have cocultured PHHs with primary KCs or macrophages derived from a monocyte cell line and showed cytokine release from the KCs or macrophages following stimulation with LPS or other cytokines. Nguyen et al. demonstrated from LPS-stimulated MPCCs the increased secretion of six different cytokines that scaled with the number of primary KCs incorporated into the cocultures [73]; Sarkar et al. demonstrated the increased secretion of 11 different cytokines following LPS stimulation of PHH-KC cocultures in the perfused LiverChip platform [105]; and, Vernetti et al. demonstrated that increasing doses of LPS caused increased secretion of TNFα from microfluidic cocultures containing PHHs and U937-derived macrophages [112]. Liver cocultures with activated KCs or macrophages have been shown to display reduced activities of CYP450 enzymes (i.e., 3A4) [73, 104], which can lead to drug–drug interactions and enhanced toxicity of certain pharmaceuticals. Indeed, both trovafloxacin [112] and ranitidine [101] have been shown to display increased hepatotoxicity in cocultures containing activated KCs or macrophages as compared to quiescent control cocultures.

Malaria, caused by the *Plasmodium* parasite, causes ~3000 deaths every day from ~250 million reported cases globally. Continued development of antimalarial drugs and vaccines against the liver stage of *Plasmodium* can potentially interrupt the life cycle of the parasite at a critical stage and prevent relapse. Due to species-specific differences in antigenic variation and mechanisms of host cell invasion [126, 127], human liver models of malaria infection are needed for developing efficacious and safe therapeutics. Human MPCCs have been successfully infected with *Plasmodium* sporozoites [45], and the infection efficiency can be enhanced when the cultures are subjected to hypoxia [63]. Infected MPCCs can be used with HCS to determine the effects of antimalarial drugs and vaccines on the sporozoite size and number [50], as well as the potential for toxicity [61]. The infection of iHeps with *Plasmodium* now allows the ability to investigate inter-individual drug responses [128].

Hepatitis B and C viruses (HBV and HCV) chronically infect the liver of 130–170 million and 400 million people worldwide, respectively. Conventional PHH monolayers can be infected with both viruses [129, 130], but the rapid decline in CYP450 activities in monolayers makes screening for drug efficacy and toxicity difficult. On the other hand, higher functioning and longer-lasting engineered liver models infected with HCV/HBV can mitigate such a limitation with conventional PHH monolayers. For instance, Kang et al. infected their abovementioned rat hepatocyte/endothelial microfluidic coculture with a recombinant adenovirus containing a replication competent copy of the HBV genome, and detected cell-secreted HBV DNA in the device for 8 days [109]. However, the use of the adenovirus to circumvent the inability of rat hepatocytes to be infected with a human pathogen like HBV does not capture the dynamics of a human-specific viral infection event. In contrast, phenotypically stable MPCCs containing PHHs can be infected with both HCV [43] and HBV [44]. Interestingly, randomly distributed cocultures of the same two cell types (PHHs and 3T3-J2 fibroblasts) do not support viral infection, likely due to an incomplete polarization and lower functionality of the hepatocytes than in MPCCs. Infection of iHeps with HCV [131] and HBV [44] enables the investigation of the effects of donor genotype and host genes on infection efficiency, propagation, and resistance to drug therapies.

Nonalcoholic fatty liver disease (NAFLD) is on an epidemic rise (~1 in 4 individuals in the USA), and is a major risk factor for type 2 diabetes mellitus (T2DM) [132] and nonalcoholic steatohepatitis (NASH) that can progress to liver cancer, which is a virtually untreatable disease [133]. Animal models of such diseases do not suffice for drug development due to significant species-specific differences in NAFLD [134] and drug metabolism [135] pathways; thus, human liver models are essential. Davidson et al. showed that human MPCCs exposed to a hyperglycemic culture medium for 3 weeks developed fatty liver (steatosis) and became resistant to insulin-mediated suppression of gluconeogenesis concomitantly, but CYP450 activities, albumin secretion, and urea synthesis were not affected [64]. Treating the steatotic MPCCs with the antidiabetic drug metformin reduced gluconeogenesis. Thus, a diet-induced "fatty" MPCC model that displays a disease-relevant phenotype but still maintains stable drug metabolism enzymes can be used to screen for the efficacy and toxicity of drug candidates that cause a reduction in hepatic glucose output and steatosis. In another example, the LiverChip model containing PHHs described above was incubated for 14 days with excess free fatty acids (FFA) containing palmitic and oleic acids [136]. As in the study by Davidson et al. using MPCCs [65], steatotic PHHs in the LiverChip did not experience hepatotoxicity; however, genes associated with NAFLD and albumin secretion were increased, while CYP3A4 and CYP2C9 enzyme activities were significantly reduced. Treating the cultures with FFAs in the presence of metformin caused a reduction in cellular fat content as compared to untreated controls.

Once NAFLD progresses to NASH, however, HSCs become activated into myofibroblasts that secrete proinflammatory cytokines and deposit excessive collagen that can lead to fibrosis [133]. Reversing such fibrosis using pharmaceutical drugs can potentially halt the progression of NASH into cirrhosis and hepatocellular carcinoma. Engineered human liver cocultures can be used to model aspects of NASH and fibrosis for utility in phenotypic drug discovery. For example, Davidson et al. recently developed a micropatterned triculture (MPTC) platform in which (a) micropatterned PHHs were functionally stabilized using the 3T3-J2 fibroblasts (as in MPCCs described above), and (b) the PHH phenotype was modulated by culturing activated HSCs within the fibroblast monolayer at physiologically relevant ratios with PHHs; such a triculture configuration was used since the HSCs were not able to stabilize the PHH phenotype to the same magnitude and longevity as the fibroblasts [74]. While albumin and urea secretions were relatively similar in MPTCs and MPCCs (suggesting well-differentiated PHHs), over the course of 2 weeks, increasing HSC numbers within MPTCs (a) downregulated hepatic CYP450 (2A6, 3A4) and transporter activities, (b) caused hepatic steatosis, and (c) enhanced the secretion of pro-inflammatory IL-6 and CRP; effects that are consistent with clinical findings in patients with the early stages of NASH/fibrosis [137, 138]. Perhaps more importantly, inhibition of NADPH oxidase (NOX) and/or activation of farnesoid X receptor (FXR) using clinically relevant drugs, GKT137831 and obeticholic acid (OCA), respectively, alleviated hepatic dysfunctions in MPTCs at nontoxic concentrations, thereby suggesting MPTC utility for screening the efficacy and toxicity of anti-NASH/fibrosis drugs.

In another example of an engineered NASH human liver model, Feaver et al. created a platform in which PHHs were cultured in a collagen gel on one surface of a polycarbonate transwell membrane, while HSCs and macrophages were cultured on the other surface [139]. The HSC/macrophage side was subjected to liver sinusoidal-like hemodynamic flow via a cone-and-plate viscometer, while the hepatocyte side was subjected to continuous perfusion to recapitulate interstitial flow. When exposed for 10 days to a lipotoxic milieu (high insulin and glucose, and free fatty acids), PHHs in this coculture model accumulated lipids, increased glucose output, and displayed reduced insulin sensitivity. Furthermore, inflammatory markers (i.e., IL-6 and ALT) were secreted at higher levels, and HSCs displayed increased activation as assessed via alpha-SMA staining. More importantly, correlation was demonstrated between transcriptomic and lipidomic data obtained in vitro and in human liver NASH biopsies. Finally, treating the in vitro diseased cocultures with OCA led to improvements in the lipidomic signature, and a reduction in inflammatory and fibrotic secreted factors.

Besides diet, some drugs can also cause fibrosis-like effects in the liver, which represents a type of DILI; therefore, modeling such effects in engineered human liver models is important for preclinical drug development. For instance, Norona et al. demonstrated drug-induced fibrogenesis in Organovo's bioprinted human liver tissues [93]. Specifically, treating the bioprinting liver tissues with methotrexate and thioacetamide for up to 14 days caused increased LDH release relative to vehicle controls, enhanced deposition of fibrillar collagen I, and a surge in proinflammatory cytokines initially followed by alterations in immunomodulatory cytokines at subsequent time-points. Similarly, Vernetti et al. showed the migration of activated HSCs to the hepatocyte layer in layered microfluidic human liver cocultures treated with methotrexate [112]. We anticipate that other liver coculture models will be utilized for modeling drug-induced fibrosis now with the proof-of-concept established in the abovementioned studies.

8   Practical Considerations in Using Cocultures for Drug Toxicity Studies

An important consideration in the design and use of engineered liver cocultures for drug screening is the type of material used (i.e., scaffold type and tubing for microfluidics) to interface with the cells. Drugs can often bind to the material(s) in a culture platform and not reach the cells, which necessitates cell-free experiments to trouble-shoot any issues. Thus, using materials that do not significantly bind lipophilic molecules, such as drugs and hormones that the cells need to function optimally, is critical for building culture platforms for liver and other tissues [140]. An interesting strategy is to coat microchannels in a culture device with endothelial cells [141], thereby preventing drug-related material from binding to the underlying material.

The throughput of a platform is also an important consideration for testing more than just a few compounds, especially in the early stages of drug development with tight timelines. Adapting engineered liver cocultures to a multiwell footprint that can be interfaced with robotic fluid handlers is thus useful to meet throughput demands. For instance, MPCCs from human [53] and animal [142] hepatocytes are all presented in an industry-standard multiwell plate format (up to 384-well plates) that seamlessly integrates with both robotic fluidic handlers and HCS instruments [61]. Similarly, the InSphero [78] and LiverChip [104] platforms have both been adapted to multiwell plate formats for increasing the throughput of spheroidal liver cocultures. While increasing the throughput of a platform can potentially help reduce the cost of testing each drug, the use of animal liver cells and/or cancerous cell lines within culture models can also aid in cost reduction as well as mitigate the inherent donor-to-donor variability with primary cells. However, the use of such "alternative" cell sources due to constraints of cost during drug development is ultimately a compromise over primary cells in human physiological relevance.

9 Conclusions and Future Outlook

Over many high-profile drug failures in clinical trials and in the marketplace [125], it has become increasingly clear that animals are not fully predictive of human DILI [3], which necessitates the utilization of in vitro models of the human liver during preclinical drug development [4]. The development of human liver models began several decades ago with the isolation [143, 144] and culture of hepatocytes on ECM protein-coated plastic [10–12, 24]. Today, the use of sophisticated engineering tools, such as micropatterning [42], microfluidics [98, 112], specialized plates [78, 81], biomaterials scaffolds [145], and 3D bioprinting [93], has allowed more precise control over the liver cell microenvironment, which has led to stabilized liver functions for several weeks. Such longevity of functions has proven highly useful for chronic treatment with drugs to significantly enhance the sensitivity for DILI prediction over short-term (<48 h) drug treatment of conventional monolayers (Table 1) [4]. Most of the liver models that display high levels of functions cocultivate hepatocytes with NPCs; surprisingly, even non-liver-derived NPC types (i.e., 3T3-J2 murine embryonic fibroblasts) can induce high levels of functions in hepatocytes from multiple species, including humans, which suggests that the molecular mediators underlying the "coculture effect" are relatively well-conserved across species [5]. Often, the exact liver architecture is not fully recapitulated in engineered liver cocultures (i.e., disorganized spheroidal cultures and circular islands in MPCCs), but still leads to healthy and functioning liver cells, which suggests that the biochemical and biophysical microenvironment around the cells is ultimately more important for generating high-fidelity human liver models than mimicking the macroarchitecture of the native liver. Furthermore, optimizing the homotypic and heterotypic cell–cell interactions using technology (i.e., micropatterning, specialized plates to create controlled sized spheroids, and bioprinting) is important to enhance liver functions and enable reproducible data sets across many experiments. Lastly, while liver NPCs such as KCs, HSCs, and LSECs have all been incorporated into engineered liver cocultures to study how DILI is modulated by these cell types, it remains unclear how to incorporate biliary epithelial cells in models in such a way that they can form bile ducts that drain the contents of the hepatic bile canaliculi into a separate flow compartment than that used to mimic blood flow.

Table 1
Benefits and potential limitations of liver coculture platforms for DILI screening

Model	Benefits	Potential limitations
Randomly distributed (conventional) cocultures	• Can be cultured in high-throughput plate formats • No specialized system needed to establish cocultures • Different NPC types can be used to support hepatocytes • Easily compatible with high content imaging readouts	• Can display variability in induction of hepatocyte functions with the choice of specific NPC type • Can display morphological and functional instability due to regions of suboptimal cell–cell interactions within the monolayer • Are not able to sustain infection with HBV/HCV and malaria due to potential lack of complete hepatocyte polarity
Micropatterned cocultures	• Controlled cell–cell interactions allow for higher and stable functions for 4–6 weeks than randomly distributed cocultures • Modular design allows for the use of different NPC types without significantly altering hepatocyte homotypic interactions • Can be infected with HBV, HCV, and malaria • Display fatty liver phenotype when treated with hyperglycemic and/or high fatty acid containing culture medium • Compatible with high content imaging readouts	• Currently rely on collagen alone for hepatocyte attachment as opposed to more complex liver-inspired ECM • Currently lack all liver stromal cells • Use nonhuman supporting fibroblasts • Require specialized equipment and devices for patterning collagen
Spheroidal cocultures	• Can be created using a variety of different methods/plates • Cell-secreted ECM protein matrix forms around the spheroids • Multicellular interactions can be studied • Maintenance of major liver functions for several weeks • Have been shown to be compatible with multiple applications within the drug development pipeline	• Can be difficult to control disorganized cell type interactions over time • Necrosis can occur in the center of larger spheroids • Size variability can occur with some methods • High content imaging for entire spheroid may require expensive confocal microscopy depending on the spheroid size

(continued)

Table 1
(continued)

Model	Benefits	Potential limitations
Bioprinted cocultures	• Precise control of cell placement allows formation of separate hepatocyte and NPC compartments • Versatile method to create diverse architectures as desired • Multicellular interactions can be studied • Maintenance of major liver functions for 1 month • Compatible with DILI screening and to model drug-induced fibrosis	• Printing resolution does not always allow placement of individual cells • Low-throughput • Requires complex and expensive equipment • Requires significantly more cells than other higher-throughput/miniaturized methods • Potential heterogeneous drug distribution across large printed tissues
Perfused cocultures	• Dynamic fluid flow for nutrient and waste exchange • Several commercial configurable devices available for cell culture and perfusion • Layered architectures can be created with single chamber or multichamber microfluidic device designs • Sustained functionality for 2–4 weeks • Gradients of oxygen/hormones can be created to model zonal liver phenotypes	• Potential binding of drugs to tubing and materials used • Large dead volume requiring higher quantities of novel compounds for treatment of cell cultures • Low-throughput • Shear stress may cause lower hepatic functions • May wash away built-up beneficial molecules with perfusion

Some key issues that pertain to engineered liver cocultures will need to be addressed moving forward. First, it will be useful to rely on similar endpoints and data normalization schemes (i.e., based on cell number, protein, and/or RNA levels) when showing functionality and stability of an engineered liver coculture so that the data can be compared across different laboratories. Second, consortia led by pharmaceutical companies and regulatory agencies will be important to evaluate multiple engineered liver cocultures using a consistent set of drugs and endpoints. Currently, it remains unclear which of the engineered liver coculture platforms outperforms the others due to a lack of standardized comparisons by the same personnel in the same laboratories using the same cell donors. Third, engineered liver cocultures will need to mimic aspects of innate and adaptive immunity as well as different liver diseases to better predict idiosyncratic toxicity in the clinic. Nonetheless, engineered liver cocultures coupled with cellular stress markers have been shown to accurately detect the DILI potential of hepatotoxins that were previously thought to be idiosyncratic (i.e., troglitazone, diclofenac, and clozapine) [62, 72, 93, 112]. However, it is not currently possible to predict with in vitro approaches which *specific* individuals will adapt to cell stress and which individual will experience progressive and severe DILI. The differentiation of iPSCs from thousands of human patients with different genetic backgrounds into multiple types of liver cells may potentially be useful to elucidate inter-individual variations in DILI outcomes [71, 146]. When cultured in an advanced platform like MPCCs, human iHeps display sensitivity/specificity for DILI detection that now approaches that measured in stable PHHs [72]. However, further improvements in the functional maturity of iHeps and other iPSC-derived liver NPC types will be needed to enable the routine use of these cells for investigating DILI during drug development.

In conclusion, different types of engineered liver cocultures are available for investigating DILI potential in multiple phases of drug development based on the posed hypotheses, throughput requirements, and budgetary constraints. The continued development and validation of engineered cocultures using both primary and iPSC-derived human liver cells will ultimately provide a better understanding of idiosyncratic DILI, reduce the usage of animals in preclinical drug development, and mitigate the risk of DILI to patients.

Acknowledgments

The authors would like to thank Christine Lin and Brenton Ware for their helpful discussions. This work was funded by the National Institutes of Health (1R21ES027622-01 to S.R.K.). Salman R. Khetani is an equity holder in Ascendance Biotechnology, which has licensed the MPCC system from MIT and MPTC system from Colorado State University for commercial distribution.

References

1. Kaplowitz N (2005) Idiosyncratic drug hepatotoxicity. Nat Rev Drug Discov 4(6):489–499. https://doi.org/10.1038/nrd1750

2. Abboud G, Kaplowitz N (2007) Drug-induced liver injury. Drug Saf 30(4):277–294

3. Olson H, Betton G, Robinson D, Thomas K, Monro A, Kolaja G, Lilly P, Sanders J, Sipes G, Bracken W, Dorato M, Van Deun K, Smith P, Berger B, Heller A (2000) Concordance of the toxicity of pharmaceuticals in humans and in animals. Regul Toxicol Pharmacol 32(1):56–67. https://doi.org/10.1006/rtph.2000.1399

4. Lin C, Khetani SR (2016) Advances in engineered liver models for investigating drug-induced liver injury. Biomed Res Int 2016:1829148. https://doi.org/10.1155/2016/1829148

5. Bhatia SN, Balis UJ, Yarmush ML, Toner M (1999) Effect of cell-cell interactions in preservation of cellular phenotype: cocultivation of hepatocytes and nonparenchymal cells. FASEB J 13(14):1883–1900

6. Bezerra JA (1998) Liver development: a paradigm for hepatobiliary disease in later life.

Semin Liver Dis 18(3):203–216. https://doi.org/10.1055/s-2007-1007157

7. Cereghini S (1996) Liver-enriched transcription factors and hepatocyte differentiation. FASEB J 10(2):267–282

8. Kmieć Z (2001) Cooperation of liver cells in health and disease. Adv Anat Embryol Cell Biol 161:III–XIII. 1–151

9. Guillouzo A (1998) Liver cell models in in vitro toxicology. Environ Health Perspect 106(Suppl 2):511–532

10. Langenbach R, Malick L, Tompa A, Kuszynski C, Freed H, Huberman E (1979) Maintenance of adult rat hepatocytes on C3H/10T1/2 cells. Cancer Res 39(9):3509–3514

11. Michalopoulos G, Russell F, Biles C (1979) Primary cultures of hepatocytes on human fibroblasts. In Vitro 15(10):796–806

12. Guguen-Guillouzo C, Clément B, Baffet G, Beaumont C, Morel-Chany E, Glaise D, Guillouzo A (1983) Maintenance and reversibility of active albumin secretion by adult rat hepatocytes co-cultured with another liver epithelial cell type. Exp Cell Res 143(1):47–54

13. Clement B, Guguen-Guillouzo C, Campion JP, Glaise D, Bourel M, Guillouzo A (1984) Long-term co-cultures of adult human hepatocytes with rat liver epithelial cells: modulation of albumin secretion and accumulation of extracellular material. Hepatology 4(3):373–380

14. Loreal O, Levavasseur F, Fromaget C, Gros D, Guillouzo A, Clement B (1993) Cooperation of Ito cells and hepatocytes in the deposition of an extracellular matrix in vitro. Am J Pathol 143(2):538–544

15. Morin O, Normand C (1986) Long-term maintenance of hepatocyte functional activity in co-culture: requirements for sinusoidal endothelial cells and dexamethasone. J Cell Physiol 129(1):103–110. https://doi.org/10.1002/jcp.1041290115

16. Billiar TR, Curran RD, Stuehr DJ, West MA, Bentz BG, Simmons RL (1989) An L-arginine-dependent mechanism mediates Kupffer cell inhibition of hepatocyte protein synthesis in vitro. J Exp Med 169(4):1467–1472

17. Shimaoka S, Nakamura T, Ichihara A (1987) Stimulation of growth of primary cultured adult rat hepatocytes without growth factors by coculture with nonparenchymal liver cells. Exp Cell Res 172(1):228–242

18. Bhatia SN, Balis UJ, Yarmush ML, Toner M (1998) Probing heterotypic cell interactions: hepatocyte function in microfabricated co-cultures. J Biomater Sci Polym Ed 9(11):1137–1160

19. Goulet F, Normand C, Morin O (1988) Cellular interactions promote tissue-specific function, biomatrix deposition and junctional communication of primary cultured hepatocytes. Hepatology 8(5):1010–1018

20. Khetani SR, Chen AA, Ranscht B, Bhatia SN (2008) T-cadherin modulates hepatocyte functions in vitro. FASEB J 22(11):3768–3775. https://doi.org/10.1096/fj.07-105155

21. Di L, Brown KE, Gómez-Lechón MJ, Sohara N, Cusi K, Jones CN, Vickers JA, Cho CH, Hengstler JG, Liu Tsang V, Yarmush ML, Shoelson SE, Doshi U, Feng B, Brunt EM, Jover R, Znoyko I, Tuleuova N, Caulum MM, Berthiaume F, Brulport M, Chen AA, Toner M, Lee J, Li AP, Goosen TC, Heinecke JW, Donato MT, Levy MT, Lee JY, Henry CS, Tilles AW, Schormann W, Cho LM, Dunn JC, Goldfine AB, Lai Y, Trojanowska M, Ramanculov E, Yarmush ML, Bauer A, Jadin KD, Rotem A, Steyn SJ, Reuben A, Reddi AH, Hermes M, Sah RL, Hubel A, Varma MV, Zern MA, Nussler AK, DeLong S, Tompkins RG, Obach RS, Revzin A, Fandrich F, West JL, Ruhnke M, Bhatia SN, Ungefroren H, Griffin L, Bockamp E, Oesch F, von Mach M-A (2013) A perspective on the prediction of drug pharmacokinetics and disposition in drug research and development. Drug Metab Dispos 41(12):1975–1993. https://doi.org/10.1124/dmd.113.054031

22. Griffith LG, Wu B, Cima MJ, Powers MJ, Chaignaud B, Vacanti JP (1997) In vitro organogenesis of liver tissue. Ann N Y Acad Sci 831:382–397

23. Donato MT, Castell JV, Gomez-Lechon MJ (1991) Co-cultures of hepatocytes with epithelial-like cell lines: expression of drug-biotransformation activities by hepatocytes. Cell Biol Toxicol 7(1):1–14

24. Guguen-Guillouzo C, Clement B, Lescoat G, Glaise D, Guillouzo A (1984) Modulation of human fetal hepatocyte survival and differentiation by interactions with a rat liver epithelial cell line. Dev Biol 105(1):211–220

25. Lescoat G, Theze N, Clement B, Guillouzo A, Guguen-Guillouzo C (1985) Modulation of fetal and neonatal rat hepatocyte functional activity by glucocorticoids in co-culture. Cell Differ 16(4):259–268

26. Jongen WM, Sijtsma SR, Zwijsen RM, Temmink JH (1987) A co-cultivation system consisting of primary chick embryo hepatocytes and V79 Chinese hamster cells as a model for metabolic cooperation studies. Carcinogenesis 8(6):767–772

27. Talbot NC, Pursel VG, Rexroad CE Jr, Caperna TJ, Powell AM, Stone RT (1994) Colony isolation and secondary culture of fetal porcine hepatocytes on STO feeder cells. In Vitro Cell Dev Biol Anim 30A(12):851–858

28. Kuri-Harcuch W, Mendoza-Figueroa T (1989) Cultivation of adult rat hepatocytes on 3T3 cells: expression of various liver differentiated functions. Differentiation 41(2):148–157

29. Villafuerte BC, Koop BL, Pao CI, Gu L, Birdsong GG, Phillips LS (1994) Coculture of primary rat hepatocytes and nonparenchymal cells permits expression of insulin-like growth factor binding protein-3 in vitro. Endocrinology 134(5):2044–2050. https://doi.org/10.1210/endo.134.5.7512496

30. Hui EE, Bhatia SN (2007) Micromechanical control of cell-cell interactions. Proc Natl Acad Sci U S A 104(14):5722–5726. https://doi.org/10.1073/pnas.0608660104

31. Khetani SR, Szulgit G, Del Rio JA, Barlow C, Bhatia SN (2004) Exploring interactions between rat hepatocytes and nonparenchymal cells using gene expression profiling. Hepatology 40(3):545–554. https://doi.org/10.1002/hep.20351

32. Mesnil M, Fraslin JM, Piccoli C, Yamasaki H, Guguen-Guillouzo C (1987) Cell contact but not junctional communication (dye coupling) with biliary epithelial cells is required for hepatocytes to maintain differentiated functions. Exp Cell Res 173(2):524–533

33. Corlu A, Kneip B, Lhadi C, Leray G, Glaise D, Baffet G, Bourel D, Guguen-Guillouzo C (1991) A plasma membrane protein is involved in cell contact-mediated regulation of tissue-specific genes in adult hepatocytes. J Cell Biol 115(2):505–515

34. Donato MT, Gomez-Lechon MJ, Castell JV (1990) Drug metabolizing enzymes in rat hepatocytes co-cultured with cell lines. In Vitro Cell Dev Biol 26(11):1057–1062

35. West MA, Manthei R, Bubrick MP (1993) Autoregulation of hepatic macrophage activation in sepsis. J Trauma 34(4):473–479. discussion 479–480

36. Michalopoulos G, Strom SC, Kligerman AD, Irons GP, Novicki DL (1981) Mutagenesis induced by procarcinogens at the hypoxanthine-guanine phosphoribosyl transferase locus of human fibroblasts cocultured with rat hepatocytes. Cancer Res 41(5):1873–1878

37. Guillouzo A, Morel F, Fardel O, Meunier B (1993) Use of human hepatocyte cultures for drug metabolism studies. Toxicology 82(1–3):209–219

38. Mertens K, Rogiers V, Vercruysse A (1993) Glutathione dependent detoxication in adult rat hepatocytes under various culture conditions. Arch Toxicol 67(10):680–685

39. De La Vega FM, Mendoza-Figueroa T (1991) Dimethyl sulfoxide enhances lipid synthesis and secretion by long-term cultures of adult rat hepatocytes. Biochimie 73(5):621–624

40. Lebreton JP, Daveau M, Hiron M, Fontaine M, Biou D, Gilbert D, Guguen-Guillouzo C (1986) Long-term biosynthesis of complement component C3 and alpha-1 acid glycoprotein by adult rat hepatocytes in a co-culture system with an epithelial liver cell-type. Biochem J 235(2):421–427

41. Allen JW, Hassanein T, Bhatia SN (2001) Advances in bioartificial liver devices. Hepatology 34(3):447–455. https://doi.org/10.1053/jhep.2001.26753

42. Khetani SR, Bhatia SN (2008) Microscale culture of human liver cells for drug development. Nat Biotechnol 26(1):120–126. https://doi.org/10.1038/nbt1361

43. Ploss A, Khetani SR, Jones CT, Syder AJ, Trehan K, Gaysinskaya VA, Mu K, Ritola K, Rice CM, Bhatia SN (2010) Persistent hepatitis C virus infection in microscale primary human hepatocyte cultures. Proc Natl Acad Sci U S A 107(7):3141–3145. https://doi.org/10.1073/pnas.0915130107

44. Shlomai A, Schwartz RE, Ramanan V, Bhatta A, de Jong YP, Bhatia SN, Rice CM (2014) Modeling host interactions with hepatitis B virus using primary and induced pluripotent stem cell-derived hepatocellular systems. Proc Natl Acad Sci U S A 111(33):12193–12198. https://doi.org/10.1073/pnas.1412631111

45. March S, Ng S, Velmurugan S, Galstian A, Shan J, Logan DJ, Carpenter AE, Thomas D, Sim BKL, Mota MM, Hoffman SL, Bhatia SN (2013) A microscale human liver platform that supports the hepatic stages of Plasmodium falciparum and vivax. Cell Host Microbe 14(1):104–115. https://doi.org/10.1016/j.chom.2013.06.005

46. Qin D, Xia Y, Whitesides GM (2010) Soft lithography for micro- and nanoscale patterning. Nat Protoc 5(3):491–502. https://doi.org/10.1038/nprot.2009.234

47. Singhvi R, Kumar A, Lopez GP, Stephanopoulos GN, Wang DI, Whitesides GM, Ingber DE (1994) Engineering cell shape and function. Science (New York, NY) 264(5159):696–698

48. Bhatia SN, Balis UJ, Yarmush ML, Toner M (1998) Microfabrication of hepatocyte/

fibroblast co-cultures: role of homotypic cell interactions. Biotechnol Prog 14(3):378–387. https://doi.org/10.1021/bp980036j

49. Rheinwald JG, Green H (1975) Serial cultivation of strains of human epidermal keratinocytes: the formation of keratinizing colonies from single cells. Cell 6(3):331–343

50. March S, Ramanan V, Trehan K, Ng S, Galstian A, Gural N, Scull MA, Shlomai A, Mota MM, Fleming HE, Khetani SR, Rice CM, Bhatia SN (2015) Micropatterned coculture of primary human hepatocytes and supportive cells for the study of hepatotropic pathogens. Nat Protoc 10(12):2027–2053. https://doi.org/10.1038/nprot.2015.128

51. Lin C, Khetani SR (2017) Micropatterned co-cultures of human hepatocytes and stromal cells for the assessment of drug clearance and drug-drug interactions. Curr Protoc Toxicol 72:14.17.11–14.17.23. https://doi.org/10.1002/cptx.23

52. Chan TS, Yu H, Moore A, Khetani SR, Tweedie D (2013) Meeting the challenge of predicting hepatic clearance of compounds slowly metabolized by cytochrome P450 using a novel hepatocyte model, HepatoPac. Drug Metab Dispos 41(12):2024–2032. https://doi.org/10.1124/dmd.113.053397

53. Lin C, Shi J, Moore A, Khetani SR (2016) Prediction of drug clearance and drug-drug interactions in microscale cultures of human hepatocytes. Drug Metab Dispos 44(1):127–136. https://doi.org/10.1124/dmd.115.066027

54. Kratochwil NA, Meille C, Fowler S, Klammers F, Ekiciler A, Molitor B, Simon S, Walter I, McGinnis C, Walther J, Leonard B, Triyatni M, Javanbakht H, Funk C, Schuler F, Lave T, Parrott NJ (2017) Metabolic profiling of human long-term liver models and hepatic clearance predictions from in vitro data using nonlinear mixed-effects modeling. AAPS J 19(2):534–550. https://doi.org/10.1208/s12248-016-0019-7

55. Dixit V, Moore A, Tsao H, Hariparsad N (2016) Application of micropatterned cocultured hepatocytes to evaluate the inductive potential and degradation rate of major xenobiotic metabolizing enzymes. Drug Metab Dispos 44(2):250–261. https://doi.org/10.1124/dmd.115.067173

56. Moore A, Chothe PP, Tsao H, Hariparsad N (2016) Evaluation of the interplay between uptake transport and CYP3A4 induction in micropatterned cocultured hepatocytes. Drug Metab Dispos 44(12):1910–1919. https://doi.org/10.1124/dmd.116.072660

57. Ballard TE, Wang S, Cox LM, Moen MA, Krzyzewski S, Ukairo O, Obach RS (2016) Application of a micropatterned cocultured hepatocyte system to predict preclinical and human-specific drug metabolism. Drug Metab Dispos 44(2):172–179. https://doi.org/10.1124/dmd.115.066688

58. Wang WW, Khetani SR, Krzyzewski S, Duignan DB, Obach RS (2010) Assessment of a micropatterned hepatocyte coculture system to generate major human excretory and circulating drug metabolites. Drug Metab Dispos 38(10):1900–1905. https://doi.org/10.1124/dmd.110.034876

59. Ramsden D, Tweedie DJ, St George R, Chen LZ, Li Y (2014) Generating an in vitro-in vivo correlation for metabolism and liver enrichment of a hepatitis C virus drug, faldaprevir, using a rat hepatocyte model (HepatoPac). Drug Metab Dispos 42(3):407–414. https://doi.org/10.1124/dmd.113.055947

60. Ramsden D, Tweedie DJ, Chan TS, Taub ME, Li Y (2014) Bridging in vitro and in vivo metabolism and transport of faldaprevir in human using a novel cocultured human hepatocyte system, HepatoPac. Drug Metab Dispos 42(3):394–406. https://doi.org/10.1124/dmd.113.055897

61. Trask OJ, Moore A, LeCluyse EL (2014) A micropatterned hepatocyte coculture model for assessment of liver toxicity using high content imaging analysis. Assay Drug Dev Technol 12(1):16–27. https://doi.org/10.1089/adt.2013.525

62. Khetani SR, Kanchagar C, Ukairo O, Krzyzewski S, Moore A, Shi J, Aoyama S, Aleo M, Will Y (2013) Use of micropatterned cocultures to detect compounds that cause drug-induced liver injury in humans. Toxicol Sci 132(1):107–117. https://doi.org/10.1093/toxsci/kfs326

63. Ng S, March S, Galstian A, Hanson K, Carvalho T, Mota MM, Bhatia SN (2013) Hypoxia promotes liver stage malaria infection in primary human hepatocytes in vitro. Dis Model Mech. https://doi.org/10.1242/dmm.013490

64. Davidson MD, Ballinger KR, Khetani SR (2016) Long-term exposure to abnormal glucose levels alters drug metabolism pathways and insulin sensitivity in primary human hepatocytes. Sci Rep 6:28178. https://doi.org/10.1038/srep28178

65. Davidson MD, Lehrer M, Khetani SR (2015) Hormone and drug-mediated modulation of glucose metabolism in a microscale model of the human liver. Tissue Eng Part C Methods

21(7):716–725. https://doi.org/10.1089/ten.TEC.2014.0512

66. Xu JJ, Henstock PV, Dunn MC, Smith AR, Chabot JR, de Graaf D (2008) Cellular imaging predictions of clinical drug-induced liver injury. Toxicol Sci 105(1):97–105. https://doi.org/10.1093/toxsci/kfn109

67. Trials IoMUCtRtFFFC, Manning FJ, Swartz M (1995) Review of the Fialuridine (FIAU) Clinical Trials. https://doi.org/10.17226/4887

68. Krzyzewski S, Khetani SR, Barros S (2011) Assessing chronic toxicity of fialuridine in a micropatterned hepatocyte co-culture model. In: The toxicologist, supplement to toxicological sciences, vol 120, Suppl 2. p 540 (abstract #2523)

69. Ware BR, McVay M, Sunada WY, Khetani SR (2017) Exploring chronic drug effects on microengineered human liver cultures using global gene expression profiling. Toxicol Sci. https://doi.org/10.1093/toxsci/kfx059

70. Berger DR, Ware BR, Davidson MD, Allsup SR, Khetani SR (2015) Enhancing the functional maturity of induced pluripotent stem cell-derived human hepatocytes by controlled presentation of cell-cell interactions in vitro. Hepatology 61(4):1370–1381. https://doi.org/10.1002/hep.27621

71. Davidson MD, Ware BR, Khetani SR (2015) Stem cell-derived liver cells for drug testing and disease modeling. Discov Med 19(106):349–358

72. Ware BR, Berger DR, Khetani SR (2015) Prediction of drug-induced liver injury in micropatterned co-cultures containing iPSC-derived human hepatocytes. Toxicol Sci 145(2):252–262. https://doi.org/10.1093/toxsci/kfv048

73. Nguyen TV, Ukairo O, Khetani SR, McVay M, Kanchagar C, Seghezzi W, Ayanoglu G, Irrechukwu O, Evers R (2015) Establishment of a hepatocyte-kupffer cell coculture model for assessment of proinflammatory cytokine effects on metabolizing enzymes and drug transporters. Drug Metab Dispos 43(5):774–785. https://doi.org/10.1124/dmd.114.061317

74. Davidson MD, Kukla D, Khetani SR (2017) Microengineered cultures containing human hepatic stellate cells and hepatocytes for drug development. Integr Biol (Camb). https://doi.org/10.1039/C7IB00027H

75. Godoy P, Hewitt NJ, Albrecht U, Andersen ME, Ansari N, Bhattacharya S, Bode JG, Bolleyn J, Borner C, Böttger J, Braeuning A, Budinsky RA, Burkhardt B, Cameron NR, Camussi G, Cho C-S, Choi Y-J, Craig Rowlands J, Dahmen U, Damm G, Dirsch O, Donato MT, Dong J, Dooley S, Drasdo D, Eakins R, Ferreira KS, Fonsato V, Fraczek J, Gebhardt R, Gibson A, Glanemann M, Goldring CEP, Gómez-Lechón MJ, Groothuis GMM, Gustavsson L, Guyot C, Hallifax D, Hammad S, Hayward A, Häussinger D, Hellerbrand C, Hewitt P, Hoehme S, Holzhütter H-G, Houston JB, Hrach J, Ito K, Jaeschke H, Keitel V, Kelm JM, Kevin Park B, Kordes C, Kullak-Ublick GA, LeCluyse EL, Lu P, Luebke-Wheeler J, Lutz A, Maltman DJ, Matz-Soja M, McMullen P, Merfort I, Messner S, Meyer C, Mwinyi J, Naisbitt DJ, Nussler AK, Olinga P, Pampaloni F, Pi J, Pluta L, Przyborski SA, Ramachandran A, Rogiers V, Rowe C, Schelcher C, Schmich K, Schwarz M, Singh B, Stelzer EHK, Stieger B, Stöber R, Sugiyama Y, Tetta C, Thasler WE, Vanhaecke T, Vinken M, Weiss TS, Widera A, Woods CG, Xu JJ, Yarborough KM, Hengstler JG (2013) Recent advances in 2D and 3D in vitro systems using primary hepatocytes, alternative hepatocyte sources and non-parenchymal liver cells and their use in investigating mechanisms of hepatotoxicity, cell signaling and ADME. Arch Toxicol 87(8):1315–1530. https://doi.org/10.1007/s00204-013-1078-5

76. Acikgoz A, Giri S, Cho MG, Bader A (2013) Morphological and functional analysis of hepatocyte spheroids generated on poly-HEMA-treated surfaces under the influence of fetal calf serum and nonparenchymal cells. Biomol Ther 3(1):242–269. https://doi.org/10.3390/biom3010242

77. Bell CC, Hendriks DFG, Moro SML, Ellis E, Walsh J, Renblom A, Fredriksson Puigvert L, Dankers ACA, Jacobs F, Snoeys J, Sison-Young RL, Jenkins RE, Nordling Å, Mkrtchian S, Park BK, Kitteringham NR, Goldring CEP, Lauschke VM, Ingelman-Sundberg M (2016) Characterization of primary human hepatocyte spheroids as a model system for drug-induced liver injury, liver function and disease. Sci Rep 6:25187. https://doi.org/10.1038/srep25187

78. Messner S, Agarkova I, Moritz W, Kelm JM (2013) Multi-cell type human liver microtissues for hepatotoxicity testing. Arch Toxicol 87(1):209–213. https://doi.org/10.1007/s00204-012-0968-2

79. Proctor WR, Foster AJ, Vogt J, Summers C, Middleton B, Pilling MA, Shienson D, Kijanska M, Strobel S, Kelm JM, Morgan P, Messner S, Williams D (2017) Utility of spherical human liver microtissues for prediction of clinical drug-induced liver injury. Arch Toxicol. https://doi.org/10.1007/s00204-017-2002-1

80. Kostadinova R, Boess F, Applegate D, Suter L, Weiser T, Singer T, Naughton B, Roth A (2013) A long-term three dimensional liver co-culture system for improved prediction of clinically relevant drug-induced hepatotoxicity. Toxicol Appl Pharmacol 268(1):1–16. https://doi.org/10.1016/j.taap.2013.01.012

81. Miyamoto Y, Ikeuchi M, Noguchi H, Yagi T, Hayashi S (2015) Spheroid formation and evaluation of hepatic cells in a three-dimensional culture device. Cell Med 8(1–2):47–56. https://doi.org/10.3727/21551 7915X689056

82. Tong WH, Fang Y, Yan J, Hong X, Hari Singh N, Wang SR, Nugraha B, Xia L, Fong ELS, Iliescu C, Yu H (2016) Constrained spheroids for prolonged hepatocyte culture. Biomaterials 80:106–120. https://doi.org/10.1016/j.biomaterials.2015.11.036

83. No da Y, Lee SA, Choi YY, Park D, Jang JY, Kim DS, Lee SH (2012) Functional 3D human primary hepatocyte spheroids made by co-culturing hepatocytes from partial hepatectomy specimens and human adipose-derived stem cells. PLoS One 7(12):e50723. https://doi.org/10.1371/journal.pone.0050723

84. Rebelo SP, Costa R, Silva MM, Marcelino P, Brito C, Alves PM (2015) Three-dimensional co-culture of human hepatocytes and mesenchymal stem cells: improved functionality in long-term bioreactor cultures. J Tissue Eng Regen Med. https://doi.org/10.1002/term.2099

85. Takayama K, Kawabata K, Nagamoto Y, Kishimoto K, Tashiro K, Sakurai F, Tachibana M, Kanda K, Hayakawa T, Furue MK, Mizuguchi H (2013) 3D spheroid culture of hESC/hiPSC-derived hepatocyte-like cells for drug toxicity testing. Biomaterials 34(7):1781–1789. https://doi.org/10.1016/j.biomaterials.2012.11.029

86. Liu Y, Wei J, Lu J, Lei D, Yan S, Li X (2016) Micropatterned coculture of hepatocytes on electrospun fibers as a potential in vitro model for predictive drug metabolism. Mater Sci Eng C Mater Biol Appl 63:475–484. https://doi.org/10.1016/j.msec.2016.03.025

87. Lutolf MP, Hubbell JA (2005) Synthetic biomaterials as instructive extracellular microenvironments for morphogenesis in tissue engineering. Nat Biotechnol 23(1):47–55. https://doi.org/10.1038/nbt1055

88. Chen AA, Thomas DK, Ong LL, Schwartz RE, Golub TR, Bhatia SN (2011) Humanized mice with ectopic artificial liver tissues. Proc Natl Acad Sci U S A 108(29):11842–11847. https://doi.org/10.1073/pnas.1101791108

89. Li CY, Stevens KR, Schwartz RE, Alejandro BS, Huang JH, Bhatia SN (2014) Micropatterned cell-cell interactions enable functional encapsulation of primary hepatocytes in hydrogel microtissues. Tissue Eng A 20(15–16):2200–2212. https://doi.org/10.1089/ten.tea.2013.0667

90. Tasnim F, Toh Y-C, Qu Y, Li H, Phan D, Narmada BC, Ananthanarayanan A, Mittal N, Meng RQ, Yu H (2016) Functionally enhanced human stem cell derived hepatocytes in galactosylated cellulosic sponges for hepatotoxicity testing. Mol Pharm 13(6):1947–1957. https://doi.org/10.1021/acs.molpharmaceut.6b00119

91. Larkin AL, Rodrigues RR, Murali TM, Rajagopalan P (2013) Designing a multicellular organotypic 3D liver model with a detachable, nanoscale polymeric Space of Disse. Tissue Eng Part C Methods 19(11):875–884. https://doi.org/10.1089/ten.tec.2012.0700

92. Orbach SM, Cassin ME, Ehrich MF, Rajagopalan P (2017) Investigating acetaminophen hepatotoxicity in multi-cellular organotypic liver models. Toxicol In Vitro 42:10–20. https://doi.org/10.1016/j.tiv.2017.03.008

93. Norona LM, Nguyen DG, Gerber DA, Presnell SC, LeCluyse EL (2016) Editor's highlight: modeling compound-induced fibrogenesis in vitro using three-dimensional bioprinted human liver tissues. Toxicol Sci 154(2):354–367. https://doi.org/10.1093/toxsci/kfw169

94. Jeon H, Kang K, Park SA, Kim WD, Paik SS, Lee SH, Jeong J, Choi D (2017) Generation of multilayered 3D structures of HepG2 cells using a bio-printing technique. Gut Liver 11(1):121–128. https://doi.org/10.5009/gnl16010

95. Ma X, Qu X, Zhu W, Li Y-S, Yuan S, Zhang H, Liu J, Wang P, Lai CSE, Zanella F, Feng G-S, Sheikh F, Chien S, Chen S (2016) Deterministically patterned biomimetic human iPSC-derived hepatic model via rapid 3D bioprinting. Proc Natl Acad Sci U S A 113(8):2206–2211. https://doi.org/10.1073/pnas.1524510113

96. Powers MJ, Domansky K, Kaazempur-Mofrad MR, Kalezi A, Capitano A, Upadhyaya A, Kurzawski P, Wack KE, Stolz DB, Kamm R, Griffith LG (2002) A microfabricated array bioreactor for perfused 3D liver culture. Biotechnol Bioeng 78(3):257–269

97. Powers MJ, Janigian DM, Wack KE, Baker CS, Beer Stolz D, Griffith LG (2002) Functional behavior of primary rat liver cells in a three-dimensional perfused microarray bioreactor. Tissue Eng 8(3):499–513. https://doi.org/10.1089/1076327027 60184745

98. Sivaraman A, Leach JK, Townsend S, Iida T, Hogan BJ, Stolz DB, Fry R, Samson LD, Tannenbaum SR, Griffith LG (2005) A microscale in vitro physiological model of the liver: predictive screens for drug metabolism and enzyme induction. Curr Drug Metab 6(6):569–591

99. Hwa AJ, Fry RC, Sivaraman A, So PT, Samson LD, Stolz DB, Griffith LG (2007) Rat liver sinusoidal endothelial cells survive without exogenous VEGF in 3D perfused co-cultures with hepatocytes. FASEB J 21(10):2564–2579. https://doi.org/10.1096/fj.06-7473com

100. Domansky K, Inman W, Serdy J, Dash A, Lim MH, Griffith LG (2010) Perfused multiwell plate for 3D liver tissue engineering. Lab Chip 10(1):51–58. https://doi.org/10.1039/b913221j

101. Dash A, Inman W, Hoffmaster K, Sevidal S, Kelly J, Obach RS, Griffith LG, Tannenbaum SR (2009) Liver tissue engineering in the evaluation of drug safety. Expert Opin Drug Metab Toxicol 5(10):1159–1174. https://doi.org/10.1517/17425250903160664

102. Tsamandouras N, Kostrzewski T, Stokes CL, Griffith LG, Hughes DJ, Cirit M (2017) Quantitative assessment of population variability in hepatic drug metabolism using a perfused three-dimensional human liver microphysiological system. J Pharmacol Exp Ther 360(1):95–105. https://doi.org/10.1124/jpet.116.237495

103. Sarkar U, Rivera-Burgos D, Large EM, Hughes DJ, Ravindra KC, Dyer RL, Ebrahimkhani MR, Wishnok JS, Griffith LG, Tannenbaum SR (2015) Metabolite profiling and pharmacokinetic evaluation of hydrocortisone in a perfused three-dimensional human liver bioreactor. Drug Metab Dispos 43(7):1091–1099. https://doi.org/10.1124/dmd.115.063495

104. Long TJ, Cosgrove PA, Dunn RT 2nd, Stolz DB, Hamadeh H, Afshari C, McBride H, Griffith LG (2016) Modeling therapeutic antibody-small molecule drug-drug interactions using a three-dimensional perfusable human liver coculture platform. Drug Metab Dispos 44(12):1940–1948. https://doi.org/10.1124/dmd.116.071456

105. Sarkar U, Ravindra KC, Large E, Young CL, Rivera-Burgos D, Yu J, Cirit M, Hughes DJ, Wishnok JS, Lauffenburger DA, Griffith LG, Tannenbaum SR (2017) Integrated assessment of diclofenac biotransformation, pharmacokinetics, and omics-based toxicity in a 3D human liver-immunocompetent co-culture system. Drug Metab Dispos. https://doi.org/10.1124/dmd.116.074005

106. Kane BJ, Zinner MJ, Yarmush ML, Toner M (2006) Liver-specific functional studies in a microfluidic array of primary mammalian hepatocytes. Anal Chem 78(13):4291–4298. https://doi.org/10.1021/ac051856v

107. Novik E, Maguire TJ, Chao P, Cheng KC, Yarmush ML (2010) A microfluidic hepatic coculture platform for cell-based drug metabolism studies. Biochem Pharmacol 79(7):1036–1044. https://doi.org/10.1016/j.bcp.2009.11.010

108. Esch MB, Prot JM, Wang YI, Miller P, Llamas-Vidales JR, Naughton BA, Applegate DR, Shuler ML (2015) Multi-cellular 3D human primary liver cell culture elevates metabolic activity under fluidic flow. Lab Chip 15(10):2269–2277. https://doi.org/10.1039/c5lc00237k

109. Kang YBA, Sodunke TR, Lamontagne J, Cirillo J, Rajiv C, Bouchard MJ, Noh M (2015) Liver sinusoid on a chip: long-term layered co-culture of primary rat hepatocytes and endothelial cells in microfluidic platforms. Biotechnol Bioeng 112(12):2571–2582. https://doi.org/10.1002/bit.25659

110. Rennert K, Steinborn S, Gröger M, Ungerböck B, Jank A-M, Ehgartner J, Nietzsche S, Dinger J, Kiehntopf M, Funke H, Peters FT, Lupp A, Gärtner C, Mayr T, Bauer M, Huber O, Mosig AS (2015) A microfluidically perfused three dimensional human liver model. Biomaterials 71:119–131. https://doi.org/10.1016/j.biomaterials.2015.08.043

111. Prodanov L, Jindal R, Bale SS, Hegde M, McCarty WJ, Golberg I, Bhushan A, Yarmush ML, Usta OB (2016) Long-term maintenance of a microfluidic 3D human liver sinusoid. Biotechnol Bioeng 113(1):241–246. https://doi.org/10.1002/bit.25700

112. Vernetti LA, Senutovitch N, Boltz R, Debiasio R, Shun TY, Gough A, Taylor DL (2016) A human liver microphysiology platform for investigating physiology, drug safety, and disease models. Exp Biol Med (Maywood) 241(1):101–114. https://doi.org/10.1177/1535370215592121

113. Lee-Montiel FT, George SM, Gough AH, Sharma AD, Wu J, DeBiasio R, Vernetti LA, Taylor DL (2017) Control of oxygen tension recapitulates zone-specific functions in human liver microphysiology systems. Exp Biol Med (Maywood) 242:1617–1632. https://doi.org/10.1177/1535370217703978

114. Kietzmann T (2017) Metabolic zonation of the liver: the oxygen gradient revisited. Redox Biol 11:622–630. https://doi.org/10.1016/j.redox.2017.01.012

115. Jungermann K, Kietzmann T (1996) Zonation of parenchymal and nonparenchymal metabolism in liver. Annu Rev Nutr 16:179–203. https://doi.org/10.1146/annurev.nu.16.070196.001143

116. Anundi I, Lähteenmäki T, Rundgren M, Moldeus P, Lindros KO (1993) Zonation of acetaminophen metabolism and cytochrome P450 2E1-mediated toxicity studied in isolated periportal and perivenous hepatocytes. Biochem Pharmacol 45(6):1251–1259

117. Soto-Gutierrez A, Gough A, Vernetti LA, Taylor DL, Monga SP (2017) Pre-clinical and clinical investigations of metabolic zonation in liver diseases: the potential of microphysiology systems. Exp Biol Med (Maywood) 242:1605–1616. https://doi.org/10.1177/1535370217707731

118. Allen JW, Bhatia SN (2003) Formation of steady-state oxygen gradients in vitro: application to liver zonation. Biotechnol Bioeng 82(3):253–262. https://doi.org/10.1002/bit.10569

119. Allen JW, Khetani SR, Bhatia SN (2005) In vitro zonation and toxicity in a hepatocyte bioreactor. Toxicol Sci 84(1):110–119. https://doi.org/10.1093/toxsci/kfi052

120. McCarty WJ, Usta OB, Yarmush ML (2016) A microfabricated platform for generating physiologically-relevant hepatocyte zonation. Sci Rep 6:26868. https://doi.org/10.1038/srep26868

121. Khetani SR, Berger DR, Ballinger KR, Davidson MD, Lin C, Ware BR (2015) Microengineered liver tissues for drug testing. J Lab Autom 20(3):216–250. https://doi.org/10.1177/2211068214566939

122. O'Brien PJ, Irwin W, Diaz D, Howard-Cofield E, Krejsa CM, Slaughter MR, Gao B, Kaludercic N, Angeline A, Bernardi P, Brain P, Hougham C (2006) High concordance of drug-induced human hepatotoxicity with in vitro cytotoxicity measured in a novel cell-based model using high content screening. Arch Toxicol 80(9):580–604. https://doi.org/10.1007/s00204-006-0091-3

123. Tolosa L, Gómez-Lechón MJ, Donato MT (2015) High-content screening technology for studying drug-induced hepatotoxicity in cell models. Arch Toxicol 89(7):1007–1022. https://doi.org/10.1007/s00204-015-1503-z

124. Tolosa L, Pinto S, Donato MT, Lahoz A, Castell JV, O'Connor JE, Gómez-Lechón MJ (2012) Development of a multiparametric cell-based protocol to screen and classify the hepatotoxicity potential of drugs. Toxicol Sci 127(1):187–198. https://doi.org/10.1093/toxsci/kfs083

125. Corsini A, Ganey P, Ju C, Kaplowitz N, Pessayre D, Roth R, Watkins PB, Albassam M, Liu B, Stancic S, Suter L, Bortolini M (2012) Current challenges and controversies in drug-induced liver injury. Drug Saf 35(12):1099–1117. https://doi.org/10.2165/11632970-000000000-00000

126. Carlton JM, Angiuoli SV, Suh BB, Kooij TW, Pertea M, Silva JC, Ermolaeva MD, Allen JE, Selengut JD, Koo HL, Peterson JD, Pop M, Kosack DS, Shumway MF, Bidwell SL, Shallom SJ, van Aken SE, Riedmuller SB, Feldblyum TV, Cho JK, Quackenbush J, Sedegah M, Shoaibi A, Cummings LM, Florens L, Yates JR, Raine JD, Sinden RE, Harris MA, Cunningham DA, Preiser PR, Bergman LW, Vaidya AB, van Lin LH, Janse CJ, Waters AP, Smith HO, White OR, Salzberg SL, Venter JC, Fraser CM, Hoffman SL, Gardner MJ, Carucci DJ (2002) Genome sequence and comparative analysis of the model rodent malaria parasite Plasmodium yoelii yoelii. Nature 419(6906):512–519. https://doi.org/10.1038/nature01099

127. McCutchan TF, Lal AA, de la Cruz VF, Miller LH, Maloy WL, Charoenvit Y, Beaudoin RL, Guerry P, Wistar R, Hoffman SL (1985) Sequence of the immunodominant epitope for the surface protein on sporozoites of Plasmodium vivax. Science (New York, NY) 230(4732):1381–1383

128. Ng S, Schwartz RE, March S, Galstian A, Gural N, Shan J, Prabhu M, Mota MM, Bhatia SN (2015) Human iPSC-derived hepatocyte-like cells support plasmodium liver-stage infection in vitro. Stem Cell Reports 4(3):348–359. https://doi.org/10.1016/j.stemcr.2015.01.002

129. Gripon P, Diot C, Thézé N, Fourel I, Loreal O, Brechot C, Guguen-Guillouzo C (1988) Hepatitis B virus infection of adult human hepatocytes cultured in the presence of dimethyl sulfoxide. J Virol 62(11):4136–4143

130. Fournier C, Sureau C, Coste J, Ducos J, Pageaux G, Larrey D, Domergue J, Maurel P (1998) In vitro infection of adult normal human hepatocytes in primary culture by hepatitis C virus. J Gen Virol 79(Pt 10): 2367–2374

131. Schwartz RE, Trehan K, Andrus L, Sheahan TP, Ploss A, Duncan SA, Rice CM, Bhatia SN (2012) Modeling hepatitis C virus infection using human induced pluripotent stem cells. Proc Natl Acad Sci U S A 109(7):2544–2548. https://doi.org/10.1073/pnas.1121400109

132. Calzadilla Bertot L, Adams LA (2016) The natural course of non-alcoholic fatty liver disease. Int J Mol Sci 17(5). https://doi.org/10.3390/ijms17050774

133. Jahn D, Rau M, Wohlfahrt J, Hermanns HM, Geier A (2016) Non-alcoholic steatohepatitis: from pathophysiology to novel therapies. Dig Dis 34(4):356–363. https://doi.org/10.1159/000444547

134. Teufel A, Itzel T, Erhart W, Brosch M, Wang XY, Kim YO, von Schönfels W, Herrmann A, Brückner S, Stickel F, Dufour J-F, Chavakis T, Hellerbrand C, Spang R, Maass T, Becker T, Schreiber S, Schafmayer C, Schuppan D, Hampe J (2016) Comparison of gene expression patterns between mouse models of non-alcoholic fatty liver disease and liver tissues from patients. Gastroenterology. https://doi.org/10.1053/j.gastro.2016.05.051

135. Shih H, Pickwell GV, Guenette DK, Bilir B, Quattrochi LC (1999) Species differences in hepatocyte induction of CYP1A1 and CYP1A2 by omeprazole. Hum Exp Toxicol 18(2):95–105

136. Kostrzewski T, Cornforth T, Snow SA, Ouro-Gnao L, Rowe C, Large EM, Hughes DJ (2017) Three-dimensional perfused human in vitro model of non-alcoholic fatty liver disease. World J Gastroenterol 23(2):204–215. https://doi.org/10.3748/wjg.v23.i2.204

137. Hardwick RN, Fisher CD, Canet MJ, Scheffer GL, Cherrington NJ (2011) Variations in ATP-binding cassette transporter regulation during the progression of human nonalcoholic fatty liver disease. Drug Metab Dispos 39(12):2395–2402. https://doi.org/10.1124/dmd.111.041012

138. Merrell MD, Cherrington NJ (2011) Drug metabolism alterations in nonalcoholic fatty liver disease. Drug Metab Rev 43(3):317–334. https://doi.org/10.3109/03602532.2011.577781

139. Feaver RE, Cole BK, Lawson MJ, Hoang SA, Marukian S, Blackman BR, Figler RA, Sanyal AJ, Wamhoff BR, Dash A (2016) Development of an in vitro human liver system for interrogating nonalcoholic steatohepatitis. JCI Insight 1(20):e90954. https://doi.org/10.1172/jci.insight.90954

140. Hughes DJ, Kostrzewski T, Sceats EL (2017) Opportunities and challenges in the wider adoption of liver and interconnected microphysiological systems. Exp Biol Med (Maywood) 242:1593–1604. https://doi.org/10.1177/1535370217708976

141. Schimek K, Busek M, Brincker S, Groth B, Hoffmann S, Lauster R, Lindner G, Lorenz A, Menzel U, Sonntag F, Walles H, Marx U, Horland R (2013) Integrating biological vasculature into a multi-organ-chip microsystem. Lab Chip 13(18):3588–3598. https://doi.org/10.1039/c3lc50217a

142. Ukairo O, Kanchagar C, Moore A, Shi J, Gaffney J, Aoyama S, Rose K, Krzyzewski S, McGeehan J, Andersen ME, Khetani SR, LeCluyse EL (2013) Long-term stability of primary rat hepatocytes in micropatterned cocultures. J Biochem Mol Toxicol 27(3):204–212. https://doi.org/10.1002/jbt.21469

143. Seglen PO (1976) Preparation of isolated rat liver cells. Methods Cell Biol 13:29–83

144. Seglen PO (1972) Preparation of rat liver cells. I. Effect of Ca^{2+} on enzymatic dispersion of isolated, perfused liver. Exp Cell Res 74(2):450–454

145. Liu Tsang V, Chen AA, Cho LM, Jadin KD, Sah RL, DeLong S, West JL, Bhatia SN (2007) Fabrication of 3D hepatic tissues by additive photopatterning of cellular hydrogels. FASEB J 21(3):790–801. https://doi.org/10.1096/fj.06-7117com

146. Scott CW, Peters MF, Dragan YP (2013) Human induced pluripotent stem cells and their use in drug discovery for toxicity testing. Toxicol Lett 219(1):49–58. https://doi.org/10.1016/j.toxlet.2013.02.020

Chapter 12

Status and Future of 3D Cell Culture in Toxicity Testing

Monicah A. Otieno, Jinping Gan, and William Proctor

Abstract

Drug-induced liver injury is a major reason for safety-related attrition in the pharmaceutical industry. There is continued search for in vitro models that can be used to consistently and reliably select compounds with reduced liability for liver injury. 2D in vitro models, such as liver cell lines and primary hepatocytes have been used for many decades prior to advancement to micropatterned 2D liver models; the latter have improved metabolic activity and can be cultured for long periods without loss of function/viability. The emergence of 3D liver models, including spheroids, 3D bioprinted livers, and liver-on-chip have the potential to revolutionize in vitro liver toxicity testing. These models have been collectively coined as microphysiological systems (MPS). The MPS models can be maintained in culture for at least 1-month during which they retain significant drug metabolism capability. Some MPS models can also be cocultured with other nonparenchymal supporting cells, such as endothelial, Kupffer, and stellate cells, which increases the versatility of the models for toxicity assessment. An added benefit of some MPS models is the ability to sample supernatant for biomarker measurements. There are several contexts of use for which MPS models can be applied, and the most likely use will be for candidate drug screening and mechanistic studies.

Key words 3D models, Liver, Microphysiological systems, MPS, Spheroids, Liver-on-chip, Bioprinted

1 Introduction

Drug-induced liver injury (DILI) is a major contributor to drug attrition in the pharmaceutical industry [1], and is the major cause of acute liver failure leading to death or requiring liver transplantation [2]. DILI can be categorized as intrinsic or idiosyncratic [3]. Intrinsic DILI is exemplified by acetaminophen where liver injury is predictable and can be monitored with serum biochemical markers. In contrast, idiosyncratic DILI (iDILI) occurs in a few individuals in large populations exposed to drugs, and is often not predicted by animal toxicology studies [3]. There are several in silico, in vitro, and in vivo approaches (Fig. 1) that can be taken to de-risk DILI during drug discovery and development. These approaches can be applied proactively to select candidates with reduced risk for DILI or retrospectively for mechanistic

Minjun Chen and Yvonne Will (eds.), *Drug-Induced Liver Toxicity*, Methods in Pharmacology and Toxicology,
https://doi.org/10.1007/978-1-4939-7677-5_12, © Springer Science+Business Media, LLC, part of Springer Nature 2018

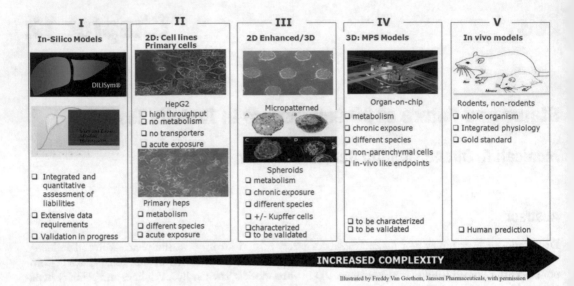

Fig. 1 Current approaches for assessing drug-induced liver injury

understanding of liver findings in the clinic or in animal studies. Traditionally, in vitro studies have been conducted in primary hepatocytes or liver-derived cell lines, such as HepG2 or THLE cells transfected with cytochrome P450s [4–7]. More recently, cytotoxicity has been combined with additional mechanistic end points, such as inhibition of hepatic transporters, most commonly the bile salt efflux pump (BSEP), and assessment of mitochondrial dysfunction for an integrated assessment of DILI risk [8–11]. The term of two-dimentional (2D) models has recently been coined to describe these traditional hepatocyte models, to distinguish from the newer three-dimenional (3D) liver models [12]. In this chapter, we describe various 3D liver models, current progress in the characterization and use of these models, and the challenges and opportunities in improving predictive values of these models.

2   Advantages and Limitations of Traditional 2D Hepatocyte Models

Traditional 2D hepatocyte models mentioned here refers to those cells grown in monolayers, such as primary hepatocytes and liver-derived cell lines. These models can be used early in the drug discovery process for hazard identification. An advantage of these models is their amenability to high throughput screening and high-content image analyses [7]. Use of 2D systems are discussed in more detail in Chaps. 8 and 9. A major disadvantage is they either lack metabolic capability or the enzymatic activity deteriorate with time during culture [13, 14], and these defects lead to loss of hepatocyte phenotype, e.g., albumin secretion and morphology, in culture [13]. The gaps in these traditional 2D models have led to innovative approaches, such as enhanced 2D models and 3D models, which have generated more complex models that retain hepatocyte-like phenotypes, physiology, and functions. The most commonly used enhanced 2D model is the matrix overlay hepatocyte sandwich culture model usually used for assessing transporter function [15]. Other models include the micropatterned cocultures of hepatocytes, fibroblasts, and Kupffer cells [16, 17] and iPSC-derived hepatocytes [18, 19]. The micropatterned models have the advantage of maintaining viability and hepatocyte function for prolonged incubation times of at least 7 days, and are useful for assessing the metabolic clearance of compounds with low turnover, studying transporter mechanisms, and assessing cytotoxicity. These models have been detailed in Chaps. 10 and 11 of this volume.

3 Characteristics of 3D Liver Models

3D liver models include the self-aggregated spheroids, 3D printed tissues, and fluidic-based 3D models that can be cultured as mono-cultures of hepatocytes or as cocultures with nonparencyhmal cells including sinusoidal endothelial cells, Kupffer cells, or stellate cells [12, 20–22]. These models are improved over 2D models because they can be maintained in culture for prolonged periods (>2 weeks) while remaining viable and retaining enhanced metabolic activity during this culture period, and some models that are cocultured with nonparenchymal cells allow for detection of toxicities caused by compounds that may target these cells. The term of microphysi-ological systems (MPS) has been coined to describe the enhanced 3D models, i.e., 3D spheroids, 3D bioprinted tissues, and fluidic-based organs-on-chip. Methods for preparation and characterization of these models are described in detail below.

3.1 3D Spheroids

Spheroids are generated from self-aggregating liver-derived cell lines [23, 24], primary hepatocytes [25], or iPSC-derived hepato-cytes [22] with or without supporting nonparenchymal cells. Ideally, the size of the spheroids should be optimized to prevent necrotic centers and culture conditions are usually controlled to prevent disaggregation, which at times may be caused by turbu-lence when manipulating the cells during handling. The following part describe three methods used for developing and characteriz-ing spheroid cultures.

3.1.1 Primary Hepatocyte Spheroid Cocultured with Nonparenchymal Cells

This method, adapted from Bell et al. [25], describes the simplest approach for culturing spheroids. Cryopreserved primary hepatocytes and nonparenchymal cells are seeded at a ratio of 2:1 into ultralow attachment 96-well plates at 2000 cells per well in hepatocyte media containing 10% FBS and centrifuged at $100 \times g$

for 2 min. Spheroids form by self-aggregation of the cells, and on Days 4 or 5, 50% of the media is exchanged with serum-free media every 2–3 days, and the spheroids can be maintained in culture for at least 1 month. The hepatocyte spheroids prepared with this method were characteristically similar to human liver based on their transcriptomic and proteomic signatures; they also maintained hepatocyte functionality and showed increased sensitivity to liver toxicants compared to 2D hepatocytes (Fig. 2).

Berger et al. [23]. also describes an equally simple approach for a hepatocyte/fibroblast spheroid coculture. In this method 3T3 fibroblasts are seeded at 8000 cells/well into a micropatterned 96-well plate (40,000 cells/well in 24-well plates), and the cells incubated in standard Dulbecco's Modified Eagle's culture medium for 2 days. Cryopreserved human hepatocytes at 25,000 cells/well are added to the fibroblasts in the 96-well plate (or 125,000 cells/well in 24-well plates) in conventional hepatocyte media, and the coculture incubated for at least 2 days to allow for spheroid formation. Cytochrome P450 activities in the hepatocyte/fibroblast spheroid coculture were significantly improved over standard 2D hepatocytes and HepG2 cells, but was marginally improved over HepaRG cells (Fig. 3).

3.1.2 Primary Hepatocyte Spheroid Cocultured with Endothelial Cells in a Collagen Matrix

This method, adapted from Okudaira et al. [26], includes additional complexity compared to the simple method described previously (vide supra) by controlling the size of formed spheroids, coating the hepatocytes with endothelial cells (HUVECs), and forming the spheroids in a collagen matrix. Controlling the size of the spheroids prevents formation of large spheroid aggregates, which can form necrotic centers due to poor perfusion of nutrients and oxygen. In this method (Fig. 4), primary hepatocytes were cultured in a 6-well plate at 7.5×10^6 cells/well in 1.5 mL hepatocyte culture media and centrifuged at low speed (80 rpm) in a humidified CO_2 incubator. Self-aggregating hepatocyte spheroids were collected on Day 2 and sieved through a wire mesh to generated 50–150 μm aggregates that were suspended in 1 mL hepatocyte media. Reconstituted collagen (Cell matrix Type 1A) was added to the spheroid suspension for a final collagen concentration of 1.2 mg/mL; the suspension was incubated for 1 h at 4 °C, washed with 10 mL cold hepatocyte media, and then centrifuged for 1 min at $40 \times g$. The collagen coated hepatocyte/HUVEC spheroids were suspended in 12 mL hepatocyte culture medium and plated on a 100 mm cell culture dish coated with 4% agarose. The medium (6 mL per dish) was replaced on Day 2 of coculture and HUVEC-covered hepatocytes spheroids were collected on Day 4 of coculture for experiments. The spheroid coculture of hepatocytes with HUVECs significantly improved urea and albumin synthesis compared to spheroid cultures of hepatocytes only or the standard 2D culture.

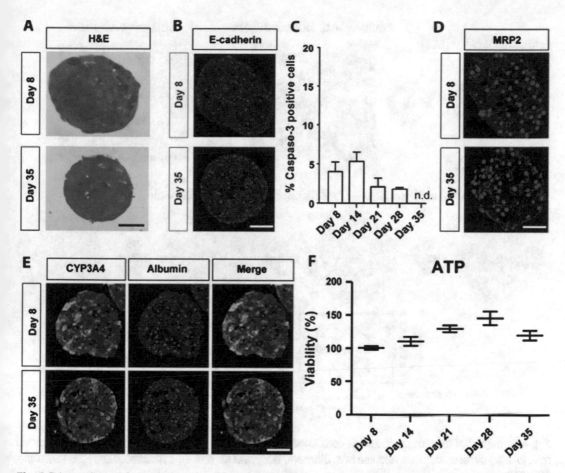

Fig. 2 Primary human hepatocyte spheroids. (**a**) H&E staining, (**b**) E-Cadherin staining, (**c**) Caspase 3 expression, (**d, e**) MRP2, CYP3A4, and Albumin staining (**f**) ATP levels. Adapted from Bell, Catherine et al., (2016) *Science Reports*, **6**, 25,187

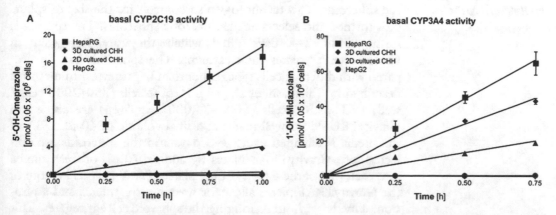

Fig. 3 Basal activity of CYP2C19 (**a**) and CYP3A4 (**b**) in HepG2, HepaRG, 2D- and 3D cultured primary cryopreserved human hepatocytes. Adapted from Berger, B et al., (2016), Frontiers in Pharmacology, 7, 443

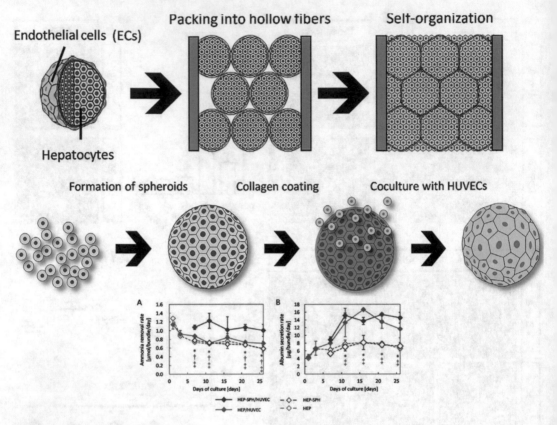

Fig. 4 Formation of hepatocyte spheroids cocultured with endothelial cells (HUVECs). (**a**) Ammonium removal rate, (**b**) albumin secretion rate. Adapted from Okudaira, Tatsuya et al., (2016), *J. Bioscience and Bioengineering*, **122**, 213

3.1.3 Primary Hepatocyte and Liver-Derived Cell Lines Spheroids Using the Hanging Drop System

In this method, gravitational force is utilized to allow cells to assemble into spheroids in a hanging droplet using proprietary plates (GravityPLUS™). This is a scaffold-free system because the cells form de novo extracellular matrix, e.g., collagen, as they form the spheroids. This technology also controls for the size of spheroids formed and selects against necrotic spheroids. The spheroids form within 2–4 days after which they are harvested in GravityTRAP™ plates for treatment. The spheroids can be prepared with different cells types other than hepatocytes. In methods described by Takahashi et al. [24], HepG2 cells (250–2000 cells/well) or HepaRG cells (8000–24,000 cells/well) are seeded in GravityPLUS™ 96-well plates at a final volume of 40 μL. 75% of the media is changed every 1–3 days and the spheroids are collected into GravityTRAP plates by adding 70 μL of fresh media into each well of the GravityPLUS plates. The V-shaped bottom of the GravityTRAP plates allow for washing, treatment, and aspiration of media without dislodging the spheroid cell aggregates. This technology can also be used to develop spheroid cocultures with other nonparenchymal cells, e.g., Kupffer cells.

Methods for formation of 3D spheroids are easily amenable for treatment in a 96-well format, ranging from very simple techniques to more complex proprietary approaches. In addition to measurement of markers released in the media, the spheroids are also amenable for immunohistochemical staining for cellular markers of interest.

3.2 3D Bioprinted Liver

3D printing is a process whereby biological materials are printed onto 3D scaffolds. Significant strides have been made with the technology in tissue engineering and medicine [27], including advances to print medical devices. The common 3D bioprinting approaches are inkjet bioprinting, microextrusion bioprinting, and laser-assisted bioprinting [28]. Inkjet bioprinting has been adapted from 2D inkjet printing where the ink in cartridges is replaced by biomaterials and the paper is replaced by a predefined 3D location. In microextrusion bioprinting, the printers extrude biological materials onto a substrate using a microextrusion head. As the name suggests, laser-assisted bioprinting uses laser technology to transfer biological material to a substrate. This technology has been applied to develop bioprinted 3D liver tissues [29]; the tissues are manufactured with the proprietary Novagen® bioprinting technology that uses NovoGel® bio inks to print hepatocytes and nonparenchymal cells onto inserts of 24-well transwell culture plates using proprietary media and matrix. The tissues are fed with hepatocyte media (600 μL) and allowed to mature for 3 days in a humidified CO_2 incubator prior to treatment with compounds for durations of at least 1 month. The 3D tissues are dense, making them amenable to microscopic processing techniques typically used for native liver tissues, such as tissue sectioning and staining. The bioprinted livers maintain normal hepatocyte function, detected by albumin secretion, and viability for prolonged culture periods of up to 28 days (Fig. 5). The 3D bioprinted liver comprised of hepatocytes and stellate cells, has been used to model fibrosis with agents such as monocrotaline [30] and methotrexate [31], where fibrosis was detected by tissue staining for α-smooth actin, a marker for activated cells, and was accompanied by release of cytokines. This model shows potential for use and application in toxicity testing.

3.3 Liver-on-Chip

Advances in microfluidic engineering have recently made it possible to create miniaturized in vitro cell culture systems, known as organs-on-chips [32, 33], in which human cells and tissues are subjected to fluid flow and mechanical stress in well-controlled microenvironments. These attributes allow cells to flourish and maintain their in vivo-like phenotypic properties. Fluidic flow allows for replenishment of nutrients and removal of waste, which enhances cell viability and normal functioning of the cells. Collectively, these properties seem conducive for hepatocytes to retain their differentiated phenotype, i.e., albumin secretion and morphology.

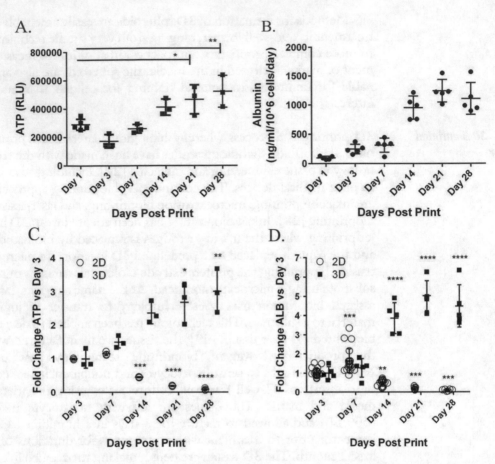

Fig. 5 Measurement of tissue ATP and secreted albumin from 3D bioprinted liver tissues over 28 days. Adapted from Nguyen, Deborah, G et al. (2016), *PLoS ONE*, **11**, e0158674

A fluidic-based liver-on-chip microdevice based on a platform developed by Nortis (Fig. 6) prepared with primary hepatocytes cocultured with endothelial (Eahy.926), differentiated macrophages (U397), and stellate (LX-2) cell lines has recently been described [34]. Cells remained viable in the microdevice for at least 25 days based on lack of release of leakage enzymes; active secretion of albumin and urea demonstrated normal functioning of hepatocytes. Metabolic competency was confirmed based on formation of oxidative and glucuronide metabolites using probe substrates for CYP3A4 (testosterone), CYP 2C9 (diclofenac), and UDP-glucuronyltransferase (phenolphthalein). The model also incorporated the use of biosensors [35] for reactive oxygen species, mitochondrial functions and hepatic transport inhibition to characterize adverse outcome pathways for hepatotoxicants.

Another fluidic-based liver microdevice built based on the platform developed at the Wyss Institute [32] has recently been reported [36]. This model is composed of an upper chamber seeded with primary human hepatocytes sandwiched in a collagen

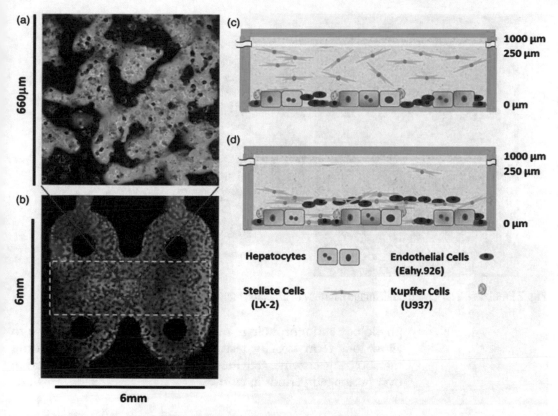

Fig. 6 (a, b) Self-organization of hepatocytes and supporting nonparenchyma cells in liver-on-chip, **(c)** diagram based on confocal image of cells on Day 1 after seeding and **(d)** on Day 7, showing self-organization. Adapted from Vernetti Lawrence, A. et al. (2016), Experimental Biology & Medicine, 241, 101

matrix that is separated by a porous membrane from a lower chamber containing nonparenchymal cells (Fig. 7). Continuous media flow is maintained in both chambers, which enhances hepatocyte function and viability.

4   Properties to Consider During Characterization of MPS Liver Models

The 3D microphysiological liver models hold great promise as the next generation in vitro models. However, because these models are in the early stages of development with limited application in drug development, some properties that should be considered during their development and characterization to qualify them for use in testing compounds. These include (1) showing superiority over current standard models, such as traditional 2D hepatocytes, (2) identifying the relevant adverse outcome pathways known to be perturbed during the development of DILI, e.g., formation of reactive oxygen species, perturbation of bile acid homeostasis or mitochondrial function, (3) maintenance of normal hepatocyte

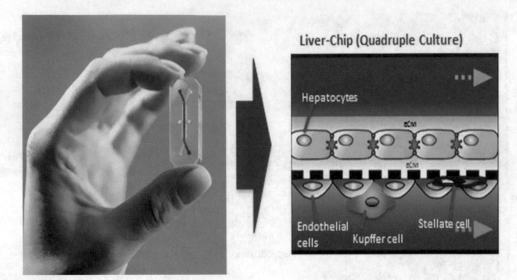

Fig. 7 Emulate's liver-chip model. Image courtesy of Emulate, Inc.

physiology and morphology over prolonged periods in culture to allow long-term toxicity testing, and (4) maintenance of drug metabolizing enzyme activities and hepatic transporter function over prolonged periods in culture.

5   Potential Biomarkers to Measure in 3D MPS Liver Models

Because of the liver-like functionality of the 3D MPS liver models conventional and novel markers for liver injury, such as transaminases (ALT, AST), glutamate dehydrogenase (GLDH), miR122, cytokeratin 18, and high mobility group box 1 protein (HMGB1) [37] may be incorporated as end points in these models. Systems that contain nonparenchymal cells, such as endothelial, Kupffer and stellate cells, can be used to characterize compound-mediated changes in innate immune response, and some end points, such as cytokines have already been incorporated into the MPS models [31].

6   3D MPS Liver Models Context of Use

The specific context of use for which the MPS models can be applied will need to be carefully crafted. Some areas where MPS models may facilitate decision making during drug discovery and development are: (1) candidate drug screening, i.e., MPS models could be used to prioritize new candidates prior to toxicity testing in animals, (2) human risk assessment, i.e., the MPS models could inform on human relevance of liver findings in the case of conflicted observations when compounds are tested in multiple species, (3) mechanistic studies, i.e., to investigate mechanisms for toxicities encountered in nonclinical studies or in the clinic, and (4) prediction of human clearance for compounds that are metabolized slowly and have low turnover in human microsomes or hepatocytes.

Acknowledgments

The authors acknowledge the Innovation and Quality (IQ) Microphysiological (MPS) Working Group members and the participation of Brett Howell of DILIsym, Inc. and Paul Watkins of University of North Carolina in discussions on MPS standards for liver models.

References

1. Tujios S, Fontana RJ (2011) Mechanisms of drug-induced liver injury: from bedside to bench. Nat Rev Gastroenterol Hepatol 8(4):202–211. https://doi.org/10.1038/nrgastro.2011.22

2. Fontana RJ, Hayashi PH, Gu J, Reddy KR, Barnhart H, Watkins PB, Serrano J, Lee WM, Chalasani N, Stolz A, Davern T, Talwakar JA, Network D (2014) Idiosyncratic drug-induced liver injury is associated with substantial morbidity and mortality within 6 months from onset. Gastroenterology 147(1):96–108. e104. https://doi.org/10.1053/j.gastro.2014.03.045

3. Fontana RJ (2014) Pathogenesis of idiosyncratic drug-induced liver injury and clinical perspectives. Gastroenterology 146(4):914–928. https://doi.org/10.1053/j.gastro.2013.12.032

4. Gustafsson F, Foster AJ, Sarda S, Bridgland-Taylor MH, Kenna JG (2014) A correlation between the in vitro drug toxicity of drugs to cell lines that express human P450s and their propensity to cause liver injury in humans. Toxicol Sci 137(1):189–211. https://doi.org/10.1093/toxsci/kft223

5. Soltanpour Y, Hilgendorf C, Ahlstrom MM, Foster AJ, Kenna JG, Petersen A, Ungell AL (2012) Characterization of THLE-cytochrome P450 (P450) cell lines: gene expression background and relationship to P450-enzyme activity. Drug Metab Dispos 40(11):2054–2058. https://doi.org/10.1124/dmd.112.045815

6. Dambach DM, Andrews BA, Moulin F (2005) New technologies and screening strategies for hepatotoxicity: use of in vitro models. Toxicol Pathol 33(1):17–26. https://doi.org/10.1080/01926230590522284

7. O'Brien PJ, Irwin W, Diaz D, Howard-Cofield E, Krejsa CM, Slaughter MR, Gao B, Kaludercic N, Angeline A, Bernardi P, Brain P, Hougham C (2006) High concordance of drug-induced human hepatotoxicity with in vitro cytotoxicity measured in a novel cell-based model using high content screening. Arch Toxicol 80(9):580–604. https://doi.org/10.1007/s00204-006-0091-3

8. Schadt S, Simon S, Kustermann S, Boess F, McGinnis C, Brink A, Lieven R, Fowler S, Youdim K, Ullah M, Marschmann M, Zihlmann C, Siegrist YM, Cascais AC, Di Lenarda E, Durr E, Schaub N, Ang X, Starke V, Singer T, Alvarez-Sanchez R, Roth AB, Schuler F, Funk C (2015) Minimizing DILI risk in drug discovery – a screening tool for drug candidates. Toxicol In Vitro 30(1 Pt B):429–437. https://doi.org/10.1016/j.tiv.2015.09.019

9. Shah F, Leung L, Barton HA, Will Y, Rodrigues AD, Greene N, Aleo MD (2015) Setting clinical exposure levels of concern for drug-induced liver injury (DILI) using mechanistic in vitro assays. Toxicol Sci 147(2):500–514. https://doi.org/10.1093/toxsci/kfv152

10. Otieno MA, Snoeys J, Lam W, Ghosh A, Player MR, Pocai A, Salter R, Simic D, Skaggs H, Singh B, Heng-Keang L (2017) Fasiglifam (TAK-875): mechanistic investigation and retrospective identification of hazards for drug induced liver injury (DILI). Toxicol Sci. https://doi.org/10.1093/toxsci/kfx040

11. Thompson RA, Isin EM, Li Y, Weidolf L, Page K, Wilson I, Swallow S, Middleton B, Stahl S, Foster AJ, Dolgos H, Weaver R, Kenna JG (2012) In vitro approach to assess the potential for risk of idiosyncratic adverse reactions caused by candidate drugs. Chem Res Toxicol 25(8):1616–1632. https://doi.org/10.1021/tx300091x

12. Lauschke VM, Hendriks DF, Bell CC, Andersson TB, Ingelman-Sundberg M (2016) Novel 3D culture systems for studies of human liver function and assessments of the hepato-toxicity of drugs and drug candidates. Chem Res Toxicol 29(12):1936–1955. https://doi.org/10.1021/acs.chemrestox.6b00150

13. Shulman M, Nahmias Y (2013) Long-term culture and coculture of primary rat and human hepatocytes. Methods Mol Biol 945:287–302. https://doi.org/10.1007/978-1-62703-125-7_17

14. Wortelboer HM, de Kruif CA, van Iersel AA, Falke HE, Noordhoek J, Blaauboer BJ (1990) The isoenzyme pattern of cytochrome P450 in rat hepatocytes in primary culture, comparing different enzyme activities in microsomal incubations and in intact monolayers. Biochem Pharmacol 40(11):2525–2534

15. Kemp DC, Zamek-Gliszczynski MJ, Brouwer KL (2005) Xenobiotics inhibit hepatic uptake and biliary excretion of taurocholate in rat hepatocytes. Toxicol Sci 83(2):207–214. https://doi.org/10.1093/toxsci/kfi020

16. Trask OJ Jr, Moore A, LeCluyse EL (2014) A micropatterned hepatocyte coculture model for assessment of liver toxicity using high-content imaging analysis. Assay Drug Dev Technol 12(1):16–27. https://doi.org/10.1089/adt.2013.525

17. Lin C, Khetani SR (2016) Advances in engineered liver models for investigating drug-induced liver injury. Biomed Res Int 2016:1829148. https://doi.org/10.1155/2016/1829148

18. Ware BR, Berger DR, Khetani SR (2015) Prediction of drug-induced liver injury in micropatterned co-cultures containing iPSC-derived human hepatocytes. Toxicol Sci 145(2):252–262. https://doi.org/10.1093/toxsci/kfv048

19. Goldring C, Antoine DJ, Bonner F, Crozier J, Denning C, Fontana RJ, Hanley NA, Hay DC, Ingelman-Sundberg M, Juhila S, Kitteringham N, Silva-Lima B, Norris A, Pridgeon C, Ross JA, Young RS, Tagle D, Tornesi B, van de Water B, Weaver RJ, Zhang F, Park BK (2017) Stem cell-derived models to improve mechanistic understanding and prediction of human drug-induced liver injury. Hepatology 65(2):710–721. https://doi.org/10.1002/hep.28886

20. Xia L, Hong X, Sakban RB, Qu Y, Singh NH, McMillian M, Dallas S, Silva J, Sensenhauser C, Zhao S, Lim HK, Yu H (2016) Cytochrome P450 induction response in tethered spheroids as a three-dimensional human hepatocyte in vitro model. J Appl Toxicol 36(2):320–329. https://doi.org/10.1002/jat.3189

21. Wang Z, Luo X, Anene-Nzelu C, Yu Y, Hong X, Singh NH, Xia L, Liu S, Yu H (2015) HepaRG culture in tethered spheroids as an in vitro three-dimensional model for drug safety screening. J Appl Toxicol 35(8):909–917. https://doi.org/10.1002/jat.3090

22. Sirenko O, Hancock MK, Hesley J, Hong D, Cohen A, Gentry J, Carlson CB, Mann DA (2016) Phenotypic characterization of toxic compound effects on liver spheroids derived from iPSC using confocal imaging and three-dimensional image analysis. Assay Drug Dev Technol 14(7):381–394. https://doi.org/10.1089/adt.2016.729

23. Berger B, Donzelli M, Maseneni S, Boess F, Roth A, Krahenbuhl S, Haschke M (2016) Comparison of liver cell models using the Basel phenotyping cocktail. Front Pharmacol 7:443. https://doi.org/10.3389/fphar.2016.00443

24. Takahashi Y, Hori Y, Yamamoto T, Urashima T, Ohara Y, Tanaka H (2015) 3D spheroid cultures improve the metabolic gene expression profiles of HepaRG cells. Biosci Rep 35(3). https://doi.org/10.1042/BSR20150034

25. Bell CC, Hendriks DF, Moro SM, Ellis E, Walsh J, Renblom A, Fredriksson Puigvert L, Dankers AC, Jacobs F, Snoeys J, Sison-Young RL, Jenkins RE, Nordling A, Mkrtchian S, Park BK, Kitteringham NR, Goldring CE, Lauschke VM, Ingelman-Sundberg M (2016) Characterization of primary human hepatocyte spheroids as a model system for drug-induced liver injury, liver function and disease. Sci Rep 6:25187. https://doi.org/10.1038/srep25187

26. Okudaira T, Amimoto N, Mizumoto H, Kajiwara T (2016) Formation of three-dimensional hepatic tissue by the bottom-up method using spheroids. J Biosci Bioeng 122(2):213–218

27. Zhang GL, Fisher JP, Leong KW (2015) 3D bioprinting and nanotechnology in tissue engineering and regenerative medicine. Elsevier, London

28. Murphy SV, Atala A (2014) 3D bioprinting of tissues and organs. Nat Biotechnol 32(8):773–785. https://doi.org/10.1038/nbt.2958

29. Nguyen DG, Funk J, Robbins JB, Crogan-Grundy C, Presnell SC, Singer T, Roth AB

(2016) Bioprinted 3D primary liver tissues allow assessment of organ-level response to clinical drug induced toxicity in vitro. PLoS One 11(7):e0158674. https://doi.org/10.1371/journal.pone.0158674

30. Hanumegowda UM, Wu Y, Smith TR, Lehman-McKeeman L (2016) Monocrotaline toxicity in 3D-bioprinted human liver tissues. The Toxicologist, Supplement to Toxicological Sciences 150(1)

31. Norona LM, Nguyen DG, Gerber DA, Presnell SC, LeCluyse EL (2016) Editor's highlight: modeling compound-induced fibrogenesis in vitro using three-dimensional bioprinted human liver tissues. Toxicol Sci 154(2):354–367. https://doi.org/10.1093/toxsci/kfw169

32. Bhatia SN, Ingber DE (2014) Microfluidic organs-on-chips. Nat Biotechnol 32(8):760–772. https://doi.org/10.1038/nbt.2989

33. Ingber DE (2016) Reverse engineering human pathophysiology with organs-on-chips. Cell 164(6):1105–1109. https://doi.org/10.1016/j.cell.2016.02.049

34. Vernetti LA, Senutovitch N, Boltz R, DeBiasio R, Shun TY, Gough A, Taylor DL (2016) A human liver microphysiology platform for investigating physiology, drug safety, and disease models. Exp Biol Med 241(1):101–114. https://doi.org/10.1177/1535370215592121

35. Senutovitch N, Vernetti L, Boltz R, DeBiasio R, Gough A, Taylor DL (2015) Fluorescent protein biosensors applied to microphysiological systems. Exp Biol Med 240(6):795–808. https://doi.org/10.1177/1535370215584934

36. Hamilton G (2017) Organs-on-chips: 3D microphysiological systems for understanding mechanism of action in drug discovery and development. The Toxicologist, Supplement to Toxicological Sciences: Abstract #2350

37. Church RJ, Watkins PB (2017) The transformation in biomarker detection and management of drug-induced liver injury. Liver Int. https://doi.org/10.1111/liv.13441

Chapter 13

Reactive Metabolite Assessment in Drug Discovery and Development in Support of Safe Drug Design

Axel Pähler

Abstract

The contribution of chemically reactive metabolites to drug-induced liver injury and other immune-mediated serious adverse drug reactions has been acknowledged as an important determinant of drug failure. Reasons for individual susceptibilities of patients that result in various forms and severities of adverse drug reactions are manifold. They involve factors such as the underlying diseases, individual genotypes of the immune system, and drug specific risk factors. Likewise, the characterizing of drug metabolizing pathways leading to bioactivation and reactive metabolite formation covalently modifying cellular macromolecules alone has been proven unsuccessful in relating bioactivation to adverse drug reactions. The emergence of sensitive and specific mass spectrometry methods has led to a myriad of experimental approaches trying to establish a causal link between reactive metabolite formation and drug-induced liver injury. Many of these failed. The main two reasons are: (1) Methods are overly sensitive or unspecific and flag many drugs that show a safe history of use in a large population. (2) Reactive metabolite screening methods are too generic and fail to detect drug-specific bioactivation pathways requiring alternative experimental approaches. As a consequence, testing paradigms that integrate knowledge of bioactivation pathways based on chemical structures (structural alerts), chemotype-specific experimental tools for reactive metabolite characterization, and the quantitative assessment of bioactivation pathways relative to "safe" metabolism and dose have emerged. Such strategies that characterize bioactivation potentials in the context of drug metabolism, pharmacokinetic properties, clinical dose and additional risk factors have been proposed and successfully applied across the pharmaceutical industry. Case studies and examples for successful risk assessment strategies and general principles to guide safe drug design are discussed in this chapter.

Key words Reactive metabolites, Screening methods, Bioactivation, Idiosyncratic drug reaction, DILI, Preclinical drug optimization, Risk assessment

1 Introduction

The contribution of chemically reactive metabolites to drug-induced liver injury and other immune-mediated serious adverse drug reactions has been discussed in other chapters of this book. The bioactivation of drugs to reactive metabolites generally does not exert any biological advantage unless specifically designed for irreversible target inhibition [1, 2]. Excessive bioactivation is an unwanted drug property as cumulative evidence suggests that

Minjun Chen and Yvonne Will (eds.), *Drug-Induced Liver Toxicity*, Methods in Pharmacology and Toxicology,
https://doi.org/10.1007/978-1-4939-7677-5_13, © Springer Science+Business Media, LLC, part of Springer Nature 2018

reactive metabolites play a causal role in several forms of drug-induced toxicities. Strategies have been implemented across the pharmaceutical industry aiming at the minimization of drug bioactivation potentials [3–8].

The characterization of the risk of drug candidates to form reactive metabolites requires an understanding of underlying bioactivation pathways. These need to be rationalized for individual drugs based on structural motifs involved in these processes. In this chapter, experimental methods are described that help characterize drug bioactivation pathways by identification of chemical interactions between drug metabolites and cellular macromolecules. Trapping studies with low molecular weight nucleophiles serve as surrogate markers that help qualitatively describe potentially adverse drug metabolism features. Further, quantitative methods that relate these drug bioactivation potentials to the potential risk for adverse events are discussed within the context of the overall pharmacokinetic profile of the drug. As is becomes evident from Table 1, the majority of marketed drugs do not form appreciable amounts of reactive metabolites. Still, some of the drugs for which reactive metabolites are detected, are considered safe. The extent of reactive metabolite formation relative to the metabolic clearance and daily dose has been proven important determinants of the risk associated with reactive metabolite formation. Those drugs that are tested positive for bioactivation and that are characterized by occurrence of drug-induced liver injury (DILI) share a high dose compared to those drugs that appear to be safe despite some reactive metabolite formation in vitro. Ultimately, an integrated risk assessment approach that highlights our current understanding of reactive metabolite formation in the context of adverse drug reactions is presented that supports strategies and methodologies for the rational design of safer drugs based on acquired structure activity relationships.

2   Methods

2.1   Predicting Bioactivation Via Structural Alerts

Preclinical tools for the assessment of metabolism with regard to reactive intermediate formation are applied in most pharmaceutical companies. This systematic process might also help establish structure activity relationships at least for local systems and allows medicinal chemists to find compounds with improved reactive metabolite formation. For a few specific chemical moieties a successful prediction of reactive metabolite formation and adverse drug reactions exists. For example for certain classes of arylamines and nitrobenzenes the metabolism-dependent bioactivation toward DNA reactive intermediates leading to tumorigenicity has been established by computer modeling of activation potentials dependent on substitution pattern. Apart from these few case

Table 1
The majority of marketed drugs test negative for GSH adducts in a calibrated screening assay for reactive metabolites

Drug tested positive for GSH adducts (19/66)	Daily dose (mg)	DILI risk	Comment	Drugs tested negative for GSH adducts (47/66)
Atropine	1–3	No		Alprazolam, amantadine, amitriptyline, amlodipine, aripiprazole, atrovastatin, baclofen, buspirone, captopril, cilazapril, citalopram, dextromethorphan, diazepam, diltiazem, diphenhydramine, donepezil, enalapril, fenofibrate, fluoxetine, furosemide, gabapentin, gemfibrozil, glibenclamide, lisinopril, lorazepam, memantine, metformin, moclobemide, paroxetine, pentobarbital, phenytoin, pindolol, prazosin, probucol, quetiapine, ranitine, rimonabant, risperidone, sertraline, simvastatin, sitagliptin, sumatriptan, valsartan, venlafaxine, verapamil, warfarin, zolpidem
Carbamazepine	400–1500	Yes		
Carvedilol	12–25	No		
Chlorpromazine	75–500	No	Isolated case reports for DILI	
Clozapine	200–450	Yes	Black box warning for agranulocytosis	
Desipramine	50–150	No		
Diclofenac	100–150	Yes	DILI at high doses	
Duloxetine	20	No		
Ezetimibe	10	No		
Haloperidol	5–10	No		
Imipramine	50–150	No		
Nefazodone	400	Yes	Withdrawn	
Nifedipine	15–60	No		
Olanzapine	5–20	No		
Propanolol	40–80	No		
Pioglitazone	15–45	No	Isolated case reports for DILI	
Rosiglitazone	4–16	No		
Tienilic acid	200–600	Yes	Withdrawn	
Troglitazone	400	Yes	Withdrawn	

A positive test for reactive metabolites alone does not determine DILI outcome. GSH adduct formation in context of a high daily dose (>100 mg) appears to be a high risk for drugs to develop DILI

examples, the most commonly used approach to identify bioactivation liabilities would include the recognition of structural alerts associated with reactive metabolites formation. This approach builds on the expertise of medicinal chemists and drug metabolism scientists to prioritize compounds for testing in appropriate in vitro tools. Currently available systems such as DEREK and METEOR (Lhasa Ltd.) are available to predict chemistry-associated toxicities and metabolism processes. Most software packages (e.g., METEOR, MetabolExpert, and MetaSite) correctly predict many metabolites that are also detected experimentally; however, a relatively high incidence of false positive and false negative predictions of metabolites is still common to most computerized systems [9, 10].

Extensive literature reviews have been published that link structural motifs to drug bioactivation [1, 11–17]. Although general rules can be derived that link common functional groups with frequent cases of reactive metabolite formation, a strategy avoiding such motifs from drug design appears impractical. The sole presence of a substructure in a new chemical entity known to be metabolized to electrophiles does not automatically result in reactive metabolite formation in a newly synthesized drug molecule. Thiophenes may undergo formation of reactive S-oxides under certain conditions such as in tienilic acid resulting in time dependent P450 inactivation and formation of covalently modified proteins. A general avoidance of thiophenes would not account for the fact that thiophenes in certain chemical environments are very safe and devoid of bioactivation [18, 19]. Other examples comparing structural motifs associated with extensive reactive metabolite formation are listed in Table 2. It is worthwhile to note that most of these toxic drugs that have shown to extensively form reactive metabolites can be contrasted with newer generation of drugs that share the same structural motif. In contrast to their hepatotoxic analogs, these safe drugs show little or no evidence for reactive metabolite formation, however. This may be due to the fact that their chemical substitution pattern has been optimized by medicinal chemists to maintain pharmacological activity and selectivity. Likewise, structural modifications have rendered these molecules in a way that metabolic transformations have shifted from the original "toxicophore" to benign metabolic soft spots. Based on these reasons a general avoidance of structural motifs known to undergo bioactivation in drug design appears not to be rational.

To acknowledge the fact that general trends linking structural motifs and bioactivation exist, the expert knowledge of drug metabolism scientists, medicinal chemists and computerized expert systems should be used to prioritize compounds for testing in experiment tools to investigate bioactivation liabilities. Most of the existing applications add value to the identification of the probable sites of metabolism especially when linked to experimental data. Thus in the hand of the drug metabolism expert these software packages have a certain value in guiding the investigators to experimental approaches for the identification of drug metabolites including bioactivation products such as glutathione adducts [20, 21]. A general "ban" of functional

Table 2
Structural alerts may guide testing of drug candidates in reactive metabolite screening tools

Structural alert	Hepatotoxic drug	Safe analog	Major differentiation
Imidazo pyridine	Alpidem	Zolpidem	Safe metabolic soft spot introduced
Carboxylate	Ibufenac	Ibuprofen	Stability of acyl glucuronide
Aniline	Acetaminophen	Phenacetin	Lower rate of iminoquinone formation
Thiazolidinedione	Troglitazone	Rosiglitazone	Additional activation pathway for troglitazone; low dose for rosiglitazone
Thiophene	Tienilic acid, ticlopidine	2-Aminothiophenes	Blocked metabolic activation
		2,4-Diaminothiophenes	

Definition of toxicophores and exclusion of alerting structures from drug design appears not a valid option. Minor chemical modifications can render hepatotoxic drugs safe without losing target affinity or selectivity

groups or substituents known to be associated with bioactivation does not appear to be practical or justified. Minor chemical modifications in drug design may significantly alter physiochemical properties of new drug candidates and render them more stable toward bioactivation. Therefore the cautious use of chemical motifs commonly associated with bioactivation still should be permitted in chemical series, especially when a substitution strategy does nor proof successful without loss of pharmacological activity or off target selectivity. These new drug candidates then can be further profiled in experimental tools for the characterization of bioactivation potentials in order to ensure that they do not have a bioactivation potential that may result in excessive reactive metabolite formation. Strategies addressing these adverse properties relative to their general pharmacokinetic profile and human dose are described in this chapter.

2.2 Experimental Methods for the Detection of Reactive Metabolites

Numerous methods exist that enable characterization of the bioactivation potential of new drug molecules. These span from simple high throughput electrophile trapping studies with model nucleophiles that allow for the screening of entire chemical libraries to complex, resource-demanding in vivo studies to quantitate metabolites or altered proteins as a consequence of reactive metabolite formation. Each of these assays has their utility and justification depending on the stage in the drug discovery and development process they are applied to. Additionally, the assessment of irreversibly bound drug to hepatic proteins (covalent binding of radiolabeled drug) can quantify the extent of bioactivation processes relative to drug clearance. The extent of covalent binding relative to the drug's clearance pathways via benign biotransformation pathways aids selection of low-dose clinical candidates with acceptable bioactivation potential. Such candidates are expected to have a higher likelihood to succeed throughout the development processes resulting in safer drugs on the market.

Importantly, all of these methods have major limitations if applied in isolation for compound progression decisions. None of these assays is predictive for manifestation of toxicity in absence of additional drug characterization as it relates to dose, drug disposition and clearance as well as off target effects. Therefore, an integrated risk assessment strategy is considered critically important where reactive metabolite screening and characterization strategies should be successfully applied in today's competitive drug discovery and development setting.

In many pharmaceutical companies, optimization strategies in drug discovery focus on candidate drug design with minimized chemical liabilities for reactive metabolite formation. With the initial avoidance of excessive bioactivation potentials, further downstream consequences of reactive metabolites, such as covalent binding, detoxification pathways and involved variability in those processes do not need to be further considered. This approach relies on the rational design of drug molecules based on the underlying knowledge of the molecular features associated with bioactivation. Many cases of successful drug optimization have been described in literature that led to the generation of safe drugs with regard to bioactivation while maintenance of drug potency and favorable ADME (i.e., absorption, distribution, metabolism, and excretion) characteristics was achieved or even improved. The primary tools to assess the potential of reactive metabolite formation by hepatic bioactivation rely on reactive metabolite trapping with model electrophiles such as glutathione (GSH). Besides GSH adduct formation, other model nucleophiles that react with electrophilic metabolites can be employed. In some instances the formed reactive metabolite (electrophile) is highly reactive and cannot escape from the active site of the enzyme that catalyzed its formation. In such circumstances, direct modification of the enzyme may lead to metabolism-dependent (suicide) inactivation of the enzyme such as cytochrome P450. Thus, specific assays characterizing the potential of drug candidates to cause mechanism-dependent inactivation of P450 enzyme complement electrophilic trapping experiment and are considered as orthogonal approach to assess bioactivation liabilities [22–24].

For chemical scaffolds with reactive metabolite issues, the GSH trapping assay is typically used to develop structure–activity relationships by cycles of design, synthesis, testing, and redesign. The aim is a chemical modification of the compound that eliminates reactive metabolite formation, while maintaining potency, target specificity and favorable ADME properties. This can either be achieved by replacing the functional group involved in bioactivation, by modifying its reactivity via electron withdrawing substituents or by directing metabolism to a different metabolic soft spot [25]. Examples are described in an excellent review by Kalgutkar and Dalvie from the Pfizer group [11]. GSH adduct screening guides identification of low risk compounds, bearing in mind that the absence of GSH adducts formation does not completely safeguard against covalent binding. Conversely, a positive GSH signal should not be regarded as exclusion criteria for promising molecules. The risk–benefit assessment also takes into account the clinical indication and other treatment- and patient-related factors like the therapeutic dose, the duration and scheme of treatment (e.g., chronic versus acute), the target population, unmet medical needs, and the competitive landscape.

2.2.1 Electrophile Trapping Experiments

Many pharmaceutical companies therefore aim to minimize the potential for reactive metabolite formation in early phases of drug discovery by chemical modification and appropriate candidate selection. In conjunction the selection of highly potent and selective drugs with favorable pharmacokinetic properties ensures that predominantly low-dose candidate drugs devoid of excessive reactive metabolite formation progress into development. This process is facilitated in the discovery phase by the detection of stable trapping products of electrophilic intermediates with nucleophilic trapping reagents such as glutathione or cyanide in vitro in order to guide rational structure based drug design.

The tripeptide glutathione in Fig. 1 is the most frequently used nucleophile employed in electrophile trapping experiments.

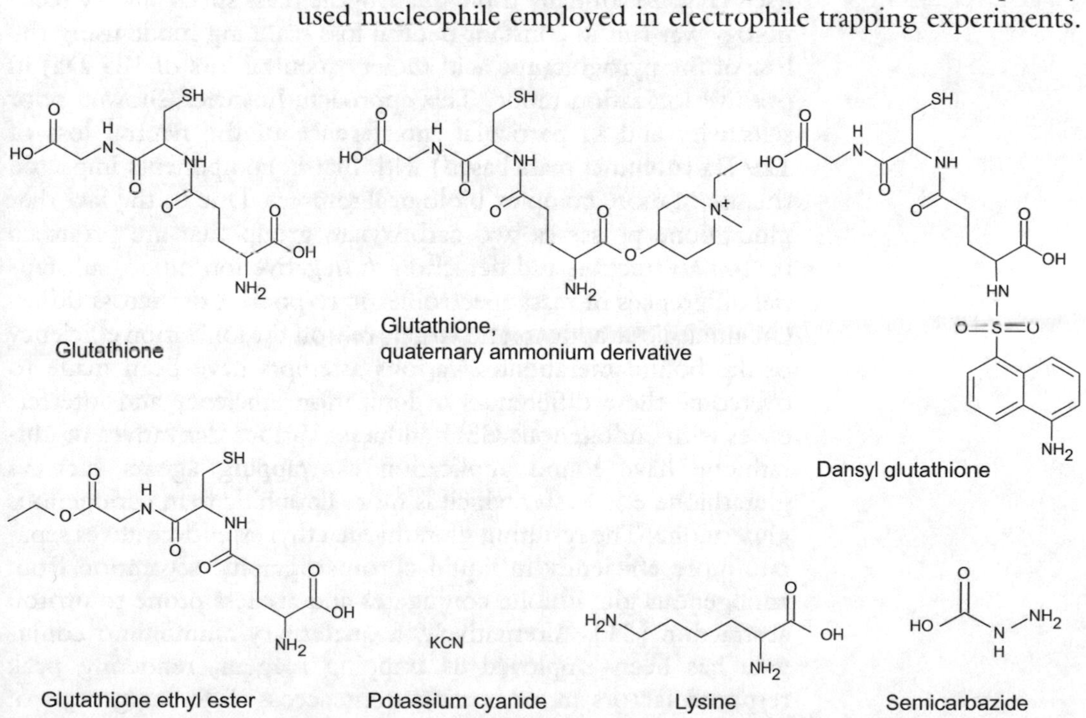

Fig. 1 Structures of nucleophilic reagents used in reactive metabolite trapping studies

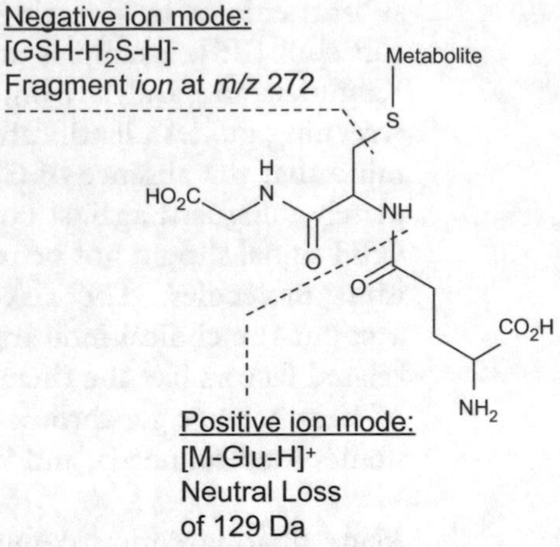

Negative ion mode:
[GSH-H₂S-H]⁻
Fragment *ion* at *m/z* 272

Positive ion mode:
[M-Glu-H]⁺
Neutral Loss
of 129 Da

Fig. 2 Structure of metabolite–glutathione adduct and major fragmentation pathways in positive and negative ionization mass spectrometry

Several specific mass spectrometry based methods employing liquid-chromatography separation methods and specific mass spectrometric workflows have been published [4, 20, 26–30]. Detection and characterization of glutathione adducts take advantage of the specific fragmentation behavior of the peptide moiety of GSH adducts and are largely independent of the conjugate itself (Fig. 2). Initially triple quadrupole mass spectrometry technology was run in constant neutral loss scanning mode using the loss of the pyroglutamic acid moiety (neutral loss of 129 Da) in positive ionization mode. This approach, however, showed poor selectivity and in particular interference of the neutral loss of 129 Da (nominal mass based) with matrix components impacted the use in more complex biological samples. Due to the fact that glutathione possesses two carboxylate group that are prone to proton abstraction and detection in negative ion mode, substantial differences in mass spectrometric response exist across different glutathione adducts and largely rely on the ionization efficiency of the bound metabolite. Various attempts have been made to overcome these differences in ionization efficiency and interferences with endogenous GSH adducts. Various derivatives of glutathione have found application as trapping agents such as glutathione ethyl-ester which is more lipophilic than endogenous glutathione. The resulting glutathione ethyl ester derivatives separate more efficiently in liquid chromatographic separation from endogenous glutathione conjugates and are less prone to proton abstraction [31]. Alternatively, a quaternary ammonium conjugate has been employed as trapping reagent, rendering peak response factors more homogenous across different groups of glutathione adducts [32].

The use of precursor ion scanning of m/z 272 in negative mode—also using triple quadrupole technology—was an improvement with regard to selectivity and is widely used as a robust alternative for the detection of known as well as unknown GSH adducts in biological matrices [33]. This generic scanning method was in particular of value if employed as a survey scan triggering enhanced resolution and enhanced product ion spectra acquisition on the precursor mass of interest in the same analytical run. The main disadvantage of the negative ionization detection and mass spectral characterization is, however, that the spectra obtained by collision induced dissociation of the $[M-H]^-$ ions of GSH adducts have limited information for structural characterization. This is due to the fact that the generated fragment ions are predominantly originating from the glutathionyl moiety of the tripeptide and are not informative on the structure of the entire conjugate [34]. In more recent years with the availably of high resolution and accurate mass instruments, the analytical GSH adduct identification was further improved and complemented with software tools for post-acquisition data analysis. In addition to the identification of GSH trapped reactive metabolites, the acquisition of accurate mass full scan and fragment ion spectra allows for the generation of empirical formulae of the adduct of concern. This enables the drug metabolism scientist to build an understanding of the biotransformation pathways yielding to adduct formation as well as for the interpretation of the site of adduction in the parent drug molecule based on interpretation of accurate mass MS/MS spectra.

Iminium ions and other hard electrophiles cannot be detected via trapping with thiol-containing nucleophiles such as glutathione or cysteine. Potassium cyanide has been used as a trapping reagent for the detection of for example iminium ions formed from alicylic amines such as in nefazodone or clozapine [35]. Cyanide adducts are readily detected by mass spectrometry based methods these but have been prone to false positive results [36]. Therefore many laboratories have established a method using ^{14}C-labeled cyanide for the quantitative determination of incorporated cyanide into the reaction product with the metabolically formed electrophile [37].

One class of reactive metabolites not covered by microsomal incubations is acyl glucuronide formation from carboxylic acid drugs. Commonly liver microsomal preparations fortified with uridine 5'-diphosphoglucuronic acid afford acyl glucuronide formation when incubated with the drug candidate under investigation. Reactivity and safety of carboxylic acid drugs that undergo glucuronidation is determined by the extend Acyl migration and acylation of proteins. This reactivity appears to be directly associated with clinical adverse effects (Fig. 3). The reactivity of acyl glucuronides can be assessed in the presence of proteins and is directly linked to their toxic effect [38, 39].

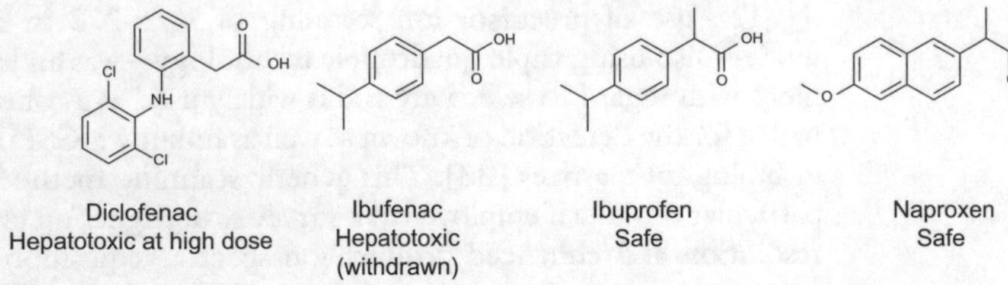

Fig. 3 Structures of hepatotoxic and safe carboxylic acid drugs

Many of the electrophile trapping experiments described in this section provide useful structural information about the nature of the adduct formed. Mass spectrometry based data evaluation allows for the characterization of bioactivation pathways leading to reactive metabolite formation and provide a rational approach to drug design. However, most of these methods lack quantitative information and provide a binary answer only. Several attempts have been made to generate quantitative reactive metabolite trapping data employing either ^{35}S-labeled glutathione or the fluorescent derivative dansyl glutathione [40, 41]. Reasonable correlations can be obtained between quantitative trapping experiments and true quantitative covalent binding studies measuring covalently modified protein. However these mostly hold true within a narrow chemical space where the chemistry of reactive metabolite formation follows a similar metabolic pathway and can rarely be generalized.

2.2.2 Mechanism Based Inhibition of Cytochrome P450 Enzymes

Mechanism-based cytochrome P450 inactivation typically involves metabolism-dependent activation of a drug to form a chemically reactive intermediate. In case this electrophile is stable enough to escape from the active site of the enzyme it may react with proteins or other cellular nucleophiles potentially causing toxic insults. These types of electrophiles can also be investigated by electrophile trapping experiments as outlined in Sect. 2.2.1. Electrophilic intermediates that are highly reactive may also directly covalently modify an active site amino acid residue in the active site of cytochrome P450 itself. Covalent modification of P450 enzymes can also lead to a neoantigen formation and can trigger an autoimmune response as one underlying mechanism in DILI. Additionally, irreversible P450 inhibition may result in nonmanageable drug–drug interactions as the inactivated P450 enzyme needs to be replaced by resynthesis. As for reactive metabolite trapping experiments, mechanism-based P450 inactivation is typically assessed in pharmaceutical industry by well-established screening methods [24, 42]. These methods determine the nonreversible inhibition of P450 enzymes upon metabolism of a drug candidate. As opposed to a competitive inhibition assay, the mechanism-based inactivation assay is a two-step assay in which the drug of interest is preincubated with a source of P450 enzymes such

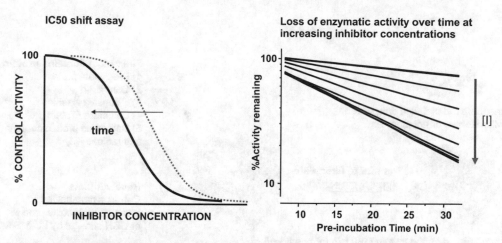

Fig. 4 Determination of mechanism-dependent cytochrome P450 inactivation resulting in a time-dependent shift in IC$_{50}$ upon preincubation. The loss of enzymatic activity over time at increasing inhibitor concentrations allows for the determination of the enzyme inactivation rate

as human liver microsomes. It is important to mention that at various time points of preincubation the test sample is then diluted to remove any competitive (reversible) inhibitor and tested for enzyme activity. As a result of these experiments and apparent shift in sensitivity toward the P450 inhibition is observed over time due to time-dependent inactivation of the enzyme. The rate of inactivation determined from these experiments serves as a readout to judge the extent of enzyme inactivation (Fig. 4).

Several groups including Nakayama et al. [5] have demonstrated that the time (or mechanism)-dependent inhibition assay is complementary tool to the GSH trapping assay in detecting reactive metabolite formation. Generally there is a tendency that compounds tested positive for time-dependent P450 inactivation also show a high degree of covalent binding. These compounds show covalent protein modification irrespective of the result of the GSH trapping assay. Thus a combination of GSH trapping studies and mechanism-based P450 inactivation appears to provide a comprehensive screening paradigm to identify covalent binding potential of drugs.

2.2.3 Covalent Binding Studies

The most direct correlation between reactive metabolite formation and DILI appears to the extent of covalent binding to human hepatic proteins. Covalent protein modification can have direct functional consequences, for example cytochrome P450 time-dependent inactivation if the reactive metabolite directly modifies the active site of the enzyme that catalyzes its formation. Originally, the determination of covalent binding properties of radiolabeled drug candidates was descried by the group at Merck. Evans et al. [3] had established an experimental protocol where human liver microsomes as enzyme source for metabolism were incubated with the radiolabeled drug

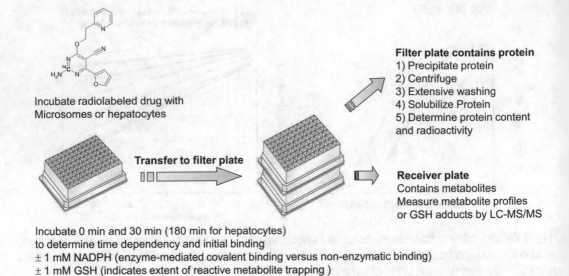

Incubate radiolabeled drug with
Microsomes or hepatocytes

Transfer to filter plate

Filter plate contains protein
1) Precipitate protein
2) Centrifuge
3) Extensive washing
4) Solubilize Protein
5) Determine protein content
and radioactivity

Receiver plate
Contains metabolites
Measure metabolite profiles
or GSH adducts by LC-MS/MS

Incubate 0 min and 30 min (180 min for hepatocytes)
to determine time dependency and initial binding
± 1 mM NADPH (enzyme-mediated covalent binding versus non-enzymatic binding)
± 1 mM GSH (indicates extent of reactive metabolite trapping)

$$CVB\left[\frac{pmol}{mgprotein}\right] = \frac{\frac{Radioactivity}{mg\ protein}(NADPH) - \frac{Radioactivity}{mg\ protein}(no\ NADPH) - \frac{Radioactivity}{mg\ protein}(initial\ binding)}{Specific\ radioactivity\ of\ drug}$$

Fig. 5 Experimental setup and workflow for the determination of covalent binding (CVB) properties of radiolabeled drugs to liver microsomes or hepatocytes

candidate and cofactors for oxidative metabolism. After quenching of the incubation with organic solvent, the protein pellet was extensively washed to remove nonirreversibly bound background radioactivity. Figure 5 depicts a modern variation of the original setup that can accommodate various control conditions to assess time-dependency of the binding, correct for nonspecific and nonenzymatic binding. In addition the covalently modified protein pellet can be analyzed separately from the incubation supernatant that contains metabolites and potential GSH adducts.

Great attention has been given to the correlation of covalent binding properties and clinical DILI outcomes since the original work by Evans et al. [3]. A lack of correlation between covalent binding data to rat liver in vitro or in vivo and the manifestation of hepatotoxicity in rat toxicology studies appears discouraging [2]. Different groups have expanded on the original data set and demonstrated that metabolism-dependent covalent binding alone cannot categorize a drug's potential to cause DILI in vivo [43–45]. However the group at Daichi-Sankyo has demonstrated that covalent binding properties, when corrected by the human dose of a drug, can classify drugs based on their potential to induce DILI [44]. Nakayama et al. and others have employed covalent binding assessment in human primary human hepatocytes as a refined tool to establish this correlation (Fig. 6). The balance between activating and detoxifying enzymes in human hepatocytes appears to be a more predictive tool than human

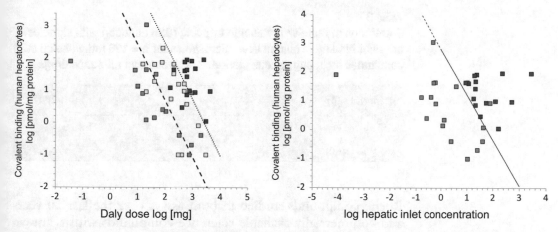

Fig. 6 Correlation between covalent binding in primary human hepatocytes and clinical DILI outcome (left, adapted from [44]). A clear separation of DILI safe compounds and those with a DILI flag can be obtained (right), when covalent binding in vitro is plotted against the hepatic inlet concentration in clinics (calculated form absorption rate constant and fraction absorbed)

liver microsomes that typically lack Phase 2 enzyme activity when incubated under standard NADPH conditions.

The association of daily dose, the formation of reactive metabolites and physicochemical properties such as log P has been investigated for a large set of Food and Drug Administration-approved oral medications. Based on these parameters of $n = 354$ drugs, an algorithm to define a clinical DILI risk was developed. When applied to an independent dataset of $n = 159$ clinical cases collected from the National Institutes of Health's LiverTox database, the DILI score correlated with the severity of clinical outcome [46].

Considering the fact that the human body burden for reactive metabolites is characterized by the amount of drug that is hepatically available after absorption, this correlation can be further refined. This analysis correlates the daily liver load (daily dose of reactive metabolites corrected for the fraction of the drug absorbed and first pass extraction) instead of daily dose against the covalent binding properties in human hepatocytes. Figure 6 shows a clear separation of high risk DILI drugs from safe drugs when applying this more physiological concept.

2.3 Data Integration and Risk Assessment Models

An integrated reactive metabolite testing strategy should acknowledge the scope and limitations of the individual assays used at different stages of drug discovery or development. Schadt et al. from Roche [47] have reported the correlation between a reactive metabolite trapping assay with GSH and the quantitative covalent binding outcome (Table 3). In this correlation the association between GSH adduct formation with significant covalent binding in human liver microsomes (>3-fold background and >30 pmol/ mg protein) has been analyzed for 136 compounds, including

Table 3
Correlation of reactive metabolite trapping (GSH adducts) with significant covalent binding in human liver microsomes for $n = 136$ radiolabeled drug candidates including various marketed or withdrawn reference drugs

HLM, $n = 136$	CVB positive	CVB negative
GSH adducts	27% (37)	5% (6)
No GSH adducts	11% (15)	57% (78)

Roche compounds studied in both assays over the last 10 years and commercially available reference compounds with a known history of DILI. In the calibrated trapping assay GSH adduct signals were called "positive" if they exceeded the signal intensity of reference drugs for which GSH adduct formation correlates with significant CVB. Table 3 shows that of all drugs, 78 did not show flags in either the GSH or the covalent binding assay (57%) and 37 (27%) showed flags in both the GSH and the covalent binding assay. A low number of compounds flag in the GSH adduct assay but not in the covalent binding assay (6, 5%) and would be considered false negative results with regard to the prediction of high covalent binding. Likewise some compounds that do not flag in the GSH adduct assay exhibit significant covalent binding (15, 11%) and are considered false negative. Fortunately false positive correlations are rare. For compounds that do not flag in the GSH adduct assay but still show significant covalent binding to microsomal protein, several explanations can be considered. For example such molecules may undergo iminium ion formation that escape trapping with GSH but would have been picked up with potassium cyanide as trapping reagent. Likewise the initially formed reactive intermediate may be so reactive that it cannot escape form the enzyme during its formation. As a consequence time dependent inactivation of cytochrome P450 may occur as outlined in Sect. 2.2.2. One of the cases is Ritonavir, a time dependent suicide inhibitor of Cyp3A4 showing no GSH adducts but significant covalent binding, which is due to binding to the heme iron rather than to protein [5].

Covalent binding assessment to human hepatic proteins with radiolabeled drug substance can occur only relatively late in drug development due to the late availability of costly radiolabeled material. At this point in development, often preclinical safety studies have already been conducted and the value of conducting reactive metabolite characterization late in development is a matter of scientific debate. Data from those companies that pioneered in the systematic assessment of covalent binding properties in context

Table 4
Correlation of reactive metabolite trapping (GSH adducts) and daily clinical dose (greater than 100 mg) with risk for clinical DILI for $n = 54$ marketed or withdrawn reference drugs

		Risk for DILI	
	$n = 54$	High	Low
GSH adducts and dose >100 mg	Yes	14	2
	No	4	34

Drugs with lack of GSH adduct formation or drugs with GSH adduct formation but daily doses less than 100 mg generally have a low DILI risk

of safety demonstrate that a general correlation between reactive metabolite formation in vitro or in vivo and manifestation of liver toxicity in preclinical animal studies does not exist. A comprehensive dataset on ~100 Merck drug candidates indicated that there was no correlation between incidence of liver toxicity observed in vivo in preclinical safety studies and level of covalent [2]. Acknowledging the fact excessive GSH adduct formation positively correlates with high in vitro covalent binding, we were interested to evaluate a reduced set of parameters for a correlation with human DILI outcome.

We classified the set of $n = 54$ compounds previously analyzed by Nakayama et al. [40] based on their human dose (≥ 100 mg or <100 mg) and their potential to form GSH adducts with the development of clinical DILI. The sensitivity of the assay conditions was 78% suggesting that 4 out of 18 DILI drugs were not correctly classified (Table 4, bottom), all of them being high dose drugs, for example ritonavir which forms reactive metabolites which directly bind to the active side of the involved enzyme. Thirteeen of the 36 low-risk drugs possess the potential to form reactive metabolites. One of these drugs is gemfibrozil whose DILI classification may have to be reviewed. The other compounds were low-dose drugs with an average dose of 36 mg per day. Based on these findings the daily dose was integrated as secondary criteria for risk assessment via GSH trapping. Applying this definition for the 54 safe and high risk drugs resulted in a vast improvement of prediction power (Table 4). With only four false negative and two false positive results (8% false classifications) a sensitivity of 78% and a specificity of 92% for this classification was achieved. Drugs with lack of GSH adduct formation or drugs with GSH adduct formation but daily doses less than 100 mg generally have a low DILI risk.

3   Conclusions and Future Directions

Proteomics approached for the identification of target proteins of chemically reactive intermediates as neoantigens triggering immune response have been proposed to bridge between reactive metabolite assessment and biological response [48–51]. An online resource on protein targets of reactive metabolites has been created by the Hanzlik group at University of Kansas [52, 53]. Chemoproteomics combined with bioinformatics approaches increase the understanding of xenobiotic posttranslational modification of proteins that might disrupt important protein–protein interactions. Functional consequences may force cells from homeostasis into cell death pathways and have consequences beyond covalent binding and antigen presentation [54].

With the advances in genome wide sequencing and the understanding of T-cell activation in immune response, several risk factors for idiosyncratic DILI have been identified. These range from direct drug antigenicity and T-cell activation [55] to drug immunogenicity reactions involving complement systems such as acquired immunity via drug-inflammation reactions. Interindividual susceptibility to idiosyncratic DILI involves various genetic variations in HLA alleles that have been associated with and increased risk for DILI. The conservation of these risk alleles across several compounds holds a promise for future risk mitigation strategies [56].

The management of reactive metabolites remains a challenge in drug discovery and is under constant debate. Consensus exists for the observation that there is a strong association between reactive metabolite formation and the manifestation of DILI. We therefore assume that avoiding reactive metabolites is the best option to reduce DILI even though the mechanistic causality between reactive metabolites and risk for DILI remains elusive. Rather than using reactive metabolite findings as isolated discontinuation criteria, the overall pharmacokinetic and pharmacodynamics profile of a new molecular entity needs to be considered to allow for a holistic risk–benefit assessment. Such candidates with a favorable dose and efficacy index have an intrinsic higher likelihood to succeed throughout the development processes leading to safer drugs for patients.

References

1. Stepan AF et al (2011) Structural alert/reactive metabolite concept as applied in medicinal chemistry to mitigate the risk of idiosyncratic drug toxicity: a perspective based on the critical examination of trends in the top 200 drugs marketed in the United States. Chem Res Toxicol 24(9):1345–1410

2. Park BK et al (2011) Managing the challenge of chemically reactive metabolites in drug development. Nat Rev Drug Discov 10(4):292–306

3. Evans DC et al (2004) Drug-protein adducts: an industry perspective on minimizing the potential for drug bioactivation in drug discovery and development. Chem Res Toxicol 17(1):3–16

4. Ma L et al (2008) Rapid screening of glutathione-trapped reactive metabolites by linear ion trap mass spectrometry with isotope pattern-dependent scanning and post-acquisition data mining. Chem Res Toxicol 21(7):1477–1483

5. Nakayama S et al (2011) Combination of GSH trapping and time-dependent inhibition assays as a predictive method of drugs generating highly reactive metabolites. Drug Metab Dispos 39(7):1247–1254

6. Sakatis MZ et al (2012) Preclinical strategy to reduce clinical hepatotoxicity using in vitro bioactivation data for >200 compounds. Chem Res Toxicol 25(10):2067–2082

7. Thompson RA et al (2012) In vitro approach to assess the potential for risk of idiosyncratic adverse reactions caused by candidate drugs. Chem Res Toxicol 25:1616–1632

8. Brink A et al (2017) Minimizing the risk of chemically reactive metabolite formation of new drug candidates: implications for preclinical drug design. Drug Discov Today 22(5):751–756

9. Caldwell GW, Yan Z (2006) Screening for reactive intermediates and toxicity assessment in drug discovery. Curr Opin Drug Discov Devel 9(1):47–60

10. Muster W et al (2008) Computational toxicology in drug development. Drug Discov Today 13(7–8):303–310

11. Dalvie D, Kalgutkar AS, Chen W (2015) Practical approaches to resolving reactive metabolite liabilities in early discovery. Drug Metab Rev 47(1):56–70

12. Kalgutkar AS (2008) Role of bioactivation in idiosyncratic drug toxicity: structure–toxicity relationship. In: Elfarra AA (ed) Advances in bioactivation research. American Association of Pharmaceutical Scientists, Arlington, VA, p 440

13. Kalgutkar AS (2011) Handling reactive metabolite positives in drug discovery: what has retrospective structure-toxicity analyses taught us? Chem Biol Interact 192(1–2):46–55

14. Kalgutkar AS (2015) Should the incorporation of structural alerts be restricted in drug design? An analysis of structure-toxicity trends with aniline-based drugs. Curr Med Chem 22(4):438–464

15. Kalgutkar AS et al (2008) Toxicophores, reactive metabolites and drug safety: when is it a cause for concern? Expert Rev Clin Pharmacol 1(4):515–531

16. Kalgutkar AS et al (2005) A comprehensive listing of bioactivation pathways of organic functional groups. Curr Drug Metab 6(3):161–225

17. Walgren JL, Mitchell MD, Thompson DC (2005) Role of metabolism in drug-induced idiosyncratic hepatotoxicity. Crit Rev Toxicol 35(4):325–361

18. Gramec D, Peterlin Masic L, Sollner Dolenc M (2014) Bioactivation potential of thiophene-containing drugs. Chem Res Toxicol 27(8):1344–1358

19. Lecoeur S et al (1994) Specificity of in vitro covalent binding of tienilic acid metabolites to human liver microsomes in relationship to the type of hepatotoxicity: comparison with two directly hepatotoxic drugs. Chem Res Toxicol 7(3):434–442

20. Brink A et al (2014) Post-acquisition analysis of untargeted accurate mass quadrupole time-of-flight MS(E) data for multiple collision-induced neutral losses and fragment ions of glutathione conjugates. Rapid Commun Mass Spectrom 28(24):2695–2703

21. Pahler A, Brink A (2013) Software aided approaches to structure-based metabolite identification in drug discovery and development. Drug Discov Today Technol 10(1):e207–e217

22. Feng S, He X (2013) Mechanism-based inhibition of CYP450: an indicator of drug-induced hepatotoxicity. Curr Drug Metab 14(9):921–945

23. Kalgutkar AS, Obach RS, Maurer TS (2007) Mechanism-based inactivation of cytochrome P450 enzymes: chemical mechanisms, structure-activity relationships and relationship to clinical drug-drug interactions and drug reactions. Curr Drug Metab 8(5):407–447

24. Orr ST et al (2012) Mechanism-based inactivation (MBI) of cytochrome P450 enzymes: structure-activity relationships and discovery strategies to mitigate drug-drug interaction risks. J Med Chem 55(11):4896–4933

25. Argikar UA, Mangold JB, Harriman SP (2011) Strategies and chemical design approaches to reduce the potential for formation of reactive metabolic species. Curr Top Med Chem 11(4):419–449

26. Baillie TA, Davis MR (1993) Mass spectrometry in the analysis of glutathione conjugates. Biol Mass Spectrom 22(6):319–325

27. Baillie TA et al (1989) The use of mass spectrometry in the study of chemically-reactive drug metabolites. Application of MS/MS and LC/MS to the analysis of glutathione- and related S-linked conjugates of N-methylformamide. J Pharm Biomed Anal 7(12):1351–1360

28. Castro-Perez J et al (2005) A high-throughput liquid chromatography/tandem mass spectrometry method for screening glutathione conjugates using exact mass neutral loss acquisition. Rapid Commun Mass Spectrom 19(6):798–804

29. Pearson PG et al (1988) Applications of tandem mass spectrometry to the characterization of derivatized glutathione conjugates. Studies with S-(N-methylcarbamoyl)glutathione, a metabolite of the antineoplastic agent N-methylformamide. Biomed Environ Mass Spectrom 16(1–12):51–56

30. Rashed MS et al (1989) Application of liquid chromatography/thermospray mass spectrometry to studies on the formation of glutathione and cysteine conjugates from monomethylcarbamate metabolites of bambuterol. Rapid Commun Mass Spectrom 3(10):360–363

31. Soglia JR et al (2004) The development of a higher throughput reactive intermediate screening assay incorporating micro-bore liquid chromatography-micro-electrospray ionization-tandem mass spectrometry and glutathione ethyl ester as an in vitro conjugating agent. J Pharm Biomed Anal 36(1):105–116

32. Soglia JR et al (2006) A semiquantitative method for the determination of reactive metabolite conjugate levels in vitro utilizing liquid chromatography-tandem mass spectrometry and novel quaternary ammonium glutathione analogues. Chem Res Toxicol 19(3):480–490

33. Dieckhaus CM et al (2005) Negative ion tandem mass spectrometry for the detection of glutathione conjugates. Chem Res Toxicol 18(4):630–638

34. Zhu M et al (2007) Detection and structural characterization of glutathione-trapped reactive metabolites using liquid chromatography-high-resolution mass spectrometry and mass defect filtering. Anal Chem 79(21):8333–8341

35. Argoti D et al (2005) Cyanide trapping of iminium ion reactive intermediates followed by detection and structure identification using liquid chromatography-tandem mass spectrometry (LC-MS/MS). Chem Res Toxicol 18(10):1537–1544

36. Rousu T, Tolonen A (2011) Characterization of cyanide-trapped methylated metabonates formed during reactive drug metabolite screening in vitro. Rapid Commun Mass Spectrom 25(10):1382–1390

37. Inoue K et al (2009) A trapping method for semi-quantitative assessment of reactive metabolite formation using [35S]cysteine and [14C]cyanide. Drug Metab Pharmacokinet 24(3):245–254

38. Stachulski AV (2011) Chemistry and reactivity of acyl glucuronides. Curr Drug Metab 12(3):215–221

39. Zhong S et al (2015) A new rapid in vitro assay for assessing reactivity of acyl glucuronides. Drug Metab Dispos 43(11):1711–1717

40. Gan J et al (2005) Dansyl glutathione as a trapping agent for the quantitative estimation and identification of reactive metabolites. Chem Res Toxicol 18(5):896–903

41. Takakusa H et al (2009) Quantitative assessment of reactive metabolite formation using 35S-labeled glutathione. Drug Metab Pharmacokinet 24(1):100–107

42. Fowler S, Zhang H (2008) In vitro evaluation of reversible and irreversible cytochrome P450 inhibition: current status on methodologies and their utility for predicting drug-drug interactions. AAPS J 10(2):410–424

43. Bauman JN et al (2009) Can in vitro metabolism-dependent covalent binding data distinguish hepatotoxic from nonhepatotoxic drugs? An analysis using human hepatocytes and liver S-9 fraction. Chem Res Toxicol 22(2):332–340

44. Nakayama S et al (2009) A zone classification system for risk assessment of idiosyncratic drug toxicity using daily dose and covalent binding. Drug Metab Dispos 37(9):1970–1977

45. Obach RS et al (2008) Can in vitro metabolism-dependent covalent binding data in liver microsomes distinguish hepatotoxic from non-hepatotoxic drugs? An analysis of 18 drugs with consideration of intrinsic clearance and daily dose. Chem Res Toxicol 21(9):1814–1822

46. Chen M, Borlak J, Tong W (2016) A model to predict severity of drug-induced liver injury in humans. Hepatology 64(3):931–940

47. Schadt S et al (2015) Minimizing DILI risk in drug discovery – a screening tool for drug candidates. Toxicol In Vitro 30(1 Pt B):429–437

48. Hong F, Freeman ML, Liebler DC (2005) Identification of sensor cysteines in human Keap1 modified by the cancer chemopreventive agent sulforaphane. Chem Res Toxicol 18(12):1917–1926

49. Hong F et al (2005) Specific patterns of electrophile adduction trigger Keap1 ubiquitination and Nrf2 activation. J Biol Chem 280(36):31768–31775

50. Shin NY et al (2007) Protein targets of reactive electrophiles in human liver microsomes. Chem Res Toxicol 20(6):859–867

51. Tzouros M, Pahler A (2009) A targeted proteomics approach to the identification of peptides modified by reactive metabolites. Chem Res Toxicol 22(5):853–862

52. Hanzlik RP, Fang J, Koen YM (2009) Filling and mining the reactive metabolite target protein database. Chem Biol Interact 179(1):38–44

53. Hanzlik RP et al (2007) The reactive metabolite target protein database (TPDB)—a web-accessible resource. BMC Bioinformatics 8:95

54. Hanzlik RP, Koen YM, Fang J (2013) Bioinformatic analysis of 302 reactive metabolite target proteins. Which ones are important for cell death? Toxicol Sci 135(2):390–401

55. Kim SH, Naisbitt DJ (2016) Update on advances in research on idiosyncratic drug-induced liver injury. Allergy Asthma Immunol Res 8(1):3–11

56. Singer JB et al (2010) A genome-wide study identifies HLA alleles associated with lumiracoxib-related liver injury. Nat Genet 42(8):711–714

In Vitro Assessment of Mitochondrial Toxicity to Predict Drug-Induced Liver Injury

Mathieu Porceddu, Nelly Buron, Pierre Rustin, Bernard Fromenty, and Annie Borgne-Sanchez

Abstract

Mitochondrial liability of drugs and other xenobiotics is a major issue for patients because such toxicity can damage different tissues and organs such as liver, heart, and muscle. Drug-induced mitochondrial toxicity is also a major concern for pharmaceutical industries. Indeed, it is now acknowledged that such mechanism of toxicity can induce severe, and sometimes fatal, liver injury which can lead to the interruption of clinical trials, or drug withdrawal after marketing, such as in the case of troglitazone. Therefore, drug-induced mitochondrial dysfunction is increasingly sought after by pharmaceutical companies by using reliable in vitro assays in order to discard potential mitochondrion-toxic drugs during drug discovery stage. This chapter presents the in vitro methods used to identify potential mitochondrion-toxic drugs. To this end, different types of biological materials are used such as isolated mouse liver mitochondria and the human hepatic HepaRG® cell line, which expresses the main enzymes and transcription factors involved in drug metabolism. The in vitro method we discussed allows to investigate several key mitochondrial parameters such as oxygen consumption, transmembrane potential, respiratory chain complex activities, and mtDNA levels. These investigations are able to detect not only direct and acute mitochondrial alterations due to parent drugs but also indirect and chronic mitochondrial liability that can be induced by secondary metabolites. Hence, it could be used to detect potential drug-induced mitochondrial liability and to understand the involved mechanisms.

Key words DILI, Drug-induced liver injury, Hepatocytes, Hepatotoxicity, Liver, Mitochondria, Mitochondrial toxicity, Oxidative stress, Respiratory chain, Transmembrane potential

1 Introduction

Mitochondrial toxicity of drugs and other xenobiotics is a major issue for patients because such toxicity can induce acute or chronic injury involving different organs and tissues such as liver, heart, muscle, kidney and adipose tissues [1–3]. In the worst scenario, these diseases can lead to long-term hospitalization and death of the patients. Ethanol consumed in excess amounts by millions of individuals all over the world is known for a long time to favor the occurrence of different liver diseases by altering mitochondrial

Minjun Chen and Yvonne Will (eds.), *Drug-Induced Liver Toxicity*, Methods in Pharmacology and Toxicology, https://doi.org/10.1007/978-1-4939-7677-5_14, © Springer Science+Business Media, LLC, part of Springer Nature 2018

function by different mechanisms [4–6]. Although still scarce, some studies also suggest that exposure to environmental contaminants such as bisphenol A and benzo[a]pyrene results in mitochondrial dysfunction [7, 8].

In addition to the public health issue, drug-induced mitochondrial toxicity is also a major concern for pharmaceutical industries. Indeed, mitochondrial liability has been pinpointed for severe adverse events and deaths in patients treated by different drugs during clinical trials and even after their marketing. Well-known examples of such drugs include for instance cerivastatin, fialuridine, perhexiline, pirprofen, and troglitazone [1, 9, 10]. For pharmaceutical industries, interruption of clinical trials or drug withdrawal after marketing can lead to huge financial loss and long-term image-tarnishing consequences [9, 11].

Whatever its cause (genetic or acquired), severe dysfunction of mitochondria is detrimental for almost all types of cells because these organelles are a turntable of cell metabolism and the major site of energy synthesis via the oxidative phosphorylation (OXPHOS) process [1, 12]. Regarding drug-induced toxicity, it is noteworthy that the list of the pharmaceuticals able to damage mitochondria is growing year after year [1, 4, 9, 13], most probably because drug-induced mitochondrial dysfunction is increasingly sought after by academic teams and pharmaceutical companies. As a matter of fact, many drugs accumulate inside mitochondria favoring their interactions with different targets including enzymes and their cofactors, and the mitochondrial genome [1, 4, 14]. In addition specific mitochondrial transporters mediate import of some drugs such as antiretroviral and anticancer nucleoside analogs [15, 16], cationic amphiphilic molecules such as amiodarone, tacrine, and perhexiline can freely enter the mitochondria by using the transmembrane potential [4, 17]. Consequently, these protonophoric drugs can transitory entail an OXPHOS uncoupling possibly followed by an OXPHOS inhibition resulting from their mitochondrial accumulation [1, 4]. In addition, some drugs can trigger mitochondrial membranes permeabilization, sometimes facilitated by calcium and ROS, leading to the cytoplasmic release of proapoptotic proteins contained in the intermembrane space [18, 19]. Other drugs, such as antiretroviral drugs, can progressively deplete mitochondrial DNA (mtDNA) by directly inhibiting the DNA polymerase γ and/or inducing mtDNA oxidative damage [1, 20, 21].

As a result, the assessment of mitochondrial toxicity is now a major issue, not only allowing to understand the mechanisms of toxicity of different xenobiotics but also to discard the most hazardous ones during drug discovery studies. Liver is one of the main targets as some drugs might preferentially accumulate in liver mitochondria because of their extensive first-pass hepatic extraction [17, 22]. Liver also contains high levels of cytochromes P450

(CYPs), which often contribute to the generation of reactive metabolites presenting mitochondrial toxicity [23, 24]. Numerous studies showed that mitochondrial dysfunction plays a primary role in drug-induced liver injury (DILI) including hepatic cytolysis, steatosis, and steatohepatitis [1, 4, 9, 20, 25, 26]. Therefore, early stage identification of mitochondrion-toxic drugs which might induce liver injury may have ethical and economic impact. Such investigations require the development of predictive in vitro assays [10, 11].

This chapter presents the methods to identify potential mitochondrion-toxic drugs in different types of biological materials. We detail in particular the in vitro methods assessing both integrity and functionality of purified mouse liver mitochondria [27] as well as cellular and mitochondrial alterations on cultured hepatic cells. Most of the assays using soluble sensors are performed in a screening mode for identification of mitochondrion-toxic drugs. However, the in vitro method we discussed here could be used to detect potential drug-induced mitochondrial liability and to understand the involved mechanisms. This chapter points out the importance of the nature of the biological model used in the mitochondrial toxicity assays and of the choice of relevant parameters to improve prediction of DILI in human and develop safer drugs.

2   Materials

2.1   Buffers and Reagents

Chemicals: Oligomycin A, rotenone, antimycin A, malonate, *m*-chlorocarbonylcyanide phenylhydrazone (*m*-Cl-CCP), $CaCl_2$, Na-glutamate, 2Na-malate, 2Na-succinate, palmitoyl-L-carnitine and reference drugs are purchased from Sigma-Aldrich (St Quentin-Fallavier, France) and kept (50–100 μL samples) in solution either in water, ethanol or DMSO at −20 °C.

Homogenization buffer: 300 mM sucrose, 5 mM TES (pH 7.2), 0.2 mM EGTA, 1 mg/mL BSA.

Swelling buffer: 200 mM sucrose, 5 mM succinate, 10 mM MOPS pH 7.4, 1 mM K_2HPO_4, 2 μM rotenone and 10 μM EGTA supplemented with 1 μM rhodamine 123 (Rh123; Molecular Probes™) for transmembrane potential assay or MitoSOX (Molecular Probes™) for mitochondrial ROS detection. Swelling of mitochondria occurs when both mitochondrial membranes are permeabilized.

Respiration buffer: medium A (250 mM sucrose, 30 mM K_2HPO_4, 1 mM EGTA, 5 mM $MgCl_2$, 15 mM KCl, and 1 mg/mL bovine serum albumin (BSA)) supplemented with respiratory substrates activating complex I (1 mM malate and 12.5 mM glutamate), complex II (25 mM succinate and 2 μM rotenone), or fatty acid oxidation (FAO) (25 µM palmitoyl-L-carnitine and 1 mM malate) and 1.65 mM ADP.

2.2 Detection Systems

2.2.1 Polarographic Oxygen Sensors

Clark type oxygen electrode (Hansatech Instruments Ltd., Norfolk, UK): The oxygen electrode allows a precise and continuous measurement of dissolved oxygen in magnetically stirred respiratory medium (medium A). The chamber made in clear cast acrylic is connected to a thermoregulated circulating water bath. The samples are incubated in 300 µL of respiratory medium A housed within a borosilicate glass reaction vessel and added with substrates, ADP (causing a sudden burst in oxygen uptake when ADP is converted to ATP), and specific respiratory chain inhibitors using Hamilton-type syringe. Typically, after inhibition by oligomycin A, oxygen consumption is restored by addition of the OXPHOS uncoupler *m*-Cl-CCP which leads to a permanently high rate of O_2 consumption due to proton leak [28].

Red-Flash technology (Pyro-Science, Aachen, Germany): O_2 consumption can be alternatively measured using the new Red-Flash technology. This technique relies on the use of an optic fiber equipped with a membrane coated with a fluorescent dye excitable with an orange-red light and showing an oxygen-dependent fluorescence in the near infrared [29, 30]. The experimental conditions are similar to O_2 consumption measurements with Clark electrode but adapted to lower incubation volumes (30–50 µL).

2.2.2 Soluble Sensors

Various fluorescent probes can be used to measure potential mitochondrial alterations.

Rhodamine 123 (Molecular Probes™, ThermoFisher Scientific, Courtaboeuf, France): Rh123 is used on isolated mitochondria to follow in real-time mitochondrial transmembrane potential changes by spectrofluorimetry ($\lambda_{Excitation}$ 485 nm; $\lambda_{Emission}$ 535 nm). Mitochondrial potential due to proton gradient induces accumulation and quenching of Rh123 fluorescence (decrease fluorescence). Conversely an increase of fluorescence (corresponding to a dye release from mitochondria) potentially brings about by addition of a drug will reflect and be proportional to a loss of the mitochondrial membrane potential. The protonophore *m*-Cl-CCP which fully dissipates the proton gradient across the inner mitochondrial membrane is used as control.

DiOC₆ (Molecular Probes™, ThermoFisher Scientific, Courtaboeuf, France): This cationic dye accumulates into mitochondria in response to electric potential across the inner mitochondrial membrane. High concentration of dye induces extensive quenching resulting in fluorescence shift that is proportional to the mitochondrial membrane potential. In the context of our platform, $DiOC_6$ is used on entire cells to measure the end-point transmembrane potential loss by flow cytometry (decrease of fluorescence; $\lambda_{Excitation}$ 488 nm, $\lambda_{Emission}$ 530 nm).

MitoXpress (Luxcel, Cork, Ireland): This phosphorescent dye is quenched by O_2, hence the amount of phosphorescence is inversely proportional to amount of extracellular O_2. When O_2 is consumed by the respiratory chain, the dye is dequenched and phosphorescence is emitted ($\lambda_{Excitation}$ 380 nm; $\lambda_{Emission}$ 650 nm). MitoXpress dye allows high throughput measurement of mitochondrial oxygen consumption in real-time by spectrofluorimetry on isolated mitochondria and cells in suspension [31, 32].

MitoSOX (Molecular Probes™, ThermoFisher Scientific, Courtaboeuf, France): MitoSOX is a cell-permeant fluorescent dye targeted to mitochondria to measure production of superoxide anions (henceforth referred to as mitochondrial reactive oxygen species or mtROS). When oxidized by superoxide anions, the dye exhibits red fluorescence which can be measured by spectrofluorimetry ($\lambda_{Excitation}$: 510 nm; $\lambda_{Emission}$: 580 nm) or flow cytometry (Fl-2: 580 nm).

2.3 Biological Models

2.3.1 Isolated Mitochondria

Liver mitochondria from 6- to 10-week-old BALB/cByf female mice (Charles River, Saint-Germain-sur-L'arbresle, France) is used to identify direct mitochondrial effects of xenobiotics. Female mice are used instead of male to reduce interindividual variability (Brenner and Borgne-Sanchez, unpublished data; [27]). Female rat liver mitochondria could also be used without significant differences in sensitivity to compounds (tested on ~20 reference drugs; [27]; unpublished data) Liver mitochondria are isolated and purified by isopycnic density-gradient centrifugation in Percoll [27, 33] allowing to obtain pure and stable mitochondrial preparations. Purified organelles resuspended in homogenization buffer (22 mg/mL of proteins) are kept on ice, and used in screening assays in the next 5 h following their preparation. Premature dilution might alter the integrity of mitochondria. To check the quality of mitochondrial preparations, samples are subjected to measurement of spontaneous swelling and transmembrane potential loss in 96-well plates at 37 °C during 30 min in presence of swelling buffer (see Sect. 3.2.1 for procedure). The preparation is considered as stable and suitable for screening assays if the spontaneous swelling and $\Delta\Psi_m$ loss are below 10% after 30 min at 37 °C (Fig. 1a). In addition, the respiratory control index (RCI) is measured by Clark electrode (see Sect. 3.1.1 for procedure) and has to be above 3 (using succinate as a substrate) to validate respiratory chain functionality (Fig. 1b) [33]. Finally, the forward scatter and side scatter (FSC/SSC) and fluorescence ($\lambda_{Excitation}$ 488 nm; $\lambda_{Emission}$ 530 nm) analysis by flow cytometry (FACSCalibur, BD Bioscience, Germany) of the mitochondrial preparation in the presence or absence of MitoTracker™ green (Molecular Probes™, ThermoFisher Scientific, Courtaboeuf, France) indicates the proportion of intact mitochondria and has to be above 95% (Fig. 1c) to ensure mitochondrial stability during the assays.

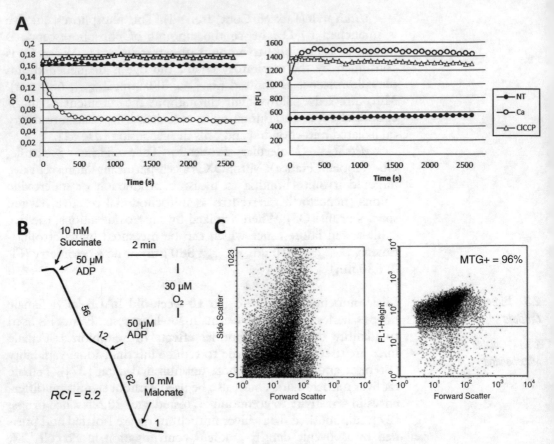

Fig. 1 Quality controls of purified mouse liver mitochondria. (**a**) Mitochondrial integrity. Spontaneous swelling (0.4%; OD at 550 nm) and $\Delta\Psi m$ loss (5%; RFU) are measured by spectrofluorimetry after 30 min incubation at 37 °C in swelling buffer as described in Sect. 3.2.1 and compared to positive controls (50 μM Ca^{2+} for swelling and 50 μM m-Cl-CCP for $\Delta\Psi_m$ loss; 100% induction). (**b**) Mitochondrial functionality. O_2 consumption by mitochondria (100 μg) is measured by Clark electrode after addition of the indicated reagents. Numbers along the trace are nmoles of O_2 consumed per minute per milligram of protein. The respiratory control index (RCI) is calculated as indicated in Sect. 3.1.1. (**c**) Purity of mitochondrial fraction. Purified mitochondria are analyzed by flow cytometry after MitoTracker Green labeling (*left panel*: size (FSC)/granulosity (SSC); *right panel*: FSC/FL-1). The percentage of labeled mitochondria (MTG+ events) reflects the purity of the mitochondrial preparation

2.3.2 HepaRG Differentiated Cells

The human hepatic HepaRG® cell line (Biopredic International, Rennes, France) is a relevant model to investigate liver mitochondrial toxicity induced by parent compounds or their metabolites. These hepatocyte-like cells express xenobiotic metabolizing activities close to those measured in primary human hepatocyte cultures [34]. Therefore, HepaRG cells possess both the metabolic performances of primary hepatocytes and the indefinite growth capacity of hepatic cell lines.

We use undifferentiated HepaRG cells cryopreserved at passage P12 (HPR101). After 2 weeks of proliferation in the HepaRG growth medium (ADD710), cells become confluent and spontaneously enter into differentiation. The HepaRG differentiation medium (ADD720) subsequently allows the cells to undergo a complete hepatocyte differentiation program within 2 weeks where two cell types (hepatocyte colonies and primitive biliary cells) are present. For compound screening, the growing cells are seeded at 2×10^4 cells/cm^2 and treated with compounds during the differentiation phase, for instance for 1, 2, 7, or 12 consecutive days. Renewal of medium and treatment is performed on days 2 and 5 for the 7 day-treatments and on days 3, 5, 7, and 10 for the 12 day-treatments.

To characterize cell metabolism, we measure lactate production (see Sect. 3.1.3) which is dependent on glycolytic activity and glucose concentration in the medium (Fig. 2a). Hence, lactate production is high in HepG2 cells cultured with 4.5 g/L glucose and reduced in HepG2 adapted to galactose. Lactate concentrations are also low in differentiated HepaRG cells grown with glucose (2 g/L). Indeed, even cultured with glucose, HepaRG cells have low glycolytic activity. Regarding mitochondrial activity, RCI measured in mitochondria isolated from HepaRG cells (see Sect. 3.1.1) is around 7 in the presence of succinate and ADP (Fig. 2b). This high RCI presumably reflects high OXPHOS capacity, thus confirming recent investigations [35]. Besides RCI, assessment of the activity of the respiratory chain complexes II and IV is informative because higher activity of complex II compared to complex IV (see Sect. 3.1.2) is characteristic of liver mitochondria [36]. Differentiated HepaRG cells show a high complex II–complex IV ratio closer to primary hepatocytes than HepG2 cells, which have high complex IV activity compared to complex II even in the presence of galactose (Fig. 2c). Hence, differentiated HepaRG cells that rely on the OXPHOS machinery for survival is a valuable model to study drug-induced hepatic mitochondrial dysfunctions [34, 37].

3   Methods

3.1   Quality Controls—Model Characterization

We set up various quality controls to validate the use of our biological models for the detection of mitochondrial dysfunction. Using purified liver mitochondria, RCI is measured to validate the functionality and stability of the mitochondrial preparation. The benefit of using HepaRG cells as a predictive model to detect drug-induced mitochondrial toxicity was validated by demonstrating that culture conditions in glucose recommended by the provider were able to detect such toxicity.

3.1.1   Respiratory Control Index (RCI)

Isolated mitochondria are incubated in a magnetically stirred 1.5 mL cell chamber with a Clark type oxygen electrode thermostated at 37 °C, in 300 µL of respiration buffer with succinate. The

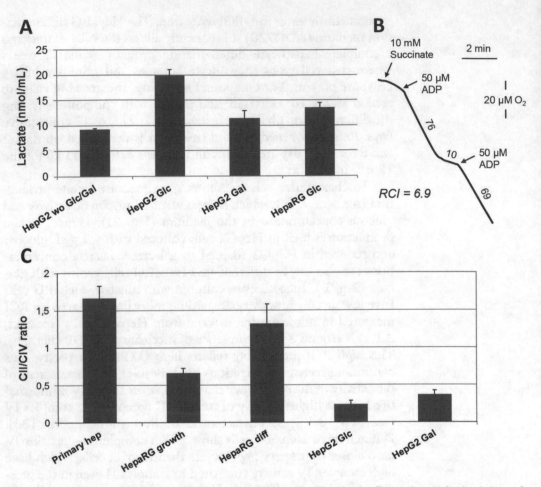

Fig. 2 Mitochondrial and glycolytic activities in HepaRG and HepG2 cells. (**a**) Glycolytic activity. Lactate production measured, as described in Sect. 3.1.3, in HepG2 cultured without glucose and galactose (HepG2 wo Glc/Gal), HepG2 cultured in glucose-rich medium (HepG2-Glc), HepG2 adapted in galactose-rich medium (HepG2-Gal) and differentiated HepaRG cells cultured with glucose (HepaRG-Glc) ($n = 3–4$, mean ± SEM, standard error of mean). (**b**) Functionality of purified HepaRG mitochondria. O_2 consumption by mitochondria (100 µg) is measured by Clark electrode after addition of the indicated reagents. Numbers along the trace are nmoles of O_2 consumed per minute per milligram of protein. The respiratory control index (RCI) is calculated as indicated in Sect. 3.1.1. (**c**) Respiratory chain activity. Ratios of complex II–complex IV (CII–CIV) activity are measured as indicated in Sect. 3.1.2 in human primary hepatocytes (frozen), cultured growing and differentiated HepaRG cells as well as cultured HepG2-Glc and HepG2-Gal cells ($n = 4–5$; mean ± SEM, standard error of mean). A CII–CIV ratio above 1 is characteristic of hepatic cells

addition of a limiting amount of ADP triggers a rapid oxygen uptake characteristic of an active phosphorylating state (state 3; conversion of added ADP to ATP) followed by a slower oxygen uptake rate when all the ADP has been phosphorylated to form ATP (state 4) inducing proton accumulation and respiratory chain inhibition. RCI, which is the [state 3 rate]–[state 4 rate] ratio, reflects the coupling between oxidizing and phosphorylating processes. Hence, a high RCI reliably indicates the integrity and functionality of the mitochondrial preparation.

3.1.2 Respiratory Chain Complex Activity

Measurements of the respiratory chain complex activity are adapted from Bénit et al. [38] to frozen primary human hepatocytes (Biopredic International, Rennes, France), growing and differentiated HepaRG cells and HepG2 cells (CRL-10741; LGC Standards, Molsheim, France) cultured in glucose or adapted to galactose. For complex II activity (EC 1.3.5.1), the cells are trypsinized, permeabilized with low digitonin and incubated at 37 °C in 10 mM KH_2PO_4 buffer (pH 7.2) with lauryl maltoside, 5 mM succinate, 100 μM oxidized decylubiquinone, 300 μM potassium cyanide, and 40 μM DCPIP (dichlorophenolindophenol sodium) in 96-well plates. Activity of this complex is measured in real-time by spectrophotometry by following the decreased absorbance of DCPIP at 600 nm (Tecan Infinite 200). For measurement of complex IV activity (EC 1.9.3.1), cells are incubated at 37 °C in KH_2PO_4 buffer (pH 7.2) with lauryl maltoside and 25 μM dithionite-reduced cytochrome c in 96-well plates. Activity of this complex is measured in real-time by spectrophotometry at 550 nm. As previously mentioned, higher activity of complex II compared to complex IV is characteristic of liver mitochondria [36].

3.1.3 Glycolytic Activity

After deproteinization of samples, 96-well plates are kept at −80 °C until use. Lactate levels are then measured by spectrofluorimetry (Tecan Infinite 200, $\lambda_{Excitation}$ 535 nm; $\lambda_{Emission}$ 580 nm) using the Lactate Fluorometric assay kit (BioVision, ENZO Life Science, Villeurbane, France) according to the supplier's recommendations.

3.2 Assessment of Acute and Direct Mitochondrial Toxicity

In order to determine whether compounds can be rapidly and directly toxic on mitochondria, we classically assess a combination of parameters in purified mouse liver mitochondria (MiToxView®) [27, 28].

3.2.1 Swelling/ Transmembrane Potential

Compounds (2× final concentrations) are distributed in 96-well plate in 100 μL/well swelling buffer. Mitochondria (22 μg) and Rh123 (2 μM) are mixed in 100 μL swelling buffer and added to each well. Absorbance (swelling; Optical Density (OD) at 550 nm) and Rh123 fluorescence ($\Delta\Psi_m$ loss; relative fluorescence unit (RFU) at $\lambda_{Excitation}$ 485 nm; $\lambda_{Emission}$ 535 nm) are recorded at 37 °C in real-time during 45 min using a spectrofluorimeter. Results are expressed in percent of induction after normalization by negative control (untreated mitochondria; 0% induction) and positive control (50 μM Ca^{2+} for swelling and 50 μM m-Cl-CCP for $\Delta\Psi_m$ loss; 100% induction).

3.2.2 Oxygen Consumption

MitoXpress dye (200 nM) is diluted in 50 μL of respiration buffer (medium A supplemented with 4× concentrated respiratory substrates and ADP) and distributed to each well of a 96-well plate. Compounds (4× final concentrations) are distributed in 96-well plate in 50 µL of medium A per well before distribution of the mitochondria (100 µg) diluted in 100 µL of medium A. Then, 100 µL of mineral oil is added to each well to avoid oxygen balance between ambient air and respiration reaction. O_2 consumption is measured in real-time during 45 min at 37 °C by spectrofluorimetry ($\lambda_{Excitation}$ 380 nm; $\lambda_{Emission}$ 650 nm). Results are expressed in percent of inhibition after normalization by negative control (untreated mitochondria; 0% inhibition) and positive control (25 mM malonate for complex II driven O_2 consumption; 2 µM rotenone for complex I and FAO driven O_2 consumption; 100% inhibition).

3.2.3 mtROS Production

Compounds (2× final concentrations) are distributed in 96-well plates in 100 µL swelling buffer per well. Mitochondria (44 µg) and MitoSOX Red dye (4 µM) are mixed in 100 µL swelling buffer and added to each well at 37 °C. Fluorescence is recorded for 45 min by spectrofluorimetry ($\lambda_{Excitation}$ 510 nm; $\lambda_{Emission}$ 590 nm). Results are expressed in percent of ROS production after normalization by negative control (untreated mitochondria; 0%) and positive control (10 µM antimycin A; 100% ROS production).

3.3 Mitochondrial Toxicity in HepaRG Cells

In order to determine whether compounds or their metabolites can be toxic on mitochondria, in particular after several days of treatment, we classically assess a combination of parameters in cultured differentiated HepaRG cells.

3.3.1 Transmembrane Potential

After treatment, the differentiation medium is removed and the cells are labeled with the $DiOC_6$ dye diluted at 10 nM in differentiation medium for 20 min at 37 °C in a humidified 5% CO_2 incubator. Cells are trypsinized for the measurement of mitochondrial membrane potential ($\Delta\Psi_m$) which is detected as an end-point measurement by flow cytometry (FACSCalibur, BD Biosciences; $\lambda_{Excitation}$ 488 nm; $\lambda_{Emission}$ 530 nm). Results are expressed in percent of potential loss after normalization by negative control (untreated cells; 0%) and positive control (1 µM staurosporine for 24 h; 100% $\Delta\Psi_m$ loss). In case of interference with the $DiOC_6$ dye, JC-1 (5,50,6,60,-tetrachloro 1,1,3,30-tetraethylbenzimidazolylca rbocyanine iodide; Molecular Probes™) can be alternatively used ($\lambda_{Excitation}$ 488 nm; $\lambda_{Emission}$ 530 and 580 nm for low and high $\Delta\Psi_m$, respectively).

3.3.2 Global Oxygen Consumption (Cell Respiration)

After treatment, cells are harvested with trypsin, loaded in 96-well plates and kept at room temperature in 50 µL differentiation medium. After addition of the MitoXpress dye (100 nM) diluted in 50 µL of respiration buffer, mineral oil is added and the oxygen consumption is immediately measured in real-time by spectrofluorimeter ($\lambda_{Excitation}$ 380 nm; $\lambda_{Emission}$ 650 nm). Results are expressed in percent of inhibition after normalization by negative control (untreated cells; 0%) and positive control (2 µM rotenone added at T0; 100% inhibition).

3.3.3   ADP/ATP Ratio

After treatment, cells are loaded in 96-well plates and permeabilized in order to measure the ATP and ADP levels using the ApoSENSOR kit (BioVision, ENZO Life Science, Villeurbane, France) according to the supplier's recommendations. The changes in ADP/ATP ratios have been used to identify metabolism imbalance and cell death [39]. The enzyme luciferase catalyzes the formation of light from ATP and luciferin. ADP levels are measured by ADP conversion to ATP that is subsequently detected using the same reaction. The light is measured using a luminometer. Results are expressed in percent of inhibition after normalization by negative control (untreated cells; 0%) and positive control (10 μM antimycin A; 100% ADP–ATP ratio alteration).

3.3.4   Quantification of mtDNA

Because drug-induced mtDNA depletion classically occurs after several days of treatment [14, 21], we measure mtDNA levels after 12 days. To this end, cells are trypsinized and pelleted before isolation of total DNA and amplification by qPCR (Mx3005 Pro thermocycler; Agilent). Primers and Taqman probes targeting mitochondrial DNA (ND1; forward primer: ccctaaaacccgccacatct; reverse primer: gagcgatggtgagagctaaggt; Taqman probe: ccatcaccctctacatcaccgccc) and nuclear DNA (GAPDH; forward primer: ctccccacacacatgcactta; reverse primer: cctagtcccagggctttgatt; Taqman probe: aaaagagctaggaaggacaggcaacttggc) are used to respectively measure mitochondrial DNA and nuclear DNA for normalization. The $2^{-\Delta\Delta Ct}$ method is used to assess the relative mtDNA levels.

3.4   Determination of Mitochondrial-Toxicity

In all assays, efficient drug concentrations inducing 20% of the effect (EC_{20}) are determined in comparison to the 100% baseline obtained with their respective positive controls. EC_{20} calculations are done on at least three replicates of treatment (three mitochondrial purifications or three cell passages) by using a nonlinear regression in Graphpad Prism4. A drug is considered as mitochondrion-toxic if the EC_{20} is $\leq 100 \times C_{max}$ (maximal plasma concentration) for at least one of the five abovementioned parameters assessed in purified mitochondria [27], or at least one parameter among transmembrane potential, global O_2 consumption, and mtDNA levels in HepaRG cells [40, 41].

3.5   Glutathione Levels in HepaRG Cells

Although it is not a mitochondrial parameter per se we can measure intracellular glutathione levels as reliable oxidative stress marker. After treatment, cells are loaded in 96-well plates in order to measure total glutathione (i.e., reduced glutathione [GSH] + oxidized glutathione [GSSG]) and only GSSG, respectively in two different wells. Difference in values obtained in both wells allows to determine GSH levels. Measurements are performed by luminescence (Tecan Infinite 200) using the GSH/GSSG-Glo™ Assay (Promega, France), according to the supplier's recommendations.

Results are expressed in percent of GSH depletion after normalization by negative control (untreated cells; 0%) and positive control (100 μM buthionine-sulfoximine; 100%).

4 Discussion/Note

4.1 Comparison with Other Detection Systems

The use of fluorescent probes is convenient to screen compounds as the assays can be done in 96- or 384-well plate-based format. It is well adapted to cell lines or isolated liver mitochondria because the biological material is not limiting. Indeed, MitoXpress requires relatively large cell amounts (around 200,000 cells/well in 96-well plates with detection by Tecan Infinite 200) in order to measure global cell respiration. Oxygraphs (Hansatech or Oroboros) require more cells (10^6 cells/measure) due to their large chamber volume (250 μL to 1 mL) but offer flexibility which allows extensive characterization of the respiratory chain activity by sequential addition of reagents in the medium during recording. The highly sensitive Red-Flash technology [29, 30] presents similar advantages although it allows measurement of O_2 consumption in less than 50 μL sample volumes. This is convenient in case of precious samples (patient tissues, primary cells, iPS-derived cells). However so far, commercially available Red-Flash devices appear better adapted to study a limited number of samples simultaneously (2–4). It is important to mention here that oxygraphy helps in case of fluorescent or colored (yellow) compounds which usually interfere with fluorescent probes, specifically with MitoXpress [27]. However, compound screening using oxygen consumption is hardly feasible by using oxygraph or Red-Flash technologies.

Finally, the extracellular flux (XF) analyzer (Agilent Technologies, Santa Clara, USA) allows real-time monitoring of the O_2 consumption rate and extracellular acidification rate in intact cells, thus combining the evaluation of OXPHOS activity and glycolysis. This technique, using a disposable sensor cartridge embedded with 96 pairs of fluorescent biosensors, thus permits a first stage identification of potential mitochondrion-toxic compounds. However, further experiments performed in isolated mitochondria should be done in order to determine whether mitochondrial dysfunction detected with this screening tool is a primary event, or only a distant consequence of upstream cellular events.

4.2 Comparison with Other Hepatic Cellular Models

The choice of the biological model is obviously of primary importance in order to study drug-induced mitochondrial dysfunction. If purified mouse liver mitochondria are useful for the identification of acute effects of parent drugs [27], long term effects or metabolite toxicity require the use of cellular assays. Primary human hepatocytes are classically used to assess mitochondrial dysfunction and cellular toxicity [32] but their use is limited due to the scarcity of liver donors, absence of cell amplification and variability between batches (for instance, secondary to different polymorphisms, preexisting liver diseases and treatments). HepG2 hepatocarcinoma cells are commonly used in toxicity assays because of their easy culture and clonal origin leading to reproducible response. However, under standard culture conditions in glucose rich-medium, HepG2 cells mainly produce ATP by glycolysis (Crabtree effect) while OXPHOS activity and FAO are maintained at a low rate [35, 42], making these cells mostly resistant to mitochondrion-toxic compounds. Their growth in galactose circumvents the Crabtree effect [43] and allows these cells to become susceptible to mitochondrial inhibition [44]. However, even when adapted to galactose medium (shift to OXPHOS machinery), they might conserve some characteristics of tumor cells, for example regarding the Bcl-2 family protein profile [33]; unpublished data) and respiratory chain activity (Fig. 2c). Indeed, tumor cells are "ready for death" and their sensitivity to compounds can be different from healthy hepatocytes. Moreover, HepG2 cells present limited biotransformation capabilities, although this feature can greatly vary between the sources of HepG2 cell lines [45]. Nonetheless, HepG2 cells express an incomplete repertoire of xenobiotic-metabolizing enzymes (XME) compared to primary human hepatocytes and HepaRG cells [37, 46]). In most cases, the Glucose-Galactose assay is based on measurement of cellular parameters such as cell growth or ATP content over short periods of treatment [44, 47]. A clear difference of response between both conditions helps to identify if mitochondrial toxicity is a dominant pathway [44]. However, this strategy fails to detect mitochondrion-toxic drugs with long-term effects and/or toxicity mediated by XME-generated metabolites [47].

Since almost 7 years, additionally to isolated mitochondria, we use the well-established HepaRG cell line in order to detect mitochondrial liability. Indeed, differentiated HepaRG cells present (even in glucose medium) low glycolytic activity (Fig. 2a) and high OXPHOS capacities with a high respiratory control index (RCI about 7) using succinate as a substrate (Fig. 2b; [35]). Moreover, the complex II–complex IV activity ratio of differentiated HepaRG cells is close to the one observed in primary hepatocytes, this being not true for HepG2 cells (even adapted to galactose) (Fig. 2c). In addition, HepaRG cells offers the advantage of a cell line with drug metabolism capacities close to those of primary hepatocytes [34, 37, 48]. Measurements of transmembrane potential, oxygen consumption, ATP/ADP ratio, GSH depletion, and mtDNA depletion during time course of treatment can help to identify drugs with moderate but significant mitochondrial toxicity but also drug-induced cytotoxicity unrelated to primary mitochondrial dysfunction (for instance, secondary to oxidative stress). These assays in HepaRG cells nicely complement screening assays on purified mitochondria on which respiratory chain complex activity can also be measured if inhibition of O_2

Table 1
Multiparametric study in purified liver mitochondria combined with time-course treatments in differentiated HepaRG cells

	Liver mitoch.	HepaRG 2d	HepaRG 7d	HepaRG 12d
Class #1				
Class #2				
Class #3				
Class #4				
Class #5				

Assessment of drug-induced toxicity in isolated mouse liver mitochondria (swelling, $\Delta\Psi_m$ loss, O_2 consumption driven by CI, CII, and FAO, mtROS production) combined with time-course treatments in differentiated HepaRG cells ($\Delta\Psi_m$ loss, global O_2 consumption, ADP–ATP ratio, GSH, mtDNA) can allow the identification of mitochondrion-toxic compounds with DILI risk. Mitochondrial toxicity was determined as indicated in Sect. 3.4. When taking into account all these parameters, compounds can tentatively be classified in five classes: Class #1: compounds with direct and acute mitochondrial toxicity due to the parent drug (i.e., amiodarone, lovastatin, lumiracoxib, perhexiline, saquinavir, and troglitazone); Class #2: compounds with direct mitochondrial toxicity of a reactive metabolite (i.e., acetaminophen, mercaptopurine); Class #3: compounds with direct but long-term mitochondrial toxicity (i.e., fialuridine, zalcitabine, and zidovudine); Class #4: compounds with rapid cytotoxic effect inducing downstream mitochondrial damages; Class #5: compounds with no apparent mitochondrial toxicity (i.e., amantadine). Color code: red: strong effect (toxicity $\geq$ 50% of the respective positive control of mitochondrial liability); pink: moderate effect (20% < toxicity < 50%); orange: low effect (toxicity $\leq$ 20%); white: no effect. 2, 7, and 12 days correspond to 2, 7, and 12 day-treatment, respectively

consumption is detected. Table 1 provides an illustration of what can be obtained in term of identification of mitochondrial toxicants and understanding of their mechanisms of toxicity by using this strategy. Indeed, the multiparametric screen in mouse liver mitochondria combined with time-course treatment in HepaRG cells may allow the distinction between: (1) direct and acute mitochondrial toxicity of the parent drug, (2) direct mitochondrial toxicity of a reactive metabolite, (3) direct but long-term mitochondrial toxicity, and (4) rapid cytotoxic effect with downstream mitochondrial damages. Such strategy can be used in order to detect drug-induced mitochondrial toxicity at drug discovery stage or during preclinical development, thus being useful to adapt drug development strategy (modifications of drug chemical structure, use of specific mouse models, …).

5   Conclusion and Future Directions

Given the importance of drug-induced mitochondrial toxicity in DILI [49], a great deal of efforts has been made in the last decade to develop predictive tools and assays to study drug-induced mitochondrial dysfunction in vitro [10]. The use of fluorescent probes and commercial devices helped to set up screening assays, and thus nowadays a combination of read-out and biological models improves the prediction of drug toxicity risk in human [47, 50].

Our platform combines multiparametric assays on both purified hepatic mitochondria and cultured HepaRG differentiated cells. This strategy allows the detection of direct and acute mitochondrial toxicity of parent drug, their metabolites and/or long-term induced mitochondrial toxicity. Whereas the use of purified mitochondria allows medium-throughput screening (200 compounds/months, at four concentrations in triplicate on five parameters), studies in HepaRG cells are, at the moment, performed in low throughput, i.e., ~22 compounds per month (excluding cell growth period) at four concentrations, three time-points, 4–5 parameters in triplicate. Future development might consist in the combination of 2–3 readouts on the same sample as well as the use of more sensitive probes to reduce cell number per point. To respect the 3R principle, we have developed assays in purified HepaRG mitochondria, which also have the advantage to be close to the human metabolism. Investigation of a large panel of reference drugs on this system might be useful to challenge the sensitivity of human versus rodent mitochondria to drug-induced toxicity. Finally, it will be interesting to measure other mitochondrial parameters in order to better understand the mechanisms whereby drugs can alter mitochondrial function. For instance, we plan to study the mitochondrial FAO pathway with different fatty acids as some drugs can differentially inhibit the oxidation of short-chain, medium chain and long-chain fatty acids [51, 52].

Acknowledgments

This review was supported by a grant from the Agence Nationale de la Recherche (ANR-16-CE18-0010-03 MITOXDRUGS). We are very grateful to Biopredic International (Rennes, France) and especially Dr. Christophe Chesné for providing HepaRG cells for the characterization experiments and Sandrine Camus for recommendations on HepaRG cell culture.

References

1. Begriche K, Massart J, Robin MA, Borgne-Sanchez A, Fromenty B (2011) Drug-induced toxicity on mitochondria and lipid metabolism: mechanistic diversity and deleterious consequences for the liver. J Hepatol 54:773–794

2. Gougeon ML, Penicaud L, Fromenty B, Leclercq P, Viard JP, Capeau J (2004) Adipocytes targets and actors in the pathogenesis of HIV-associated lipodystrophy and metabolic alterations. Antivir Ther 9:161–177

3. Varga ZV, Ferdinandy P, Liaudet L, Pacher P (2015) Drug-induced mitochondrial dysfunction and cardiotoxicity. Am J Physiol Heart Circ Physiol 309:H1453–H1467

4. Fromenty B, Pessayre D (1995) Inhibition of mitochondrial beta-oxidation as a mechanism of hepatotoxicity. Pharmacol Ther 67:101–154

5. Knockaert L, Descatoire V, Vadrot N, Fromenty B, Robin MA (2011) Mitochondrial

CYP2E1 is sufficient to mediate oxidative stress and cytotoxicity induced by ethanol and acetaminophen. Toxicol In Vitro 25:475–484

6. Lieber CS, DeCarli L, Rubin E (1975) Sequential production of fatty liver, hepatitis, and cirrhosis in sub-human primates fed ethanol with adequate diets. Proc Natl Acad Sci U S A 72:437–441

7. Hardonniere K, Saunier E, Lemarie A, Fernier M, Gallais I, Helies-Toussaint C, Mograbi B, Antonio S, Benit P, Rustin P, Janin M, Habarou F, Ottolenghi C, Lavault MT, Benelli C, Sergent O, Huc L, Bortoli S, Lagadic-Gossmann D (2016) The environmental carcinogen benzo[a]pyrene induces a Warburg-like metabolic reprogramming dependent on NHE1 and associated with cell survival. Sci Rep 6:30776

8. Jiang Y, Xia W, Yang J, Zhu Y, Chang H, Liu J, Huo W, Xu B, Chen X, Li Y, Xu S (2015) BPA-induced DNA hypermethylation of the master mitochondrial gene PGC-1alpha contributes to cardiomyopathy in male rats. Toxicology 329:21–31

9. Labbe G, Pessayre D, Fromenty B (2008) Drug-induced liver injury through mitochondrial dysfunction: mechanisms and detection during preclinical safety studies. Fundam Clin Pharmacol 22:335–353

10. Will Y, Dykens J (2014) Mitochondrial toxicity assessment in industry—a decade of technology development and insight. Expert Opin Drug Metab Toxicol 10:1061–1067

11. Nadanaciva S, Will Y (2011) Investigating mitochondrial dysfunction to increase drug safety in the pharmaceutical industry. Curr Drug Targets 12:774–782

12. Wallace DC, Fan W, Procaccio V (2010) Mitochondrial energetics and therapeutics. Annu Rev Pathol 5:297–348

13. Naven RT, Swiss R, Klug-McLeod J, Will Y, Greene N (2013) The development of structure-activity relationships for mitochondrial dysfunction: uncoupling of oxidative phosphorylation. Toxicol Sci 131:271–278

14. Schon E, Fromenty B (2015) Alteration of mitochondrial DNA in liver diseases, vol 150. Taylor & Francis, New-York

15. Govindarajan R, Leung GP, Zhou M, Tse CM, Wang J, Unadkat JD (2009) Facilitated mitochondrial import of antiviral and anticancer nucleoside drugs by human equilibrative nucleoside transporter-3. Am J Physiol Gastrointest Liver Physiol 296:G910–G922

16. Lee EW, Lai Y, Zhang H, Unadkat JD (2006) Identification of the mitochondrial targeting signal of the human equilibrative nucleoside transporter 1 (hENT1): implications for inter-species differences in mitochondrial toxicity of fialuridine. J Biol Chem 281:16700–16706

17. Berson A, Renault S, Letteron P, Robin MA, Fromenty B, Fau D, Le Bot MA, Riche C, Durand-Schneider AM, Feldmann G, Pessayre D (1996) Uncoupling of rat and human mitochondria: a possible explanation for tacrine-induced liver dysfunction. Gastroenterology 110:1878–1890

18. Al Maruf A, O'Brien PJ, Naserzadeh P, Fathian R, Salimi A, Pourahmad J (2017) Methotrexate induced mitochondrial injury and cytochrome c release in rat liver hepatocytes. Drug Chem Toxicol:1–11

19. Kowaltowski AJ, Castilho RF, Vercesi AE (2001) Mitochondrial permeability transition and oxidative stress. FEBS Lett 495:12–15

20. Pessayre D, Mansouri A, Berson A, Fromenty B (2010) Mitochondrial involvement in drug-induced liver injury. Handb Exp Pharmacol:311–365

21. Gardner K, Hall PA, Chinnery PF, Payne BA (2014) HIV treatment and associated mitochondrial pathology: review of 25 years of in vitro, animal, and human studies. Toxicol Pathol 42:811–822

22. Mansouri A, Haouzi D, Descatoire V, Demeilliers C, Sutton A, Vadrot N, Fromenty B, Feldmann G, Pessayre D, Berson A (2003) Tacrine inhibits topoisomerases and DNA synthesis to cause mitochondrial DNA depletion and apoptosis in mouse liver. Hepatology 38:715–725

23. Antherieu S, Rogue A, Fromenty B, Guillouzo A, Robin MA (2011) Induction of vesicular steatosis by amiodarone and tetracycline is associated with up-regulation of lipogenic genes in HepaRG cells. Hepatology 53:1895–1905

24. Aubert J, Begriche K, Knockaert L, Robin MA, Fromenty B (2011) Increased expression of cytochrome P450 2E1 in nonalcoholic fatty liver disease: mechanisms and pathophysiological role. Clin Res Hepatol Gastroenterol 35:630–637

25. Lee WM (2003) Drug-induced hepatotoxicity. N Engl J Med 349:474–485

26. Russmann S, Kullak-Ublick GA, Grattagliano I (2009) Current concepts of mechanisms in drug-induced hepatotoxicity. Curr Med Chem 16:3041–3053

27. Porceddu M, Buron N, Roussel C, Labbe G, Fromenty B, Borgne-Sanchez A (2012) Prediction of liver injury induced by chemicals in human with a multiparametric assay on isolated mouse liver mitochondria. Toxicol Sci 129:332–345

28. Buron N, Porceddu M, Roussel C, Begriche K, Trak-Smayra V, Gicquel T, Fromenty B, Borgne-Sanchez A (2017) Chronic and low exposure to a pharmaceutical cocktail induces mitochondrial dysfunction in liver and hyperglycemia: differential responses between lean and obese mice. Environ Toxicol 32: 1375–1389

29. El-Khoury R, Dufour E, Rak M, Ramanantsoa N, Grandchamp N, Csaba Z, Duvillie B, Benit P, Gallego J, Gressens P, Sarkis C, Jacobs HT, Rustin P (2013) Alternative oxidase expression in the mouse enables bypassing cytochrome c oxidase blockade and limits mitochondrial ROS overproduction. PLoS Genet 9:e1003182

30. Bénit P, Chrétien D, Porceddu M, Rustin P, Rak M (2017) A performing, versatile and inexpensive device for oxygen uptake measurement. J Clin Med 6(6), pii: E58. doi:10.3390/jcm6060058

31. Will Y, Hynes J, Ogurtsov VI, Papkovsky DB (2006) Analysis of mitochondrial function using phosphorescent oxygen-sensitive probes. Nat Protoc 1:2563–2572

32. Dykens JA, Jamieson JD, Marroquin LD, Nadanaciva S, Xu JJ, Dunn MC, Smith AR, Will Y (2008) In vitro assessment of mitochondrial dysfunction and cytotoxicity of nefazodone, trazodone, and buspirone. Toxicol Sci 103:335–345

33. Buron N, Porceddu M, Brabant M, Desgue D, Racoeur C, Lassalle M, Pechoux C, Rustin P, Jacotot E, Borgne-Sanchez A (2010) Use of human cancer cell lines mitochondria to explore the mechanisms of BH3 peptides and ABT-737-induced mitochondrial membrane permeabilization. PLoS One 5:e9924

34. Guillouzo A, Corlu A, Aninat C, Glaise D, Morel F, Guguen-Guillouzo C (2007) The human hepatoma HepaRG cells: a highly differentiated model for studies of liver metabolism and toxicity of xenobiotics. Chem Biol Interact 168:66–73

35. Peyta L, Jarnouen K, Pinault M, Guimaraes C, Pais de Barros JP, Chevalier S, Dumas JF, Maillot F, Hatch GM, Loyer P, Servais S (2016) Reduced cardiolipin content decreases respiratory chain capacities and increases ATP synthesis yield in the human HepaRG cells. Biochim Biophys Acta 1857:443–453

36. Chretien D, Rustin P, Bourgeron T, Rotig A, Saudubray JM, Munnich A (1994) Reference charts for respiratory chain activities in human tissues. Clin Chim Acta 228:53–70

37. Aninat C, Piton A, Glaise D, Le Charpentier T, Langouet S, Morel F, Guguen-Guillouzo C, Guillouzo A (2006) Expression of cytochromes P450, conjugating enzymes and nuclear receptors in human hepatoma HepaRG cells. Drug Metab Dispos 34:75–83

38. Benit P, Goncalves S, Philippe Dassa E, Briere JJ, Martin G, Rustin P (2006) Three spectrophotometric assays for the measurement of the five respiratory chain complexes in minuscule biological samples. Clin Chim Acta 374:81–86

39. Bradbury DA, Simmons TD, Slater KJ, Crouch SP (2000) Measurement of the ADP:ATP ratio in human leukaemic cell lines can be used as an indicator of cell viability, necrosis and apoptosis. J Immunol Methods 240:79–92

40. Pertuiset C, Porceddu M, Buron N, Camus S, Chesné C, Borgne-Sanchez A (2015) Identification of drug-induced mitochondrial alterations using HepaRG cell line. Toxicol Lett 238:S316–S317

41. Porceddu M, Pertuiset C, Camus S, Chesné C, Buron N, Borgne-Sanchez A (2016) In vitro prediction of antiretroviral drug-induced hepatotoxicicty by using mitochondrial MiToxView screening platform. Toxicol Sci 150:S598

42. Igoudjil A, Massart J, Begriche K, Descatoire V, Robin MA, Fromenty B (2008) High concentrations of stavudine impair fatty acid oxidation without depleting mitochondrial DNA in cultured rat hepatocytes. Toxicol In Vitro 22:887–898

43. Rossignol R, Gilkerson R, Aggeler R, Yamagata K, Remington SJ, Capaldi RA (2004) Energy substrate modulates mitochondrial structure and oxidative capacity in cancer cells. Cancer Res 64:985–993

44. Marroquin LD, Hynes J, Dykens JA, Jamieson JD, Will Y (2007) Circumventing the Crabtree effect: replacing media glucose with galactose increases susceptibility of HepG2 cells to mitochondrial toxicants. Toxicol Sci 97:539–547

45. Hewitt NJ, Hewitt P (2004) Phase I and II enzyme characterization of two sources of HepG2 cell lines. Xenobiotica 34:243–256

46. Guo L, Dial S, Shi L, Branham W, Liu J, Fang JL, Green B, Deng H, Kaput J, Ning B (2011) Similarities and differences in the expression of drug-metabolizing enzymes between human hepatic cell lines and primary human hepatocytes. Drug Metab Dispos 39:528–538

47. Hynes J, Nadanaciva S, Swiss R, Carey C, Kirwan S, Will Y (2013) A high-throughput dual parameter assay for assessing drug-induced mitochondrial dysfunction provides additional predictivity over two established mitochondrial toxicity assays. Toxicol In Vitro 27:560–569

48. Michaut A, Le Guillou D, Moreau C, Bucher S, McGill MR, Martinais S, Gicquel T, Morel I, Robin MA, Jaeschke H, Fromenty B (2016) A cellular model to study drug-induced liver

injury in nonalcoholic fatty liver disease: application to acetaminophen. Toxicol Appl Pharmacol 292:40–55

49. Pessayre D, Fromenty B, Berson A, Robin MA, Letteron P, Moreau R, Mansouri A (2012) Central role of mitochondria in drug-induced liver injury. Drug Metab Rev 44:34–87

50. Nadanaciva S, Rana P, Beeson GC, Chen D, Ferrick DA, Beeson CC, Will Y (2012) Assessment of drug-induced mitochondrial dysfunction via altered cellular respiration and acidification measured in a 96-well platform. J Bioenerg Biomembr 44:421–437

51. Fromenty B, Freneaux E, Labbe G, Deschamps D, Larrey D, Letteron P, Pessayre D (1989) Tianeptine, a new tricyclic antidepressant metabolized by beta-oxidation of its heptanoic side chain, inhibits the mitochondrial oxidation of medium and short chain fatty acids in mice. Biochem Pharmacol 38:3743–3751

52. Freneaux E, Fromenty B, Berson A, Labbe G, Degott C, Letteron P, Larrey D, Pessayre D (1990) Stereoselective and nonstereoselective effects of ibuprofen enantiomers on mitochondrial beta-oxidation of fatty acids. J Pharmacol Exp Ther 255:529–535

Chapter 15

Bile Salt Export Pump: Drug-Induced Liver Injury and Assessment Approaches

Ruitang Deng

Abstract

Bile acid homeostasis is maintained through the tightly regulated enterohepatic circulation of bile acids. Biliary excretion of bile acids by bile salt export pump (BSEP) is the rate-limiting step in the circulation. Impairment of BSEP function and expression results in excessive accumulation of hepatic bile acids, which are toxic to hepatocytes. Indeed, genetic deficiencies in BSEP resulting in diminished or reduced BSEP activity or cell surface expression directly cause cholestatic liver diseases including progressive familial intra-hepatic cholestasis type II (PFICII) and benign intrahepatic cholestasis (BRIC) or predispose to intrahe-patic cholestasis of pregnancy and drug-induced cholestasis. Drugs or compounds inhibiting BSEP activity, repressing BSEP transcription, or reducing cell surface expression of BSEP protein have the potential to induce cholestatic liver injury. Accumulating evidences reveal that inhibition of BSEP activity is one of the mechanisms for drug-induced liver injury (DILI). Studies also show that repression of BSEP transcription or reduction of its canalicular membrane expression contribute to a spectrum of cholestatic injuries. Currently, a number of in vitro methods are employed to assess the cholestatic potentials of drugs or com-pounds. These methods can be divided into three categories based on the mechanisms of action of the test drugs or compounds: (1) inhibition of BSEP activity; (2) repression of BSEP transcription; and (3) reduc-tion of cell surface expression of BSEP protein. Here, applications, advantages, and limitations of these in vitro approaches are described and discussed.

Key words Bile salt export pump, BSEP, Cholestasis, Drug-induced liver injury, DILI, Drug-induced cholestasis, BSEP activity, BSEP transcription, BSEP expression

1 Introduction

Bile acids are the metabolites of cholesterol and are synthesized in the liver. Approximately 0.5 g of bile acids are produced daily in human liver. Bile acid homeostasis is maintained through a tightly regulated enterohepatic circulation of bile acids. After synthesis in hepatocytes in the liver, bile acids are excreted into bile and stored in the gallbladder. After each meal, bile acids are released from the gall-bladder into the small intestine where the majority of bile acids (95%) are reabsorbed. Through portal blood circulation, bile acids are returned to the liver, completing the enterohepatic circulation [1–4].

Minjun Chen and Yvonne Will (eds.), *Drug-Induced Liver Toxicity*, Methods in Pharmacology and Toxicology, https://doi.org/10.1007/978-1-4939-7677-5_15, © Springer Science+Business Media, LLC, part of Springer Nature 2018

Biliary secretion of bile acids from hepatocytes into bile is the rate-limiting step in the enterohepatic circulation of bile acids and is mainly mediated by the canalicular member transporter, bile salt export pump (BSEP) [5–10].

As the canalicular transporter of bile acids, BSEP plays an essential role in maintaining hepatic as well as systemic bile acid homeostasis. Impairment of BSEP expression and function results in decreased biliary excretion of bile acids with concurrent accumulation of excessive bile acids in the liver, which is toxic to hepatocytes. Genetic deficiencies in BSEP cause progressive familial intrahepatic cholestasis type 2 (PFIC2) [11–23], benign recurrent intrahepatic cholestasis type 2 (BRIC2) [23–25] and contribute to intrahepatic cholestasis of pregnancy [26–30] and drug-induced cholestasis [31, 32].

Under cholestatic conditions, high levels of hepatic bile acids, especially hydrophobic bile acids, such as chenodeoxycholic acid (CDCA), have been implicated in causing liver damage [33–40]. Studies in vitro and in vivo reveal several possible mechanisms by which bile aids induce hepatic cytotoxicity. First, elevated bile acids damage the integrity of cell membranes through their detergent property [33–35]. Second, bile acids cause mitochondrial stress and promote the generation of reactive oxygen species, which in turn cause damage to the cells [36–39]. Third, bile acids induce endoplasmic reticulum stress, contributing to cell death [40–42]. Finally, bile acids may induce inflammatory responses to contribute cell damage [43–45]. Through those mechanisms, bile acids eventually cause cell death in two distinct pathways, apoptosis and necrosis [46–49]. Relatively lower concentrations of bile acids appear to lead to apoptosis while higher concentrations of bile acids cause cell death through necrosis [39, 50, 51]. Although both types of cell death are observed under cholestatic conditions, necrosis is the predominant form of cell death in the cholestatic mouse model [49, 52].

Drug-induced liver injury (DILI) is a major cause of serious liver illness in humans and has at times resulted in drug withdrawal from the market [53–58]. As the major bile acid transporter, BSEP has been long recognized as a potential mechanism contributing to DILI (Fig. 1). In humans, certain BSEP variants have been associated with drug-induced cholestasis [31, 32]. Accumulating evidence suggests that inhibition of BSEP is one of the mechanisms for drug-induced liver toxicity [59–74]. A close correlation has been established between the potency of BSEP inhibition by drugs or compounds and the severity of DILI [61–64, 72–74]. Many in vitro methods have been developed to evaluate the inhibitory potency of BSEP activity by drugs or compounds [59–77]. Screening drug candidates or compounds for inhibition of BSEP activity has become a more widely used approach during drug discovery.

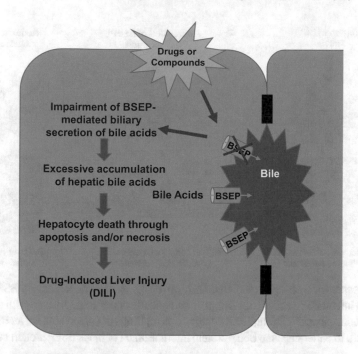

Fig. 1 BSEP-associated drug-induced liver injury. Drugs or compounds act on BSEP, impairing BSEP function or expression. As a result, biliary excretion of bile acids is reduced with concurrent accumulation of excessive bile acids in hepatocytes. Elevation of hepatic bile acids causes cell death through apoptosis and/or necrosis, and subsequently leads to cholestatic liver injury

In contrast to our current understanding on inhibition of BSEP activity as a possible mechanism contributing to DILI, much less attention and efforts have been given to investigating the disruption of BSEP expression caused by drugs or compounds. Disruption of BSEP expression can be at the transcriptional and/or posttranscriptional level. Limited studies have demonstrated that repression of BSEP transcription by endobiotics, such as estrogens, and xenobiotics, including drugs, contributes to intrahepatic cholestasis or DILI [78–82]. Consistently, studies have shown that BSEP expression levels are reduced in cholestatic patients [83–85]. As a canalicular membrane transporter, BSEP activity is directly correlated with its cell surface expression levels. Under physiological condition, the expression levels of BSEP on the canalicular membrane are determined by a balance between cell surface targeting and internalization of BSEP protein [4, 86, 87]. Blockage of cell surface targeting or enhanced internalization leads to reduced cell surface expression, consequently causing cholestatic liver injury [4, 10, 87]. Such posttranscriptional effects on BSEP cell surface expression have been demonstrated in various cholestatic conditions [88–96]. Although there are various methods for assessing drug or compound disruption of BSEP expression, they are not fully utilized in drug candidate screening.

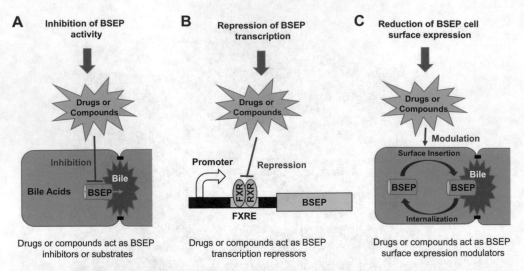

Fig. 2 Mechanisms of BSEP-mediated DILI. (**a**) Drugs or compounds act as BSEP inhibitors or weak substrates to inhibit BSEP activity. (**b**) Drugs or compounds act as BSEP transcription repressors to repress BSEP transcription, especially through FXR antagonism. (**c**) Drugs or compounds act as BSEP cell surface expression modulators to either enhance BSEP protein internalization or block BSEP protein cell surface insertion

Taken together, a drug or compound can potentially induce cholestatic liver injury through: (1) inhibiting BSEP activity; (2) repressing BSEP transcription; and (3) reducing BSEP cell surface expression (Fig. 2). Here, we describe the methods to assess the cholestatic potentials of drugs or compounds through those three mechanisms and discuss their advantages and limitations.

2   Measuring BSEP Inhibition

Direct inhibition of BSEP activity by drugs has been proposed as a major mechanism for drug-induced cholestasis [59–74]. Extensive evaluation of drugs or compounds with or without potential to cause cholestatic injury reveals a direct correlation between BSEP inhibition and drug-induced cholestasis [61–64, 72–74]. Theoretically, BSEP-mediated biliary excretion of bile acids can be inhibited by drugs or compounds that serve as either BSEP substrates or inhibitors. As a specialized bile acid transporter, BSEP has a very narrow substrate spectrum, exhibiting high affinity and selectivity toward conjugated bile salts with highest affinity for taurine-conjugated CDCA and cholic acid (CA) [5, 6, 70, 97]. No drugs or compounds have been identified as BSEP substrates with high affinity. Therefore, most of identified drugs to cause cholestatic injury are BSEP inhibitors, and it remains to be determined how these drugs or compounds bind to BSEP and interfere with its activity. Currently, there are many in vitro methods available to screen drugs or chemicals that inhibit BSEP activity. Based on cellular components used for the assays, those methods can be divided into two major categories: (1) vesicular membrane-based and (2) whole cell-based assays.

2.1 Vesicular Membrane-Based Assays

As an efflux transporter, functional BSEP proteins are localized on the canalicular membrane. Before inserted into canalicular membranes or immediately following internalization, BSEP proteins are present in small membrane vesicles within the cytoplasm. Two types of assays, i.e., vesicular transport [98–102] and ATPase assays [103], have been established based on vesicular membranes prepared from BSEP-expressing cells. Membrane fractions prepared from BSEP-expressing cells contain three types of membrane structures: (1) vesicles that originated from plasma membranes containing BSEP proteins in the right orientation, called right-side-out vesicles; (2) vesicles derived from intracellular membranes containing BSEP proteins in an orientation opposite to those on cell surface, called inside-out vesicles; and (3) open membrane fragments that originated from either plasma or intracellular membranes. Not all three membrane structures are employed in vesicular membrane-based assays. Inside-out vesicles are exclusively used for vesicular transport assays while ATPase assays involve both inside-out vesicles and open membrane fragments. It should be pointed out that the presence of right-side-out vesicles in the vesicular membrane preparations does not seem to interfere with either assay.

2.1.1 Vesicular Transport Assays

Vesicular transport is one of the most widely used assays for in vitro screening of drugs or compounds [77, 98, 99]. In inside-out vesicles, BSEP substrate and ATP binding sites are located on the outer face of the vesicle. Thus, vesicular transport is carried out similarly to transporter uptake assays, with the substrates being translocated from the reaction medium to the inside of the vesicle in the presence of ATP. The assays can be carried out in two formats, directly or indirectly. Direct vesicular transport assay is designed to screen BSEP substrates while indirect vesicular transport assay is formatted to screen both BSEP inhibitors and substrates in the presence of a standard BSEP substrate or probe.

Most commonly used vesicular membranes are prepared as crude membranes from either liver tissues [100–102] or BSEP-overexpressing cells [5, 13, 70, 96, 103–106]. For preparation of membrane vesicles from human or rodent liver, liver tissues are homogenized, followed by isolation of crude membrane fractions through a series of differential centrifugations. Canalicular membrane fractions can be further purified by sucrose gradient centrifugations. Insect cells overexpressing BSEP, such as *Spodoptera frugiperda* 9 (sf9) and sf21, are the most commonly used host cells for preparing BSEP-containing vesicular membranes [5, 13, 70, 106, 107], and are currently commercially available from different vendors. Other host cells including various mammalian cell lines overexpressing BSEP have also been used to prepare BSEP-containing vesicular membranes, such as HEK, CHO, LLC-PK1, MDCK, and HeLa cells [13, 96, 104, 105, 108]. Overexpression of BSEP in insect sf9 or sf21 cells is achieved by infection of the cells with human BSEP cDNA-containing baculoviruses. In mammalian cells, BSEP is overexpressed by either transient transfection (transduction) or stable expression of BSEP. For preparation of vesicular membranes from cell lines, BSEP-expressing cells are homogenized and crude membrane fractions are collected after removing nuclear, mitochondrial and other cell debris with centrifugation. The crude membrane suspensions are then passed through a 27-gauge needle to facilitate the assembly of membrane vesicles from open membrane fragments. The vesicle suspension can be used immediately or stored at −80 °C.

BSEP activity in the vesicles is directly impacted by the expression levels of BSEP and the composition of the membranes. Vesicles isolated from liver tissues contain physiologically relevant levels of BSEP proteins while the BSEP protein levels in vesicles prepared from cell lines overexpressing BSEP vary widely depending on the host cells and overexpression approaches. Compared to mammalian cells, insect sf9 or sf21 cells express much more abundant BSEP protein due to the use of a strong promoter derived from baculovirus. BSEP protein levels in vesicles prepared from stable BSEP-expressing cells are relatively higher than in vesicles isolated from transient transfected cells and are relatively consistent from batch to batch. The compositions of vesicular membranes differ among vesicles prepared from liver tissues, insect cells, or mammalian cell lines. Vesicular membranes from insect cells contain less cholesterol. Studies have shown that the cholesterol content of the vesicular membranes has marked effects on BSEP activity [107, 109]. The changes in membrane fluidity due to difference in cholesterol content are speculated to be the possible reason for the effects on BSEP activity.

Vesicles prepared from liver tissues contain many other membrane transporters in addition to BSEP, which may complicate the interpretation of the screening results. Lack of BSEP specificity coupled with the complexities in preparing the vesicles from liver tissues limits their utility as routine screening assays. Therefore, vesicles with high levels of BSEP protein that are isolated from insect cells using a relatively simple production procedure have become the most commonly used reagent for routine screening of BSEP inhibitors.

Before carrying out the indirect (inhibition) vesicular transport assays, direct (uptake) vesicular transport assays with a standard BSEP substrate or probe are usually performed to establish the optimal assay conditions, including appropriate vesicle concentrations, incubation time linearity and substrate concentrations.

For performing the inhibition vesicle transport assays, vesicles are incubated with increasing concentrations of test drugs or compounds in the presence of the BSEP substrate taurocholate (radiolabeled or cold) for a predetermined period of time. Since ATP is required for BSEP to transport taurocholate, ATP is also added into the incubation buffer. Parallel assays with AMP in the incubation buffer are included in the experiments to serve as negative controls to evaluate possible passive diffusion, non-BSEP related transport and nonspecific binding of the test drugs or compounds to the vesicles. A positive control of BSEP inhibitors, such as cyclosporin A and ketoconazole, should be included in the assays. The reactions are stopped by adding 3× reaction volume of cold buffer. Vesicles are retained through filtration with glass or membrane filters. The amount of taurocholate inside the vesicles is quantified by liquid scintillation counter for radiolabeled taurocholate or LC-MS/MS for cold taurocholate.

Inhibition potencies of the test drugs or compounds on BSEP activity are determined by the reduction of taurocholate uptake into the vesicles in the presence of the test drug or compound. ATP-dependent uptake activity (active transport) is calculated by subtracting the uptake activity with AMP (passive diffusion) from uptake activity with ATP. The IC_{50} is calculated from the percentage activity remaining using commercially available curve fitting software.

The advantages of vesicular transport assays are multifold. The assay is relatively simple to carry out and can be run in a high-throughput format, such as in a 96-well plate. It is also advantageous that the assays directly measure the actual disposition of the substrates across the cell membrane. However, the assay is not suitable for screening drugs or chemical compounds with medium to high passive permeability, which will not be well retained inside the vesicles. In addition, high nonspecific binding of some test drugs or compounds in this assay can potentially be problematic, indicating the importance of appropriate controls in the assays.

2.1.2 ATPase Assays

As an ATP-binding cassette (ABC) transporter, BSEP requires ATP as an energy source to transport its substrates. Substrate binding to BSEP activates the ATPase enzyme to hydrolyze ATP, releasing energy and inorganic phosphate. Inorganic phosphate can be detected by a simple colorimetric reaction. The amount of inorganic phosphate released is directly correlated to the BSEP activity. BSEP proteins in both inside-out vesicles and open membrane fragments contribute to the ATPase activity detected [103]. Since high levels of BSEP expression is required for carrying out the assays, crude vesicular membranes prepared from insect cells are preferred over preparations from liver tissues or mammalian cells. However, vesicular membranes prepared from insect cells contain less cholesterol which has a negative impact on the ATPase activity of BSEP. Studies showed that modification of insect cell-derived vesicular membranes by cholesterol loading during the preparation decreases the basal ATPase activity and enhances substrate-stimulated ATPase activity of BSEP [110]. Therefore, cholesterol-loaded membranes from insect cells are commonly used for the ATPase assays.

Similar to vesicular transport assays, ATPase assays can be performed in both direct (activation) and indirect (inhibition) formats. It is not uncommon that both activation and inhibition assays are carried out in parallel. ATPase activation detected in the direct assays indicates that the test drug or compound is a substrate of BSEP. The inhibition of ATPase activity detected in the indirect assays indicates that the test drug or compound is either a slowly transported substrate or inhibitor of BSEP. Prior to carrying out the assays, optimal assay conditions should be established with the standard BSEP substrate taurocholate or taurochenodeoxycholate to obtain the best signal-to-noise ratio, including membrane vesicle protein contents, ATP concentrations and reaction times.

For the inhibition assays, vesicular membranes are incubated with increasing concentrations of test drugs or compounds in the presence of a standard BSEP substrate (activator), taurocholate or taurochenodeoxycholate, for a defined period of time. The reactions are stopped by adding 12% sodium dodecyl sulfate. Appropriate controls should be included in the assays. First, due to some contaminated inorganic phosphate in assay suspension and presence of nonenzymatic ATP hydrolysis, the baseline organic phosphate levels should be detected and subtracted from the total ATPase activity. Second, some ATPase activities unrelated to BSEP are always present in membrane preparations. A background control for baseline ATPase activity of the host cell membranes should be included and subtracted from the total ATPase activity. Third, as an ABC transporter, BSEP ATPase activity is effectively inhibited by orthovanadate. Membrane preparations often contain a small amount of orthovanadate-insensitive ATPase activity. Detection and subtraction of the orthovanadate-insensitive ATPase activity is essential. Fourth, a positive control with known BSEP inhibitor, such as cyclosporin A, should be included in the assays.

The advantages of the ATPase assay include its feasibility for high-throughput screening, its great reproducibility, and its ability to evaluate test drugs or compounds with medium to high permeability. In addition, no radiolabeling of the BSEP probes and test drugs or compounds are required. However, the ATPase assay is an indirect method and does not provide precise information on the transport rate of the substrates. The assay is not BSEP ATPase-specific and membrane vesicles containing other ATPase-related proteins result in a high assay background. In addition, test drugs or compounds that are slowly translocated by BSEP often give a false negative reading due to such a slow rate of ATP hydrolysis that the inorganic phosphate released is too low to be detected by the assay.

Taken together, both vesicular transport and ATPase assays have advantages and limitations. Therefore, in some cases, use of both assays is required to accurately assess the BSEP transport and inhibition profiles of the test drugs or compounds.

2.2 Whole Cell-Based Assays

In hepatocytes, bile acid uptake is mediated primarily by the basolateral membrane transporter sodium/taurocholate cotransporting polypeptide (NTCP) and excreted by the canalicular efflux transporter BSEP. Cell-based assays provide much more accurate prediction than vesicular membrane-based assays alone. The results derived from the cell-based approaches are more relevant pharmacologically and toxicologically to the status in vivo. In addition, cell-based assays also allow for investigating the inhibitory effects of test drug or compound's metabolites on BSEP activity and biliary bile acid excretion. Currently, several cell-based assays with distinct features and applications are established using either BSEP-overexpressing cell lines or primary hepatocytes. Primary hepatocytes are still the gold standard for evaluating a drug or compound's inhibitory effects on BSEP activity and biliary bile acid excretion. There are three main types of assay formats that use hepatocytes, including hepatocytes in suspension, sandwich cultured hepatocytes, and hepatocytes in coculture.

2.2.1 BSEP-Overexpressing Cells

Transient or stable BSEP-overexpressing cells are used in this assay. The assay can be run in both direct and indirect format. The direct (transport) assay is carried out to screen whether the test drugs or compounds are BSEP substrates while indirect (inhibition) assays are run to determine whether test drugs or compounds inhibit BSEP mediated transport of its substrate or probe [104, 105, 111]. Cells are seeded in transwell plates with a permeable membrane insert. After cultured for a couple of days allowing cells to form tight junction, those cells are polarized with apical membrane exposing to the upper compartment while the basolateral membrane exposing to the lower compartment. For screening the potency of test drugs or compounds for inhibiting BSEP activity, test drugs or compounds at various concentrations are added into the lower compartment medium containing the standard BSEP substrate taurocholate (radiolabeled or cold). The amount of taurocholate in the upper compartment medium over time is determined by liquid scintillation counter for radiolabeled taurocholate or by LC-MS/MS for cold taurocholate. The inhibition potency of the test drug or compound is calculated by the reduction of transported BSEP substrate taurocholate in the presence of the test drug or compound. The IC_{50} values are determined with various concentrations of the drugs or compounds tested.

The assay is a useful tool to screen drugs or compounds for BSEP substrates with medium or high membrane permeability. However, the assay is not suitable for screening test drugs or compounds with low or little membrane permeability. Most of the BSEP-overexpressing cells are not suitable for the inhibition assays since uptake of BSEP substrate taurocholate is minimal in those cell lines due to low or no expression of bile acid uptake transporters. To overcome such limitation, cell lines overexpressing both BSEP and NTCP have been generated. In those double-transfected cells taurocholate is rapidly taken up. Currently, two such cell lines have been established including HeLa and LLC-PK1 cells [104, 108]. Since both HeLa and LLC-PK1 host cells are not liver-derived and lack hepatic metabolic enzymes, use of these cells is limited to investigating the effects of the parental drugs or compounds but not the drug or compound metabolites.

2.2.2 Hepatocytes in Suspension

Hepatocytes have been widely used for assessing various liver functions including drug uptake, metabolism, clearance, and drug-mediated modulation of gene expression. However, hepatocytes in suspension are not considered a good model for evaluating canalicular bile acid excretion since BSEP protein and other transporters on the canalicular membrane are internalized upon isolation. Currently, it is still debatable whether BSEP protein is expressed on the cell surface of hepatocytes in suspension. However, recent studies using hepatocytes in suspension demonstrated that bile acids were taken up and effluxed to the medium [65, 112]. Using this model, drugs to cause cholestatic injury were found to inhibit bile acid efflux and the data generated correlated well with the results from studies using other methods, thus providing a validation for using hepatocytes in suspension for evaluating biliary bile acid excretion.

The assay is relatively easy to carry out. Freshly isolated or cryopreserved hepatocytes are incubated in suspension with increasing concentrations of test drugs or compounds in the presence of a BSEP substrate (CA or CDCA), for a defined period of time. Bile acids (CA or CDCA) are taken up by hepatocytes and conjugated with taurine or glycine within the cells. Newly conjugated cholic acid or chenodeoxycholic acid are not membrane permeable and are excreted into the medium by active transporters, including BSEP. The amounts of conjugated bile acids in the medium are quantified by LC-MS/MS. The reduced efflux rates of conjugated bile acids in the presence of test drugs or compounds indicate the inhibitory effects of the test drugs or compounds on biliary bile acid excretion.

The advantages of the assay include its easiness to perform, short period of hepatocyte culturing, and its ability to be run in a high-throughput format. However, the assay is still not thoroughly validated. In addition, the assay by no means is BSEP-specific because other hepatic transporters may also be involved in efflux of conjugated bile acids.

2.2.3 *Sandwich Cultured Hepatocytes*

Sandwich cultured hepatocytes are well-established and widely used for evaluating biliary excretion of bile acids [62, 64, 113–121]. The assay mimics most closely the biliary clearance of bile acids in vivo. Primary hepatocytes freshly isolated or cryopreserved from human or animals can be used in the assay. Upon isolation and cultivation in regular culture, hepatocytes lose certain characteristic functions and structural features, such as reduced hepatic transporter expression, decreased metabolism capacity, and failure to form canalicular structure. However, when cultured between two layers of gelled collagen (sandwich) for extended period of time (3–10 days depending on the species), hepatocytes retain or regain many in vivo functional and structural features, including improved transporter and metabolism enzyme expression, prolonging survival in vitro, retained cuboidal morphology and polarization of canalicular and basolateral membrane, and formation of functional bile networks (canaliculi).

The ability of sandwich cultured hepatocytes to form functional canalicular network and retain canalicular expression of BSEP makes the assay a unique tool to evaluate biliary excretion of test drugs or compounds and their ability to inhibit biliary excretion of BSEP substrates. Substrates transported by BSEP are accumulated in the canalicular network and can be quantified by modulating the tight junctions using medium with or without Ca^{2+} [122, 123]. In the presence of Ca^{2+}, sandwich cultured hepatocytes develop tight junctions to form canaliculi. However, when replaced with Ca^{2+}-free medium or buffer, the tight junctions between hepatocytes fragment and the BSEP substrates in the canaliculi are released.

Freshly isolated or cryopreserved hepatocytes are cultured on collagen I coated plates, and then overlaid with a Matrigel matrix. Canalicular networks normally take 3–10 days to form depending on the species and should be morphologically confirmed under reverse phase contrast microscopy or high-content imaging. After formation of canalicular network, either biliary excretion assays or excretion inhibition assays can be carried out. For excretion inhibition assays, test drugs or compounds can be either preloaded or incubated together with a BSEP substrate probe. Briefly, sandwich cultured hepatocytes are preincubated with Hanks' balanced salts solution (HBSS) containing Ca^{2+} (maintaining tight junctions and canalicular network) or Ca^{2+}-free HBSS (disrupting tight junctions and opening canaliculi) in the absence or presence of increasing concentrations of test drugs or compounds for 10 min. Following the preincubation, cells are incubated with the BSEP substrate taurocholate (radiolabeled or cold) in the presence or absence of increasing concentrations of test drugs or compounds in

Ca^{2+}-containing HBSS for a predefined period of time (normally no longer than 30 min). The transport process is stopped by washing the cells with an ice-cold buffer. Cells are lysed for BSEP substrate quantitation by scintillation counting for radiolabeled taurocholate or LC/MS/MS for cold taurocholate. The excretion rate of taurocholate is determined by the difference between the Ca^{2+} buffer (intracellular and canalicular taurocholate) and Ca^{2+}-free buffer (intracellular taurocholate). The biliary excretion index (BEI) is calculated using the percentage of a test compound excreted in the canalicular pocket compared to the total amount in both intracellular and canalicular compartments. The inhibitory effects of a test drug or compound on biliary excretion of taurocholate are determined by the difference in the absence and presence of the test drug or compound. The IC_{50} values are calculated based on the regression of BSEP substrate biliary clearance over several test-compound concentrations.

As the gold standard for evaluating the inhibitory effects of test drugs or compounds on biliary bile acid excretion, sandwich cultured hepatocyte assays have several advantageous features. First, the assays most closely mimic the biliary excretion of bile acids in vivo, providing a more accurate prediction of the inhibitory activities of the test drug and compound in vivo. Second, since sandwich cultured hepatocytes largely maintain the metabolic function, the assays can evaluate the inhibitory effects of both parent drugs or compounds and their metabolites. Third, the assays have the ability to evaluate the combined effects of the test drugs or compounds on BSEP activity as well as on BSEP expression if the drugs or compounds have modulating effects on BSEP expression (see BSEP expression-associated methods).

However, several limitations have to be considered in performing the assays and interpreting the data. First, a test drug or compound may inhibit BSEP substrate uptake and such effects should be determined by comparing the BSEP substrate uptake in the absence and presence of the test drug or compound. Second, the canalicular network may gradually be reestablished during the incubation period after preincubation in Ca^{2+}-free buffer. Thus measurable substrate may begin to accumulate in canaliculi during the incubation period with Ca^{2+}-containing HBSS. Third, the culture medium of sandwich cultured hepatocytes is usually supplemented with cytokines to improve cell survival. It is possible that those cytokines have measurable effects on BSEP transcription and cell surface expression [124], which may complicate the interpretation of the data. Fourth, certain test drugs or compounds may damage the canalicular network. The integrity of the cell morphology and canalicular network should be closely monitored and the testing concentration range should be adjusted accordingly. Fifth, although BSEP is the major bile acid efflux transporter, other hepatic transporters at both canalicular and basolateral membranes are also involved in certain bile acids transport. Therefore, strictly speaking, the sandwich cultured hepatocyte assay is not BSEP-specific. Using other transporter-specific inhibitors or hepatocytes from gene-knockout animal may overcome this limitation.

2.2.4 Hepatocytes in Coculture

Another cell model for liver is cocultured hepatocytes with stromal cells or fibroblasts [125–127]. Micropatterned hepatocytes grow as hepatocyte islands which are surrounded by supportive stromal cells or fibroblasts, a characteristic architecture of liver tissue. The advantage of this approach is that co-culture of supportive stromal cells or fibroblasts improves hepatocyte longevity and functions for up to 4 weeks [128]. Currently, the assay reagents are commercially available as HepatoPac from Hepregen. It combines the B-CLEAR technology [121] and transporter certified human hepatocytes with HepatoPac micro-patterned co-cultures. Similar to sandwich cultured hepatocyte, a functional canalicular network is formed in the hepatocyte islands and biliary excretion of bile acids can be evaluated by the assay. After establishment of canalicular network, the inhibitory effects of test drugs or compounds on biliary bile acid excretion are evaluated in the presence of increasing concentrations of test drugs or compounds and BSEP substrate probe taurocholate (radiolabeled or cold). Decreased efflux of taurocholate into the canalicular pockets represents the inhibitory activity of the test drugs or compounds on biliary bile acid excretion. BEI and IC_{50} values are calculated as described in sandwich cultured hepatocyte assays. Due to the relative complexity of the approach, the assay has not been widely used for evaluating the cholestatic potentials of test drugs or compounds.

3 Methodology Based on Repression of BSEP Transcription

BSEP expression is transcriptionally regulated through several signaling pathways, notably the farnesoid X receptor (FXR) pathway [129–133]. Activation of FXR by bile acids induces BSEP expression [129, 130]. Such feed-forward regulation of BSEP by bile acids/FXR is the main mechanism by which hepatic bile acid homeostasis is maintained, preventing excessive accumulation of bile acids in the liver. Drugs or compounds that act as FXR antagonist or weak agonist have the potential to repress BSEP expression causing DILI. For example, the antidiabetic drug troglitazone, which causes DILI and was withdrawn from the market, acts as a weak agonist of FXR and antagonizes bile acid-mediated activation of FXR, repressing BSEP expression [78]. Estrogen 17β-estradiol-mediated repression of BSEP expression contributes to the pathogenesis of intrahepatic cholestasis of pregnancy [79]. Studies also show that repression of BSEP expression is a possible mechanism for drug-induced cholestasis [81, 82]. Drugs with dual inhibitory effects on BSEP activity and expression are often associated with severe clinically reported DILI [82]. Several in vitro methods have been reported to screen drugs or compounds with potential for repressing BSEP expression, including FXR antagonism-based reporter assays [78, 79, 134, 135], real-time PCR [78, 79, 82], and Western blotting [79, 82, 91, 136].

3.1 FXR Antagonism-Based BSEP Promoter Report Assays

The human or rodent BSEP approximate promoter, located usually 2–2.5 kb upstream of the transcription start site, is cloned into a luciferase reporter vector, such as the GL4.10 vector [134, 135]. The native BSEP promoter contains two FXR responsive elements, which exhibit FXR isoform-specificity in human, but not rodent, BSEP [135]. In the presence of FXR, drugs or compounds with FXR agonistic activity induce BSEP transcription, increasing luciferase expression and activity. In contrast, drugs or compounds with FXR antagonistic activity repress BSEP transcription, decreasing luciferase expression and activity. The effects of test drugs or compounds on FXR-mediated transcription of BSEP promoter are evaluated in the absence and presence of a standard FXR agonist, such as the most potent endogenous FXR agonist chenodeoxycholic acid or potent synthetic FXR agonist GW4064. The reporter assays can be performed in 24-, 48-, or 96-well plate formats.

Human hepatoma cell line Huh 7 cells are commonly used as host cells to carry out the assays [78, 79, 134, 135]. The BSEP promoter reporter is transiently cotransfected with the FXR plasmid and the null-Renilla luciferase plasmid as an internal control, followed by incubation of the transfected cells overnight. The next day, transfected cells are treated with increasing concentrations of test drugs or compounds in the absence and presence of chenodeoxycholic acid or GW4064. After treatment for a defined period (usually 24–48 h), dual luciferase reporter assays are performed. Luciferase activities are measured using a Luminometer. The firefly luminescence is normalized based on the Renilla luminescence signal and the ratio of treatment over control serves as fold activation. Both half maximal effective concentration (EC_{50}) for FXR agonistic activity and IC_{50} for FXR antagonistic activity are determined with data from several concentrations of test drugs or compound.

3.2 Real-Time PCR Assay

Real-time PCR assay is carried out to detect and quantify BSEP mRNA levels following treatment of cells with test drugs or compounds [78, 79, 82]. Both primary hepatocytes (human or rodents) and hepatocyte-derived cell lines can be used for the assays. Among cell lines, endogenous BSEP expression levels vary significantly. Huh 7 cells express more abundant BSEP than other cells such as HepG2 and are commonly used for the assay. Huh 7 cells or primary hepatocytes seeded in 12-well plates are treated with increasing concentrations of test drugs or compounds for 24–48 h in the absence or presence of a BSEP expression inducer, chenodeoxycholic acid or GW4064. Total RNAs are isolated from treated cells and subjected to synthesis of the first strand cDNA with random primers and reverse transcriptase. Real-time PCR assays using BSEP-specific probes or primers are carried out. The expression levels of housekeeping genes serve as internal standards. Commonly used housekeeping genes include glyceraldehydes-3-phosphate dehydrogenase (GAPDH), β2-microglobulin, β-actin or 18S rRNA. At least two internal standard genes should be included in the assays to improve the accuracy and reproducibility of the assays. The expression levels of BSEP mRNA are determined and normalized against the expression levels of internal standard genes. The values of EC_{50} and IC_{50} of the test drugs or compounds are calculated based on the results with various concentrations of the test drugs or compounds.

3.3 *Western Blotting*   Cells treated with test drugs or compounds as described in real-time PCR assays are lysed and crude membrane fractions are prepared through differential centrifugation, which are then subjected to Western blotting [79, 82, 91, 136]. After transfer, the membrane is split and the top portion is blotted for BSEP (~175 kDa) with anti-BSEP antibodies and the bottom portion is blotted for housekeeping proteins such as GAPDH (37 kDa) or β-actin (42 kDa) with anti-GAPDH or b-actin antibodies. BSEP and housekeeping proteins are quantified by densitometric analysis. The expression levels of housekeeping genes are used to normalize BSEP expression. The values of EC_{50} and IC_{50} of the test drugs or compounds are determined.

Among the three assays for BSEP transcription and expression, FXR antagonism-based BSEP promoter reporter assay is most suitable for screening large numbers of test drugs or compounds since the assay is relative simple and can be formatted in a high-throughput fashion. However, the modulating effects of test drugs or compounds detected in the assay may not accurately reflect their effects on endogenous BSEP expression. On the other hand, real-time PCR and Western blotting are relatively complicated and time-consuming, thus limiting their use in the initial screening of a large sample of drugs or compounds. However, both assays directly measure the modulating effects of the test drugs or compounds on endogenous BSEP expression. They are thus physiologically and pharmacologically more relevant than BSEP promoter reporter assay. Therefore, it is recommended that BSEP promoter reporter assay is performed for initial screening while real-time PCR and Western blotting are carried out to confirm the modulating effects of the drugs or compounds detected by the BSEP promoter reporter assay.

4   Methodology Based on Cell Surface Expression of BSEP Protein

As a canalicular membrane transporter, BSEP expression levels on the canalicular membrane dictate biliary excretion of bile acids. BSEP deficiencies due to mutations cause inherent as well as acquired forms of cholestasis [11–32]. A common feature of these BSEP mutations is the reduction or total loss of BSEP protein expression at the canalicular membrane while BSEP function may not be affected [17]. For example, BSEP V444A variant, a common mutation associated with PFIC2, intrahepatic cholestasis of pregnancy, and drug-induced cholestasis, exhibits markedly reduced canalicular membrane expression while its activity is normal [31]. The clinical severity of these mutations tends to correlate inversely with the amount of BSEP protein expressed on the cell surface [89].

Consistent with reduced canalicular membrane expression of BSEP in cholestatic patients, decreased expression of BSEP protein at the canalicular membrane is also a characteristic of experimental cholestasis induced by estradiol-17β-D-glucuronide [93], taurolithocholic acid [92] or cyclosporine A [90] in rodents. Upon treatment with those cholestatic agents, BSEP protein is redistributed from canalicular membrane to the subapical cytoplasm. Conversely, ursodeoxycholic acid [137], 4-phenylbutyrate [138–140], and silymarin [141] exert their anticholestatic effects through enhancing cell surface expression of BSEP protein.

Under physiological conditions, the cell surface expression level of BSEP protein is maintained through a recycling mechanism, a balance between membrane insertion and internalization of BSEP protein [86, 87]. Membrane localization of BSEP protein is regulated through various posttranslational processes including glycosylation [142], phosphorylation [143] and ubiquitination [144, 145]. Drugs or compounds that modulate any of those posttranscriptional processes have significant impact on the cell surface expression of BSEP, potentially causing DILI. Several in vitro methods are currently available to screen drugs or compounds with potential for reducing cell surface expression of BSEP protein, including Western blot following biotin labeling, flow cytometry, and immunofluorescence.

4.1   Western Blot Following Biotin Labeling

Primary hepatocytes or Huh 7 cells are treated with increasing concentrations of test drugs or compounds for 24–48 h in the absence or presence of a BSEP inducer, chenodeoxycholic acid or GW4064. Cell surface proteins are labeled with membrane-impermeable biotin [89, 108, 138, 144]. After cells are lysed, biotin-labeled proteins are captured with immobilized streptavidin beads. The captured proteins are released from the beads with an elution buffer and subjected to Western blotting using anti-BSEP antibodies. The cell surface expression of a housekeeping gene

Na/K-ATPase is detected as an internal control. Protein bands on the Western blot are quantified by densitometric analysis. BSEP protein expression levels are normalized with Na/K-ATPase expression. The inhibitory effects are determined by the reduction of BSEP protein levels in the presence of the test drug or compound. The values of IC_{50} are calculated.

4.2 Flow Cytometry Analysis

Flow cytometry is a well-established tool for the reliable detection of cell surface proteins or markers [146, 147]. The assay has not been widely used for the detection of cell surface expression of BSEP. The assay can be carried out in primary hepatocytes or cell lines such as Huh 7 cells. Cells are treated with various doses of test drugs or compounds for 24–48 h in the absence or presence of a BSEP inducer, chenodeoxycholic acid or GW4064. Single cell suspensions are prepared with one of the following methods, using cell scraper, EDTA solution, trypsin digestion or commercial cell detachment solution (such as Accutase solution from Bio-Rad). The advantages of using EDTA solution or cell scraper to detach cells from the plates and making single cell suspensions include preservation of BSEP antigenicity. However, some of the cells are physically damaged during preparation. On the other hand, digestion with trypsin or cell detachment solution has little damage to the cells. However, the antigenicity of BSEP protein may be compromised by the enzyme digestion. Therefore, preliminary experiments for testing those methods should be carried out in untreated cells to determine the appropriate methods for preparing single cell suspension. Cells are stained with BSEP-specific, fluorescein isothiocyanate (FITC)-labeled antibodies or with unlabeled primary anti-BSEP antibodies, followed by staining with FITC-labeled secondary antibodies. After extensive washing away unbound antibodies, cell suspensions are subjected to flow cytometry analysis. For short-term storage, cells can be fixed in 1% paraformaldehyde and flow cytometry analyses of the fixed cells should be carried out within 24 h after fixation. The inhibitory activity of the test drug or compound is determined by the reduced fluorescence staining in the presence of the test drug or compound. The IC_{50} values are calculated.

It should be noted that several factors can interfere with the results of the assays. First, cell death should be minimized during the procedure since dead cells can produce artifacts due to nonspecific binding and increasing autofluorescence levels. Second, negative controls should be included without staining to eliminate possible autofluorescence of the cells. Third, to eliminate the possible effects of nonspecific antibody binding, normal IgG or non-immunized serum should be included as negative controls for primary or secondary antibodies. In addition, appropriate dilution of the primary and secondary antibodies should be determined to achieve the highest signal-to-noise ratio prior to the assay application.

4.3 Immuno-fluorescence Assays

This assay has been used to detect canalicular membrane expression of BSEP [85, 108, 148–150]. Both primary hepatocytes and cell lines such as Huh 7 cells are used for the assay. Cells are treated with increasing concentrations of test drugs or compounds for 24–48 h in the absence or presence of a BSEP inducer, chenodeoxycholic acid or GW4064. Cells are fixed with cold methanol or 4% paraformaldehyde, followed by treatment of the fixed cells with 0.05% Triton X-100 to permeabilize the cell membrane. The cells are incubated in a buffer containing primary anti-BSEP antibodies, followed by detection of primary antibodies by fluorescence-conjugated secondary antibodies. Nucleuses are stained with 4',6-diamidino-2-phenylindole (DAPI) or other agents. BSEP staining is visualized under a confocal microscope. Similar controls as described in flow cytometry analysis should be included in the assays.

Among the three approaches to detect cell surface expression of BSEP, flow cytometry analysis has long been a robust tool for reliable detection of cell surface proteins, and has several advantages over Western blotting and immunofluorescence. First, it has the potential to format as a high-throughput screening assay. Second, the results are more quantitative and reproducible than Western blot and immunofluorescence. Third, the assays are relatively simple and cost effective. One advantage of the immunofluorescence assay is its ability to visualize the entire cellular distribution of BSEP protein in addition to canalicular membrane localization. Furthermore, high-content imaging and analysis can be applied to the assay, gaining additional information on cell morphology changes and other phenotypic perturbations by test drugs or compounds [151–153].

5 Summary and Discussion

As the canalicular transporter of bile acids, impairments of BSEP activity and expression are implicated in various cholestatic liver disorders [11–32]. Compelling evidence has established that BSEP inhibition is one of the mechanisms for drug-induced cholestasis or DILI [59–77]. Screening of drug candidates or compounds with BSEP inhibition assays leads to early identification of drug candidates or compounds with cholestatic potentials in drug development. However, the predictability for drug-induced cholestasis or DILI using BSEP inhibition data is characterized by high incidence of false negative, with 30–40% noninhibitors of BSEP causing cholestasis or DILI [64, 72, 154]. The data indicated that factors or mechanisms other than BSEP inhibition are involved in the development of drug-induced cholestasis or DILI. Among other factors or mechanisms, repression of BSEP transcription, especially through FXR antagonism, and reduced BSEP expression on canalicular membrane by drugs or compounds may play important roles in drug-induced cholestasis or DILI [4, 10, 78–82, 87]. To fully understand the effects of drug candidates or compounds on BSEP and consequently BSEP-associated cholestasis or DILI, assays for BSEP activity, transcription as well as cell surface expression should be carried out. Recent investigations demonstrate that in addition to BSEP-related mechanisms, other factors or mechanisms, such as mitochondrial dysfunction, are also implicated in the development of DILI [57, 155, 156].

Among various in vitro BSEP assays described, there are advantages and limitations for individual assays (Table 1). Considering

Table 1

Advantages and limitations of the BSEP assays

Assays	Advantages	Limitations
Inhibition of BSEP activity		
Vesicular transport assay	The assay is relatively simple to carry out and can be run in a high-throughput format. The assays directly measure the actual disposition of the substrates across the cell membranes	The assay is not suitable for screening drugs or compounds with medium to high passive permeability. High nonspecific binding of some test drugs or compounds can potentially be problematic, requiring appropriate controls in the assays
ATPase assay	The assay is suitable for high-throughput screening with great reproducibility. The assay can be used to evaluate test drugs or compounds with medium to high permeability. No radiolabeling of the BSEP probes, and test drugs or compounds is required	The assay does not provide precise information on the transport rate of the substrates. The assay is not BSEP ATPase-specific since membrane vesicles containing other ATPase-related proteins resulting in a high assay background. The assay is not suitable for evaluating test drugs or compounds that are slowly translocated by BSEP
BSEP-overexpressing cells	The assay is a useful tool to screen drugs or compounds for BSEP substrates with medium or high membrane permeability. Cell lines overexpressing both BSEP and NTCP are capable of taking up taurocholate probe and can be used in BSEP inhibition assays	The assay is not suitable for screening test drugs or compounds with low or little membrane permeability. Most of the BSEP-overexpressing cells are not suitable for the inhibition assays since uptake of BSEP substrate taurocholate is minimal in those cell lines due to low or no expression of bile acid uptake transporters

(continued)

Table 1
(continued)

Assays	Advantages	Limitations
Hepatocytes in suspension	The assay is relatively easy to carry out. It requires a short period of hepatocyte culturing. The assay can be run in a high-throughput format	The assay is still not thoroughly validated. The assay by no means is BSEP-specific because other hepatic transporters may also be involved in efflux of conjugated bile acids
Sandwich cultural hepatocytes	The assay is considered as the gold standard for evaluating the inhibitory effects of test drugs or compounds on biliary bile acid excretion. The assay most closely mimics the biliary excretion of bile acids in vivo, providing a more accurate prediction of the inhibitory activities of the test drugs and compounds in vivo. The assay can evaluate the inhibitory effects of both parent drugs or compounds and their metabolites. The assay has the ability to evaluate the combined effects of the test drugs or compounds on BSEP activity as well as on BSEP transcription and expression	Test drugs or compounds may inhibit BSEP substrate uptake, which complicates interpretation of the data. The supplemented cytokines in hepatocytes culture medium may have modulatory effects on BSEP transcription and cell surface expression. Certain test drugs or compounds may damage the canalicular network, limiting the assay to testing low concentrations of the drugs or compounds. The assay, strictly speaking, is not BSEP-specific since other hepatic transporters at both canalicular and basolateral membranes are also involved in certain bile acids transport
Hepatocytes in coculture	Coculture of hepatocytes with supportive stromal cells or fibroblasts retains the characteristic architecture of liver tissue, improving hepatocyte longevity and functions for up to 4 weeks	Due to the relative complexity of the approach, the assay has not been widely used for evaluating the cholestatic potentials of test drugs or compounds
Repression of BSEP transcription		
BSEP promoter report assays	BSEP promoter reporter assay is most suitable for screening large numbers of test drugs or compounds since the assay is relative simple and can be formatted in a high-throughput fashion. It is recommended that BSEP promoter reporter assay is performed for initial screening	The modulating effects of test drugs or compounds detected in the report assay may not accurately reflect their effects on endogenous BSEP expression

(continued)

Table 1
(continued)

Assays	Advantages	Limitations
Real-time PCR	The assay directly detects the modulating effects of the test drugs or compounds on endogenous BSEP transcription with mRNA levels being detected. It is thus physiologically and pharmacologically more relevant than BSEP promoter reporter assay	The assay is relatively complicated and time consuming, thus limiting to its use in screening relatively small sizes of samples or as a confirmation assay for the BSEP promoter report data
Western blot	The assay is physiologically and pharmacologically more relevant than the BSEP promoter reporter and real-time PCR assay since BSEP protein levels are detected	The assay is most complicated among the three methods. The success of the assay is heavily relied on the availability of high quality BSEP antibodies. The assay is less quantitative than the other two assays. It is limited to evaluating relatively small size of samples or as a confirmation assay for the results obtained with BSEP promoter report and real-time PCR assays
Reduction of BSEP cell surface expression		
Western blot following biotin-labeling	The assay takes advantages of a strong interaction between biotin and streptavidin, which makes it possible to specifically isolate and enrich cell surface proteins	The assay is relatively complicated and time consuming, which limits its use to screening small number of drugs or compounds
Flow cytometry analysis	The assay is relatively simple and cost effective. It has the potential to format as a high-throughput screening assay. The results obtained from the assay are more quantitative and reproducible than western blot and immunofluorescence assay	The assay requires high quality BSEP antibodies that specifically recognize the extra cellular portion of the protein, which can be challenging considering that only small portion of BSEP protein is exposed on extracellular surface
Immunofluorescent assay	The assay has ability to visualize the entire cellular distribution of BSEP protein in addition to canalicular membrane. High content imaging can be applied to the assay	The assay is relatively time consuming and not readily for screening large amounts of samples. The assay requires high quality BSEP antibodies with high specificity

the diverse properties in cell permeability, metabolism and disposition of the drug candidates or compounds, it is impractical to use one set of assays to fully evaluate the cholestatic potentials of the drugs candidates or compounds. However, as a general guidance, the assays with the capability of high-throughput should be carried out for initial screening of a large size of samples. Specifically, vesicular transport assays for identifying BSEP inhibitors or substrates, BSEP promoter reporter assays for detecting BSEP transcription repressors, and flow cytometry assays for screening BSEP cell surface expression modulators are performed for initial screening. Positive hits from those assays can then be further evaluated and confirmed by sandwich cultured hepatocytes, Western blotting, or immunofluorescent assays. For drug candidates or compounds with high permeability, ATPase assays are recommended for initial screening for BSEP inhibitors or substrates. For drug candidates or compounds with active metabolites which potentially impair BSEP activity and/or expression, hepatocytes-based assays, such as sandwich cultured hepatocytes, should be preferably carried out.

References

1. Russell DW (2003) The enzymes, regulation, and genetics of bile acid synthesis. Annu Rev Biochem 72:137–174
2. Trauner M, Boyer JL (2003) Bile salt transporters: molecular characterization, function, and regulation. Physiol Rev 83:633–671
3. Chiang JY (2004) Regulation of bile acid synthesis: pathways, nuclear receptors, and mechanisms. J Hepatol 40:539–551
4. Soroka CJ, Boyer JL (2014) Biosynthesis and trafficking of the bile salt export pump, BSEP: therapeutic implications of BSEP mutations. Mol Asp Med 37:3–14. https://doi.org/10.1016/j.mam.2013.05.001.
5. Gerloff T, Stieger B, Hagenbuch B et al (1998) The sister of P-glycoprotein represents the canalicular bile salt export pump of mammalian liver. J Biol Chem 273:10046–10050
6. Green RM, Hoda F, Ward KL (2000) Molecular cloning and characterization of the murine bile salt export pump. Gene 241:117–123
7. Kullak-Ublick GA, Stieger B, Hagenbuch B et al (2000) Hepatic transport of bile salts. Semin Liver Dis 20:273–292
8. Meier PJ, Stieger B (2002) Bile salt transporters. Annu Rev Physiol 64:635–661
9. Kullak-Ublick GA, Stieger B, Meier PJ (2004) Enterohepatic bile salt transporters in normal physiology and liver disease. Gastroenterology 126:322–342
10. Lam P, Soroka CJ, Boyer JL (2010) The bile salt export pump: clinical and experimental aspects of genetic and acquired cholestatic liver disease. Semin Liver Dis 30:125–133. https://doi.org/10.1055/s-0030-1253222
11. Strautnieks SS, Bull LN, Knisely AS et al (1998) A gene encoding a liver-specific ABC transporter is mutated in progressive familial intrahepatic cholestasis. Nat Genet 20:233–238
12. Jansen PL, Strautnieks SS, Jacquemin E et al (1999) Hepatocanalicular bile salt export pump deficiency in patients with progressive familial intrahepatic cholestasis. Gastroenterology 117:1370–1379
13. Wang L, Soroka CJ, Boyer JL (2002) The role of bile salt export pump mutations in progressive familial intrahepatic cholestasis type II. J Clin Invest 110:965–972
14. Scheimann AO, Strautnieks SS, Knisely AS et al (2007) Mutations in bile salt export pump (ABCB11) in two children with progressive familial intrahepatic cholestasis and cholangiocarcinoma. J Pediatr 150:556–559
15. Hayashi H, Takada T, Suzuki H et al (2005) Two common PFIC2 mutations are associated with the impaired membrane trafficking of BSEP/ABCB11. Hepatology 41:916–924
16. Plass JR, Mol O, Heegsma J et al (2004) A progressive familial intrahepatic cholestasis type 2 mutation causes an unstable,

temperature-sensitive bile salt export pump. J Hepatol 40:24–30

17. Strautnieks SS, Byrne JA, Pawlikowska L et al (2008) Severe bile salt export pump deficiency: 82 different ABCB11 mutations in 109 families. Gastroenterology 134:1203–1214

18. Treepongkaruna S, Gaensan A, Pienvichit P et al (2009) Novel ABCB11 mutations in a Thai infant with progressive familial intrahepatic cholestasis. World J Gastroenterol 15:4339–4342

19. Davit-Spraul A, Fabre M, Branchereau S et al (2010) ATP8B1 and ABCB11 analysis in 62 children with normal gamma-glutamyl transferase progressive familial intrahepatic cholestasis (PFIC): phenotypic differences between PFIC1 and PFIC2 and natural history. Hepatology 51:1645–1655. https://doi.org/10.1002/hep.23539

20. Saber S, Vazifehmand R, Bagherizadeh I et al (2013) A novel ABCB11 mutation in an Iranian girl with progressive familial intrahepatic cholestasis. Indian J Hum Genet 19:366–368. https://doi.org/10.4103/0971-6866.120813

21. Francalanci P, Giovannoni I, Candusso M et al (2013) Bile salt export pump deficiency: a de novo mutation in a child compound heterozygous for ABCB11. Laboratory investigation to study pathogenic role and transmission of two novel ABCB11 mutations. Hepatol Res 43:315–319. https://doi.org/10.1111/j.1872-034X.2012.01061.x

22. Vitale G, Pirillo M, Mantovani V et al (2016) Bile salt export pump deficiency disease: two novel, late onset, ABCB11 mutations identified by next generation sequencing. Ann Hepatol 15:795–800. https://doi.org/10.5604/16652681.1212618.

23. Lam CW, Cheung KM, Tsui MS et al (2006) A patient with novel ABCB11 gene mutations with phenotypic transition between BRIC2 and PFIC2. J Hepatol 44:240–242

24. van Mil SW, van der Woerd WL, van der Brugge G et al (2004) Benign recurrent intrahepatic cholestasis type 2 is caused by mutations in ABCB11. Gastroenterology 127:379–384

25. Kubitz R, Keitel V, Scheuring S et al (2006) Benign recurrent intrahepatic cholestasis associated with mutations of the bile salt export pump. J Clin Gastroenterol 40:171–175

26. Eloranta ML, Häkli T, Hiltunen M et al (2003) Association of single nucleotide polymorphisms of the bile salt export pump gene with intrahepatic cholestasis of pregnancy. Scand J Gastroenterol 38:648–652

27. Keitel V, Vogt C, Häussinger D et al (2006) Combined mutations of canalicular transporter proteins cause severe intrahepatic cholestasis of pregnancy. Gastroenterology 131:624–629

28. Meier Y, Zodan T, Lang C et al (2008) Increased susceptibility for intrahepatic cholestasis of pregnancy and contraceptive-induced cholestasis in carriers of the 1331T>C polymorphism in the bile salt export pump. World J Gastroenterol 14:38–45

29. Dixon PH, van Mil SW, Chambers J et al (2009) Contribution of variant alleles of ABCB11 to susceptibility to intrahepatic cholestasis of pregnancy. Gut 58:537–544. https://doi.org/10.1136/gut.2008.159541

30. Pauli-Magnus C, Lang T, Meier Y et al (2004) Sequence analysis of bile salt export pump (ABCB11) and multidrug resistance p-glycoprotein 3 (ABCB4, MDR3) in patients with intrahepatic cholestasis of pregnancy. Pharmacogenetics 14:91–102

31. Lang C, Meier Y, Stieger B et al (2007) Mutations and polymorphisms in the bile salt export pump and the multidrug resistance protein 3 associated with drug-induced liver injury. Pharmacogenet Genomics 17:47–60

32. Ulzurrun E, Stephens C, Crespo E et al (2013) Role of chemical structures and the 1331T>C bile salt export pump polymorphism in idiosyncratic drug-induced liver injury. Liver Int 33:1378–1385

33. Schubert R, Schmidt KH (1988) Structural changes in vesicle membranes and mixed micelles of various lipid compositions after binding of different bile salts. Biochemistry 27:8787–8794

34. Sagawa H, Tazuma S, Kajiyama G (1993) Protection against hydrophobic bile salt-induced cell membrane damage by liposomes and hydrophilic bile salts. Am J Phys 264:G835–G839

35. Billington D, Evans CE, Godfrey PP et al (1980) Effects of bile salts on the plasma membranes of isolated rat hepatocytes. Biochem J 188:321–327

36. Palmeira CM, Rolo AP (2004) Mitochondrially-mediated toxicity of bile acids. Toxicology 203:1–15

37. Sokol RJ, Dahl R, Devereaux MW et al (2005) Human hepatic mitochondria generate reactive oxygen species and undergo the permeability transition in response to hydrophobic bile acids. J Pediatr Gastroenterol Nutr 41:235–243

38. Rolo AP, Palmeira CM, Wallace KB (2003) Mitochondrially mediated synergistic cell killing by bile acids. Biochim Biophys Acta 1637:127–132

39. Sokol RJ, Winklhofer-Roob BM, Devereaux MW et al (1995) Generation of hydroperoxides in isolated rat hepatocytes and hepatic mitochondria exposed to hydrophobic bile acids. Gastroenterology 109:1249–1256

40. Iizaka T, Tsuji M, Oyamada H et al (2007) Interaction between caspase-8 activation and endoplasmic reticulum stress in glycochenodeoxycholic acid-induced apoptotic HepG2 cells. Toxicology 241:146–156

41. Adachi T, Kaminaga T, Yasuda H et al (2014) The involvement of endoplasmic reticulum stress in bile acid-induced hepatocellular injury. J Clin Biochem Nutr 54:129–135. https://doi.org/10.3164/jcbn.13-46

42. Tsuchiya S, Tsuji M, Morio Y et al (2006) Involvement of endoplasmic reticulum in glycochenodeoxycholic acid-induced apoptosis in rat hepatocytes. Toxicol Lett 166: 140–169

43. Gujral JS, Farhood A, Bajt ML et al (2003) Neutrophils aggravate acute liver injury during obstructive cholestasis in bile duct-ligated mice. Hepatology 38:355–363

44. Gujral JS, Liu J, Farhood A et al (2004) Functional importance of ICAM-1 in the mechanism of neutrophil-induced liver injury in bile duct-ligated mice. Am J Physiol Gastrointest Liver Physiol 286:G499–G507

45. Allen K, Jaeschke H, Copple BL (2011) Bile acids induce inflammatory genes in hepatocytes: a novel mechanism of inflammation during obstructive cholestasis. Am J Pathol 178:175–186

46. Spivey JR, Bronk SF, Gores GJ (1993) Glycochenodeoxycholate-induced lethal hepatocellular injury in rat hepatocytes. Role of ATP depletion and cytosolic free calcium. J Clin Invest 92:17–24

47. Yerushalmi B, Dahl R, Devereaux MW et al (2001) Bile acid-induced rat hepatocyte apoptosis is inhibited by antioxidants and blockers of the mitochondrial permeability transition. Hepatology 33:616–626

48. Rust C, Wild N, Bernt C et al (2009) Bile acid-induced apoptosis in hepatocytes is caspase-6-dependent. J Biol Chem 284:2908–2916

49. Perez MJ, Briz O (2009) Bile-acid-induced cell injury and protection. World J Gastroenterol 15:1677–1689

50. Galle PR, Theilmann L, Raedsch R et al (1990) Ursodeoxycholate reduces hepatotoxicity of bile salts in primary human hepatocytes. Hepatology 12:486–491

51. Woolbright BL, Dorko K, Antoine DJ et al (2015) Bile acid-induced necrosis in primary human hepatocytes and in patients with obstructive cholestasis. Toxicol Appl Pharmacol 283:168–177

52. Fickert P, Trauner M, Fuchsbichler A et al (2005) Oncosis represents the main type of cell death in mouse models of cholestasis. J Hepatol 42:378–385

53. Reuben A, Koch DG, Lee WM et al (2010) Acute Liver Failure Study Group. Drug-induced acute liver failure: results of a U.S. multicenter, prospective study. Hepatology 52:2065–2076

54. Sarges P, Steinberg JM, Lewis JH (2016) Drug-induced liver injury: highlights from a review of the 2015 literature. Drug Saf 39:801–821

55. Lewis JH (2015) The art and science of diagnosing and managing drug-induced liver injury in 2015 and beyond. Clin Gastroenterol Hepatol 13:2173–2189.e8

56. Vuppalanchi R, Liangpunsakul S, Chalasani N (2007) Etiology of new-onset jaundice: how often is it caused by idiosyncratic drug-induced liver injury in the United States? Am J Gastroenterol 102:558–562

57. Kim SH, Naisbitt DJ (2016) Update on advances in research on idiosyncratic drug-induced liver injury. Allergy Asthma Immunol Res 8:3–11. https://doi.org/10.4168/aair.2016.8.1.3

58. Abboud G, Kaplowitz N (2007) Drug-induced liver injury. Drug Saf 30:277–294

59. Fattinger K, Funk C, Pantze M et al (2001) The endothelin antagonist bosentan inhibits the canalicular bile salt export pump: a potential mechanism for hepatic adverse reactions. Clin Pharmacol Ther 69:223–231

60. Kostrubsky SE, Strom SC, Kalgutkar AS et al (2006) Inhibition of hepatobiliary transport as a predictive method for clinical hepatotoxicity of nefazodone. Toxicol Sci 90:451–459

61. Morgan RE, Trauner M, van Staden CJ et al (2010) Interference with bile salt export pump function is a susceptibility factor for human liver injury in drug development. Toxicol Sci 118:485–500

62. Ogimura E, Sekine S, Horie T (2011) Bile salt export pump inhibitors are associated with bile acid-dependent drug-induced toxicity in sandwich-cultured hepatocytes. Biochem Biophys Res Commun 416:313–317. https://doi.org/10.1016/j.bbrc.2011.11.032

63. Guo YX, Xu XF, Zhang QZ et al (2015) The inhibition of hepatic bile acids transporters Ntcp and Bsep is involved in the pathogenesis of isoniazid/rifampicin-induced hepatotoxicity. Toxicol Mech Methods 25:382–387. https://doi.org/10.3109/15376516.2015.1033074

64. Pedersen JM, Matsson P, Bergström CA et al (2013) Early identification of clinically relevant drug interactions with the human bile salt export pump (BSEP/ABCB11). Toxicol Sci 136:328–343. https://doi.org/10.1093/toxsci/kft197

65. Zhang J, He K, Cai L et al (2016) Inhibition of bile salt transport by drugs associated with liver injury in primary hepatocytes from human, monkey, dog, rat, and mouse. Chem Biol Interact 255:45–54. https://doi.org/10.1016/j.cbi.2016.03.019

66. Kenna JG (2014) Current concepts in drug-induced bile salt export pump (BSEP) interference. Curr Protoc Toxicol 61:23.7.1–23.715. https://doi.org/10.1002/0471140856.tx2307s61

67. Funk C, Ponelle C, Scheuermann G et al (2001) Cholestatic potential of troglitazone as a possible factor contributing to troglitazone-induced hepatotoxicity: in vivo and in vitro interaction at the canalicular bile salt export pump (Bsep) in the rat. Mol Pharmacol 59:627–635

68. Stieger B, Fattinger K, Madon J et al (2000) Drug- and estrogen-induced cholestasis through inhibition of the hepatocellular bile salt export pump (Bsep) of rat liver. Gastroenterology 118:422–430

69. Rodrigues AD, Lai Y, Cvijic ME et al (2014) Drug-induced perturbations of the bile acid pool, cholestasis, and hepatotoxicity: mechanistic considerations beyond the direct inhibition of the bile salt export pump. Drug Metab Dispos 42:566–574. https://doi.org/10.1124/dmd.113.054205

70. Byrne JA, Strautnieks SS, Mieli-Vergani G et al (2002) The human bile salt export pump: characterization of substrate specificity and identification of inhibitors. Gastroenterology 123:1649–1658

71. Wolf KK, Vora S, Webster LO et al (2010) Use of cassette dosing in sandwich-cultured rat and human hepatocytes to identify drugs that inhibit bile acid transport. Toxicol In Vitro 24:297–309. https://doi.org/10.1016/j.tiv.2009.08.009

72. Dawson S, Stahl S, Paul N et al (2012) In vitro inhibition of the bile salt export pump correlates with risk of cholestatic drug-induced liver injury in humans. Drug Metab Dispos 40:130–138

73. Cheng Y, Woolf TF, Gan J et al (2016) In vitro model systems to investigate bile salt export pump (BSEP) activity and drug interactions: a review. Chem Biol Interact 255:23–30. https://doi.org/10.1016/j.cbi.2015.11.029

74. Aleo MD, Luo Y, Swiss R et al (2014) Human drug-induced liver injury severity is highly associated with dual inhibition of liver mitochondrial function and bile salt export pump. Hepatology 60:1015–1022. https://doi.org/10.1002/hep.27206

75. Sakurai A, Kurata A, Onishi Y et al (2007) Prediction of drug-induced intrahepatic cholestasis: in vitro screening and QSAR analysis of drugs inhibiting the human bile salt export pump. Expert Opin Drug Saf 6:71–86

76. Kis E, Ioja E, Rajnai Z et al (2012) BSEP inhibition: in vitro screens to assess cholestatic potential of drugs. Toxicol In Vitro 26:1294–1299. https://doi.org/10.1016/j.tiv.2011.11.002

77. Tang H, Shen DR, Han YH et al (2013) Development of novel, 384-well high-throughput assay panels for human drug transporters: drug interaction and safety assessment in support of discovery research. J Biomol Screen 18:1072–1083. https://doi.org/10.1177/1087057113494807

78. Kaimal R, Song X, Yan B et al (2009) Differential modulation of farnesoid X receptor signaling pathway by the thiazolidinediones. J Pharmacol Exp Ther 330:125–134. https://doi.org/10.1124/jpet.109.151233

79. Song X, Vasilenko A, Chen Y et al (2014) Transcriptional dynamics of bile salt export pump during pregnancy: mechanisms and implications in intrahepatic cholestasis of pregnancy. Hepatology 60:1993–2007. https://doi.org/10.1002/hep.27171

80. Yu J, Lo JL, Huang L et al (2002) Lithocholic acid decreases expression of bile salt export pump through farnesoid X receptor antagonist activity. J Biol Chem 277:31441–31447

81. Donato MT, López-Riera M, Castell JV et al (2016) Both cholestatic and steatotic drugs trigger extensive alterations in the mRNA level of biliary transporters in rat hepatocytes: application to develop new predictive biomarkers for early drug development. Toxicol Lett 263:58–67. https://doi.org/10.1016/j.toxlet.2016.10.008

82. Garzel B, Yang H, Zhang L et al (2014) The role of bile salt export pump gene repression in drug-induced cholestatic liver toxicity. Drug Metab Dispos 42:318–122. https://doi.org/10.1124/dmd.113.054189

83. Zollner G, Thueringer A, Lackner C et al (2014) Alterations of canalicular ATP-binding cassette transporter expression in drug-induced liver injury. Digestion 90:81–88. https://doi.org/10.1159/000365003

84. Shoda J, Kano M, Oda K et al (2001) The expression levels of plasma membrane transporters in the cholestatic liver of patients undergoing biliary drainage and their association with the impairment of biliary secretory function. Am J Gastroenterol 96:3368–3378

85. Zollner G, Fickert P, Zenz R et al (2001) Hepatobiliary transporter expression in percutaneous liver biopsies of patients with cholestatic liver diseases. Hepatology 33: 633–646

86. Kipp H, Arias IM (2000) Intracellular trafficking and regulation of canalicular ATP-binding cassette transporters. Semin Liver Dis 20:339–351

87. Hayashi H, Sugiyama Y (2013) Bile salt export pump (BSEP/ABCB11): trafficking and sorting disturbances. Curr Mol Pharmacol 6:95–103

88. Elferink MG, Olinga P, Draaisma AL et al (2004) LPS-induced downregulation of MRP2 and BSEP in human liver is due to a posttranscriptional process. Am J Physiol Gastrointest Liver Physiol 287: G1008–G1016

89. Lam P, Pearson CL, Soroka CJ et al (2007) Levels of plasma membrane expression in progressive and benign mutations of the bile salt export pump (Bsep/Abcb11) correlate with severity of cholestatic diseases. Am J Physiol Cell Physiol 293:C1709–C1716

90. Román ID, Fernández-Moreno MD, Fueyo JA, Roma MG, Coleman R (2003) Cyclosporin A induced internalization of the bile salt export pump in isolated rat hepatocyte couplets. Toxicol Sci 71:276–281

91. Micheline D, Emmanuel J, Serge E (2002) Effect of ursodeoxycholic acid on the expression of the hepatocellular bile acid transporters (Ntcp and bsep) in rats with estrogen-induced cholestasis. J Pediatr Gastroenterol Nutr 35:185–191

92. Crocenzi FA, Mottino AD, Sanchez Pozzi EJ et al (2003) Impaired localisation and transport function of canalicular Bsep in taurolithocholate induced cholestasis in the rat. Gut 52:1170–1177

93. Crocenzi FA, Mottino AD, Cao J et al (2003) Estradiol-17beta-D-glucuronide induces endocytic internalization of Bsep in rats. Am J Physiol Gastrointest Liver Physiol 285: G449–G459

94. Zinchuk V, Zinchuk O, Okada T (2005) Experimental LPS-induced cholestasis alters subcellular distribution and affects colocalization of Mrp2 and Bsep proteins: a quantitative colocalization study. Microsc Res Tech 67:65–70

95. Roma MG, Crocenzi FA, Mottino AD (2008) Dynamic localization of hepatocellular transporters in health and disease. World J Gastroenterol 14:6786–6801

96. Byrne JA, Strautnieks SS, Ihrke G et al (2009) Missense mutations and single nucleotide polymorphisms in ABCB11 impair bile salt export pump processing and function or disrupt pre-messenger RNA splicing. Hepatology 49:553–567

97. Noé J, Stieger B, Meier PJ (2002) Functional expression of the canalicular bile salt export pump of human liver. Gastroenterology 123:1659–1666

98. Marroquin LD, Bonin PD, Keefer J et al (2017) Assessment of bile salt export pump (BSEP) inhibition in membrane vesicles using radioactive and LC/MS-based detection methods. Curr Protoc Toxicol 71:14.14.1–14.14.20. https://doi.org/10.1002/cptx.15

99. van Staden CJ, Morgan RE, Ramachandran B et al (2012) Membrane vesicle ABC transporter assays for drug safety assessment. Curr Protoc Toxicol. Chapter 23:Unit 23.5. https://doi.org/10.1002/0471140856.tx2305s54.

100. Stieger B, O'Neill B, Meier PJ (1992) ATP-dependent bile-salt transport in canalicular rat liver plasma-membrane vesicles. Biochem J 284:67–74

101. Adachi Y, Kobayashi H, Kurumi Y et al (1991) ATP-dependent taurocholate transport by rat liver canalicular membrane vesicles. Hepatology 14:655–659

102. Nishida T, Gatmaitan Z, Che M et al (1991) Rat liver canalicular membrane vesicles contain an ATP-dependent bile acid transport system. Proc Natl Acad Sci U S A 88:6590–6594

103. Kis E, Rajnai Z, Ioja E et al (2009) Mouse Bsep ATPase assay: a nonradioactive tool for assessment of the cholestatic potential of drugs. J Biomol Screen 14:10–15. https://doi.org/10.1177/1087057108326145

104. Mita S, Suzuki H, Akita H et al (2006) Inhibition of bile acid transport across Na+/taurocholate cotransporting polypeptide (SLC10A1) and bile salt export pump (ABCB11)-coexpressing LLC-PK1 cells by cholestasis-inducing drugs. Drug Metab Dispos 34:1575–1581

105. Mita S, Suzuki H, Akita H et al (2006) Vectorial transport of unconjugated and conjugated bile salts by monolayers of LLC-PK1 cells doubly transfected with human NTCP and BSEP or with rat Ntcp and Bsep. Am J Physiol Gastrointest Liver Physiol 290:G550–G556

106. Cai SY, Wang L, Ballatori N et al (2001) Bile salt export pump is highly conserved during vertebrate evolution and its expression is inhibited by PFIC type II mutations. Am J Physiol Gastrointest Liver Physiol 281:G316–G322

107. Kis E, Ioja E, Nagy T et al (2009) Effect of membrane cholesterol on BSEP/Bsep activity: species specificity studies for substrates and inhibitors. Drug Metab Dispos 37:1878–1886

108. Ho RH, Leake BF, Kilkenny DM et al (2010) Polymorphic variants in the human bile salt export pump (BSEP; ABCB11): functional characterization and interindividual variability. Pharmacogenet Genomics 20:45–57

109. Guyot C, Hofstetter L, Stieger B (2014) Differential effects of membrane cholesterol content on the transport activity of multidrug resistance-associated protein 2 (ABCC2) and of the bile salt export pump (ABCB11). Mol Pharmacol 85:909–920. https://doi.org/10.1124/mol.114.092262

110. Janossy J (2009) PREDEASY™ Mouse Bsep ATPase assay. http://www.solvobiotech.com/science-letter/predeasy-mouse-bsep-atpase-assay

111. Harris MJ, Kagawa T, Dawson PA et al (2004) Taurocholate transport by hepatic and intestinal bile acid transporters is independent of FIC1 overexpression in Madin-Darby canine kidney cells. J Gastroenterol Hepatol 19:819–825

112. He K, Zhang J, Cai L et al (2014) Inhibition of bile salt export by marketed drugs in primary hepatocytes from human, monkey, dog, rat, and mouse, toxicol supplement. Toxicol Sci 138(1)

113. LeCluyse EL, Audus KL, Hochman JH (1994) Formation of extensive canalicular networks by rat hepatocytes cultured in collagen-sandwich configuration. Am J Phys 266:C1764–C1774

114. Liu X, LeCluyse EL, Brouwer KR et al (1999) Biliary excretion in primary rat hepatocytes cultured in a collagen-sandwich configuration. Am J Phys 277:G12–G21

115. Chandra P, LeCluyse EL, Brouwer KL (2001) Optimization of culture conditions for determining hepatobiliary disposition of taurocholate in sandwich-cultured rat hepatocytes. In Vitro Cell Dev Biol Anim 37:380–385

116. Swift B, Pfeifer ND, Brouwer KL (2010) Sandwich-cultured hepatocytes: an in vitro model to evaluate hepatobiliary transporter-based drug interactions and hepatotoxicity. Drug Metab Rev 42:446–471

117. Swift B, Brouwer KL (2010) Influence of seeding density and extracellular matrix on bile acid transport and mrp4 expression in sandwich-cultured mouse hepatocytes. Mol Pharm 7:491–500

118. Bi YA, Kazolias D, Duignan DB (2006) Use of cryopreserved human hepatocytes in sandwich culture to measure hepatobiliary transport. Drug Metab Dispos 34:1658–1665

119. Lepist EI, Gillies H, Smith W et al (2014) Evaluation of the endothelin receptor antagonists ambrisentan, bosentan, macitentan, and sitaxsentan as hepatobiliary transporter inhibitors and substrates in sandwich-cultured human hepatocytes. PLoS One 9:e87548. https://doi.org/10.1371/journal.pone.0087548

120. Yang K, Pfeifer ND, Köck K et al (2015) Species differences in hepatobiliary disposition of taurocholic acid in human and rat sandwich-cultured hepatocytes: implications for drug-induced liver injury. J Pharmacol Exp Ther 353:415–423. https://doi.org/10.1124/jpet.114.221564

121. Perry CH, Smith WR, St Claire RL 3rd et al (2011) Automated applications of sandwich-cultured hepatocytes in the evaluation of hepatic drug transport. J Biomol Screen 16:427–435. https://doi.org/10.1177/1087057111400192

122. Liu X, LeCluyse EL, Brouwer KR et al (1999) Use of Ca2þ modulation to evaluate biliary excretion in sandwich-cultured rat hepatocytes. J Pharmacol Exp Ther 289:1592–1599

123. Reed DJ, Pascoe GA, Thomas CE (1990) Extracellular calcium effects on cell viability and thiol homeostasis. Environ Health Perspect 84:113–120

124. Diao L, Li N, Brayman TG et al (2010) Regulation of MRP2/ABCC2 and BSEP/ABCB11 expression in sandwich cultured human and rat hepatocytes exposed to inflammatory cytokines TNF-alpha, IL-6, and IL-1beta. J Biol Chem 285:31185–31192. https://doi.org/10.1074/jbc.M110.107805.

125. Ware BR, Berger DR, Khetani SR (2015) Prediction of drug-induced liver injury in micropatterned co-cultures containing iPSC-derived human hepatocytes. Toxicol Sci 145:252–262. https://doi.org/10.1093/toxsci/kfv048

126. Trask OJ Jr, Moore A, LeCluyse EL (2014) A micropatterned hepatocyte coculture model for assessment of liver toxicity using high-content imaging analysis. Assay Drug Dev Technol 12:16–27. https://doi.org/10.1089/adt.2013.525

127. Khetani SR, Kanchagar C, Ukairo O et al (2013) Use of micropatterned cocultures to detect compounds that cause drug-induced liver injury in humans. Toxicol Sci 132:107–117. https://doi.org/10.1093/toxsci/kfs326

128. Shulman M, Nahmias Y (2013) Long-term culture and coculture of primary rat and human hepatocytes. Methods Mol Biol 945:287–302. https://doi.org/10.1007/978-1-62703-125-7_17

129. Ananthanarayanan M, Balasubramanian N, Makishima M et al (2001) Human bile salt export pump promoter is transactivated by the farnesoid X receptor/bile acid receptor. J Biol Chem 276:28857–28865

130. Plass JR, Mol O, Heegsma J et al (2002) Farnesoid X receptor and bile salts are involved in transcriptional regulation of the gene encoding the human bile salt export pump. Hepatology 35:589–596

131. Deng R, Yang D, Radke A et al (2007) Hypolipidemic agent guggulsterone regulates the expression of human bile salt export pump: dominance of transactivation over FXR-mediated antagonism. J Pharmacol Exp Ther 320:1153–1162

132. Song X, Kaimal R, Yan B et al (2008) Liver receptor homolog 1 transcriptionally regulates human bile salt export pump expression. J Lipid Res 49:973–984

133. Weerachayaphorn J, Cai SY, Soroka CJ et al (2009) Nuclear factor erythroid 2-related factor 2 is a positive regulator of human bile salt export pump expression. Hepatology 50:1588–1596

134. Deng R, Yang D, Yang J et al (2006) Oxysterol 22(R)-hydroxycholesterol induces the expression of the bile salt export pump through nuclear receptor farsenoid X receptor but not liver X receptor. J Pharmacol Exp Ther 317:317–325

135. Song X, Chen Y, Valanejad L et al (2013) Mechanistic insights into isoform-dependent and species-specific regulation of bile salt export pump by farnesoid X receptor. J Lipid Res 54:3030–3044. https://doi.org/10.1194/jlr.M038323

136. Chen Y, Song X, Valanejad L et al (2013) Bile salt export pump is dysregulated with altered farnesoid X receptor isoform expression in patients with hepatocellular carcinoma. Hepatology 57:1530–1541. https://doi.org/10.1002/hep.26187

137. Dombrowski F, Stieger B, Beuers U (2006) Tauroursodeoxycholic acid inserts the bile salt export pump into canalicular membranes of cholestatic rat liver. Lab Investig 86:166–174

138. Hayashi H, Sugiyama Y (2007) 4-Phenylbutyrate enhances the cell surface expression and the transport capacity of wild-type and mutated bile salt export pumps. Hepatology 45:1506–1516

139. Gonzales E, Grosse B, Schuller B et al (2015) Targeted pharmacotherapy in progressive familial intrahepatic cholestasis type 2: evidence for improvement of cholestasis with 4-phenylbutyrate. Hepatology 62:558–566. https://doi.org/10.1002/hep.27767

140. Hayashi H, Naoi S, Hirose Y et al (2016) Successful treatment with 4-phenylbutyrate in a patient with benign recurrent intrahepatic cholestasis type 2 refractory to biliary drainage and bilirubin absorption. Hepatol Res 46:192–200. https://doi.org/10.1111/hepr.12561

141. Crocenzi FA, Basiglio CL, Pérez LM et al (2005) Silibinin prevents cholestasis-associated retrieval of the bile salt export pump, Bsep, in isolated rat hepatocyte couplets: possible involvement of cAMP. Biochem Pharmacol 69:1113–1120

142. Mochizuki K, Kagawa T, Numari A et al (2007) Two N-linked glycans are required to maintain the transport activity of the bile salt export pump (ABCB11) in MDCK II cells. Am J Physiol Gastrointest Liver Physiol 292:G818–G828

143. Kubitz R, Sütfels G, Kühlkamp T et al (2004) Trafficking of the bile salt export pump from the Golgi to the canalicular membrane is regulated by the p38 MAP kinase. Gastroenterology 126:541–553

144. Hayashi H, Sugiyama Y (2009) Short-chain ubiquitination is associated with the degradation rate of a cell-surface-resident bile salt export pump (BSEP/ABCB11). Mol Pharmacol 75:143–150

145. Wang L, Dong H, Soroka CJ et al (2008) Degradation of the bile salt export pump at endoplasmic reticulum in progressive familial intrahepatic cholestasis type II. Hepatology 48:1558–1569

146. Black CB, Duensing TD, Trinkle LS et al (2011) Cell-based screening using high-throughput flow cytometry. Assay Drug Dev Technol 9:13–20. https://doi.org/10.1089/adt.2010.0308

147. Gedye CA, Hussain A, Paterson J et al (2014) Cell surface profiling using high-throughput flow cytometry: a platform for biomarker discovery and analysis of cellular heterogeneity. PLoS One 9:e105602. https://doi.org/10.1371/journal.pone.0105602

148. Imagawa K, Takayama K, Isoyama S, Tanikawa K, Shinkai M, Harada K, Tachibana M, Sakurai F, Noguchi E, Hirata K, Kage M, Kawabata K, Sumazaki R, Mizuguchi H (2017) Generation of a bile salt export pump deficiency model using patient-specific induced pluripotent stem cell-derived hepatocyte-like cells. Sci Rep 7:41806. https://doi.org/10.1038/srep41806.

149. Lundquist P, Englund G, Skogastierna C et al (2014) Functional ATP-binding cassette drug efflux transporters in isolated human and rat hepatocytes significantly affect assessment of drug disposition. Drug Metab Dispos 42:448–458. https://doi.org/10.1124/dmd.113.054528

150. Kruglov EA, Gautam S, Guerra MT et al (2011) Type 2 inositol 1,4,5-trisphosphate receptor modulates bile salt export pump activity in rat hepatocytes. Hepatology 54:1790–1999. https://doi.org/10.1002/hep.24548

151. Barber JA, Stahl SH, Summers C et al (2015) Quantification of drug-induced inhibition of canalicular cholyl-l-lysyl-fluorescein excretion from hepatocytes by high content cell imaging. Toxicol Sci 148:48–59. https://doi.org/10.1093/toxsci/kfv159

152. Qiu L, Finley J, Taimi M et al (2015) High-content imaging in human and rat hepatocytes using the fluorescent dyes CLF and CMFDA is not specific enough to assess BSEP/Bsep and/or MRP2/Mrp2 inhibition by cholestatic drugs. Appl In Vitro Toxicol 1:198–212

153. Boutros M, Heigwer F, Laufer C (2015) Microscopy-based high-content screening. Cell 163:1314–1325. https://doi.org/10.1016/j.cell.2015.11.007

154. Morgan RE, van Staden CJ, Chen Y et al (2013) A multifactorial approach to hepatobiliary transporter assessment enables improved therapeutic compound development. Toxicol Sci 136:216–241. https://doi.org/10.1093/toxsci/kft176

155. Mosedale M, Watkins PB (2017) Drug-induced liver injury: advances in mechanistic understanding that will inform risk management. Clin Pharmacol Ther 101:469–480. https://doi.org/10.1002/cpt.564

156. Schadt HS, Wolf A, Pognan F et al (2016) Bile acids in drug induced liver injury: key players and surrogate markers. Clin Res Hepatol Gastroenterol 40:257–266. https://doi.org/10.1016/j.clinre.2015.12.017

Chapter 16

High Content Screening for Prediction of Human Drug-Induced Liver Injury

Mikael Persson

Abstract

High content screening (HCS) has emerged as a powerful tool for predicting drug-induced liver injury (DILI) in the early phases of drug discovery. It combines automated imaging with image analysis to assess cell health and customized parameters in a multiparametric fashion, enabling coverage over several mechanisms important for DILI. In simple two-dimensional cell models, various HCS assays typically show a sensitivity of ~50% with a high specificity of >90%. With relatively high throughput and short turn-around times, this makes it ideal for early decision making in drug discovery. HCS for DILI has lately expanded into complex three-dimensional models to further improve predictivity. The wealth of HCS data make it particularly amenable for machine learning and systems biology approaches for building rational models for prediction of DILI.

Key words Imaging, Multiparametric, DILI, High content, Predictivity

1 Introduction

1.1 Basics of High Content Screening

High content screening (HCS) combines automated microscopy with image analysis to assess biological end points ranging from relatively simple cell-based readouts to complex multiparametric phenotypes, sometimes also in heterogeneous multicell type cultures. It has emerged as a powerful tool to assess spatial, temporal, and complex biological changes induced by small molecules, biologics, or other modalities, which are typically hard to assess using traditional biochemical assays. HCS enables analysis not only at the single cell level but also on cell populations or whole organisms, with or without targeting of cells or areas of interest. The ability to acquire multiparametric information at the individual cell level aids in gaining more mechanistic insight into the actions of compounds or molecules. As more informed decisions can be made based on increased biological understanding, HCS has been developed into an important tool for predictive toxicology and safety assessments during early stages of drug discovery, as well as for problem solving

Minjun Chen and Yvonne Will (eds.), *Drug-Induced Liver Toxicity*, Methods in Pharmacology and Toxicology,
https://doi.org/10.1007/978-1-4939-7677-5_16, © Springer Science+Business Media, LLC, part of Springer Nature 2018

in later stages of drug development, with several applications for drug-induced liver injury (DILI) [1–4].

Since HCS is based on automated imaging of cells or tissue, it typically makes use of fluorescent dyes or fluorescently labeled antibodies to identify and quantify various biological processes, pathways, molecules, organelles, and other cellular functions. Additionally, engineered reporter cell lines can be used for assessing particular pathways of interest. These tools allow the user to customize multiple endpoints for the biology and toxicology of interest, and the endpoints can be analyzed by HCS as long as they can be accurately imaged. The limitations of the assays are the need for good spectral separation in the fluorescent channels as well as the specificity of the probes or biosensors, and the ability of imaging algorithms to accurately detect and quantify the relevant biological phenotypes. Independent of whether assays are performed using wide field or confocal imaging, on living or fixed cells, the key to successful assays is the image quality. Unlike the human mind, the current HCS algorithms are unable to make any inference beyond what is depicted, and thus the images must be of sufficient quality such that the biological phenotypes or process of interest are accurately displayed.

In addition to image quality, a crucial component of successful application of high content analysis is the image analysis algorithms. They have to produce robust data and accurately describe the biological phenomena or phenotypes that are subject of the study. Several high content imaging providers offer basic software for image analysis, dedicated software suits are available from independent providers, and specific algorithms can be developed as stand-alone applications in existing software packages. The real benefit of the image algorithms is that they analyze the images in a truly objective manner with high content of data compared to the manual scoring by independent human operators. For example, a relatively simple multiplexed assay using four different spectrally separated probes can easily generate hundreds of data features which can be used for phenotypic profiling.

Independent on whether the data comes from simple two-dimensional models or three-dimensional microphysiological systems, the wealth of HCA data makes it very amenable to machine learning and systems biology approaches [5, 6]. A single experiment may yield hundreds of parameters describing the phenotypes induced by compound treatment. Several of these parameters may be interdependent, and, when viewed as single entities they are potentially of relatively low own value. However, when using "big data" approaches typically used in other omics techniques, new patterns and less obvious phenotypes can emerge. Instead of extracting only parameters the biologist have an intrinsic understanding of (e.g., 4–6 parameters describing crude biology), it is now becoming more and more usual to extract all possible features (e.g., hundreds of parameters) from an experiment in an unbiased manner and then sort out biological phenotypes by computational pattern recognition approaches. Such approaches have been successfully used for predicting nephrotoxic toxic compounds [7] and is well on the way for DILI predictions.

1.2 HCS for Prediction of DILI

Whereas HCS and cell toxicity can be employed to predict various types of animal and human toxicities and adverse effects such as cardiac toxicity, kidney toxicity, neurotoxicity to name a few [4], even showing high concordance with systemic tolerance and the severity of general organ toxicity [8], most validations in literature have been toward human clinical DILI. HCS for prediction of DILI in early drug discovery has evolved into a standard tool in the pharmaceutical industry because the commonly used end points are relatively sensitive, can be assessed simultaneously, and in sufficient throughput to be amenable to the large amounts of compounds coming out of primary efficacy screens. Typical approaches make use of liver-derived cell lines or primary hepatocytes and apply multiparametric imaging of cytotoxicity and mitochondrial toxicity-related end points after incubation with test article. Predictivity for human clinical hepatotoxicity has been established based on validation studies with relatively large compounds sets of marketed drugs with known clinical propensity for DILI. HCS hepatotoxicity assays typically show 40–60% sensitivity, depending on the endpoints assessed and concentration ranges tested, and >90% specificity (i.e., <10% false positives) on average [9–17]. These values have been confirmed across several pharmaceutical companies through a collaborative effort in the Innovative Medicines Initiative's Mechanism-Based Integrated Systems for Prediction of Drug-Induced Liver Injury (IMI MIP-DILI) consortium [18]. Using each company's own version of an HCS assay for DILI predictions but with the very same compounds and test concentrations, a test set of ~90 compounds were tested across end points and cell models, including HepG2, HepaRG, primary human hepatocytes, and induced pluripotent stem cell derived hepatocytes. It was shown that, in a pharmaceutical industry setting, most of the assays and models showed ~50% sensitivity and >90% specificity. Most importantly, it was shown that the pharmaceutical companies made the same decisions on the same compounds, e.g., showing the same false positives and false negatives. This highlights the utility and robustness of HCS for DILI predictions in early drug discovery. One of the reasons for the similar predictivity values is that virtually all of the HCS assays derive much of their predictivity from basic cell health measurements such as cytotoxicity and mitochondrial toxicity derived parameters. Although the assays do not identify all hepatotoxic compounds (due to for example lack of full hepatic metabolism, the absence of immune responses, and cell to cell contacts), the relatively high throughput and low costs makes them very fit for purpose as early screening tools, with the high specificity ensuring that promising compounds are not unnecessarily discarded.

Not surprisingly, it has shown that taking the human therapeutic maximum concentration (C_{max}) into account greatly reduces the amount of false positives [9]. This fits well with the concept that it is the exposure that determines the toxicity, with safer compounds having larger safety margins. Although the C_{max} is seldom known in early drug discovery, the safety margins from the validations can often be used to estimate what exposures would carry a relatively low risk for hepatotoxicity. Safety margins of 30–100× between human therapeutic C_{max} and the in vitro toxicity is generally recommended depending on the assay [9–11]. For the data sets in MIP-DILI, a safety margin of 75× was statistically found to be the most optimal [18]. Without accounting for C_{max} as a generic guide for human exposures, larger validations in HepG2 typically show similar sensitivity but with more false positives [9, 16]. The HCS assays can be geared toward working in absence of using C_{max}, but typically with a loss in sensitivity as the required safety margins need to be lowered.

Besides the most common HCS assay that assess cell health and mitochondrial parameters, there are also several other phenotypical screens that can predict adverse effects in the liver. HCS has been used for predictions of cholestasis through inhibition of canalicular transport through visualization of fluorescent bile salt derivatives, induction of steatosis and phospholipidosis using specific probes, and adaptation and survival responses using reporter cell lines for stress signaling pathways such as Nrf2 and NFκB just to name a few [1, 19–21]. More endpoints related to hepatotoxicity should ultimately lead to increased predictivity or increased understanding of underlying mechanism; however, it is equally important to include end points that rule out false positives. One such example is assessment of cell cycle state as otherwise compounds that inhibit the cell cycle progression may be mistaken for cytotoxic compounds when only counting nuclei [22, 23]. A list of some of the most popular probes for HCS assessment of DILI potential is presented in Table 1.

1.3 HCS in Complex Models

While the very early phases of drug discovery often typically restricts HCS screening to simple two-dimensional cell cultures because of the need for high throughput and rapid turnaround times in order to drive fast design–make–test cycles in medicinal chemistry, there is room for more complex and sophisticated models in later phases of the screening cascade. The less sophisticated models simply do not provide the same level of complexity, and thereby more relevance for DILI, as the more physiological models do. The lack of "complete" sensitivity toward DILI is most often attributed to lack of full physiological metabolism capacity, low

Table 1
Assortment of some of the most common dyes for DILI predictions using HCS

Probe	Excitation	Emission	Function	Usage	Live	Fixed
Hoechst 33342, Hoechst 33258, DAPI	350	450	Cell-permeant nucleic acid probe binding to the minor groove of DNA	Counting and morphological assessment of nuclei	X	X
MitoTracker Orange	550	575	Voltage dependent mitochondrial dye	Assessment of mitochondrial membrane potential and amount of mitochondria	X	X
MitoTracker Red	575	600	Voltage dependent mitochondrial dye	Assessment of mitochondrial membrane potential and amount of mitochondria	X	X
MitoTracker Green	488	510	Voltage independent mitochondrial dye	Assessment of mitochondrial morphology and amount	X	X
Tetramethylrhodamine	550	575	Voltage dependent mitochondrial dye	Assessment of mitochondrial membrane potential and amount of mitochondria	X	
TOTO-3	640	660	Non-cell-permeant nucleic acid probe binding to minor groove of DNA	Counting of necrotic and late apoptotic nuclei	X	(X)
CellROX Green	500	520	Oxidative stress dye which fluoresces upon oxidation	Assessment of reactive oxygen species and oxidative stress	X	X
CellROX Orange	550	570	Oxidative stress dye which fluoresces upon oxidation	Assessment of reactive oxygen species and oxidative stress	X	X

(continued)

Table 1
(continued)

Probe	Excitation	Emission	Function	Usage	Live	Fixed
LipidTox Red Neutral Stain	575	630	Probe which interacts with neutral lipid droplets	Assessment of steatosis	X	X
LipidTox Green Phospholipidosis Stain	495	525	Probe which interacts with phospholipid droplets	Assessment of phospholipidosis	X	X
LysoTracker Green	505	510	Probe with affinity for acidic organelles	Assessment of lysosomal activity	X	X
LysoTracker Red	575	590	Probe with affinity for acidic organelles	Assessment of lysosomal activity	X	X
Fluo-4	495	505	Probe which increases fluorescence upon binding of Ca2+	Assessment of calcium homeostasis	X	
Monochlorobimane	395	490	Probe which fluoresces upon binding of glutathione	Assessment of glutathione levels	X	X
CellEvent Caspase 3/7	505	530	Peptide which fluoresces after cleavage by Caspase 3 and 7	Assessment of early apoptosis	X	X
Cholyl-lysyl-fluorescein	488	520	Fluorescent labeled probe transported by BSEP	Assessment of cholestasis potential through BSEP	X	
5-Chloromethylfluorescein diacetate	488	520	Fluorescent labeled probe transported by MRP2	Assessment of cholestasis potential through MRP2	X	

Depending on the mechanisms of interest, probes can be selected for multiparametric imaging as long as they are spectrally separated and methodological compatible

tissue-like morphology, low inter cell communication, lack of transporters, lack of immune cells and other cell types, and limited possibilities for repeat-dose testing to name a few. Several more complex models have been generated in an attempt to correct or circumvent these issues. None of these systems are ideal and able to address all the shortcomings of the simple models, but each one has its own strength and weaknesses. The choice will come down to the mechanism which is trying to be addressed or predicted.

In vitro models constantly continue to evolve to more closely mimic true physiological systems that should deliver more insightful and relevant information. However, as the in vitro model systems become more complex, going from three-dimensional cell cultures to true microphyisological systems, so does the requirements for imaging. Whereas HCS is relatively straightforward for in two-dimensional cell cultures, it is more complex and technically challenging in three-dimensional systems, and one is usually restricted to using confocal systems. Experimental challenges include suboptimal diffusion of probes and antibodies into the biological system, lower level of light penetration to obtain sufficient imaging depth, limitations in microscope z-axis travel to assess the entire organoid, and the need for automated targeting algorithms. Still, the potential for increased predictivity for DILI due to the higher physiological relevance continues to drive the advancement of HCS in complex models. While several contract research organizations offer imaging based assays in spheroids for DILI prediction, there are currently not many validations in the literature. The concept has been shown beyond doubt in terms of enhanced functional transporter expression and increased metabolic capacity, but due to the complexity of HCS in spheroids, most validations for DILI predictions are made using biochemical end points [24–27]. Recognized as the future of advanced phenotypical drug testing, three-dimensional cell cultures, microphysiological systems, and organ-on-a-chip models are rapidly being adopted and developed by the pharmaceutical industries for predictions of adverse effects, including hepatotoxicity, often with multiparametric imaging as an endpoint.

2 A Generalized Protocol for HCS Prediction of DILI Using Simple Cell Cultures

As there are several imaging equipment and analysis software, each with its own preferred ways of working, here we represent a generalized protocol that can be easily adapted to each software.

2.1 Cell Culturing

The typical standard HCS assay for use in early drug discovery typically employs either hepatic cell lines such as HepG2 and HepaRG, or stem cell derived hepatocytes, or primary hepatocytes. This protocol will assume the use of HepG2 cells as they can be argued to be the most common and cost-effective. The cells are typically plated in 96-well plates at 15,000 cells/well the day before compound addition. Care should be taken to properly separate cells from each other as the HCS performs best when cells are growing separately and in a single layer. This can be achieved by passing the cells through an 18 G needle prior to plating. The C3a clone of HepG2 has proven to be well suited for HCS since it is not as prone to grow in aggregates as other HepG2 clones are. Coated plates may help in achieving a flattened out cell morphology, enabling easier focusing for the imaging platform.

2.2 Compound Addition and Incubation

Compounds of interest are typically diluted in tenfold concentration response, either in multiples of known C_{max}, or as is more usual in the pharmaceutical industry, in a fixed concentration range (going from low nanomolar to high micromolar) in order to be compliant with screening paradigms in early drug discovery. The duration of compound incubation is usually 24 or 72 h, but shorter term incubations are also possible. In general, shorter incubations are usually better for more mechanistic insight (e.g., mitochondrial perturbations) whereas longer incubations are better for assessing cytotoxicity related end points but with less information about the cause. For screening purposes, 24-h incubation time appears to be practical and a good compromise.

2.3 Staining of Cells and Cellular Organelles

Several different probes can be used and multiplexed, with the only limitation that they need to be specific, preferably with a functional end point, and have good spectral separation. While the probes may be tailored to the specific biological functions of interest, almost all HCS assays for DILI predictions employ probes for staining the cell nuclei as well as potentiometric mitochondrial probes as these have been shown to provide the best sensitivity for DILI predictions. Other popular probes include the ones that target oxidative stress, glutathione, lysosomes, endoplasmatic reticulum, or lipids, to name a few. The probes are usually mixed into a cocktail for simultaneous staining and direct addition into the wells. A typical set up for the so called Quadprobe assay [9] uses a cocktail of Hoechst 33342 (final conc. 1.6 μM), MitoTracker Orange (final conc. 50 nM), LysoTracker Green (final conc. 50 nM) and TOTO-3 (final conc. 1 μM), for multiparametric assessment of cell counts, nuclei related parameters, mitochondria, lysosomes, and necrosis/late apoptosis after 60 min of incubation at 37 °C. Care needs to be taken when selecting the probes. Probes for live cell imaging are typically more sensitive, but probes compatible with formaldehyde fixation dramatically increase throughput. Prior to fixation or imaging, the cells need to be washed with phosphate buffered saline (PBS) to limit the presence of unbound probes in the extracellular media. Fresh 37 °C cell media is added and the cells are imaged directly unless optional cell fixation is performed.

2.4 Optional Cell Fixation

Depending on whether the employed probes are compatible with formaldehyde fixation or not, the cells can be fixed with a 4% form-aldehyde solution added directly into the wells, and incubated at room temperature for 30 min. The formaldehyde solution is then aspirated and the cells are washed with room temperature equili-brated PBS. The cells can then be imaged directly or stored at 4 °C for up to several weeks, preferably in the dark, for later imaging.

2.5 Imaging and Image Analysis

Imaging and image analysis can be performed on separate or inte-grated platforms. The procedure described here can be generalized to virtually any platform. Four channels are used for the Quadprobe assay [9]. For Hoechst 33342 (Ex. 350 nm–Em. 450 nm), the exposure should be kept low but allow clear distinction from back-ground and stained nuclei. For MitoTracker Orange (Ex. 550 nm–Em. 575 nm) the exposure should be set to allow both decreases and increases in fluorescence intensity in order to be able to assess both hypopolarization and hyperpolarization of the mitochondria. Intensities should be set according to the same principles for LysoTracker Green (Ex. 445 nm–Em. 505 nm). For TOTO-3 (Ex. 640 nm–Em. 660 nm) the exposure should be set to allow clear distinction from normal (e.g., unstained) nuclei and nuclei in dead cells with lost plasma membrane integrity. A good setup is easily achieved using positive controls (e.g., antimycin for mito-chondrial hypopolarization, chlorpromazine for cytotoxicity and loss of plasma membrane integrity). Depending on imaging plat-form, offsets may be used to allow as focused images as possible. In order to achieve a good representation of the wells, it is prudent to acquire a minimum of 3–6 fields of view per well when using 20× magnification. Lesser magnification is not recommended as it does not allow distinction of organelles such as the mitochondria. The image analysis is typically set up to first detect and count nuclei to target the rest of the analysis. Thresholds should be set so that the nuclei are clearly outlined, intensity variances measureable, and segmentation should be performed to allow proper counting of nuclei localized close together. For mitochondrial parameters, the thresholds should be set up to clearly outline the mitochondrial morphology in an area either defined by the shape of the cells or an artificial ring (representing the cytoplasm) depending on what the software allows. Optimally, the algorithm should be able to assess both increases (mitochondrial hyperpolarization) and decreases (mitochondrial hypopolarization) while still being able to outline the mitochondrial area as a surrogate measure of the mitochondrial mass (see Fig. 1 for an example). The lysosomal parameters should be set up according to similar criteria using. For analysis of loss of plasma membrane integrity, the algorithm should only assess stain-ing in the nuclei as outlined by the Hoechst stain. Imaging algo-rithms as the one briefly outlined can easily generate hundreds or thousands of parameters for each cell. All of it can be used for true

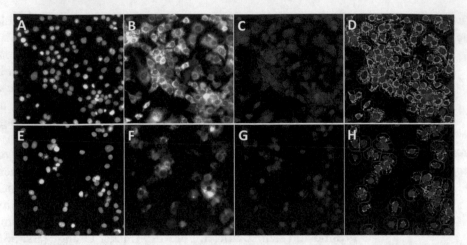

Fig. 1 (**a**)–(**d**) shows a typical image from a control well with staining of cell nuclei (**a**), mitochondria (**b**), the merged image with blue nuclei and red mitochondria (**c**), and image algorithm performance with nuclei outlined in blue, cell outlined in dark green, and mitochondria detected in green. (**e**)–(**h**) shows a similar layout but for a toxic compound that shows cytotoxicity by reduction of nuclei, including appearance of smaller and more intense nuclei, typically representing necrotic cells (**e**), and mitochondrial toxicity through hypopolarization, seen as decreased intensity (**f**). This appears as blue nuclei and limited red mitochondrial staining in the merged image (**g**) and apparent also in how the image algorithm analysis the image (**h**)

high content analysis, or selected parameters of high biological understanding may be selected for more targeted phenotypes. The results may then be used in connection with validation sets in order to predict propensity for DILI as outlined previously.

3　A Case Study

Compound X was being developed for a psychiatric indication but showed liver enzyme elevations in 4 week rodent toxicity studies, precluding it from further development. The HCS Quadprobe assay was employed on the compound, and it was found to cause mitochondrial hypopolarization and mild cytotoxicity, which had previously been missed in the traditional biochemical ATP assays where the compound appeared devoid of adverse effects. Compound X had a predicted human C_{max} of 3 μM and could be plotted against other drugs with known DILI propensity and was shown to be in the risk zone for human DILI, confirming the results from the rodent studies (Fig. 2). Furthermore, Compound X could be phenotypically interrogated against the company's database of HCS results for hundreds of compounds with known clinical DILI outcome in order to provide a more quantitative risk assessment. Compound X clustered together with efavirenz, ketoconazole, amytryptiline, and amiodarone, and could be predicted to show a similar profile in terms of DILI propensity in man. An HCS campaign was conducted on the chemical series from where

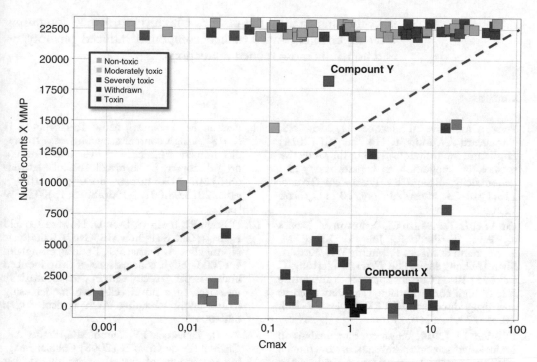

Fig. 2 Compound X, which showed adverse liver enzyme elevations in 4 week rodent toxicity studies, is plotted against the zone classification system previously presented [9], and is predicted to be in a zone of populated only by drugs associated with clinical hepatotoxicity. Compound Y is a derived from further screening in the chemical series, and is predicted to be a non-liver toxic compound. The figure is adapted from the zone classification system presented in Persson et al., 2013

Compound X was derived, and Compound Y was identified. Although not completely clean, the compound showed milder effects together with a slightly lower predicted C_{max}, making it end up in the zone where compounds are predicted to be safe. Advancement of the compound into a 4-week rodent toxicity study showed that the adverse liver enzyme elevations were successfully mitigated.

4   Conclusions and Outlook

During the last decade, HCS has become a mainstream technique for predicting DILI from simple cell models, and often considered the gold standard for assessing cell health. Numerous studies and validations have shown that, using simple cell models with high throughput and short turnaround times, about 50–60% of compounds causing DILI can be predicted with low amounts of false positives. As HCS moves into more complex cell models such as cocultures and 3D systems, there are hopes that the predictivity will further increase. The potential to use all phenotypic parameters, ranging from hundreds to thousands depending on the setup, is being unlocked by the power of high performance computing clusters, enabling more refined compound induced phenotypes, and hopefully more refined predictions.

References

1. Persson M, Loye AF, Jacquet M, Mow NS, Thougaard AV, Mow T, Hornberg JJ (2014) High-content analysis/screening for predictive toxicology: application to hepatotoxicity and genotoxicity. Basic Clin Pharmacol Toxicol 115(1):18–23. https://doi.org/10.1111/bcpt.12200

2. van Vliet E, Daneshian M, Beilmann M, Davies A, Fava E, Fleck R, Jule Y, Kansy M, Kustermann S, Macko P, Mundy WR, Roth A, Shah I, Uteng M, van de Water B, Hartung T, Leist M (2014) Current approaches and future role of high content imaging in safety sciences and drug discovery. ALTEX 31(4):479–493. 10.14573/altex.1405271

3. O'Brien PJ (2014) High-content analysis in toxicology: screening substances for human toxicity potential, elucidating subcellular mechanisms and in vivo use as translational safety biomarkers. Basic Clin Pharmacol Toxicol 115(1):4–17. https://doi.org/10.1111/bcpt.12227

4. Persson M, Hornberg JJ (2016) Advances in predictive toxicology for discovery safety through high content screening. Chem Res Toxicol 29(12):1998–2007. https://doi.org/10.1021/acs.chemrestox.6b00248

5. Hartung T (2016) Making big sense from big data in toxicology by read-across. ALTEX 33(2):83–93. 10.14573/altex.1603091

6. Knudsen TB, Keller DA, Sander M, Carney EW, Doerrer NG, Eaton DL, Fitzpatrick SC, Hastings KL, Mendrick DL, Tice RR, Watkins PB, Whelan M (2015) FutureTox II: in vitro data and in silico models for predictive toxicology. Toxicol Sci 143(2):256–267. https://doi.org/10.1093/toxsci/kfu234

7. Adler M, Ramm S, Hafner M, Muhlich JL, Gottwald EM, Weber E, Jaklic A, Ajay AK, Svoboda D, Auerbach S, Kelly EJ, Himmelfarb J, Vaidya VS (2016) A quantitative approach to screen for nephrotoxic compounds in vitro. J Am Soc Nephrol 27(4):1015–1028. https://doi.org/10.1681/ASN.2015010060

8. Benbow JW, Aubrecht J, Banker MJ, Nettleton D, Aleo MD (2010) Predicting safety toleration of pharmaceutical chemical leads: cytotoxicity correlations to exploratory toxicity studies. Toxicol Lett 197(3):175–182

9. Persson M, Loye AF, Mow T, Hornberg JJ (2013) A high content screening assay to predict human drug-induced liver injury during drug discovery. J Pharmacol Toxicol Methods 68(3):302–313. https://doi.org/10.1016/j.vascn.2013.08.001. S1056-8719(13)00283-9 [pii]

10. O'Brien PJ, Irwin W, Diaz D, Howard-Cofield E, Krejsa CM, Slaughter MR, Gao B, Kaludercic N, Angeline A, Bernardi P, Brain P, Hougham C (2006) High concordance of drug-induced human hepatotoxicity with in vitro cytotoxicity measured in a novel cell-based model using high content screening. Arch Toxicol 80(9):580–604

11. Xu JJ, Henstock PV, Dunn MC, Smith AR, Chabot JR, de Graaf D (2008) Cellular imaging predictions of clinical drug-induced liver injury. Toxicol Sci 105(1):97–105

12. Tolosa L, Pinto S, Donato MT, Lahoz A, Castell JV, O'Connor JE, Gomez-Lechon MJ (2012) Development of a multiparametric cell-based protocol to screen and classify the hepatotoxicity potential of drugs. Toxicol Sci 127(1):187–198. https://doi.org/10.1093/toxsci/kfs083. kfs083 [pii]

13. Peyre L, de Sousa G, Barcellini-Couget S, Luzy AP, Zucchini-Pascal N, Rahmani R (2015) High-content screening imaging and real-time cellular impedance monitoring for the assessment of chemical's bio-activation with regards hepatotoxicity. Toxicol In Vitro 29(7):1916–1931. https://doi.org/10.1016/j.tiv.2015.07.024

14. Trask OJ Jr, Moore A, LeCluyse EL (2014) A micropatterned hepatocyte coculture model for assessment of liver toxicity using high-content imaging analysis. Assay Drug Dev Technol 12(1):16–27. https://doi.org/10.1089/adt.2013.525

15. Sirenko O, Hesley J, Rusyn I, Cromwell EF (2014) High-content assays for hepatotoxicity using induced pluripotent stem cell-derived cells. Assay Drug Dev Technol 12(1):43–54. https://doi.org/10.1089/adt.2013.520

16. Garside H, Marcoe KF, Chesnut-Speelman J, Foster AJ, Muthas D, Kenna JG, Warrior U, Bowes J, Baumgartner J (2014) Evaluation of the use of imaging parameters for the detection

of compound-induced hepatotoxicity in 384-well cultures of HepG2 cells and cryopreserved primary human hepatocytes. Toxicol In Vitro 28(2):171–181. https://doi.org/10.1016/j.tiv.2013.10.015

17. Saito J, Okamura A, Takeuchi K, Hanioka K, Okada A, Ohata T (2016) High content analysis assay for prediction of human hepatotoxicity in HepaRG and HepG2 cells. Toxicol In Vitro 33:63–70. https://doi.org/10.1016/j.tiv.2016.02.019

18. Persson M, Aerts H, Edsbagge J, Gerets H, Hewitt P, Hornberg J, Juhila S, Karjalainen M, Lowatt C, Mesens N, Newham P, Richert L, Thelin A, Weaver R (2016) High content analysis for prediction of human druginduced liver injury across several pharmaceutical companies within the innovative medicines initiative MIP-DILI consortium. Paper presented at the Society of Toxicology, New Orleans, 2016

19. Barber JA, Stahl SH, Summers C, Barrett G, Park BK, Foster JR, Kenna JG (2015) Quantification of drug-induced inhibition of canalicular cholyl-L-lysyl-fluorescein excretion from hepatocytes by high content cell imaging. Toxicol Sci 148(1):48–59. https://doi.org/10.1093/toxsci/kfv159

20. Pradip A, Steel D, Jacobsson S, Holmgren G, Ingelman-Sundberg M, Sartipy P, Bjorquist P, Johansson I, Edsbagge J (2016) High content analysis of human pluripotent stem cell derived hepatocytes reveals drug induced steatosis and phospholipidosis. Stem Cells Int 2016:2475631. https://doi.org/10.1155/2016/2475631

21. Herpers B, Wink S, Fredriksson L, Di Z, Hendriks G, Vrieling H, de Bont H, van de Water B (2016) Activation of the Nrf2 response by intrinsic hepatotoxic drugs correlates with suppression of NF-kappaB activation and sensitizes toward TNFalpha induced cytotoxicity. Arch Toxicol 90(5):1163–1179. https://doi.org/10.1007/s00204-015-1536-3

22. Schorpp K, Rothenaigner I, Maier J, Traenkle B, Rothbauer U, Hadian K (2016) A multi-plexed high-content screening approach using the chromobody technology to identify cell cycle modulators in living cells. J Biomol Screen. https://doi.org/10.1177/1087057116641935

23. Massey AJ (2015) Multiparametric cell cycle analysis using the operetta high-content imager and harmony software with PhenoLOGIC. PLoS One 10(7):e0134306. https://doi.org/10.1371/journal.pone.0134306

24. Bell CC, Hendriks DF, Moro SM, Ellis E, Walsh J, Renblom A, Fredriksson Puigvert L, Dankers AC, Jacobs F, Snoeys J, Sison-Young RL, Jenkins RE, Nordling A, Mkrtchian S, Park BK, Kitteringham NR, Goldring CE, Lauschke VM, Ingelman-Sundberg M (2016) Characterization of primary human hepatocyte spheroids as a model system for drug-induced liver injury, liver function and disease. Sci Rep 6:25187. https://doi.org/10.1038/srep25187

25. Richert L, Baze A, Parmentier C, Gerets HH, Sison-Young R, Dorau M, Lovatt C, Czich A, Goldring C, Park BK, Juhila S, Foster AJ, Williams DP (2016) Cytotoxicity evaluation using cryopreserved primary human hepatocytes in various culture formats. Toxicol Lett 258:207–215. https://doi.org/10.1016/j.toxlet.2016.06.1127

26. Kostadinova R, Boess F, Applegate D, Suter L, Weiser T, Singer T, Naughton B, Roth A (2013) A long-term three dimensional liver co-culture system for improved prediction of clinically relevant drug-induced hepatotoxicity. Toxicol Appl Pharmacol 268(1):1–16. https://doi.org/10.1016/j.taap.2013.01.012

27. Ramaiahgari SC, den Braver MW, Herpers B, Terpstra V, Commandeur JN, van de Water B, Price LS (2014) A 3D in vitro model of differentiated HepG2 cell spheroids with improved liver-like properties for repeated dose high-throughput toxicity studies. Arch Toxicol 88(5):1083–1095. https://doi.org/10.1007/s00204-014-1215-9

Chapter 17

Interpretation, Integration, and Implementation of In Vitro Assay Data: The Predictive Toxicity Challenge

Deborah S. Light, Michael D. Aleo, and J. Gerry Kenna

Abstract

Human drug-induced liver injury (DILI) is still a leading cause of attrition in drug development and for adverse outcomes in the marketplace. Identifying DILI risk for humans in standard animal safety testing conducted before clinical trials, in advance of the drug regulatory review and approval process is sometimes elusive. Numerous mechanisms of small molecule driven hepatotoxicity have been elucidated (e.g., reactive metabolite formation, oxidative stress, mitochondrial inhibition, bile salt export pump inhibition) and are amenable to high-throughput screening approaches. It is possible to highlight and distinguish hazard gradations of risk for human DILI when these assays are consolidated into a single point of view. In some instances, these in vitro assays highlight the potential clinical hazard without animal safety studies confirming this view. Scientifically, the idea of developing a hazard matrix approach as a better option to animal studies requires a paradigm shift that challenges the status quo. Altering opinions and traditions to effect enduring change in this area require organizational effort and commitment. Utilizing a flexible, business-disciplined framework such as Accelerating Implementation Methodology (AIM), offers structure to implement organizational change. Common barriers associated with bringing lasting change are: inappropriate sponsorship (e.g., level, commitment, and influence), organizational commitment, lack of understanding of organizational culture, resistance to change, and not identifying key stakeholders, or not hearing stakeholders' opposing views. Given time and appropriate scientific evidence, a hazard matrix approach to identifying compounds with higher potential to cause severe DILI in the clinic can be institutionalized within the pharmaceutical industry.

Key words AIM, DILI, In vitro assays, Screening approaches

1 Paradigm Shifts in Science

The Structure of Scientific Revolutions [1] by Thomas Kuhn has long stood as a critical treatise on the nature of scientific progress. In his discourse, scientific revelation and progress is not a smooth and steady accumulation of knowledge and insights, but rather comprised of a series of mini "revolutions." These mini revolutions are based on paradigm shifts in science, in which a new scientific thought was sufficiently unprecedented to attract a group of adherents away from the competing modes of scientific activity while, simultaneously, it was sufficiently open-ended to leave all sorts of

Minjun Chen and Yvonne Will (eds.), *Drug-Induced Liver Toxicity*, Methods in Pharmacology and Toxicology,
https://doi.org/10.1007/978-1-4939-7677-5_17, © Springer Science+Business Media, LLC, part of Springer Nature 2018

problems for the group of adherents to resolve" ([1], p. 10) Paradigm shifts are new model systems or theories that seek to resolve old problems or inaccuracies. They inadvertently create new issues to resolve since they are still under investigation. The proverbial "problem" is how best to determine, from the existing facts, a new cornerstone on which one can build a new paradigm that further enlightens and focusses science. Paradigm shifts acquire their status because they are more successful than their previous competitors in solving problems that the group of new practitioners has come to realize as acute ([1], p. 23). "Though a generation is sometimes required to effect the change, scientific communities have again and again been converted to new paradigms [with time].... Though some scientists, particularly the older and more experienced ones, may resist indefinitely, most of them can be reached in one way or another. Conversions will occur a few at a time until, after the last holdouts have died, the whole profession will again be practicing under a single, but now different paradigm. We must therefore ask how conversion is induced and how resisted" ([1], p. 152).

Even though Kuhn's first publication regarding the philosophical treatment of scientific revolutions occurred over 50 years ago, the basic principles and underlying issues he identified continue to be relevant to change in modern day scientifically based organizations. By nature, humans are inherently resistant to the idea of major change (i.e., paradigm shift), so it should not be surprising that such change only occurs in organizations when it is recognized that the need for change is greater than the need to stay the same.

Kuhn's insight into the nature of scientific revolutions and resistance to change is especially germane to today's issues within the field of discovery toxicology, where the single most important aim is to "predict" accurately the toxicological outcome of xenobiotic exposure in humans before humans are actually exposed to the agent. Yogi Berra purportedly quipped "It's tough to make predictions, especially about the future". Even a so-called "expert" requires vast amounts of knowledge and insight to make good "predictions" using existing tools and insight. Yet Niels Bohr cautions that "an expert is a man who has made all the mistakes that can be made in a very narrow field".

2 Predictions in Toxicology

In the physical sciences, predictions (like planetary movements) can be made with mathematical precision. Conversely, only some biological and toxicological responses are influenced predominantly by molecular interactions that can be assessed using relatively simple in vitro model systems in isolation. A good example is the use of the Ames assay to assess the in vitro mutagenic potential of xenobiotics [2]. A positive finding in this assay is considered by scientists and regulatory agencies as sufficient to identify a carcinogenic compound, in the absence of any animal test data. In other cases, in silico/in vitro models can inform experimental design in animal or human studies, or may provide valuable supplementary information that can aid the interpretation of data obtained from directed experiments in animals or humans. An example of this would be investigating the translational effects of a mitochondrial uncoupler on animal body temperature [3].

On the contrary, the study of undesirable side effects caused by prescription drugs (i.e., human adverse drug reactions) is rather more challenging. Some adverse drug reactions can be attributed to exaggerated primary pharmacology (e.g., bleeding caused by anticoagulants, blood pressure lowering caused by antihypertensives), while others arise due to off-target secondary pharmacology (e.g., anti-androgen-induced imbalance of estrogen/androgen leading to gynecomastia) [4]. However, many clinically important adverse drug reactions are unrelated to either primary or secondary pharmacology. One of the most frequent and concerning is drug-induced liver injury (DILI). For a few licensed drugs (e.g., acetaminophen), DILI is highly reproducible and dose-dependent ("Type A") and occurs in both animals and humans. However, a retrospective analysis by numerous pharmaceutical companies of compounds progressed into clinical trials revealed that whereas mild human liver injury was evident for many different compounds, only 55% of compounds that caused human liver injury had caused liver abnormalities when evaluated preclinically using standard animal models [5, 6]. Furthermore, this analysis is likely to have underestimated the true frequency of this occurrence since many drug candidates that cause DILI in animals are not progressed into clinical trials. Exceptions can arise when the anticipated human exposure is sufficiently larger compared to minor liver effects in animals (e.g., mild, reversible elevations in liver transaminases without any corresponding histopathology changes) or the anticipated risk-to-benefit ratio is considered sufficient to warrant clinical evaluation of the compound (e.g., oncology agents). To this day, human DILI continues to be an important cause of compound attrition early in clinical drug development [6–8].

In addition, many licensed drugs cause human DILI, yet do not cause adverse liver injury in nonclinical safety testing of new medicines. Typically, such apparently "human specific" DILI is not overtly dose-dependent and occurs only rarely in humans, i.e., it is an idiosyncratic toxicity that arises only in certain susceptible individuals and can be detected only when large numbers of patients have been exposed to the culprit drug, either late in clinical development (phase III) or after marketing approval (phase IV) [9]. Because idiosyncratic DILI is caused by so many different drugs, it is an important cause of serious human ill health and can result in life threatening liver failure. In addition, idiosyncratic DILI is a leading cause of compound attrition in late drug development, of failed drug registration, of cautionary labeling and of withdrawal of previously licensed drugs. In combination, Type A and idiosyncratic DILI are major reasons for compound attrition due to toxicity in the pharmaceutical industry [8].

The risks posed by DILI can be tackled and managed in three distinct and complementary ways. The first is to devise and implement strategies that enable compounds with desirable efficacy and other properties, but only low propensity to cause DILI, to be designed and selected during drug discovery. This increases the likelihood that compounds progressed into the clinic will have good hepatic safety profiles. Useful methods must be able to identify compounds that can predict risk of both Type A and idiosyncratic DILI with good specificity and sensitivity and be applicable throughout drug discovery, when chemical choices are available. This necessitates a major paradigm shift from use of traditional regulatory animal studies to evaluate human DILI risk, which is based on a prevailing assumption (i.e., "old paradigm") that the complexity of integrated biological responses can always be measured and observed most effectively in vivo. The second way to tackle and manage human DILI risk is to differentiate between high risk and low risk patient groups and/or individuals, enabling targeting of potentially problematic drugs to patients most likely to derive clinical benefit from them as part of a personalized healthcare strategy. The third approach is to develop better ways to detect and manage DILI that arises in susceptible patients. Although the second and third approaches are outside the scope of this chapter, they have been reviewed by others [10].

The purpose of this chapter is to discuss how the predictive toxicology challenge can be tackled, to summarize the promising progress already made in developing a "new paradigm" which integrates multiple in silico and in vitro data types, and to highlight key future opportunities and difficulties. In particular, we address the obstacles that need to be surmounted when seeking to adopt and implement the new paradigm within large pharmaceutical companies.

3   DILI In Vitro Hazard/Liability Matrix Development and Validation

Currently there is no consensus within pharma on the most appropriate way to derisk DILI during drug discovery and a variety of different approaches have been proposed. For example, Dambach et al. [11] described a tiered cascade developed by Bristol-Myers Squibb, in which initial compound screening and optimization was undertaken using T-antigen immortalized human liver epithelial (THLE) cell lines that expressed various human cytochrome (CYP) enzymes and in vitro toxicity testing in human hepatocytes was undertaken prior to compound progression [11]. Other investigators have described different in vitro toxicity screening approaches [12, 13] or have instead focused on minimization of both drug dose plus reactive metabolite formation [14–16]. A focus on metabolic bioactivation as a DILI risk factor is well justified [17], although it is important to recognize that DILI can also arise via other mechanisms.

3.1 AstraZeneca Approach

A strategy developed within one leading pharmaceutical company (AstraZeneca) has been published in the peer reviewed scientific literature [18, 19] and highlights many of the issues that need to be incorporated and resolved when attempting to de-risk DILI in drug discovery. Initially, the intention of the strategy was to provide consistent guidance to project teams on how best to assess and interpret data on reactive metabolite formation. However, it was also recognized that other potentially relevant mechanisms also needed to be addressed, for example drug induced mitochondrial injury [20]. An additional important driver was that DILI and other toxicities were observed in animals and humans for many project compounds and were a leading cause of project failure [21, 22]. Consequently, the goals of the strategy were to identify methods that could be used in drug discovery to aid selection of compounds with the least possible human DILI liabilities, to develop guidance to project teams on how best to use the methods, and in particular to provide quantitative criteria that could enable decisions to be made on whether it was appropriate to progress compounds or more advisable to design and select alternative molecules.

Initially, the strategy was developed with "top down" strong support from senior management (vice president level) in drug safety and drug metabolism/pharmacokinetics departments. As the work progressed, it became increasingly clear that medicinal chemists needed to be fully engaged as stakeholders and strategy team members. Also, open communication with all disease areas and their many cross-functional project teams was required. The final roll-out of the strategy required its endorsement by all research areas across global drug discovery, plus drug development. This necessitated detailed face to face meetings at all global research sites. Success was achieved by setting out the scientific rationale for the approach, the validation data that had been obtained, and the opportunity to use the strategy to reduce markedly the likelihood of project failure due to DILI in clinical development. In addition, it was important to recognize that different projects teams could have quite different target product profiles for patient safety (e.g., non-insulin-dependent diabetes vs. advanced oncology), which influenced their judgment of whether the anticipated clinical benefit could justify progression into humans of compounds with in vitro safety signals.

The strategy focused on in vitro quantitative evaluation of several key mechanisms by which DILI can be initiated. In addition to reactive metabolite formation, the mechanisms evaluated were: inhibition of mitochondrial function, intrinsic cell cytotoxicity in the presence and absence of CYP450 3A4 activity, and inhibition of the Bile Salt Export Pump (BSEP). The scientific rationale that underpinned selection of these mechanisms has been discussed elsewhere [18, 19]. In addition, the test cascade evaluated inhibition of the Multidrug Resistance Protein Type 2 (MRP2). Inhibition by drugs of MRP2 is not in itself considered to be a mechanism by which DILI can be initiated, but is an important biliary efflux transporter whose activity could play a hepatoprotective role when BSEP activity is inhibited [23]. Hence this could be an additive DILI risk factor, especially since MPR2 inhibition may result in elevated concentrations within hepatocytes of drugs and/ or drug metabolites that are excreted into bile via MRP2.

A single model system could not be identified which could be used to quantify effects of test compounds on each of the selected mechanisms, and was suitable for routine high volume use during drug discovery. Therefore a multiassay in vitro test cascade was developed, which is summarized in Table 1. Since the primary purpose was to identify drugs that can cause DILI in humans, the assays focused on human liver biology and utilized either human liver cells or human liver transporters. Apart from the covalent binding studies, which required use of human hepatocytes and synthesis of radiolabeled test compounds, the selected assays could be undertaken in high throughput format. This enabled assessment of their

Table 1
In vitro assays used to construct in vitro DILI hazard matrix

Mechanism	Assay	References
1. Reactive metabolite formation	Human hepatocyte covalent binding (of radiolabeled drugs)	[19]
2. Mitochondrial inhibition	HepG2 cell cytotoxicity ratio in galactose vs. glucose media	[19]
3. Cell cytotoxicity	THLE cell cytotoxicity	[25]
4. CYP3A4-potentiated cell cytotoxicity	THLE-3A4 cell cytotoxicity	[25]
5. BSEP inhibition	BSEP inhibition in inverted membrane vesicles	[24]
6. MRP2 inhibition	MRP2 inhibition in inverted membrane vesicles	[19]

predictive value for human DILI by testing of substantial numbers of hepatotoxic and nonhepatotoxic test drugs (>80 for each assay), and determining in vitro compound concentrations that caused 50% reductions when compared with vehicle control values, i.e., IC_{50} or EC_{50} values [24, 25]. None of the assays provided high DILI sensitivity and specificity when evaluated in isolation, even when drug doses and drug concentrations in plasma were taken into account. Therefore the data provided by all of the assays was integrated and analyzed in combination. Potencies of the effects observed in the five in vitro safety assays were assigned binary scores of 0 or 1, depending upon whether or not these were below or above threshold values of concern that had been determined following evaluation of reference "DILI" and "no DILI" drugs. Summation of these binary values yielded aggregated in vitro assay scores for each drug (see Fig. 1). Human hepatocyte covalent binding (CVB) binding data were adjusted for the extent of in vitro compound turnover, resulting in fractional CVB (f_{cvb}) values that were multiplied by the maximum recommended daily therapeutic doses of the drugs to estimate daily CVB burden (Fig. 1). A two-dimensional plot of aggregated in vitro assay scores vs CVB burden for each drug produced the "hazard matrix," which is illustrated in Figs. 1 and 2 [19].

The hazard matrix was developed using data obtained from 36 test pharmaceuticals, of which 27 caused clinically concerning DILI (plus various other idiosyncratic adverse reactions), one caused severe hypersensitivities that led to discontinuation of its development and nine did not cause clinically concerning idiosyncratic adverse reactions. Seven of the nine "safe" drugs exhibited aggregated in vitro panel scores <2 and CVB burden

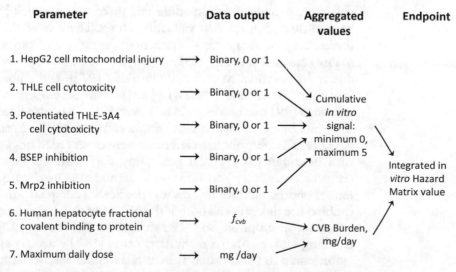

Fig. 1 Process used to generate integrated in vitro hazard matrix values for test drugs

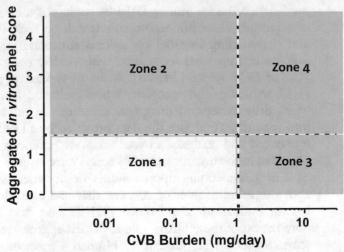

Excellent discrimination between 27 toxic drugs and 9 non-toxic drugs (100% sensitivity, 78% specificity)

Fig. 2 Integrated in vitro hazard matrix

<1 mg/day (zone 1 of Fig. 2; specificity 78%). All of the 27 "idio-syncratic concern" drugs exhibited aggregated in vitro panel scores ≥2 and/or CVB burden ≥1 mg/day (sensitivity 100%), although the number and magnitude of in vitro signals that were detected varied markedly between these drugs. CVB burden was ≥1 mg/day and aggregated in vitro assay scores were one or zero (zone 3) for 15 drugs; whereas aggregated in vitro scores were ≥2 and CVB burden was <1 mg/day (zone 2) for six drugs; and aggregated in vitro scores were ≥2 and CVB burden was ≥1 mg/day (zone 4) for eight drugs.

To assess further the predictive value of the Hazard Matrix, data were generated for an additional three drugs, which had not been evaluated in the first validation study. These were the endo-thelin receptor antagonists: sitaxsentan (withdrawn from use due to rare causes of acute liver failure [26]), bosentan (usage restricted due to its potential to cause human DILI [27]), and ambrisentan (not found to cause human DILI [28]). Neither sitaxsentan in rats and dogs [29] nor bosentan in rats were found to cause liver toxic-ity, while bile duct hyperplasia, single cell necrosis, and transami-nase/alkaline phosphatase elevations were observed in dogs treated with bosentan [30]. When generating data with the endothelin receptor antagonists, an improved method was used to quantify mitochondrial inhibition. This was the Seahorse™ platform, which enabled the direct evaluation of the effects of the drugs on cellular oxygen consumption and extracellular acidification [31]. The resulting Hazard Matrix from AstraZeneca [32] correctly assigned ambrisentan to "safe" zone 1. Both sitaxsentan and bosentan were assigned to zone 4, although the potencies of the signals observed with sitaxsentan were markedly greater than the signals observed with bosentan. This distinction became especially clear when the potencies of effects observed in each of the individual in vitro toxicity assays were adjusted to account the human plasma concentrations of the drugs. This was achieved by dividing the maximum human drug plasma concentrations by the in vitro IC_{50} or EC_{50} values. In accordance with recommendations for the interpretation of in vitro drug-drug interaction data [33], values ≥ 0.1 were assigned binary scores of 1, and values <0.1 were given scores of 0. Using this approach, sitaxsentan exhibited positive exposure adjusted signals in all five in vitro assays and a high CVB burden, whereas bosentan exhibited a positive exposure adjusted signal in only one assay (BSEP inhibition) and a moderate CVB burden [32]. This analysis indicates that human plasma exposure data have the potential to improve markedly the interpretation of in vitro safety data.

However, since robust plasma exposure data are available only once clinical trials have been performed and the desired clinical dose has been defined, it is important to recognize that exposure adjustment of in vitro toxicity data is not a realistic option before progression of a new test compound into humans. Therefore the Hazard Matrix illustrated in Fig. 1 is more suitable for use during drug discovery, when chemical choice is available.

The potential value of the Hazard Matrix for predicting DILI in animals was not evaluated. Therefore it is unclear whether or not it can reliably identify compounds that will cause DILI in animals that would prevent progression into humans. Hence the Hazard Matrix does not replace the need for animal safety studies prior to clinical trials. However, the approach can be expected to increase the likelihood that compounds progressed into clinical trials will not cause idiosyncratic DILI in humans. Therefore it should reduce the need for in vivo animal safety testing of compounds that have unsuitable human safety profiles. This is a significant potential 3Rs benefit.

At the time that this work was undertaken, the process of selection and annotation of tested drugs posed a major problem and required extracting relevant information from the published scientific literature and from drug labels. This was a laborious and time consuming process. Since then, the US FDA has published relevant data in the Liver Toxicity Knowledgebase (LTKB) [34] and it is recommended that this database should be used to aid future evaluation of alternative assays.

3.2 Pfizer Approach   An analogous approach was developed at Pfizer after sitaxsentan was voluntarily withdrawn from approved marketplaces and discontinued from ongoing clinical development [35]. With this event there was renewed interest in developing a more comprehensive screening strategy to avoid acquiring or developing compounds with significant DILI potential. In vitro assays which were similar to those described above for AstraZeneca, were incorporated into the Pfizer matrix approach for detecting DILI compounds with a high degree of specificity and sensitivity. The Pfizer matrix aggregated multiple DILI liability factors. These were: inhibition of both liver mitochondria and BSEP [36], human dose (total dose >100 mg), systemic C_{max} exposure (>1.1 µM), cytotoxic potential in liver cell lines, and certain chemical property descriptors such as PSA and clogP values [37]. This multifactorial compound stratification approach vastly improved upon the in vitro human liver hazard detection method published previously by Xu et al. [38]. The DILI predictive value of the Pfizer matrix was demonstrated in part by use of the LTKB categorization system of DILI risks to assign test drugs to either MOST-, LESS-, or NO-DILI concern categories; this classification was based on review of FDA drug labeling and causality evidence [39]. The initial LTKB list of 287 drugs [39] has now been expanded to 1036 drugs [40] and represents an improvement over previous annotations [38, 41], which were more limited in scope both in terms of numbers of drugs as well as annotations based on case and literature reviews. Despite the great attention and time spent annotating a large list of over 1000 drugs for DILI risk in humans, this is a relatively small list compared to the expectations of medicinal chemistry designers where data needs tend to be extremely large. For example, in the field of QSAR (quantitative structure–activity relationships) modeling it is unlikely that a few thousand compounds – or even tens of thousands of compounds in a training data set – will confidently represent the entire pharmaceutical chemistry space [42]. As a consensus-driven organization these and many other challenges were faced during the conception and implementation of this new screening paradigm, the principles of which are outlined below.

4 Implementation

Enabling a research organization to develop and implement complex, long-term, predictive investigations when the outcome and value of the work are not likely to come to fruition for several years is very challenging. Careful planning and strong sponsorship are key contributing factors to success of any long-term endeavor. The first critical step is to gain (and retain) commitment from leadership and resources holders (e.g., people, funding) for the length of the project. It is also important to remember that resistance to change is normal and past problems are likely to be repeated, thus careful stakeholder management throughout the project is critical. Stakeholders need to understand key questions: (1) what is the proposed change, (2) what is the benefit of changing vs staying the same, and (3) how success will be measured. Educating and building an understanding among key stakeholders is necessary to driving change throughout the life cycle of the project.

How a project is launched can vary. A directive from leadership setting the expectation that a project will be undertaken and completed is perceived differently than a project brought up through scientific lines and managed by influence. Both approaches have advantages and challenges. The former might get results faster at the start but could drive dissenters underground. Those not fully convinced of the value of the project may disrupt implementation later in the timeline, causing delays and creating unanticipated complications. If the latter is solely consensus driven, progress may be slow and tedious but this provides an opportunity to bring about universal change. However, the latter can also create an opt-in/-out mentality if key groups or leaders do not prioritize the project and clearly communicate that. When a key sponsor or discipline leader is not an advocate or wants additional parameters added, implementation can be delayed or even halted while the issues are addressed. If the project is for the broader organization but does not directly improve or add value to a particular group that must be involved in the work, additional education and reinforcement may be needed to gain that leadership acceptance.

The success of a project is also dependent on an organization's culture and risk tolerance. In any organization, it is important to have clear objectives and milestones agreed by the team and management at the project start. Implementation generally consumes a large amount of time and resource to be successful. Many organizations do not allow time for the implementation phase of a project. A key to executing and implementing a successful project within a large, matrix organization is utilization of good project management practices and tools such as Accelerating Implementation Methodology (AIM) [43]. AIM provides a framework for planning, execution, and implementation of any project to increase the likelihood of success. To facilitate the implementation of a successful project, the most important factor is strong sponsorship. The sponsor should have the authority to make decisions and provide resources such as people and funding. Without sponsors at the senior level and sponsors or advocates at the mid-management level, it is difficult to retain an organization's attention and energy. There is a risk of an "opt out" mentality for a project if there is not clear management buy-in and encouragement.

The project also needs a Scientific Lead who is a subject matter expert (SME) and will act as advocate for the project. An experienced project manager is necessary to employ tools and techniques to manage and drive the objectives forward. The Scientific Lead and the Project Manager should not be the same individual as both roles are demanding. Another key to success is to build the project team by involving engaged experts with specific roles who can commit to conducting the actual work.

For complex, cross-disciplinary projects, core team members should actively engage their disciplines early in the project life cycle to build an understanding of the project objectives. The team must identify their key stakeholders. The Sponsor and/or Scientific Lead should help those targets understand how the project outcomes will be of benefit to them/the organization and how it will change the way they work. Building an understanding and obtaining acceptance early helps to develop project advocates before it fully rolls out. Educating and gaining feedback and perspectives from stakeholders (e.g., end-users, colleagues who will be doing the work, leadership) early and at set project milestones is essential to offer the team an opportunity to correct or improve the new process, and to find out if/how new processes are understood and being utilized. This also allows the team to refine their objectives and outcomes and avoid changes later in the project when change can be more difficult or more expensive. Tools such as interviews or surveys allow feedback to be gained directly from the users.

In reality, there is likely to be turnover in personnel and possibly in organizational structure during a multiyear projects' life cycle. If multiple, key team members and/or sponsor(s) or other influencers leave the company, the team may need to reeducate new sponsors or leaders and incorporate their thinking or changes. This can cause project delays and creates the risks of disengaging team members. Loss of SMEs or key scientific opinion leaders within the company can also slow a project, as finding talented colleagues with very specific expertise and gaining agreement for their time commitment can be time-consuming. Continually needing to reengage or reeducate stakeholders can create a loss of motivation or energy drain for the SMEs. This needs to be managed carefully, through reinforcement from sponsors/leaders.

Additional challenges to a long-term project can be changes in organizational structure or philosophy within lines/disciplines, that can create new barriers to keeping resources committed to the project (people or funding). Once again, discussions with leadership and organizational sponsors by the Scientific Lead or Project Lead will be needed to get the project back on track.

During a project life cycle, keeping the sponsor(s) and stakeholders informed of progress is important in order to keep these key colleagues engaged. Once results are available, they should be shared with the sponsor and key stakeholders. A communication plan should be developed in advance of close out of the project, to enable the team to provide outcomes and measures of success (or failure) to the organization.

Experience shows that choosing the right targets to be the first to use any new tools or assays is another key to success. At AstraZeneca, being able to develop new in vitro assays which aided the selection of drug candidates with low DILI liabilities was very positively received. However, initial attempts to roll out the assays to discovery project teams that were already in a mature state, and ready to progress to the next milestone, was difficult. Having to go back and reintroduce new assays meant that these teams had to move their milestones further out and because of this the teams pushed back. After the project team held discussions with management, it was decided that it was preferable to focus the roll out of new in vitro assays on projects in early discovery, where there was abundant chemical choice. This was a positive outcome from feedback received.

Long-term initiatives are difficult and complex. However, when they have positive outcomes that shift us to a new, improved paradigm of being better able to predict safety and bring safer medicines to patients faster, it is hard to argue against their value.

5   Specific Challenges in Industry

The need to develop new paradigms that can solve old problems is extremely important in science, but is riddled with challenges that are organizationally specific based on historical context, individual perspectives and scientific merit. In large pharmaceutical organizations a new scientific approach for derisking of toxicity would likely come out of some sort of an investigative line function within a drug safety and/or pharmacokinetic and drug metabolism department. However, effective utilization of any such approach requires its adoption by medicinal chemists and regulatory toxicologists, who are situated in different parts of the organization and might be expected to question, underappreciate or even negate its value. In particular, from a regulatory perspective animal testing or early human clinical data may well not reinforce the hazard perspective gained from in vitro testing for idiosyncratic human liver injury. The outcome of progression of a compound that exhibits one or more DILI signals can either be a false positive or true positive, depending upon whether the deleterious liver effect is observed in animals or humans and the phase at which in vivo liver injury was observed. For example, nefazodone did not exemplify aspects of DILI in preclinical or clinical trials, while its injurious potential in humans was really defined after-market authorization [44]. Therefore, an in vitro assay that raised DILI concern for nefazodone might be interpreted (incorrectly) as a false positive if compared with animal safety data or clinical trial data, or (correctly) as a true positive if compared with postmarketing clinical safety data.

Furthermore, other possible shortcomings of a new predictive toxicity paradigm might quickly be perceived as negating its potential value. Since the evaluation of any new proposed approach will be based on retrospective analysis of old drugs, it may not adequately represent issues with future drugs that are not represented in the retrospective analysis. This is a common issue with in silico modeling of in vitro assay results, where continued testing has to be conducted in order to refresh the in silico model with new and innovative chemical space (e.g., chemical space and targets covered). Consequently it is reasonable to expect that any proposed safety hazard matrix (e.g., that outlined in Figs. 1 and 2) may suffer from false negatives. A particular difficulty is that this limitation may only become apparent over many years, once large numbers of compounds have been tested and broad coverage of chemical space has been achieved. In contrast, in silico models of in vitro assays can be refreshed quite quickly and do not require years to resolve. Another issue is the false negative space that will arise since not all mechanisms of DILI are tested in any pragmatic, high volume test cascade. The effects of this could be large or small. For example, the liver injury potential caused by the triphosphate metabolite of zaclitabine could be missed unless a specific screen for mitochondrial DNA polymerase gamma replication has been developed and utilized [45].

Retrospective testing can lead to the identification of animal models that enable much improved prediction of clinical DILI than the species used in conventional drug safety studies. An example is panadiplon, which caused transaminase elevations in healthy volunteers that were not predicted by standard preclinical studies using rats, dogs or monkeys. Only after the clinical adverse effect was noted was it found that Dutch-belted rabbits were observed to be sensitive to liver injury, whereas other animals were not [46]. The same issue is true for fialuridine, where five people died in the phase II clinical trial due to fatal DILI. An analysis by the US National Academy of Sciences of all preclinical fialuridine toxicity tests, which included studies in mice, rats, dogs, and monkeys, concluded that the available animal data provided no indication that the drug would cause liver failure in humans. Two decades later a chimeric mouse model, that replaced murine liver cells with human liver cells, was able to reproduce the type of injury observed clinically (jaundice and lethargy); laboratory tests (elevated transaminase and lactic acidosis), and changes to the liver in the drug-treated mice mirrored those observed in human participants in the fialuridine trial [47]. It should be noted that the human DILI potential of fialuridine was also demonstrated in the woodchuck [48] (an uncommon nonclinical species used in testing) and in a specialized human in vitro liver culture system [49].

Although time eventually brings additional information and tools to bear, the current issue is how to utilize in vitro information that is relevant to clinical outcomes for compounds that do not display adverse liver effects in animal studies. A big advancement to this challenging area is provided by DILIsym® software as described in Chap. 6 in this volume. This proprietary software program uses computational systems biology to integrate in vitro toxicity assay data and drug exposure data, and thereby simulate and thereby "anticipate" in vivo liver adverse effects in animals and humans exposed to test drugs. The model was built initially by analysis of data obtained from the literature, or experimentally, for exemplar compounds that caused liver injury in vivo via a variety of mechanisms plus chemically similar nontoxic compounds. The mechanisms of liver injury (and exemplar compounds) were: reactive metabolite formation (acetaminophen, 3′-hydroxyacetanilide, methapyrilene, furosemide, aflatoxin B1, and lapatinib), inhibition of bile acid efflux from hepatocytes via BSEP (lapatinib, bosentan, telmisartan, CP-724714, and glibenclamide), mitochondrial toxicity (tolcapone, buprenorphine, and etomoxir) and mitochondrial DNA depletion (fialuridine). After building the integrated models, recent clinical candidates that failed in clinical development due to unexpected liver injury signals (TAK875 (Takeda), MK0536 (Merck), and AMG009 (Amgen)) were examined to determine the effectiveness of the model for simulating and thereby anticipating human DILI potential, and/or to build refinements into the modeling software.

The established clinical perspective on risk of fatal injury was based on observations by Hy Zimmerman [50] and coined by Robert Temple as Hy's law [51]. The premise is that causality justified drug-induced hepatocellular injury which occurs in the presence of jaundice is clinically concerning, since it is indicative of marked liver injury that in some susceptible patients may progress to life-threatening acute liver failure [50–52]. This observation was later codified by the FDA, which has provided the following guidance on how cases of drug-induced liver injury can be detected in clinical trials:

- The drug causes hepatocellular injury, generally shown by a higher incidence of threefold or greater elevations above the upper level of normal (ULN) of alanine aminotransferase or aspartate aminotransferase than the control drug or placebo.

- Among trial subjects showing such aminotransferase elevations, often with aminotransferases much greater than 3×ULN, one or more also show elevation of serum total bilirubin to >2×ULN, without initial findings of cholestasis (elevated serum alkaline phosphatase).

- No other likely reason can be found to explain the combination of increased aminotransferases and total bilirubin, such as viral hepatitis A, B, or C; preexisting or acute liver disease; or coadministration of another drug capable of causing the observed injury.

Due to the low frequency of idiosyncratic human DILI caused by many drugs, cases observed during clinical trials can be expected to arise only rarely. Finding one justified Hy's law case in the clinical trial database of a drug is worrisome; finding two is considered highly predictive that the drug has the potential to cause severe DILI when given to a larger population [53]. The assessment of risk for serious, life-threatening drug-induced liver injury associated with a drug, at present is an iterative process based on accumulation of clinical data [54]. Assessment of risk-to-benefit ratios regarding a novel agent with hepatotoxicity issues (especially one for a life-threatening condition) requires considerable judgment and education on the part of prescribers and patients. The spectrum of drug-induced liver injury is broad and is similar to liver disorders arising via other causes [55]. Because serious cases are typically rare, it is difficult to define a priori which patient is most at risk. The determination of actual risk is at the individual level at first and then accumulated with time across numerous treated patients. Many individual patients can benefit from a drug with a black box warning for liver injury without any adverse consequences. For example, there are reports where patients experienced transaminase elevations when treated with bosentan, but had no evidence of liver injury after they were switched to sitaxsentan [56]. Conversely, there are also examples were patients tolerated sitaxsentan without any signs of liver injury but developed transaminase elevations when switched to bosentan after the withdrawal of sitaxsentan [57]. A better understanding of liver injury causality is achieved only after the event has occurred through a thorough retrospective analysis, and the adjudication of each case can highlight the need for clinical samples consented and retained from trials for additional analyses. The most effective way to manage the human clinical risk posed by idiosyncratic DILI is to advance compounds into clinical development that have low propensity to cause known mechanisms of toxicity. Hence, there is a need for a new predictive screening paradigm that can enable this to be achieved.

When deciding whether or not to progress an individual compound into development, it necessary to undertake a risk–benefit assessment that takes account of safety liabilities and numerous other considerations. These will include the available chemical space (which typically is restricted), the anticipated clinical dose and exposure, the severity of the disease state, plus known clinical adverse outcomes caused by preexisting drugs used to treat that clinical indication. When assessing safety liability, we think that it is appropriate to use a hazard matrix approach for highlighting potential human liver injury risks. This can be performed prior to nonclinical animal safety studies and clinical trials, when it is important to select a molecule that is likely to be safe in humans. At this stage, key rhetorical questions which should be asked are: Am I better than... my previous chemical series; my previous lead compound; a competitor in development or the marketplace with liver injury? Such comparisons can be expected to ensure that clinical candidates in a program are sufficiently differentiated from each other in terms of potential hazard, thereby reducing the risk of failure of the entire program due to toxicity.

At the present time we think that use of the hazard matrix approach to aid internal decision making within projects and companies is justified. However, we recognize that the approach has not been evaluated and validated sufficiently rigorously to be used for regulatory decision making. Current gaps, which hopefully can be tackled in the near future, include a need to standardize individual assay protocols in multiple laboratories and to develop rigorous performance/acceptance criteria for the assays. It will be important also to test large numbers of hepatotoxic and nonhepatotoxic drugs, in order to gain more robust insight into sensitivity and specificity of the hazard matrix for assessing DILI risk and to establish whether the matrix can reliably distinguish between pharmaceutical agents with the potential to cause fatal human liver injury and those that may cause less clinically concerning types of liver injury [58].

References

1. Kuhn TS (1970) The structure of scientific revolutions. International encyclopedia of unified science foundations of the unity of science, vol 2, no 2, 2nd edn. University of Chicago Press, Chicago

2. U.S. Department of Health and Human Services, Food and Drug Administration, Center for Drug Evaluation and Research (CDER) (June 2012) Guidance for industry on: S2(R1) Genotoxicity testing and data interpretation for pharmaceuticals intended for human use. Available at: https://www.fda.gov/downloads/drugs/-guidancecomplianceregulatoryinformation/guidances/ucm074931.pdf

3. Haasio K, Koponen A, Penttila KE, Nissinen E (2002) Effects of entacapone and tolcapone on mitochondrial membrane potential. Eur J Pharmacol 453(1):21–26

4. Yun GY, Kim SH, Kim SW, Joo JS, Kim JS, Lee ES, Lee BS, Kang SH, Moon HS, Sung JK, Lee HY, Kim KH (2016) Atypical onset of bicalutamide-induced liver injury. World J Gastroenterol 22(15):4062–4065. https://doi.org/10.3748/wjg.v22.i15.4062

5. Greaves P, Williams A, Eve M (2004) First dose of potential new medicines to humans: how animals help. Nat Rev Drug Discov 3(3):226–236. https://doi.org/10.1038/nrd1329

6. Olson H, Betton G, Robinson D, Thomas K, Monro A, Kolaja G, Lilly P, Sanders J, Sipes G, Bracken W, Dorato M, Van Deun K, Smith P, Berger B, Heller A (2000) Concordance of the toxicity of pharmaceuticals in humans and in animals. Regul Toxicol Pharmacol 32(1):56–67.https://doi.org/10.1006/rtph.2000.1399

7. Laverty H, Benson C, Cartwright E, Cross M, Garland C, Hammond T, Holloway C, McMahon N, Milligan J, Park B, Pirmohamed M, Pollard C, Radford J, Roome N, Sager P, Singh S, Suter T, Suter W, Trafford A, Volders P, Wallis R, Weaver R, York M, Valentin J (2011) How can we improve our understanding of cardiovascular safety liabilities to develop safer medicines? Br J Pharmacol 163(4):675–693. https://doi.org/10.1111/j.1476-5381.2011.01255.x

8. Waring MJ, Arrowsmith J, Leach AR, Leeson PD, Mandrell S, Owen RM, Pairaudeau G, Pennie WD, Pickett SD, Wang J, Wallace O, Weir A (2015) An analysis of the attrition of drug candidates from four major pharmaceutical companies. Nat Rev Drug Discov 14(7):475–486. https://doi.org/10.1038/nrd4609

9. Kaplowitz N (2005) Idiosyncratic drug hepatotoxicity. Nat Rev Drug Discov 4(6):489–499. https://doi.org/10.1038/nrd1750

10. Lewis JH (2015) The art and science of diagnosing and managing drug-induced liver injury in 2015 and beyond. Clin Gastroenterol Hepatol 13(12):2173–2189.e8. https://doi.org/10.1016/j.cgh.2015.06.017

11. Dambach DM, Andrews BA, Moulin F (2005) New technologies and screening strategies for hepatotoxicity: use of in vitro models. Toxicol Pathol 33(1):17–26. https://doi.org/10.1080/01926230590522284

12. Gomez-Lechon MJ, Tolosa L, Donato MT (2016) Metabolic activation and drug-induced liver injury: in vitro approaches for the safety risk assessment of new drugs. J Appl Toxicol 36(6):752–768. https://doi.org/10.1002/jat.3277

13. Zhang J, Doshi U, Suzuki A, Chang CW, Borlak J, Li AP, Tong W (2016) Evaluation of multiple mechanism-based toxicity endpoints in primary cultured human hepatocytes for the identification of drugs with clinical hepatotoxicity: results from 152 marketed drugs with known liver injury profiles. Chem Biol Interact 255:3–11. https://doi.org/10.1016/j.cbi.2015.11.008

14. Nakayama S, Atsumi R, Takakusa H, Kobayashi Y, Kurihara A, Nagai Y, Nakai D, Okazaki O (2009) A zone classification system for risk assessment of idiosyncratic drug toxicity using daily dose and covalent binding. Drug Metab Dispos 37(9):1970–1977. https://doi.org/10.1124/dmd.109.027797

15. Sakatis MZ, Reese MJ, Harrell AW, Taylor MA, Baines IA, Chen L, Bloomer JC, Yang EY, Ellens HM, Ambroso JL, Lovatt CA, Ayrton AD, Clarke SE (2012) Preclinical strategy to reduce clinical hepatotoxicity using in vitro bioactivation data for >200 compounds. Chem Res Toxicol 25(10):2067–2082. https://doi.org/10.1021/tx300075j

16. Usui T, Mise M, Hashizume T, Yabuki M, Komuro S (2009) Evaluation of the potential for drug-induced liver injury based on in vitro covalent binding to human liver proteins. Drug Metab Dispos 37(12):2383–2392. https://doi.org/10.1124/dmd.109.028860

17. Park BK, Boobis A, Clarke S, Goldring CE, Jones D, Kenna JG, Lambert C, Laverty HG, Naisbitt DJ, Nelson S, Nicoll-Griffith DA, Obach RS, Routledge P, Smith DA, Tweedie DJ, Vermeulen N, Williams DP, Wilson ID, Baillie TA (2011) Managing the challenge of chemically reactive metabolites in drug development. Nat Rev Drug Discov 10(4):292–306. https://doi.org/10.1038/nrd3408

18. Thompson RA, Isin EM, Li Y, Weaver R, Weidolf L, Wilson I, Claesson A, Page K, Dolgos H, Kenna JG (2011) Risk assessment and mitigation strategies for reactive metabolites in drug discovery and development. Chem Biol Interact 192(1–2):65–71. https://doi.org/10.1016/j.cbi.2010.11.002

19. Thompson RA, Isin EM, Li Y, Weidolf L, Page K, Wilson I, Swallow S, Middleton B, Stahl S, Foster AJ, Dolgos H, Weaver R, Kenna JG (2012) In vitro approach to assess the potential for risk of idiosyncratic adverse reactions caused by candidate drugs. Chem Res Toxicol 25(8):1616–1632. https://doi.org/10.1021/tx300091x

20. Dykens JA, Will Y (2007) The significance of mitochondrial toxicity testing in drug development. Drug Discov Today 12(17–18):777–785. https://doi.org/10.1016/j.drudis.2007.07.013

21. Cook D, Brown D, Alexander R, March R, Morgan P, Satterthwaite G, Pangalos MN (2014) Lessons learned from the fate of AstraZeneca's drug pipeline: a five-dimensional framework. Nat Rev Drug Discov 13(6):419–431. https://doi.org/10.1038/nrd4309

22. Keisu M, Andersson TB (2010) Drug-induced liver injury in humans: the case of ximelagatran. Handb Exp Pharmacol 196:407–418. https://doi.org/10.1007/978-3-642-00663-0_13

23. Kenna JG (2014) Current concepts in drug-induced bile salt export pump (BSEP) interference. Curr Protoc Toxicol 61:23.7.1–23.7.15. https://doi.org/10.1002/0471140856.tx2307s61

24. Dawson S, Stahl S, Paul N, Barber J, Kenna JG (2012) In vitro inhibition of the bile salt export pump correlates with risk of cholestatic drug-induced liver injury in humans. Drug Metab Dispos 40(1):130–138. https://doi.org/10.1124/dmd.111.040758

25. Gustafsson F, Foster AJ, Sarda S, Bridgland-Taylor MH, Kenna JG (2014) A correlation between the in vitro drug toxicity of drugs to cell lines that express human P450s and their propensity to cause liver injury in humans. Toxicol Sci 137(1):189–211. https://doi.org/10.1093/toxsci/kft223

26. Galie N, Hoeper MM, Gibbs JS, Simonneau G (2011) Liver toxicity of sitaxentan in pulmonary arterial hypertension. Eur Respir J 37(2):475–476. https://doi.org/10.1183/09031936.00194810

27. Humbert M, Segal ES, Kiely DG, Carlsen J, Schwierin B, Hoeper MM (2007) Results of European post-marketing surveillance of bosentan in pulmonary hypertension. Eur Respir J 30(2):338–344. https://doi.org/10.1183/09031936.00138706

28. McGoon MD, Frost AE, Oudiz RJ, Badesch DB, Galie N, Olschewski H, McLaughlin VV, Gerber MJ, Dufton C, Despain DJ, Rubin LJ (2009) Ambrisentan therapy in patients with pulmonary arterial hypertension who discontinued bosentan or sitaxsentan due to liver function test abnormalities. Chest 135(1):122–129. https://doi.org/10.1378/chest.08-1028

29. Owen K, Cross DM, Derzi M, Horsley E, Stavros FL (2012) An overview of the preclinical

toxicity and potential carcinogenicity of sitaxentan (Thelin®), a potent endothelin receptor antagonist developed for pulmonary arterial hypertension. Regul Toxicol Pharmacol 64(1):95–103. https://doi.org/10.1016/j.yrtph.2012.05.017

30. U.S. Department of Health and Human Services, Food and Drug Administration, Center for Drug Evaluation and Research (CDER) (2001) Overall summary and evaluation of preclinical pharmacodynamics, toxicokinetics and toxicology. Available at: https://www.fda.gov/ohrms/dockets/ac/01/briefing/3775b2_07_PharmToxReview.htm

31. Brand MD, Nicholls DG (2011) Assessing mitochondrial dysfunction in cells. Biochem J 435(2):297–312. https://doi.org/10.1042/BJ20110162

32. Kenna JG, Stahl SH, Eakins JA, Foster AJ, Andersson LC, Bergare J, Billger M, Elebring M, Elmore CS, Thompson RA (2015) Multiple compound-related adverse properties contribute to liver injury caused by endothelin receptor antagonists. J Pharmacol Exp Ther 352(2):281–290. https://doi.org/10.1124/jpet.114.220491

33. U.S. Department of Health and Human Services, Food and Drug Administration, Center for Drug Evaluation and Research (CDER) (Feb 2012) Guidance for industry on: Drug interaction studies-study design, data analysis, implications for dosing, and labeling recommendations. Available at: https://www.fda.gov/downloads/drugs/guidancecomplianceregulatoryinformation/guidances/ucm292362.pdf

34. Chen M, Zhang J, Wang Y, Liu Z, Kelly R, Zhou G, Fang H, Borlak J, Tong W (2013) The liver toxicity knowledge base: a systems approach to a complex end point. Clin Pharmacol Ther 93(5):409–412. https://doi.org/10.1038/clpt.2013.16

35. Pfizer (Dec 2010) Pfizer stops clinical trials of Thelin® and initiates voluntary product withdrawal in the interest of patient safety. Available at: http://www.pfizer.com/news/press-release/press-release-detail/pfizer_stops_clinical_trials_of_thelin_and_initiates_voluntary_product_withdrawal_in_the_interest_of_patient_safety

36. Aleo MD, Luo Y, Swiss R, Bonin PD, Potter DM, Will Y (2014) Human drug-induced liver injury severity is highly associated with dual inhibition of liver mitochondrial function and bile salt export pump. Hepatology 60(3):1015–1022. https://doi.org/10.1002/hep.27206

37. Shah F, Leung L, Barton HA, Will Y, Rodrigues AD, Greene N, Aleo MD (2015) Setting clinical exposure levels of concern for drug-induced liver injury (DILI) using mechanistic in vitro assays. Toxicol Sci 147(2):500–514. https://doi.org/10.1093/toxsci/kfv152

38. Xu JJ, Henstock PV, Dunn MC, Smith AR, Chabot JR, de Graaf D (2008) Cellular imaging predictions of clinical drug-induced liver injury. Toxicol Sci 105(1):97–105. https://doi.org/10.1093/toxsci/kfn109

39. Chen M, Vijay V, Shi Q, Liu Z, Fang H, Tong W (2011) FDA-approved drug labeling for the study of drug-induced liver injury. Drug Discov Today 16(15–16):697–703. https://doi.org/10.1016/j.drudis.2011.05.007

40. Chen M, Suzuki A, Thakkar S, Yu K, Hu C, Tong W (2016) DILIrank: the largest reference drug list ranked by the risk for developing drug-induced liver injury in humans. Drug Discov Today 21(4):648–653. https://doi.org/10.1016/j.drudis.2016.02.015

41. Greene N, Fisk L, Naven RT, Note RR, Patel ML, Pelletier DJ (2010) Developing structure-activity relationships for the prediction of hepatotoxicity. Chem Res Toxicol 23(7):1215–1222. https://doi.org/10.1021/tx1000865

42. Cumming JG, Davis AM, Muresan S, Haeberlein M, Chen H (2013) Chemical predictive modelling to improve compound quality. Nat Rev Drug Discov 12(12):948–962. https://doi.org/10.1038/nrd4128

43. Implementation Management Associates (2016) Accelerating Implementation Methodology (AIM). Available at: http://www.imaworldwide.com/

44. Choi S (2003) Nefazodone (Serzone) withdrawn because of hepatotoxicity. Can Med Assoc J 169(11):1187

45. Kakuda TN (2000) Pharmacology of nucleoside and nucleotide reverse transcriptase inhibitor-induced mitochondrial toxicity. Clin Ther 22(6):685–708. https://doi.org/10.1016/S0149-2918(00)90004-3

46. Ulrich RG, Bacon JA, Branstetter DG, Cramer CT, Funk GM, Hunt CE, Petrella DK, Sun EL (1995) Induction of a hepatic toxic syndrome in the Dutch-belted rabbit by a quinoxalinone anxiolytic. Toxicology 98(1–3):187–198

47. Xu D, Nishimura T, Nishimura S, Zhang H, Zheng M, Guo YY, Masek M, Michie SA, Glenn J, Peltz G (2014) Fialuridine induces acute liver failure in chimeric TK-NOG mice: a model for detecting hepatic drug toxicity prior to human testing. PLoS Med 11(4):e1001628. https://doi.org/10.1371/journal.pmed.1001628

48. Tennant BC, Baldwin BH, Graham LA, Ascenzi MA, Hornbuckle WE, Rowland PH,

Tochkov IA, Yeager AE, Erb HN, Colacino JM, Lopez C, Engelhardt JA, Bowsher RR, Richardson FC, Lewis W, Cote PJ, Korba BE, Gerin JL (1998) Antiviral activity and toxicity of fialuridine in the woodchuck model of hepatitis B virus infection. Hepatology 28(1):179–191. https://doi.org/10.1002/hep.510280124

49. Krzyzewski S, Khetani SR, Barros S (2011) Assessing chronic toxicity of fialuridine in a micropatterned hepatocyte co-culture model (Abstract 2523). Toxicologist Suppl Toxicol Sci 120(2):540

50. Zimmerman HJ (1999) Hepatotoxicity: the adverse effects of drugs and other chemicals on the liver, 2nd edn. Lippincott Williams & Wilkins, Philadelphia, PA

51. Reuben A (2004) Hy's law. Hepatology 39(2):574–578

52. Reuben A (2008) Hy's law explained. Available at: http://www.documentshare.org/general-reference/hys-law-explained/

53. U.S. Department of Health and Human Services, Food and Drug Adeministration, Center for Drug Evaluation and Research (CDER) (July 2009) Guidance for industry on: drug-induced liver injury: premarketing clinical evaluation. Available at: https://www.fda.gov/downloads/Drugs/…/guidances/UCM174090.pdf

54. Temple R (2006) Hy's law: predicting serious hepatotoxicity. Pharmacoepidemiol Drug Saf 15(4):241–243. https://doi.org/10.1002/pds.1211

55. Maddrey WC (2005) Drug-induced hepatotoxicity: 2005. J Clin Gastroenterol 39(4 Suppl 2):S83–S89

56. Benza RL, Mehta S, Keogh A, Lawrence EC, Oudiz RJ, Barst RJ (2007) Sitaxsentan treatment for patients with pulmonary arterial hypertension discontinuing bosentan. J Heart Lung Transplant 26(1):63–69. https://doi.org/10.1016/j.healun.2006.10.019

57. Don GW, Joseph F, Celermajer DS, Corte TJ (2012) Ironic case of hepatic dysfunction following the global withdrawal of sitaxentan. Intern Med J 42(12):1351–1354. https://doi.org/10.1111/imj.12007

58. Avigan MI (2014) DILI and drug development: a regulatory perspective. Semin Liver Dis 34(2):215–226. https://doi.org/10.1055/s-0034-1375961

Part IV

Methodologies Applied in Regulatory Science

Chapter 18

Perspectives on the Regulatory and Clinical Science of Drug-Induced Liver Injury (DILI)

Mark I. Avigan and Monica A. Muñoz

Abstract

This chapter provides a regulatory framework of drug-induced liver injury (DILI) risk assessment, whose foundation is the understanding, identification, and evaluation of different forms of hepatotoxicity caused by a drug or biological agent. Regulatory scientists strive to translate evolving knowledge into an accurate and efficient prediction of DILI risk in humans as early as possible in a product's life cycle. In addition, better characterization of factors that underlie individual susceptibility can lead to improved risk minimization, and ultimately enhance the balance between treatment-associated benefits and risks. Heightened DILI risk plays a critical role in the trajectory of approval for a therapeutic product. Compound development may be terminated when a signal of potentially serious DILI emerges given the theoretical risks to trial subjects and potential opportunity cost that may be incurred. The limitations of currently available analytical tools to quantify DILI risk undoubtedly have resulted in the premature discontinuation of compounds that ultimately may have been associated with negligible or acceptable levels of risk for the intended treatment population. For other compounds, an associated DILI risk may go unrecognized in the premarket setting, and only shows an unacceptable benefit–risk balance in the postmarketing setting. No drug or biological agent has been withdrawn in the US market following approval due to hepatotoxicity since the publication of the FDA Guidance for Industry on DILI Premarketing Clinical Evaluation in 2009. Nonetheless, some recently approved agents have been linked to an increased risk for DILI in vulnerable patients, resulting in the inclusion of Boxed Warnings or Warnings of hepatotoxicity in several of their product labels.

Key words Drug-induced liver injury, Hepatotoxicity, Clinical trials, Risk–benefit, Surveillance

1 Framework for DILI Risk Assessment

A broad range of pathologic phenotypes and clinical patterns of hepatotoxicity have been causally associated with specific therapeutic drugs and biologic agents [1]. These include both acute as well as chronic forms of liver injury, reflecting a diverse set of toxic effects of drugs that target specific components of the liver—an organ that is comprised of intricate anatomical and developmental interactions between different cell types and lineages. Because of the robust regenerative and cytoprotective capacity of the

Minjun Chen and Yvonne Will (eds.), *Drug-Induced Liver Toxicity*, Methods in Pharmacology and Toxicology, https://doi.org/10.1007/978-1-4939-7677-5_18, © Springer Science+Business Media, LLC, part of Springer Nature 2018

liver, many acute and subacute forms of DILI are fully reversible. Recovery of the organ may occur as a consequence of adaptation of the liver cells in the face of continued exposure to the agent responsible for the initial liver disturbance (e.g., acetaminophen-induced damage of hepatocytes in the centrolobular region of the hepatic lobules, and amoxicillin-clavulanate-induced damage of cholangiocytes in biliary ductules) [2, 3]. In other instances, discontinuation of treatment appears to be a prerequisite to set the liver on a path toward full recovery, irrespective of the liver cell populations that are primarily damaged. Nonetheless, there are important scenarios connected to specific treatment agents when an idiosyncratic liver injury will progress beyond a mild transient disturbance of the organ to a higher level of severity in susceptible patients. They include the following: (1) progression of DILI when adaptation fails and the treatment has not been discontinued in a timely manner, (2) rapid acceleration of liver injury to a stage of severe necrosis and/or acute liver failure, irrespective whether treatment with the hepatotoxic agent has been discontinued, (3) induction of permanent histopathologic changes such as collagen deposition, bile duct ablation, sinusoidal obstruction as complications of chronic or subacute forms of DILI, (4) induction of long-standing autoimmune hepatitis (AIH) initiated by treatment-induced changes in T-cell homeostasis. So far, the specific host and environmental factors that underlie idiosyncratic liver injury susceptibility in each of these circumstances to particular drugs or biological agents are not fully understood.

2 FDA Guidance on the Premarketing Assessment of DILI Risk and Hy's Law

From a regulatory perspective, predicting the risk for idiosyncratic and serious hepatotoxic events is especially important as the benefits and risks of a new drug or biological agent are being weighed to determine both its approvability for marketing and appropriate indications of use [4]. Among the various DILI phenotypes that have been identified, in recent years there has been a concentrated effort to improve the identification and evaluation of agents that pose a risk for severe or life-threatening acute hepatocellular injury and acute liver failure (ALF) with a risk for death or liver transplant. This important milestone in the regulatory science of DILI is based largely on a seminal observation by Hyman Zimmerman in the 1970s that drug-induced hepatocellular injury marked by elevations of liver aminotransferases accompanied by jaundice (i.e., elevated serum bilirubin levels) has a significant probability of progression to liver failure that can lead to death (or liver transplant) [5, 6]. It should be emphasized that the rises in bilirubin must not be the result of benign unrelated causes, including Gilbert's syndrome and hemolysis. In contrast to drug-induced cholestatic liver injury which is marked by high early peak alkaline phosphatase (ALP) levels >2X the Upper Limit of Normal (ULN) and an R value [peak serum alanine aminotransferase (ALT) XULN/ALP XULN] < 2, hepatocellular injury is marked by relatively low peak levels of ALP that are typically <2X ULN and an R value >5. Between 10% and 50% of cases of acute hepatocellular DILI associated with treatment-induced elevations of serum bilirubin (>2X ULN) have been observed to progress to ALF with death or liver transplantation as an outcome. Thus, the finding of even a single case of acute hepatocellular injury with hyperbilirubinemia that is causally associated with exposure to a suspect agent is a strong predictor that cases of ALF due to DILI are likely to occur later in a large treatment population. This phenomenon has been dubbed "Hy's law" in tribute to Dr. Zimmerman by FDA's Robert Temple [7, 8]. The "Hy's law" concept is important in the assessment of a study drug's associated hepatotoxic risk during the clinical trial phase and is a central underpinning of the guidance on the premarketing evaluation of DILI that was issued by FDA in 2009 [9]. Assuming a 10% rate of progression of Hy's law cases to liver failure, point estimates can be predicted for the risk of ALF associated with a drug in a large postmarket treatment population. The accuracy of these estimates depends on the active monitoring and thorough diagnostic assessment of cases of acute liver injury. It also depends on a complete tally of all the numerator cases of hepatocellular DILI with hyperbilirubinemia together with a measure of the denominator of all the subjects who have been treated with the study drug. For example, of the 2510 study subjects with diabetes who were treated with troglitazone during its clinical development prior to approval of the agent in 1997, two developed drug-induced hepatocellular findings consistent with Hy's law among five patients who developed ALT elevations >30X ULN [9]. Projecting these results to establish a point estimate of risk for the most severe tier of hepatocellular injury, the ALF rate due troglitazone exposure would be in the order of 1 per 12,550 treated patients. From other data, it is likely that the real incidence in diabetics treated with this agent until its withdrawal in the year of 2000 may have been even somewhat higher, and this should not be a surprise given the wide 95% statistical confidence intervals that surround such a point estimate for rare events [10–12].

According to the FDA guidance, in a drug development program, the complete absence of even one case of Hy's law across all clinical studies enables exclusion of a risk level for severe acute hepatocellular injury and ALF above a calculated rate that is defined by the "Rule-of-3." This approach applies a simple binomial calculation of a 95% upper boundary of risk, using the number of study subjects in the development program who have been treated with the test agent to divide by three [13]. To illustrate, if 3000 patients have been treated per a standard protocol and monitored carefully for changes of serum liver biochemistry, the absence of Hy's law cases supports exclusion of a risk for such injuries at a rate above 1 per 1000 and of severe acute hepatocellular injury and ALF at any rate above 1 per 10,000 (assuming that 10% of the cases would progress to the most severe tier).

It is important to note that the clinical and laboratory profiles in patients with underlying liver diseases who develop acute exacerbations in association with a suspect agent have yet to be critically considered [14–16]. The recognition of serious acute hepatocellular injury based on new biochemical and other lab test findings that are super-imposed on abnormal pretreatment baseline findings is not fully addressed in the current FDA guidance on premarketing DILI risk. This challenge for regulatory scientists is exemplified in drug development programs that are investigating new treatments for patients with chronic viral hepatitis and NASH [17–19].

There are a number of critical inter-related domains that should be analyzed in an overall assessment of risk for idiosyncratic acute hepatocellular liver injury causally associated with a suspect pharmaceutical drug or biological agent. These include (1) the incidence as well as clinical and laboratory signatures of serious or severe cases of hepatotoxicity in patients who have been treated with the product, (2) the drug-associated likelihood of causality of each clinically important treatment-associated case in the treatment population, (3) the external and biological factors and/or disease states which increase or decrease DILI susceptibility, (4) the times to onset and recovery of liver injury after initiation and discontinuation of treatment, respectively, and (5) the presence or absence of a viable strategy (ies) to mitigate serious or life-threatening outcomes upon detection of treatment-associated liver injury.

3   Preclinical Characterization of Human Idiosyncratic DILI Risk Connected to New Drugs and Biological Agents

The development of reliable preclinical approaches to accurately predict risk for serious and life-threatening forms of DILI of new drugs and biological agents remains elusive [20–27]. As described in other chapters throughout this textbook, much progress has been made in the development of a variety of tools with growing opportunities toward achieving this goal. Nonetheless, currently, each of these is marked by significant limitations and/or gaps in their utility. Some of these are listed in Table 1.

As outlined in Table 1, each of the preclinical approaches to characterize a new drug or biologic agent has a contributory role in assessing DILI risk and can impact directions taken for further investigations or scrutiny, either with other preclinical tools, in the

Table 1
Some current preclinical approaches to predict DILI risk

Methods and approaches	Test systems	Representative measures	Examples	Potential utility in risk prediction	Limitations and gaps
Structural alert modeling	Drug structures with and w/o liabilities	Programs to identify reactive components of molecules	Haloalkanes NSAIDs Enolcarboxa-mides	Can enhance drug design efficiencies and avoid agents with liability	False positives and false negatives
Toxicological stress modeling	Simulation of drug effects in liver cells and organ	In silico predictions of DILI with simulations in population	Glutathione and UDP-glucuronide levels	Can predict cut points for saturation of cytoprotective pathways	Immune-mediated mechanisms of DILI not modeled
In vitro transporter inhibition assays	Cell or vesicular systems with recombinant transporter activities	BSEP, MRP-2, MRP-3, MRP-4	Oral contraceptives; Erythromycin estolate Bosentan	Can explain hepatotoxic/ cholestatic effects of some agents	Other mechanisms of DILI not tested
In vitro mitochondrial toxicity assays	Cell test systems	ATP-dependent cellular respiration	Diclofenac Valproic acid Acetaminophen	Can explain hepatotoxic effects of some agents	Other mechanisms of DILI not tested
In vitro formation of ROS	Cell test systems	Cellular lysate analysis of ROS	Nefazodone Diclofenac Troglitazone	Can analyze important mechanism of cellular stress	Different levels of cyto-protection and recovery not considered
In vitro drug-protein adduct assays	Animal models of DILI with reactive metabolites	HPLC-based analysis of serum adducts	Acetaminophen	Can analyze exposure-related levels of toxicity	Not generalizable to other drugs and exposure conditions

(continued)

Table 1
(continued)

Methods and approaches	Test systems	Representative measures	Examples	Potential utility in risk prediction	Limitations and gaps
In vitro single cell cultures	Cell viability in presence and absence of test drug	Markers of cell death and apoptosis	Primary hepatocytes Hep-G2 cells	Highly sensitive assay for hepatotoxic parent drugs	Limited discrimination between DILI and non-DILI associated drugs
In vitro co-cultures	Cell viability in presence and absence of test drug	Markers of cell death and apoptosis	Hepatocyte and mesenchymal cell cultures	Transcellular interactions part of in vivo stimulus for hepatocyte differentiation	Co-cultures do not contain all in vivo liver factors that influence DILI
Cell viability and disruption markers	In vitro cell culture in presence of drug	Markers of cell necrosis, apoptosis, mitochondrial toxicity	DNA ladder Cytochrome c Vital stain	Pertains to multiple modes of cell loss	Limited specificity; Immune-mediated mechanisms not tested
Animal systems	In vivo hepatotoxicity findings in presence of drug	Liver tests and histopathology at different drug exposure levels	Rat Dog Monkey	Valuable in assessing exposure-related hepatotoxicity	Important Idiosyncratic elements in human DILI not present

BSEP bile salt export pump; *DILI* drug-induced liver injury; *MRP* multidrug resistance-associated protein; *NSAIDs* nonsteroidal anti-inflammatory drugs; *UDP* uridine diphosphate; *ATP* adenosine triphosphate; *HPLC* high-performance liquid chromatography; *ROS* reactive oxygen species

preapproval phases of testing, or even in a postmarket period. In some sense, no single currently used preclinical method can generate absolute predictive values of risk for serious idiosyncratic DILI. Therefore, these tools are best used to establish a "preponderance of evidence" either to support or diminish concerns surrounding hepatotoxicity connected to the new agent, as well as point to strategies or investigations to enhance overall drug development decisions and further refine predictions of DILI risk in concert with the findings of clinical trials.

4 Clinical Pharmacology and DILI Risk Characterization

In determining whether hepatotoxic risk in patients correlates with the level of pharmacological exposure to a suspect drug, there are important elements to be considered. First, standard preclinical dosing in animal models identifies threshold pharmacokinetic (PK) blood levels beyond which direct exposure-related hepatotoxicity occurs [28, 29]. PK derived measurements (e.g., Cmax levels, AUC per unit time) that best predict a threshold for toxicity vary and are influenced by a number of factors including dose response effects in liver cells and half-life of the study drug. Unfortunately, with the exception of agents that are direct hepatotoxins such as CCl_4 or acetaminophen (when misused in excessive amounts), blood levels of drugs or drug metabolites often correlate poorly with risk for serious idiosyncratic hepatotoxicity. This is due to a number of interrelated reasons. First, the discrepancy of drug concentrations in liver cells vs blood or plasma that build up over time with maintenance treatment vary depending on the drug, hepatic blood flow, and cellular uptake [30–32]. When parent drug or intermediate metabolite levels are toxic at a cellular site above threshold amounts, their distribution between the circulation and liver cells is critically important. If after multiple dosing the drug hepatocyte concentrations greatly exceed blood levels because of high cellular uptake, PK measures may not reliably predict threshold drug levels of toxicity. Second, rates of drug clearance and metabolism to nontoxic products both in the liver and other organs are determinants of residual cellular parent drug or toxic metabolite levels. Third, hepatocytes are endowed with a reservoir of cytoprotective substrates (e.g., glutathione, UDP-glucuronic acid) that are subject to depletion in certain clinical settings [33, 34]. In the case of some hepatotoxic agents, these must be saturated before toxic metabolites are able to bind and disrupt cellular molecules that are vital to sustain normal functions. Fourth, if hepatotoxicity is primarily driven by one of a number of immune mechanisms (e.g., adaptive, innate, or autoimmune processes) the drug or its metabolites may not be directly toxic to cells. In these circumstances once immune-mediated hepatocellular damage is unleashed, the course of DILI will often not be tied to PK indicators per se, but rather to steps involved in drug-related antigen presentation on the surface of liver and/or biliary epithelial cells and/or modulation of immunocyte responses.

5   Clinical Evaluation of Cases of Acute Liver Injury Associated with a Suspect Agent

In the evaluation of the severity of acute liver injury associated with a suspect agent, an approach that has been used both by the NIH Drug-induced Liver Injury Network (DILIN) and the FDA is a five-level categorical scale comprised of tiers with specified clinical and biochemical outcomes [35, 36] (Table 2). These range from very mild cases marked by transient elevations of serum liver aminotransferase levels [ALT or aspartate aminotransferase (AST)] in the absence of both significant clinical symptoms and elevations of bilirubin or other markers of liver dysfunction (Level—1 Severity) to very severe cases marked by ALF with an outcome of death or liver transplant (Level—5 Severity). Assessing the causality or likelihood of a causal association of a case of acute liver injury with exposure to the suspect agent can be especially challenging since, so far, there are no diagnostic or predictive biomarkers of DILI which are fully reliable and accurate. Therefore, the application of comprehensive

Table 2
Drug-induced Liver Injury (DILI) Severity Index [35, 36]

Score	Grade	Definition
1	Mild	Patient has elevation in ALT and/or alkaline phosphatase levels but total serum bilirubin is <2.5 mg/dL *and* INR is <1.5
2	Moderate	Patient has elevation in ALT and/or alkaline phosphatase levels *and* serum bilirubin is ≥2.5 mg/dL *or* INR is ≥1.5
3	Moderate–severe	Patient has elevation in ALT, alkaline phosphatase, bilirubin and/or INR levels *and* patient is hospitalized or an ongoing hospitalization is prolonged because of DILI
4	Severe	Patient has elevation in ALT and/or alkaline phosphatase levels *and* total serum bilirubin is ≥2.5 mg/dL and there is at least one of the following: (1) prolonged jaundice and symptoms beyond 3 months, (2) hepatic failure (INR ≥1.5, ascites or encephalopathy), or (3) other organ failure believed to be due to DILI event
5	Fatal	Patient dies or undergoes liver transplantation because of DILI event

ALT alanine aminotransferase, *INR* international normalized ratio

differential diagnosis to exclude alternative causes of liver injury other than the suspect agent underlies all the commonly described methods that are used for causality assessment of suspected DILI cases [9, 37]. The Roussel Uclaf Causality Assessment Method (RUCAM) that was developed under the auspices of the Council for International Organizations of Medical Sciences (CIOMS) in the early 1990s is one of a number of previously published DILI algorithmic scoring systems that can be applied with ease by practitioners at the bedside, often when DILI is suspected to be linked to a marketed drug [38–40]. As described in Chap. 27 in this volume, the RUCAM utilizes specified numbers of award or penalty points that are distributed in a set of domains that are designed to either support or diminish a causal link of acute hepatocellular or cholestatic liver injury with any drug or biologic agent. (The domains include point assignments based on treatment time and liver injury onset, latency after treatment discontinuation and biochemical recovery, exclusion of alternative causes, a few general risk factors, etc.) Using one common scale for the RUCAM, the measured total score for a suspect case of DILI determines a categorical level of the likelihood of causal association with the suspect agent that ranges between "highly probable" and "unlikely."

Notably, the current version of the RUCAM is a "one-size shoe fits all" algorithm with one fixed set of criteria to assess causality in the presence of acute hepatocellular injury and another in the presence of cholestatic liver injury. Unfortunately, the clinical signatures of acute idiopathic DILI as well as known risk factors for hepatotoxicity are not uniform and are influenced by a variety of different primary pathogenic mechanisms and susceptibility characteristics associated with DILI that have been implicated with exposure to particular drugs, drug classes or biological products. Thus, the ranges and weightings of point awards or penalties imposed in the RUCAM domains (e.g., time boundaries from start of treatment until liver injury, time boundaries from the discontinuation of treatment until biochemical recovery, the age range, and the use of alcohol) may not be relevant or suitable to optimally determine the likelihood of causal association of liver injury with certain suspect agents. For this reason, to preserve an algorithmic approach for causality assessment there has been a growing interest to establish a set of refined algorithms that can be selectively matched with a defined phenotype or clinical signature of acute DILI associated with a particular drug or biologic agent. Using registry data analyses, efforts are underway both in Europe and in the USA to test the utility of modifying algorithmic criteria differently for different drugs and biologic agents [41, 42].

5.1 Assessing DILI in Clinical Study Subjects

In drug development programs, a method that is typically used to assess the likelihood of causal association of cases of liver injury that occur in temporal association with exposure to the study agent relies on "expert opinion" [37, 43]. This non-algorithmic approach provides flexibility in the determination, analysis, and weighting of critical determinants for case assessment by a panel of individuals with expertise in analyzing various DILI phenotypes and clinical signatures. It is especially useful in the assessment of cases of liver injury tied to new agents when a recognized phenotype or clinical signature of hepatotoxicity has not yet been established or publicized. Although less structured compared with fixed algorithms such as the RUCAM, investigators and regulatory scientists using "expert opinion" have developed shared nomenclatures and common instruments for case assessment. One such instrument used by the NIH DILIN project as well as by FDA regulatory scientists is a categorical likelihood scale encompassing five tiers of probability of causal association of an acute liver injury event with exposure to a suspect drug or biologic agent [3, 35, 36] (Table 3).

Expert opinion provides distinct advantages in the assessment of idiosyncratic forms of acute DILI connected to mechanisms and/or clinical signatures that do not necessarily conform to the stereotypes embodied in the RUCAM. The importance of recognizing different types of acute idiosyncratic hepatocellular DILI associated with products that represent new classes of therapeutic drugs or biologic agents has been increasing in attention in recent years. Some examples described below illustrate this phenomenon.

Table 3
Categorical causality assessment scoring system based on expert opinion [3, 35, 36]

Causality score	Likelihood (%)	Description
1 = definite	>95	Liver injury is typical for the drug or herbal product ("signature" or pattern of injury, timing of onset, recovery) The evidence for causality is "beyond a reasonable doubt"
2 = highly likely	75–95	The evidence for causality is "clear and convincing" but not definite
3 = probable	50–74	The causality is supported by "the preponderance of evidence" as implicating the drug but the evidence cannot be considered definite or highly likely
4 = possible	25–49	The causality is not supported by "the preponderance of evidence"; however, one cannot definitively exclude the possibility
5 = unlikely	<25	The evidence for causality is "highly unlikely" based upon the available information
6 = insufficient data	Not applicable	Key elements of the drug exposure history, initial presentation, alternative diagnoses, and/or diagnostic evaluation prevent one from determining a causality score

5.1.1   Evaluation of Acute DILI Signals in Clinical Trials with eDISH

As described elsewhere in Chap. 20 in this volume, graphic programs that display in a multidimensional matrix peak serum liver test results of each individual study subject in a clinical trial population treated with the study agent or comparator are highly valuable to efficiently identify and focus attention on those subjects with test abnormalities of interest for further analysis. One such program is eDISH (acronym for "evaluation of Drug-Induced Serious Hepatotoxicity") [44, 45]. This two-dimensional graphic representation of peak serum ALT and bilirubin levels is divided into four domains defined by boundaries that represent a threshold multiple of the upper limits of normal for each of the indicators (ALT, 3X ULN; Bilirubin; 2X ULN). [In future generations of this program, the demarcations of these boundaries would be adjustable by analysts to interrogate changes over a subject's pretreatment baseline values or the inclusion of other liver test indicators (AST, ALP, etc.).] By clicking on a case of interest in the treatment-population-based display, the program opens a graphic timeline of liver test findings at baseline and during the treatment course of the study accompanied by a narrative with clinical and diagnostic information to support an assessment of causal association with the test agent.

6   Interpretation of DILI Case Signatures in Clinical Studies

6.1   Adaptation

In randomized clinical studies of agents that are causally linked to cases of idiosyncratic hepatotoxicity, it is not unusual to observe a higher percentage of study subjects receiving the study drug relative to the comparator agent or placebo who develop mild transient elevations of liver serum aminotransferases (AT, e.g., ALT and/or AST) early during the course of treatment. It is notable that reversal of these abnormalities often occurs even with continued dosing with the agent due to a cellular and organ-based cytoprotective and regenerative corrective response that is referred to as "adaptation" [3, 46]. With certain drugs used in dose ranges recommended in product labels (e.g., acetaminophen, tacrine), transient mild elevations of AT in exposed individuals are not uncommon, yet progression to serious liver injury virtually never occurs. Drugs associated with idiosyncratic hepatotoxicity often also induce transient AT abnormalities that reverse in many drug-exposed individuals due to adaptation. However, for reasons that remain to be elucidated, a subset of individuals with liver test abnormalities associated with each of these agents do not manifest an adaptive response, and the liver injury progresses to more severe forms connected to compromised liver function and in some instances acute liver failure. The percentages of individuals with mild transient ALT abnormalities with adaptation versus those with progression to severe liver injury depend both on the specific drug and susceptibility characteristics that are prevalent in the treatment population. To illustrate, based on different literature sources, the approximate incidences of mild transient rises of AT >3X ULN in clinical trial subjects treated with isoniazid (INH), troglitazone, and ximelagatran were ~10%, ~3%, and ~8% respectively, whereas the incidences of drug-induced ALF were <0.1%, <0.05%, and <0.05%, respectively [9, 12].

6.2 "Classic" Idiosyncratic Acute Hepatocellular DILI

Drugs and biological agents have been linked to a number of different clinical and laboratory signatures of hepatotoxicity that can be clinically serious [1, 47]. A classic form of hepatotoxicity is associated with latency periods typically ranging between 1 week and 3–6 months or even longer between start of treatment and the development of DILI marked by the onset of abnormal liver tests [48]. Although more than one inciting mechanism may be linked to classic idiosyncratic hepatotoxicity, both innate and adaptive immune responses to the accumulation of drug metabolites in hepatocytes are considered frequent drivers of liver injury.

A two-step graphic example using the eDISH instrument of this type of idiosyncratic hepatotoxicity in a phase III clinical trial of 3922 study subjects who were randomized to receive ximelagatran (X) (a direct thrombin inhibitor) or warfarin, the control drug (C), to prevent stroke and embolic events in patients with chronic non-valvular atrial fibrillation is shown in Fig. 1a and b. As shown in the right upper quadrant of Fig. 1a, there is a striking imbalance in the number of ximelagatran-treated subjects who developed elevations of both ALT and total bilirubin, compared to those treated with warfarin. A time-course of the serum liver test results together with a diagnostic analysis of one of these ximelagatran-treated individuals, excluding other causes of acute liver injury, is shown in Fig. 1b in order to exemplify findings that are consistent with "Hy's law." Ximelagatran was not approved for marketing in the USA because of its hepatotoxic profile.

6.3 Cholestatic Hepatitis

Different drug-derived antigenic molecules may form complexes with Class II HLA molecules on the surface of antigen-presenting cells, including biliary epithelial cells in biliary ductules. Immune responses to these antigenic determinants with recruitment of mononuclear cells and other inflammatory cells are likely one avenue leading to cholestatic hepatitis. This form of DILI is often marked by a prominent inflammatory infiltrate in the portal areas without significant parenchymal injury within the hepatic lobules. It is clinically associated with jaundice and pruritis, even when the hepatocellular functions of protein, clotting factor, and urea synthesis may be normally preserved. Because both cholangiocytes and/or the apical membranes of hepatocytes are selectively involved in this form of drug-associated injury, the serum ALP levels are substantially increased and R values are typically less than 2 [3].

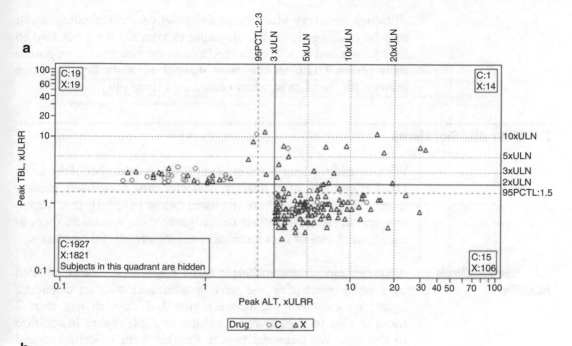

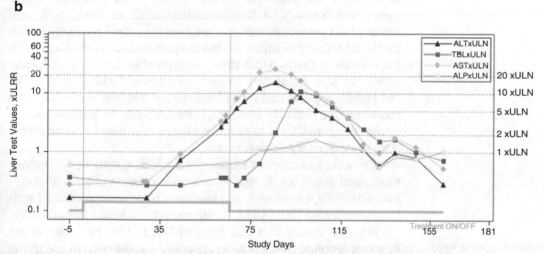

Fig. 1 (a) eDISH plot containing the peak values of serum alanine aminotransferase (ALT) activities and total bilirubin (TBL) levels of each study subject with chronic non-valvular atrial fibrillation in SPORTIF V, a phase III randomized trial of ximelagatran 36 mg bid (X, *red triangles; n* = 1960) vs warfarin (C, *green circles; n* = 1962) for the prevention of stroke and systemic embolic events [101]. The ALT and TBL values are plotted as the fold increases above the upper limit of the reference ranges (ULRR) on the *x* axis and *y* axis, respectively. (b) Time course of serum liver test results of a study subject of interest in the right upper quadrant of (a) (*ALT* alanine aminotransferase, *AST* aspartate aminotransferase, *TBL* total bilirubin, *ALP* alkaline phosphatase, *ULN* upper limit of normal, PCTL percentile) [101]. The subject is an 80 year old female randomized to receive ximelagatran. Elevated liver tests occurred 2 months after initiation of ximelagatran in the absence of symptoms, leading to its discontinuation 4 days later and a switch to treatment with warfarin. Serological test results for Hepatitis A, B, and C, CMV and EBV, as well as ANA and SMA, at the time of the liver injury were all negative. The liver tests eventually returned to normal. This case of acute hepatocellular DILI demonstrates findings that are consistent with "Hy's law"

Although recovery after discontinuation of the offending agent may be prolonged, cholestatic hepatitis typically does not lead to liver failure and is not considered as an ominous marker of potentially severe DILI, in the same manner as acute hepatocellular injury with jaundice is, when caused by a drug [49].

7   Other DILI Signatures

With expanding drug development programs a number of the acute DILI signatures with distinct characteristics have been gaining increased attention and are discussed below [47, 50]. It is important for regulatory scientists to recognize these and assess them as significant forms of hepatotoxicity that require careful evaluation.

7.1   Immunoallergic Hepatitis

Although rare, immunoallergic DILI reactions are often marked by a rapid onset after the start of treatment with an offending agent, typically ranging between just 1–2 days to less than 2 months. Due to their systemic nature, multiple organs in addition to the liver are potential targets for this form of drug-induced injury and features of hypersensitivity such as fever, rash, and eosinophilia are frequently present. Notably, rapid recurrence with increased severity of injury occurs frequently after rechallenge with the offending agent. More than one type of immunological hypersensitivity may be at play in immunoallergic DILI (Types I–IV) [51] and it appears that rechallenge either with the same drug or a cross-reactive similarly structured drug is likely to put the patient at significant risk for a hepatotoxic event that may be more severe than the earlier sensitizing event.

Of note, a number of antibiotics, including sulfa drugs, quinolones, and ketolides, as well as aromatic anticonvulsants, allopurinol, celecoxib, nevaripine, and efavirenz have been associated with immunoallergic DILI [52]. Telithromycin-induced immunoallergic hepatitis exemplifies this form of DILI. This antibiotic is the first oral ketolide that has been approved for short-term use in the USA. A review of 42 post-marketing cases of acute liver injury in 2006 revealed a clinical signature marked by rapid acceleration of liver injury and very short latencies after treatment initiation ranging between 2 and 43 days with a median of only 10 days. Four cases had known previous telithromycin exposure pointing to the possibility of prior sensitization [53]. Some cases were also marked by the acute onset of fever, abdominal pain, and jaundice, with in some instances reported eosinophilia and/or ascites.

7.2   Autoimmune Hepatitis Associated with Immunotherapy

Immunologically based therapies encompass different products including pharmaceutical drugs, biological agents, and even some herbals. They are part of global treatment strategies under development either to *enhance* immune destruction of tumor cells in oncological diseases or *reduce* immune-mediated destruction of tissues in some autoimmune diseases. Intended treatment effects of immunotherapy may include one of the following goals: (1) increase the activities of subpopulations of T-cells or other immune cells that recognize and act to eliminate tumor cells, (2) reduce the activities of subpopulations of T-cells that directly target diseased tissues in autoimmune pathological states (e.g., the myelin sheath in multiple sclerosis), (3) change the balance of effector and regulatory cells in T-cell networks in favor of reducing autoimmune states. Molecular targets for pharmacological therapy within such a broad set of possible therapeutic objectives include specific cell surface molecules or ligands have biological roles to either modify or regulate T-cell function or proliferation.

In oncotherapy, targeted molecules for drug and biologic development by immunotherapy have been the checkpoint inhibitors [54, 55]. These include therapeutic human or humanized monoclonal antibodies directed against the cell surface molecules CTLA-4 and PD-1 (or their ligands) whose normal function is to dampen T-cell activation by costimulatory pathways when the TCR is engaged by a cognate antigen. Monoclonal products that are currently approved include ipilimumab, nivolumab, pembrolizumab, atezolizumab, avelumab, and durvalumab. When normally active, checkpoint inhibitors act as "brakes" to prevent the overactivity of autoreactive T-cells as well as the diminished suppressive functions of FOXP3+ T regulatory cells. Thus, when these pathways are inhibited by targeted therapies, antitumor immune response activities are generally enhanced, especially against immunogenic tumors including melanoma and certain lung tumors. Due to the nonselective nature and broad polyclonal hyperimmune treatment effects of checkpoint inhibitors, it is no surprise that both in animal models and in human studies the blockade of CTLA-4 and PD-1 mediated pathways by monoclonal antibodies is frequently associated with a broad range of unintended autoimmune toxicities in different organs, including the colon (which normally contains a small pool of intraepithelial lymphocytes), skin, liver, lung, and a number of endocrine organs. Although targeted for treatment, whether metastatic infiltrating tumor cells in organs, such as the liver, have a potential to exacerbate autoimmune injury due to the recruitment of increased numbers of inflammatory cells with consequent collateral damage effects is a concern that will require more study. Thus, treatment-induced AIH often presenting between 6 and 12 weeks after initiation of treatment (which can be clinically severe and lead to ALF) has been identified in clinical trials as a significant adverse event causally associated with checkpoint inhibitors [56–60].

Many cell surface molecules that are selectively targeted by immunotherapies to treat certain autoimmune diseases are expressed in different subsets of helper, effector, and regulatory cells in T-cell networks that normally demonstrate immunological homeostasis by maintaining a careful balance of the counteracting cell populations to prevent pathological states of autoimmunity. A number of immunomodulatory therapies intended to inhibit immune cell mediated damage of the myelin sheath in the treatment of MS, somewhat paradoxically have been associated with the induction of AIH. These include pegylated and non-pegylated IFN-α and IFN-β products, and glatiramer acetate [61–67]. Because the advent of immune-related diatheses including acute liver injury linked to immunomodulatory therapy may be tied to imbalances of T cell subpopulations that normally counteract one another, their clinical signatures are often different from other forms of hepatotoxicity, including "classic" idiosyncratic DILI described above. With the characteristic histopathologic features of AIH that often accompany these cases, long latencies greater than 6 months from initiation of treatment until the onset of liver injury may be present. These probably reflect gradual shifts in the proportions of autoreactive cells and regulatory T cells (Tregs) during long-term treatment or after a long washout period at the end of treatment with disparate recovery times of each T-cell subset.

Daclizumab, an IgG1 monoclonal antibody that inhibits the high affinity IL-2 receptor (CD25), has been linked to cases of treatment-induced AIH and other autoimmune adverse events in clinical trials of patients with relapsing forms of MS [68, 69]. Peak elevations of aminotransferase levels greater than 5X ULN which were often transient were observed in 4% study subjects with MS treated with Daclizumab High Yield Process (DAC HYP), compared with <1% of subjects treated with placebo in SELECT, a placebo-controlled phase IIB study to assess the efficacy and safety of the monoclonal treatment for 1 year [68, 70]. Notably, in the DAC HYP development program, one study subject developed treatment-induced ALF in an extension study. Although myelin sheath damaging CD25+ effector cells are inhibited, suppression of FOXP3+ Tregs which also express CD25 occurs and is long-lasting, possibly leading to prolonged reduced suppression of autoreactive T-cells. The recovery period of the Treg populations after administration of the last monthly DAC HYP dose upon cessation of treatment is gradual (5–6 months) and plausibly extends beyond the time of recovery of autoreactive T-cell populations [70]. Such a phenomenon may underlie a long latency with a median time to the onset of clinically significant idiosyncratic hepatotoxicity of 13 months after DAC HYP initiation observed in study subjects with MS who were treated with the monoclonal agent.

8   DILI in Patients with Underlying Liver Disease

As described above, rises of both serum liver AT (i.e., ALT and AST) levels with R values >5 are the sine qua non for hepatocellular injury. As the severity of DILI worsens with reduced liver function, there is a rise of bilirubin that reflects its reduced cellular excretion into the bile. Because patients with significant preexisting liver diseases such as chronic viral hepatitis or NASH have abnormal liver test results at baseline, it can be difficult to measure and characterize the relative effects of acute liver injury that are superimposed on chronic liver disease. Since AT levels with NASH are often increased at baseline, it has been suggested that the detection and investigation of suspected acute DILI can be driven by an observed change of serum AT, ALP, and bilirubin levels with reference to the pretreatment baseline levels of the individual, rather than a population-based upper limit of normal value [9, 71, 72]. A reliable assessment of the severity of the acute hepatotoxic injury based on quantitative changes of these indicators above their abnormal pretreatment levels is challenging. Future progress in this sphere will depend on the acquisition of patient-level longitudinal data to evaluate acute injury effects superimposed on different stages of specific preexisting liver diseases. It is notable that liver test findings of severe acute hepatocellular injury either induced by a drug or another cause in individuals with chronic liver disease complicated by moderate or severe cirrhosis can be marked by worsening liver function that may include a rising bilirubin level, an increasing INR and encephalopathy in the absence of a substantial change in ALT or AST levels [73]. In its most severe form, this signature has been referred to as acute on chronic liver failure and is associated with a high risk for poor outcomes, including death. As an example, rare forms of acute DILI with this type of signature have been reported in association with the direct antiviral agent treatment combination of dasabuvir, ombitasvir, paritaprevir, and ritonavir to treat Type C viral hepatitis [74, 75]. Hepatic decompensation and hepatic failure, including liver transplantation or fatal outcomes, have been reported postmarketing in patients treated with the components of this product. Most patients with these severe outcomes had evidence of advanced cirrhosis prior to initiating therapy. Reported cases typically occurred within 1–4 weeks of initiating therapy and were characterized by the acute onset of a rising direct serum bilirubin without further rising ALT elevations above baseline levels in association with clinical signs and symptoms of hepatic decompensation. With a paucity of studies that have enrolled substantial numbers of individuals with advanced chronic liver disease, in order to limit risk for this adverse event in susceptible patients, use of the product has been contraindicated in chronic liver disease patients with moderate and severe hepatic impairment (Child Pugh Class B and C).

As observed by Zimmerman and described in the premarketing guidance on DILI, in general terms the presence of underlying liver disease, including cirrhosis, does not appear to alter or increase an individual's risk for the development of idiosyncratic hepatotoxicity [5]. However, there are a number of important caveats or exceptions with regard to this assertion. First, because patients with moderate or severe liver disease have more limited reserve as regards biological and physiological functions that must be intact in order for the liver to optimally recover after acute liver injury, outcomes in patients with DILI may be compromised in some circumstances. For example, prior studies identified more severe idiosyncratic outcomes in patients with chronic viral hepatitis with hepatotoxicity causally associated with antituberculosis (TB) drugs compared to similarly treated patients without underlying viral hepatitis [76, 77]. In other studies, patients with Hepatitis B or C Virus (HBV or HCV) coinfected with Human Immunodeficiency Virus (HIV) who developed hepatotoxicity as a result of Highly Active Antiretroviral Therapy (HAART) were found to have more serious liver injuries [78, 79]. Second, exceptions exist in which certain underlying liver diseases that may be silent are likely to increase susceptibility to the development of DILI after exposure to specific treatment agents. A recent example is a concern that patients with quiescent or subclinical idiopathic AIH have increased susceptibility to clinically significant acute liver injury induced by immunomodulatory agents. To illustrate, as described above, daclizumab has been linked in clinical trials both to the induction of de novo AIH, as well as an unmasking of subclinical idiopathic AIH by a treatment-induced shift in T-cell homeostasis that is associated with the suppression of FOXP3+ Tregs [80].

9   Risk Factors for Idiosyncratic DILI

Different risk factors for DILI have been identified and are described in Chap. 23 in this volume. None of these have proven universal for any drug that is linked to DILI in all patient populations. Nonetheless, some appear to be more generalizable to multiple agents, compared with others. Among these, as listed in the RUCAM are geriatric age, chronic alcohol usage, and pregnancy. DILI risk factors may be associated with a change in hepatocellular uptake, metabolism, transport, and/or a reduction in renal clearance of the parent drug or its metabolites [33, 81]. By increasing levels of hepatocellular or subcellular exposure to these molecules, these changes may lead to liver injury or cholestasis in susceptible individuals. It is notable that a few drugs appear to be associated with a higher risk for hepatotoxicity in infants and children, rather than in the elderly. One example, valproic acid (VPA) appears to be linked to an increased risk for idiosyncratic severe liver injury in pediatric patients less than 2 years, through one or more mechanisms of mitochondrial toxicity including the production of reactive metabolites in mitochondria that are derived from 4-ene-VPA, a metabolite of the parent molecule [82, 83]. Other risk factors include the presence of certain neurological disorders and concomitant use of other anticonvulsants [84].

There are certain genomic polymorphisms that are associated with an increased risk for DILI. These appear to have an impact on adaptive immune responses to a particular agent or class of agents. Categories of polymorphic molecules and examples of drugs that have been linked to an increased risk for DILI when a polymorphism is present include Class I and Class II HLA molecules (e.g., amoxicillin-clavulanate [85, 86], ximelagatran [87], lumaricoxib [88], flucloxicillin [89], ticlopidine [90], lapatinib [91]), drug-metabolizing enzymes (e.g., Cytochrome P450 isoform 2E1 and isoniazid [92, 93]), apical membrane transporters (e.g., the BSEP apical transporter and oral contraceptives [94]), and vital cellular systems subjected to toxic stress due to exposure to the xenobiotic (e.g., mitochondrial DNA Polymerase γ and valproic acid [95]). These DNA polymorphisms which serve as markers of high risk alleles for DILI have been identified by-and-large through targeted gene analysis or genome-wide association studies (GWAS), using biospecimens collected from patients who developed liver injury that was causally associated with a suspect drug, compared with patients without this adverse event, in case control studies [3, 96]. Although they differ according to the suspect drug and are connected to different pathways, the contribution of any of these to the overall risk for clinically serious idiosyncratic DILI is typically low, pointing to the combinatorial influences of other risk factors as well [97].

10   Approaches to Monitor and Manage Study Subjects for DILI in Clinical Trials

A mainstay of management of DILI is the early recognition and comprehensive evaluation of the event with a timely discontinuation of the suspect agent to avoid progression to clinically severe or irreversible hepatotoxicity. To address measurement of DILI risk, the FDA guidance on premarketing assessment of DILI has recommended that all study subjects undergo regular serum liver test monitoring and clinical evaluation with specified intervals during the course of clinical trials [9]. When ALT and/or AST levels are increased, the guidance contains guideposts for more frequent monitoring, trigger points for clinical and diagnostic evaluation, and stop rules, the latter to protect study subjects from the development of severe or life-threatening hepatotoxicity.

In the absence of reliable predictive biomarkers, the approach taken to prevent or treat DILI depends heavily on clinical considerations. Use of corticosteroids may have a role in the management of immunoallergic forms of DILI, although studies to determine the benefit of this treatment on outcomes are typically lacking [14]. However, because of the relatively high frequency of AIH as an adverse event associated with immunotherapy with checkpoint inhibitors and other immune-modulators, the use of corticosteroids has been embedded in clinical trial protocols to manage this and other autoimmune events that are triggered by treatment with these agents. As a result, product labels for these products contain recommendations for their use in the management of clinically serious AIH [69, 98]. In addition, for cases of persistent severe hepatitis not responsive to high-dose corticosteroids, some labels also describe the use of other immunosuppressive agents (e.g., mycophenolate mofetil) based on clinical trial protocols [99].

11 Methods to Refine DILI Risk Assessment with Post-Marketing Tools

A listing of post-marketing data streams used to detect, assess, and refine a risk of DILI connected to specific drugs and biologic agents is provided in Table 4. These are also described in Chap. 22 in this volume. With reference to the critically important twin goals of the early and reliable detection of cases of serious and life-threatening DILI causally associated with a marketed drug or biological agent, and the accurate quantitation of risk for such events in the "real-world" treatment population, each of these methods has both important strengths and limitations [37].

The continued DILI risk assessment may be part of routine pharmacovigilance performed by both regulators and applicants, or it may consist of a more formal surveillance given the perceived or known risks from premarketing data. These evaluations could consist of registries, enhanced pharmacovigilance (i.e., targeted follow-up), or postmarketing studies. The reliance of spontaneously reported data likely leads to detection of new risk information later in a product's life cycle given the inherent limitations of spontaneous data (e.g., underreporting, reports with limited clinical details). However, spontaneous reporting systems such as the FDA Adverse Events Reporting System (FAERS) which receives more than one million adverse event reports each year represent a relatively cost-effective approach to monitoring risk related to drugs and biologic agents. In contrast, postmarketing studies may characterize a newly marketed drug with a better quantification of the risk for DILI. These studies impose a cost on the applicant and often suffer from study design feasibility issues, particularly for orphan products. Despite these limitations, both sources of data have led to important post-market regulatory actions.

Table 4
Post marketing data streams that inform DILI risk assessment for specific marketed drugs

Data source	Examples	Benefits	Limitations
Spontaneous report databases	FAERS, VigiBase	Large repositories of reports for postmarketing DILI signaling accessible in real-time; measures of disproportionate reporting of adverse events	Underreporting; variable quality of information; reporting biases; cannot estimate DILI incidence
Peer-reviewed case reports	Journal articles describing DILI cases	Clinical DILI signatures and diagnostic tests typically described	Variable quality of information and case ascertainment; time delay until publication; publication bias
Registries	DILIN, ALFSG	Structures clinical and diagnostic assessments; real-world sampling of suspect DILI cases	Enrollees reflect referral system biases
Observational studies	CPRD, CMS	Linkages of adverse events and drug exposures to medical records enable investigations of risk	Reliant on adequate capture and coding of exposures, confounders, and outcomes; potential for unmeasured confounding; time delay in data acquisition and analysis

ALFSG Acute Liver Failure Study Group, *CMS* Centers for Medicare/Medicaid, *CPRD* Clinical Practice Research Datalink, *DILI* drug-induced liver injury, *DILIN* Drug-Induced Liver Injury Network, *FAERS* FDA Adverse Event Reporting System

While postmarketing data has frequently informed labeling modifications describing increased risks, ambrisentan is an example in which postmarketing data has informed the de-escalation of labeling. Ambrisentan was the second FDA approved endothelin receptor antagonist (ERA) approved to treat pulmonary arterial hypertension (PAH). The first ERA, bosentan, was approved in 2001 with a Risk Minimization Action Plan (RiskMAP) to manage hepatic toxicity and teratogenicity. Both the teratogenic and hepatic effects were thought to be ERA class related, although there was little preclinical or clinical trial evidence of hepatotoxicity for ambrisentan. Nonetheless, ambrisentan was approved with a similar RiskMAP, which linked drug access to patient-reported monthly liver testing. After several years of marketing experience, the totality of the postmarketing evidence surrounding ambrisentan aligned with the preclinical evidence and pointed to a relatively low hepatotoxic risk associated with this drug. Therefore, liver injury associated with ambrisentan was removed from the product label's Boxed Warning in 2011 [100].

12   Search for DILI Biomarkers and Future Directions/Opportunities

The development and validation of reliable predictors of DILI would provide an extremely valuable set of guideposts to enhance drug development and risk management. As described above, the initiation of DILI and progression to serious liver injury is a multi-step process that involves individual susceptibility factors, xenobiotic processing steps, and a host of cellular responses with adaptation or increased inflammation, necrosis and/or apoptosis resulting in either organ repair or amplified damage. At each step effective biomarkers could be leveraged as useful predictors of DILI outcomes. Overall, there is a need for biomarkers that (1) predict which drugs or biologic agents will cause idiosyncratic DILI, (2) portend serious liver cell injury before progression has taken place, and (3) identify individuals who are especially susceptible to DILI caused by a specific agent [3]. Because of the complexities and redundancies of pathways that protect the liver from xenobiotic-induced toxicity, it is not surprising that current candidate biomarkers in each of these categories fall short in their predictive powers. However, with further discovery and elucidation of the critical xenobiotic characteristics and biological pathways that impact risk for hepatotoxicity as described in Chap. 26 in this volume, our ability to model and forecast DILI during drug development is expected to improve significantly.

Disclaimer

The views expressed are those of the authors and do not necessarily represent the position of, nor imply an endorsement from, the US Food and Drug Administration or the US Government.

References

1. Fontana RJ (2014) Pathogenesis of idiosyncratic drug-induced liver injury and clinical perspectives. Gastroenterology 146(4):914–928. https://doi.org/10.1053/j.gastro.2013.12.032
2. Watkins PB, Kaplowitz N, Slattery JT, Colonese CR, Colucci SV, Stewart PW, Harris SC (2006) Aminotransferase elevations in healthy adults receiving 4 grams of acetaminophen daily: a randomized controlled trial. JAMA 296(1):87–93. https://doi.org/10.1001/jama.296.1.87
3. Avigan MI (2013) Regulatory perspectives. In: Kaplowitz N, Deleve LD (eds) Drug-induced liver disease, 3rd edn. Academic Press, London, UK, pp 689–712
4. Enhancing Benefit-Risk Assessment in Regulatory Decision-Making. Available: https://www.fda.gov/ForIndustry/UserFees/PrescriptionDrugUserFee/ucm326192.htm. Accessed 18 Mar 2017
5. Hepatotoxicity (textbook) first edition (1978) Zimmerman Chapter 16, p 349–369
6. Malchow-Moller A, Matzen P, Bjerregaard B, Hilden J, Holst-Christensen J, Staehr Johansen T, Altman L, Thomsen C, Juhl E (1981) Causes and characteristics of 500 consecutive cases of jaundice. Scand J Gastroenterol 16(1):1–6
7. Reuben A (2004) Hy's law. Hepatology 39(2):574–578. https://doi.org/10.1002/hep.20081

8. Temple R (2006) Hy's law: predicting serious hepatotoxicity. Pharmacoepidemiol Drug Saf 15(4):241–243. https://doi.org/10.1002/pds.1211

9. Guidance for Industry Drug-Induced Liver Injury: Premarketing Clinical Evaluation, Final, July 2009

10. Graham DJ, Drinkard CR, Shatin D (2003) Incidence of idiopathic acute liver failure and hospitalized liver injury in patients treated with troglitazone. Am J Gastroenterol 98(1):175–179. https://doi.org/10.1111/j.1572-0241.2003.07175.x

11. Graham DJ, Drinkard CR, Shatin D, Tsong Y, Burgess MJ (2001) Liver enzyme monitoring in patients treated with troglitazone. JAMA 286(7):831–833

12. Knowler WC, Hamman RF, Edelstein SL, Barrett-Connor E, Ehrmann DA, Walker EA, Fowler SE, Nathan DM, Kahn SE, Diabetes Prevention Program Research G (2005) Prevention of type 2 diabetes with troglitazone in the Diabetes Prevention Program. Diabetes 54(4):1150–1156

13. Rosner B (1995) The binomial distribution. In: Rosner B (ed) Fundamentals of biostatistics. Duxbury Press, Belmont, CA, pp 82–85

14. Chalasani NP, Hayashi PH, Bonkovsky HL, Navarro VJ, Lee WM, Fontana RJ, Practice Parameters Committee of the American College of Gastroenterology (2014) ACG Clinical Guideline: the diagnosis and management of idiosyncratic drug-induced liver injury. Am J Gastroenterol 109(7):950–966.; quiz 967. https://doi.org/10.1038/ajg.2014.131

15. Avigan MI, Bjornsson ES, Pasanen M, Cooper C, Andrade RJ, Watkins PB, Lewis JH, Merz M (2014) Liver safety assessment: required data elements and best practices for data collection and standardization in clinical trials. Drug Saf 37(Suppl 1):S19–S31. https://doi.org/10.1007/s40264-014-0183-6

16. Kullak-Ublick GA, Merz M, Griffel L, Kaplowitz N, Watkins PB (2014) Liver safety assessment in special populations (hepatitis B, C, and oncology trials). Drug Saf 37(Suppl 1):S57–S62. https://doi.org/10.1007/s40264-014-0186-3

17. Fried MW. Acute hepatotoxicity in HCV-cirrhotic patients treated with direct-acting antiviral agents. In: 2016 drug induced liver injury annual conference proceedings. Available: http://www.aasld.org/2016-drug-induced-liver-injury-annual-conference-proceedings

18. Fontana RJ. Diagnosis and management of DILI in NASH patients. In: 2016 drug induced liver injury annual conference proceedings. Available: http://www.aasld.org/2016-drug-induced-liver-injury-annual-conference-proceedings

19. Regev A. DILI due to cancer-immunotherapy targeting immune checkpoints: when and how to treat. In: 2016 drug induced liver injury annual conference proceedings. Available: http://www.aasld.org/2016-drug-induced-liver-injury-annual-conference-proceedings

20. Lin C, Khetani SR (2016) Advances in engineered liver models for investigating drug-induced liver injury. Biomed Res Int 2016:1829148. https://doi.org/10.1155/2016/1829148

21. Ware BR, Berger DR, Khetani SR (2015) Prediction of drug-induced liver injury in micropatterned co-cultures containing iPSC-derived human hepatocytes. Toxicol Sci 145(2):252–262. https://doi.org/10.1093/toxsci/kfv048

22. Trask OJ Jr, Moore A, LeCluyse EL (2014) A micropatterned hepatocyte coculture model for assessment of liver toxicity using high-content imaging analysis. Assay Drug Dev Technol 12(1):16–27. https://doi.org/10.1089/adt.2013.525

23. Donato MT, Gomez-Lechon MJ, Tolosa L (2017) Using high-content screening technology for studying drug-induced hepatotoxicity in preclinical studies. Expert Opin Drug Discov 12(2):201–211. https://doi.org/10.1080/17460441.2017.1271784

24. Tolosa L, Gomez-Lechon MJ, Donato MT (2015) High-content screening technology for studying drug-induced hepatotoxicity in cell models. Arch Toxicol 89(7):1007–1022. https://doi.org/10.1007/s00204-015-1503-z

25. Tolosa L, Pinto S, Donato MT, Lahoz A, Castell JV, O'Connor JE, Gomez-Lechon MJ (2012) Development of a multiparametric cell based protocol to screen and classify the hepatotoxicity potential of drugs. Toxicol Sci 127(1):187–198. https://doi.org/10.1093/toxsci/kfs083

26. Greer ML, Barber J, Eakins J, Kenna JG (2010) Cell based approaches for evaluation of drug-induced liver injury. Toxicology 268(3):125–131. https://doi.org/10.1016/j.tox.2009.08.007

27. Boelsterli UA, Lim PL (2007) Mitochondrial abnormalities—a link to idiosyncratic drug hepatotoxicity? Toxicol Appl Pharmacol 220(1):92–107. https://doi.org/10.1016/j.taap.2006.12.013

28. Maes M, Vinken M, Jaeschke H (2016) Experimental models of hepatotoxicity related

to acute liver failure. Toxicol Appl Pharmacol 290:86–97. https://doi.org/10.1016/j.taap.2015.11.016

29. Bhakuni GS, Bedi O, Bariwal J, Deshmukh R, Kumar P (2016) Animal models of hepatotoxicity. Inflamm Res 65(1):13–24. https://doi.org/10.1007/s00011-015-0883-0

30. Verbeeck RK (2008) Pharmacokinetics and dosage adjustment in patients with hepatic dysfunction. Eur J Clin Pharmacol 64(12):1147–1161. https://doi.org/10.1007/s00228-008-0553-z

31. Shah F, Leung L, Barton HA, Will Y, Rodrigues AD, Greene N, Aleo MD (2015) Setting clinical exposure levels of concern for drug-induced liver injury (DILI) using mechanistic in vitro assays. Toxicol Sci 147(2):500–514. https://doi.org/10.1093/toxsci/kfv152

32. Verbeeck RK, Horsmans Y (1998) Effect of hepatic insufficiency on pharmacokinetics and drug dosing. Pharm World Sci 20(5):183–192

33. Roth AD, Lee MY (2017) Idiosyncratic drug-induced liver injury (IDILI): potential mechanisms and predictive assays. Biomed Res Int 2017:9176937. https://doi.org/10.1155/2017/9176937

34. Mazaleuskaya LL, Sangkuhl K, Thorn CF, FitzGerald GA, Altman RB, Klein TE (2015) PharmGKB summary: pathways of acetaminophen metabolism at the therapeutic versus toxic doses. Pharmacogenet Genomics 25(8):416–426. https://doi.org/10.1097/FPC.0000000000000150

35. Fontana RJ, Watkins PB, Bonkovsky HL, Chalasani N, Davern T, Serrano J, Rochon J, Group DS (2009) Drug-Induced Liver Injury Network (DILIN) prospective study: rationale, design and conduct. Drug Saf 32(1):55–68. https://doi.org/10.2165/00002018-200932010-00005

36. Munoz MA, Kulick CG, Kortepeter CM, Levin RL, Avigan MI (2017) Liver injury associated with dimethyl fumarate in multiple sclerosis patients. Mult Scler:1352458516688351. https://doi.org/10.1177/1352458516688351

37. Avigan MI (2014) DILI and drug development: a regulatory perspective. Semin Liver Dis 34(2):215–226. https://doi.org/10.1055/s-0034-1375961

38. Danan G, Benichou C (1993) Causality assessment of adverse reactions to drugs—I. A novel method based on the conclusions of international consensus meetings: application to drug-induced liver injuries. J Clin Epidemiol 46(11):1323–1330

39. Benichou C, Danan G, Flahault A (1993) Causality assessment of adverse reactions to drugs—II. An original model for validation of drug causality assessment methods: case reports with positive rechallenge. J Clin Epidemiol 46(11):1331–1336

40. Roussel Uclaf Causality Assessment Method (RUCAM) in drug induced liver injury. LiverTox. Available: https://livertox.nih.gov/rucam.html. Accessed 18 Mar 2017

41. Danan G, Teschke R (2015) RUCAM in drug and herb induced liver injury: the update. Int J Mol Sci 17(1). https://doi.org/10.3390/ijms17010014

42. Tillmann HL, Barnhart HX, Serrano J, Rockey DC (2016) A novel computerized drug induced liver injury causality assessment tool (DILI-CAT). Hepatology 64:320A–321A

43. Hayashi PH (2016) Drug-induced liver injury network causality assessment: criteria and experience in the United States. Int J Mol Sci 17(2):201. https://doi.org/10.3390/ijms17020201

44. Watkins PB, Desai M, Berkowitz SD, Peters G, Horsmans Y, Larrey D, Maddrey W (2011) Evaluation of drug-induced serious hepatotoxicity (eDISH) application of this data organization approach to phase III clinical trials of rivaroxaban after total hip or knee replacement surgery. Drug Saf 34(3):243–252. https://doi.org/10.2165/11586600-000000000-00000

45. Senior JR (2014) Evolution of the Food and Drug Administration approach to liver safety assessment for new drugs: current status and challenges. Drug Saf 37:S9–S17. https://doi.org/10.1007/s40264-014-0182-7

46. Watkins PB (2005) Idiosyncratic liver injury: challenges and approaches. Toxicol Pathol 33(1):1–5. https://doi.org/10.1080/01926230590888306

47. Fontana RJ, Seeff LB, Andrade RJ, Bjornsson E, Day CP, Serrano J, Hoofnagle JH (2010) Standardization of nomenclature and causality assessment in drug-induced liver injury: summary of a clinical research workshop. Hepatology 52(2):730–742. https://doi.org/10.1002/hep.23696

48. Bjornsson ES, Bergmann OM, Bjornsson HK, Kvaran RB, Olafsson S (2013) Incidence, presentation, and outcomes in patients with drug-induced liver injury in the general population of Iceland. Gastroenterology 144(7):1419–1425., 1425.e1411–1413; quiz e1419–1420. https://doi.org/10.1053/j.gastro.2013.02.006

49. Zimmerman HJ (1978) Chapter 16: Drug-induced liver disease. In: Hepatotoxicity. The adverse effects of drugs and other chemicals on the liver, 1st edn. Appleton-Century-Crofts, New York, p 353

50. Castiella A, Zapata E, Lucena MI, Andrade RJ (2014) Drug-induced autoimmune liver disease: a diagnostic dilemma of an increasingly reported disease. World J Hepatol 6(4):160–168. https://doi.org/10.4254/wjh.v6.i4.160

51. Vinay K, Abbas AK, Aster JC (2015) Robbins and Cotran pathologic basis of disease, 9th edn. Elsevier/Saunders, Philadelphia, PA

52. LiverTox: clinical and research information on drug-induced liver injury. National Institute of Diabetes and Digestive and Kidney Diseases. Available: https://livertox.nih.gov/

53. Brinker AD, Wassel RT, Lyndly J, Serrano J, Avigan M, Lee WM, Seeff LB (2009) Telithromycin-associated hepatotoxicity: clinical spectrum and causality assessment of 42 cases. Hepatology 49(1):250–257. https://doi.org/10.1002/hep.22620

54. Pardoll DM (2012) The blockade of immune checkpoints in cancer immunotherapy. Nat Rev Cancer 12(4):252–264. https://doi.org/10.1038/nrc3239

55. Topalian SL, Drake CG, Pardoll DM (2015) Immune checkpoint blockade: a common denominator approach to cancer therapy. Cancer Cell 27(4):450–461. https://doi.org/10.1016/j.ccell.2015.03.001

56. Kim KW, Ramaiya NH, Krajewski KM, Jagannathan JP, Tirumani SH, Srivastava A, Ibrahim N (2013) Ipilimumab associated hepatitis: imaging and clinicopathologic findings. Investig New Drugs 31(4):1071–1077. https://doi.org/10.1007/s10637-013-9939-6

57. Kleiner DE, Berman D (2012) Pathologic changes in ipilimumab-related hepatitis in patients with metastatic melanoma. Dig Dis Sci 57(8):2233–2240. https://doi.org/10.1007/s10620-012-2140-5

58. Michot JM, Bigenwald C, Champiat S, Collins M, Carbonnel F, Postel-Vinay S, Berdelou A, Varga A, Bahleda R, Hollebecque A, Massard C, Fuerea A, Ribrag V, Gazzah A, Armand JP, Amellal N, Angevin E, Noel N, Boutros C, Mateus C, Robert C, Soria JC, Marabelle A, Lambotte O (2016) Immune-related adverse events with immune checkpoint blockade: a comprehensive review. Eur J Cancer 54:139–148. https://doi.org/10.1016/j.ejca.2015.11.016

59. Tapper EB, Volk M (2017) Strategies to reduce 30-day readmissions in patients with cirrhosis. Curr Gastroenterol Rep 19(1):1. https://doi.org/10.1007/s11894-017-0543-3

60. Ribas A, Hodi FS, Callahan M, Konto C, Wolchok J (2013) Hepatotoxicity with combination of vemurafenib and ipilimumab. N Engl J Med 368(14):1365–1366. https://doi.org/10.1056/NEJMc1302338

61. Villamil A, Mullen E, Casciato P, Gadano A (2015) Interferon beta 1a-induced severe autoimmune hepatitis in patients with multiple sclerosis: report of two cases and review of the literature. Ann Hepatol 14(2):273–280

62. Arruti M, Castillo-Trivino T, de la Riva P, Marti-Masso JF, Lopez de Munain A, Olascoaga J (2012) Autoimmune hepatitis in a patient with multiple sclerosis under treatment with glatiramer acetate. Rev Neurol 55(3):190–192

63. von Kalckreuth V, Lohse AW, Schramm C (2008) Unmasking autoimmune hepatitis under immunomodulatory treatment of multiple sclerosis—not only beta interferon. Am J Gastroenterol 103(8):2147–2148.; author reply 2148. https://doi.org/10.1111/j.1572-0241.2008.01982_9.x

64. Neumann H, Csepregi A, Sailer M, Malfertheiner P (2007) Glatiramer acetate induced acute exacerbation of autoimmune hepatitis in a patient with multiple sclerosis. J Neurol 254(6):816–817. https://doi.org/10.1007/s00415-006-0441-3

65. Garcia-Buey L, Garcia-Monzon C, Rodriguez S, Borque MJ, Garcia-Sanchez A, Iglesias R, DeCastro M, Mateos FG, Vicario JL, Balas A et al (1995) Latent autoimmune hepatitis triggered during interferon therapy in patients with chronic hepatitis C. Gastroenterology 108(6):1770–1777

66. La Gioia S, Bacis G, Sonzogni A, Frigeni B, Conti MZ, Vedovello M, Rottoli M (2014) Glatiramer acetate-induced hepatitis in a young female patient with multiple sclerosis. Mult Scler Relat Disord 3(6):732–734. https://doi.org/10.1016/j.msard.2014.08.001

67. Makhani N, Ngan BY, Kamath BM, Yeh EA (2013) Glatiramer acetate-induced acute hepatotoxicity in an adolescent with MS. Neurology 81(9):850–852. https://doi.org/10.1212/WNL.0b013e3182a2cc4a

68. Milo R (2014) The efficacy and safety of daclizumab and its potential role in the treatment of multiple sclerosis. Ther Adv Neurol Disord 7(1):7–21. https://doi.org/10.1177/1756285613504021

69. Zinbryta [Package Insert]. Biogen Inc, Cambridge, MA; 14 Dec 2016

70. Avigan M. Assessment of liver toxicity profile of DAC HYP in the clinical development program for remitting-relapsing multiple sclerosis. BLA 761029. Daclizumab High Yield Process (DAC HYP), p 164–186. Available: http://www.accessdata.fda.gov/drugsatfda_docs/nda/2016/761029Orig1s000OtherR.pdf. 5 Nov 2015

71. Chalasani N, Regev A (2016) Drug-induced liver injury in patients with preexisting chronic liver disease in drug development: how to identify and manage? Gastroenterology 151(6):1046–1051. https://doi.org/10.1053/j.gastro.2016.10.010

72. Teschke R, Danan G (2016) Diagnosis and management of drug-induced liver injury (DILI) in patients with pre-existing liver disease. Drug Saf 39(8):729–744. https://doi.org/10.1007/s40264-016-0423-z

73. Arroyo V, Moreau R, Jalan R, Gines P, Study E-CCC (2015) Acute-on-chronic liver failure: a new syndrome that will re-classify cirrhosis. J Hepatol 62(1 Suppl):S131–S143. https://doi.org/10.1016/j.jhep.2014.11.045

74. FDA Drug Safety Communication: FDA warns of .serious liver injury risk with hepatitis C treatments Viekira Pak and Technivie. Available: https://www.fda.gov/Drugs/DrugSafety/ucm468634.htm. 22 Oct 2015

75. Dyson JK, Hutchinson J, Harrison L, Rotimi O, Tiniakos D, Foster GR, Aldersley MA, McPherson S (2016) Liver toxicity associated with sofosbuvir, an NS5A inhibitor and ribavirin use. J Hepatol 64(1):234–238. https://doi.org/10.1016/j.jhep.2015.07.041

76. Saukkonen JJ, Cohn DL, Jasmer RM, Schenker S, Jereb JA, Nolan CM, Peloquin CA, Gordin FM, Nunes D, Strader DB, Bernardo J, Venkataramanan R, Sterling TR, Subcommittee ATSHoAT D (2006) An official ATS statement: hepatotoxicity of antituberculosis therapy. Am J Respir Crit Care Med 174(8):935–952. https://doi.org/10.1164/rccm.200510-1666ST

77. Ungo JR, Jones D, Ashkin D, Hollender ES, Bernstein D, Albanese AP, Pitchenik AE (1998) Antituberculosis drug-induced hepatotoxicity. The role of hepatitis C virus and the human immunodeficiency virus. Am J Respir Crit Care Med 157(6 Pt 1):1871–1876. https://doi.org/10.1164/ajrccm.157.6.9711039

78. Kramer JR, Giordano TP, Souchek J, El-Serag HB (2005) Hepatitis C coinfection increases the risk of fulminant hepatic failure in patients with HIV in the HAART era. J Hepatol 42(3):309–314. https://doi.org/10.1016/j.jhep.2004.11.017

79. Bonacini M (2004) Liver injury during highly active antiretroviral therapy: the effect of hepatitis C coinfection. Clin Infect Dis 38(Suppl 2):S104–S108. https://doi.org/10.1086/381453

80. Biologic License Application 761029. Zinbryta (daclizumab) Injection: Other Review(s), p 164–186. Available: http://www.accessdata.fda.gov/drugsatfda_docs/nda/2016/761029Orig1s000OtherR.pdf

81. Mitchell SJ, Hilmer SN (2010) Drug-induced liver injury in older adults. Ther Adv Drug Saf 1(2):65–77. https://doi.org/10.1177/2042098610386281

82. Konig SA, Siemes H, Blaker F, Boenigk E, Gross-Selbeck G, Hanefeld F, Haas N, Kohler B, Koelfen W, Korinthenberg R et al (1994) Severe hepatotoxicity during valproate therapy: an update and report of eight new fatalities. Epilepsia 35(5):1005–1015

83. Bryant AE 3rd, Dreifuss FE (1996) Valproic acid hepatic fatalities. III. U.S. experience since 1986. Neurology 46(2):465–469

84. Dreifuss FE, Santilli N, Langer DH, Sweeney KP, Moline KA, Menander KB (1987) Valproic acid hepatic fatalities: a retrospective review. Neurology 37(3):379–385

85. Hautekeete ML, Horsmans Y, Van Waeyenberge C, Demanet C, Henrion J, Verbist L, Brenard R, Sempoux C, Michielsen PP, Yap PS, Rahier J, Geubel AP (1999) HLA association of amoxicillin-clavulanate—induced hepatitis. Gastroenterology 117(5):1181–1186

86. O'Donohue J, Oien KA, Donaldson P, Underhill J, Clare M, MacSween RN, Mills PR (2000) Co-amoxiclav jaundice: clinical and histological features and HLA class II association. Gut 47(5):717–720

87. Kindmark A, Jawaid A, Harbron CG, Barratt BJ, OF B, Andersson TB, Carlsson S, Cederbrant KE, Gibson NJ, Armstrong M, Lagerstrom-Fermer ME, Dellsen A, Brown EM, Thornton M, Dukes C, Jenkins SC, Firth MA, Harrod GO, Pinel TH, Billing-Clason SM, Cardon LR, March RE (2008) Genome-wide pharmacogenetic investigation of a hepatic adverse event without clinical signs of immunopathology suggests an underlying immune pathogenesis. Pharmacogenomics J 8(3):186–195. https://doi.org/10.1038/sj.tpj.6500458

88. Singer JB, Lewitzky S, Leroy E, Yang F, Zhao X, Klickstein L, Wright TM, Meyer J, Paulding CA (2010) A genome-wide study identifies HLA alleles associated with lumiracoxib-related liver injury. Nat Genet 42(8):711–714. https://doi.org/10.1038/ng.632

89. Daly AK, Donaldson PT, Bhatnagar P, Shen Y, Pe'er I, Floratos A, Daly MJ, Goldstein DB, John S, Nelson MR, Graham J, Park BK, Dillon JF, Bernal W, Cordell HJ, Pirmohamed M, Aithal GP, Day CP, Study D, International SAEC (2009) HLA-B*5701 genotype is a major determinant of drug-induced liver injury due to flucloxacillin. Nat Genet

41(7):816–819. https://doi.org/10.1038/ng.379

90. Hirata K, Takagi H, Yamamoto M, Matsumoto T, Nishiya T, Mori K, Shimizu S, Masumoto H, Okutani Y (2008) Ticlopidine-induced hepatotoxicity is associated with specific human leukocyte antigen genomic subtypes in Japanese patients: a preliminary case-control study. Pharmacogenomics J 8(1):29–33. https://doi.org/10.1038/sj.tpj.6500442

91. Spraggs CF, Budde LR, Briley LP, Bing N, Cox CJ, King KS, Whittaker JC, Mooser VE, Preston AJ, Stein SH, Cardon LR (2011) HLA-DQA1*02:01 is a major risk factor for lapatinib-induced hepatotoxicity in women with advanced breast cancer. J Clin Oncol 29(6):667–673. https://doi.org/10.1200/JCO.2010.31.3197

92. Vuilleumier N, Rossier MF, Chiappe A, Degoumois F, Dayer P, Mermillod B, Nicod L, Desmeules J, Hochstrasser D (2006) CYP2E1 genotype and isoniazid-induced hepatotoxicity in patients treated for latent tuberculosis. Eur J Clin Pharmacol 62(6):423–429. https://doi.org/10.1007/s00228-006-0111-5

93. Lee SW, Chung LS, Huang HH, Chuang TY, Liou YH, Wu LS (2010) NAT2 and CYP2E1 polymorphisms and susceptibility to first-line anti-tuberculosis drug-induced hepatitis. Int J Tuberc Lung Dis 14(5):622–626

94. Meier Y, Zodan T, Lang C, Zimmermann R, Kullak-Ublick GA, Meier PJ, Stieger B, Pauli-Magnus C (2008) Increased susceptibility for intrahepatic cholestasis of pregnancy and contraceptive-induced cholestasis in carriers of the 1331T>C polymorphism in the bile salt export pump. World J Gastroenterol 14(1):38–45

95. Stewart JD, Horvath R, Baruffini E, Ferrero I, Bulst S, Watkins PB, Fontana RJ, Day CP, Chinnery PF (2010) Polymerase gamma gene POLG determines the risk of sodium valproate-induced liver toxicity. Hepatology 52(5):1791–1796. https://doi.org/10.1002/hep.23891

96. Urban TJ, Goldstein DB, Watkins PB (2012) Genetic basis of susceptibility to drug-induced liver injury: what have we learned and where do we go from here? Pharmacogenomics 13(7):735–738. https://doi.org/10.2217/pgs.12.45

97. McCarthy MI, Abecasis GR, Cardon LR, Goldstein DB, Little J, Ioannidis JP, Hirschhorn JN (2008) Genome-wide association studies for complex traits: consensus, uncertainty and challenges. Nat Rev Genet 9(5):356–369. https://doi.org/10.1038/nrg2344

98. Tecentriq [Package Insert]. Genentech, Inc., San Francisco, CA; 21 Oct 2016

99. Yervoy [Package Insert]. Bristol Myers Squibb, Princeton, NJ; 28 Oct 2015

100. FDA Drug Safety Communication: Liver injury warning to be removed from Letairis (ambrisentan) tablets. Available at: http://www.fda.gov/Drugs/DrugSafety/ucm245852.htm. 4 Mar 2011

101. Desai M. New Drug Application 21686 (Ximelagatran): Medical Officer Review. Available: https://www.fda.gov/ohrms/dockets/ac/04/briefing/2004-4069B1_06_FDA-Backgrounder-C-R-MOR.pdf

Chapter 19

Regulatory Toxicological Studies: Identifying Drug-Induced Liver Injury Using Nonclinical Studies

Elizabeth Hausner and Imran Khan

Abstract

This chapter presents an overview of nonclinical safety assessment and the types of information that may be generated by drug developers for review by the US Food and Drug Administration (FDA). Every new drug molecule entering clinical development undergoes the process of safety assessment, a relatively standardized series of in vitro and in vivo examinations of the intrinsic properties of the proposed therapeutic. The goals are hazard characterization, identification of target organs, and determination of a theoretical margin of safety. These studies are usually conducted according to the guidances of the FDA and International Conference on Harmonization (ICH) and to a large extent conducted to the standards of Good Laboratory Practice. The ICH and FDA's guidances allow investigators to modify safety assessment studies on a case by case basis when scientifically justified.

The components of nonclinical safety assessment include in vitro assessment of affinity for off-target receptors and enzymes, evaluation of the absorption, distribution, metabolism, and excretion (ADME), safety pharmacology, and repeat-dose animal studies and may include computer assisted analysis of the chemical structure. Standard in vivo toxicology studies alone are not sufficient to identify the potential for human drug-induced liver injury (DILI). A weight-of-evidence approach (WOE) is recommended. We discuss how each of the components of nonclinical investigation may be used in conjunction to help identify the potential for adverse hepatobiliary effects. Given the scientific flexibility offered by the FDA and ICH guidances, it is important to remember that repeat-dose animal studies may be modified to explore any identified safety signals. This allows for evaluation of possible reactive metabolites and other more subtle signals of drug-induced liver injury that might otherwise be missed in a standard single- or repeat-dose safety assessment study. Because of efforts to reduce, refine, and replace animal work, it becomes especially important to ensure that animal work is optimized. Judicious data-driven modification of the repeat-dose animal studies has the potential to increase the safety of clinical trial participants, to optimize the information obtained and to increase the translational value for the clinic.

Key words Hepatobiliary, Toxicology, GLP, Nonclinical, QSAR, Adverse, Translational, Regulatory

---

The original version of this chapter was revised. An erratum to this chapter can be found at https://doi.org/10.1007/978-1-4939-7677-5_31

Minjun Chen and Yvonne Will (eds.), *Drug-Induced Liver Toxicity*, Methods in Pharmacology and Toxicology, https://doi.org/10.1007/978-1-4939-7677-5_19, © Springer Science+Business Media, LLC, part of Springer Nature 2018

1 Introduction

Any new chemical entity in development as a human therapeutic undergoes nonclinical safety assessment to help assess and identify any potential safety signals that may be relevant to humans. This is a standardized series of both in vitro and in vivo examinations with the goals of hazard identification and characterization (intrinsic toxicity), and target organ identification. This information along with dose dependence, relationship to exposure, and, when appropriate, reversibility is used to estimate an initial safe starting dose and dose range for human studies and to identify parameters for clinical monitoring of adverse effects (ICH M3(R2) and other guidances). Usually a "margin of safety" is calculated based upon a no observed adverse effect level (NOAEL) or lowest observed adverse effect level (LOAEL) in the animals and the projected or observed therapeutic level in humans.

This overall safety assessment also applies to signals for liver toxicity. A nonclinical signal for adverse liver effects does not always cause termination of clinical trials. Depending upon the nature of the nonclinical liver effect, it may be possible to demonstrate an adequate margin of safety to allow cautious advancement in the clinical setting. This is sometimes referred to as the "low and slow" approach or low starting dose with slow increases in both dose and exposure duration. Safety assessment continues after the first in human clinical trials. New information may emerge as the in vivo animal studies move from subchronic to chronic exposure and in vitro testing may explore greater mechanistic understanding of the intended and sometimes, unexpected, pharmacology and toxicology.

The occurrence of unexpected or unpredicted serious adverse events during premarketing development or after drug approval usually requires regulators and drug sponsors to reexamine the existing data to determine if a safety signal was missed, found to be very subtle, or totally absent. Vigorous public debate exists over the predictive or translational value of nonclinical studies. Partly, these are argued from the point of view of animal welfare. No one wishes to use animals for nonpredictive or only marginally valuable research. The other side to this debate is the public health desire to decrease risk of adverse drug effects [1, 2]. A well-structured development program should minimize animal usage and maximize the safety of study participants and the public once a drug is approved.

There have been several published examinations of the correlation of nonclinical animal data with the human clinical results and liver toxicity is highlighted in these studies [3–8]. The most recent study examined 1256 adverse drug reactions (ADRs) reported from 142 drugs approved for marketing in Japan from 2001 to 2010. Overall correlation between nonclinical and clinical hepatobiliary ADRs was 57%. Correlation of hepatic function abnormality was 67%. For these drugs and events, the nonclinical safety testing was reported to be little better than a coin toss [8]. However, the focus of many of these studies is the animal data. While this is an important component of nonclinical assessment, animal studies are only one piece of the nonclinical characterization. Without consideration of the information obtained from the in vitro, pharmacokinetic, and metabolism studies, the in vivo safety assessment alone is not as informative as it could be. Given the ethical imperative to refine, reduce and replace animal work, the in vivo safety assessment studies should be viewed for where they can be modified to explore signals from the other aspects of the nonclinical work.

2   The Cyber Drawing Board

Although not required by the regulations, some Sponsors conduct a computer assisted analysis of the new drug's chemical structure. FDA reviewers also have in-house resources for computer assisted analysis and a potentially different database than drug developers for comparison. These analyses, although not yet validated for regulatory purposes, can suggest the potential for more detailed examination of the risk for hepatotoxicity. Chemical structure and properties such as lipophilicity, substituents with the potential to form reactive metabolites, induce oxidative stress, mitochondrial effects, or inhibition of hepatic transport systems may contribute to the potential for liver damage [9]. Structural alerts as identified in quantitative structure–activity relationship models (QSAR) or structure–activity relationships (SAR) analysis may raise an awareness or concern over potential hepatic damage early in the safety assessment process and prompt a sponsor to examine the possibility of reactive metabolite formation and subsequent adducts to cellular macromolecules prior to testing in animals or humans. Because the in vivo consequences of such bioactivation or adduct formation are not necessarily indicative of potential hepatotoxicity, there are two possible consequences [10]. First, a risk-averse sponsor may discontinue development of the drug at this stage. A sponsor may also use SAR data to identify a different molecule that does not form adducts, or testing may proceed to determine the in vivo effects, if any, of the bioactive metabolite. By the same token, a variety of cell culture techniques may be used proactively by sponsors to examine possible hepatic interactions. Detailed descriptions of these may be found elsewhere in this book: structural alerts (Chap. 4), QSAR modeling (Chap. 5), and in vitro technologies (Sect. 3, Chaps. 7–17).

Cell culture investigations, SAR, and QSAR may be conducted for candidate selection, or to guide development efforts, including decisions to cease development due to indications of hepatobiliary (and other) toxicity. The data used for early decision making and from drugs that are dropped early from development due to -omic, cell culture, or other data regarding liver toxicity comprise a substantial amount of data not in the public domain.

3   Safety Pharmacology

Safety pharmacology studies are usually single dose, acute studies, focused primarily on cardiovascular, neurologic, and respiratory systems. The doses used in these studies are within the range where a therapeutic exposure or effect is expected. The anticipated toxicological range of exposure is not typically used within stand-alone safety pharmacology studies. The total time for a safety pharmacology study may extend 24–72 h after the test article is administered as the purpose of these studies is to look for effects outside the expected or intended therapeutic purpose. Histopathology and clinical chemistry are not usually performed, but if there are existing concerns, perhaps from the mechanism of action, known pharmacologic class, or risk aversion, targeted tissues may be collected and examined in conjunction with focused clinical chemistry. Any effect on hepatobiliary function noticed in stand-alone safety pharmacology would have to be acute and overwhelming, and might possibly manifest as sudden unexplained death. Such a situation might halt or at least pause the development, unless there is a significant margin of safety. Given the time frame and sample size, it is likely that subtle hepatobiliary signals would not be easily detected in a safety pharmacology study. In some cases, safety pharmacology studies have been incorporated into the toxicology studies in an effort to reduce animal use. When safety pharmacology studies are embedded into repeat dose toxicology studies, toxicological doses are used rather than pharmacological doses. Instead of a single dose and the short-term exposure of a standard safety pharmacology study, the number of doses received in an embedded safety pharmacology study is the same as the encompassing toxicology study. Hepatic toxicity would be identified by a combination of clinical chemistry and histopathology as conducted in a safety assessment study.

4   Secondary Pharmacology

In addition to the intended pharmacology of the therapeutic agent, there is the potential for off-target effects. This potential is explored by in vitro evaluation of the interactions of the drug with a broad panel of receptors, transporters, ion channels, nuclear receptors, and enzymes. Given the many complex biological processes that are maintained in homeostasis with a parsimony of a few hundred receptors and other pharmacological targets, it is not surprising that any one molecule may be able to interact with multiple receptors. It is difficult to identify a truly specific pharmacotherapy given the structural range that any given molecular messaging system may be able to accommodate. Receptor binding profiles are not uniformly submitted to the FDA [11]. A major metabolite is usually tested for the intended pharmacology of the parent drug. Given the concern for active or reactive metabolites to be causative or influential in liver toxicity, it may be informative to also consider a hepatic panel of transporters for evaluation.

5 Absorption, Distribution, Metabolism, and Excretion

Evaluation of absorption, distribution, metabolism, and excretion (ADME) usually includes mass balance studies conducted in one or more of the nonclinical species, usually rodents and sometimes non-rodent species such as dogs, nonhuman primates, or rabbits. Radiolabel distribution studies provide valuable information on several levels. First is the determination of how much drug-associated radiolabel reaches the intended pharmacological target and what proportion is distributed to other tissues. This relative distribution of the drug-associated radiolabel is very important for assessing any accumulation of drug, or metabolites, and prolonged residence time of the radiolabel in any tissue, such as the liver or biliary system. Distribution is usually considered in conjunction with the proportion of drug excreted by renal, hepatobiliary (fecal), or respiratory means. Evidence that suggests accumulation of drug-associated material in the liver, enterohepatic recirculation, or prolonged residence time may call for further consideration or closer examination, especially if there is a suspect metabolite or reactive intermediate.

The liver has the remarkable metabolic capacity including the oxidative drug metabolizing enzymes (Phase I reactions), conjugative drug metabolizing enzymes (Phase II reactions), and the multitude of receptors and transport mechanisms found on hepatic and biliary cells. When the variations in metabolic capacity that are possible through numerous genetic polymorphisms are also considered, the in vitro examination of possible metabolites and the capacity for hepatotoxic metabolites takes on increased importance as a method for early signal detection [12]. The early nonclinical assessment of metabolism is conducted in cultured hepatocytes and hepatic microsomes. Both the hepatocytes and the microsomes may be from multiple nonclinical species and from humans. This allows for a primary comparison of differences in species metabolism and ascertainment that major (comprising $\geq 10\%$ of the total drug-derived species) human metabolites are represented in the animals. Identification of active metabolites requires further in vitro testing to determine whether the pharmacology of the parent or active moiety is also present in one or more of the known metabolites. A drug undergoing several metabolic pathways has the potential to produce a hepatotoxic metabolite that is minor, or less than 10% of the total, and therefore may be missed in further in vitro testing. On the other hand, only one hepatotoxic metabolite is necessary to create a scenario where drug-induced liver injury (DILI) is possible. Therefore, a drug does not need to be extensively metabolized to be potentially hepatotoxic.

Conversely, animal metabolite profiles should be examined for major drug metabolites that may not exist in humans (species-specific metabolites) and thus give rise to the possibility of species-specific effects. Species similarities or differences in rates of distribution, residence time, and clearance may signal potential toxicities or indicate factors that affect the relevance of nonclinical results for the clinic. This is another step where chemical structural analysis may be used to identify potentially hepatotoxic intermediates or reactive metabolites, e.g., the acetaminophen metabolite N-acetylimidoquinone (NAPQI) [13]. Metabolite profiles from blood and urine collected from in vivo studies, usually part of safety assessment, are also part of the developmental database for a new drug. Metabolite profiles from blood and urine collected from in vivo studies, usually part of safety assessment, are also part of the developmental database for a new drug. The in vivo pharmacokinetic profiles include parameters, such as maximum plasma concentration (C_{max}), time of maximum plasma concentration (T_{max}), volume of distribution at steady state (V_{dss}), area under the curve for the dosing interval (AUC_{0-24}) or extrapolated ($AUC_{0-\infty}$), fraction available by oral administration ($F\%$), and biological or functional half-life ($T_{1/2}$).

6   Protein Binding

Protein binding studies are also usually conducted early in development. This is an in vitro evaluation that allows for species comparisons; that is, a determination of the similarities or differences in the degree of total protein binding and qualitative differences, or to which plasma proteins the parent drug is bound. There is an assumption that only the free (non-protein bound) drug is able to interact with the intended target. In addition to the information about free versus protein-bound drug, these studies may also indicate the potential for a drug to displace other protein-bound drugs. It is infrequent that metabolites are evaluated in the protein binding studies, but this may be an area that will change. There are examples that binding of a drug or metabolite to a protein can create a drug-modified protein triggering immune-mediated hepatotoxicity [14]. These observations open the door to a new avenue of in vitro studies that could explore whether or not such drug or metabolite-modified proteins had immune stimulating properties. Some of the proposed new serum biomarkers, such as inflammosome complexes, various cytokines, and high mobility group box 1

(HMGB1) protein fit into this hypothesis [15]. While these studies are not regulatory requirements, they would seem to be prudent areas of scientific exploration if a structural alert has been detected in either parent drug or metabolite.

7 Drug–Drug Interaction Studies

Nonclinical drug–drug interaction studies are not required. However, if there are concerns for hepatotoxicity based on ADME studies or known risks for hepatotoxicity, then drug interaction studies may be helpful to clarify the potential for pharmacokinetic or pharmacodynamic interactions relevant to the hepatotoxicity. Also, if the drug under development is intended for a patient population likely to be taking multiple medications, nonclinical assessment of possible interactions may be requested if these data cannot be obtained safely in a clinical study. This allows for a nonclinical evaluation of the potential for one drug to alter the metabolism of another drug, i.e., increase or decrease.

8 Guidelines and Good Laboratory Practice

Animal safety assessment studies are conducted under ICH guidances and the guidances of the FDA[1] in the USA, the EMA[2] in the EU, or Japanese Ministry of Health and Welfare (JMHW) in Japan in accordance with Good Laboratory Practices (GLP). The Organization for Economic Development (OECD) published guidelines, internationally accepted as standard methods for safety testing. The methods are regularly updated by experts from OECD member countries. OECD guidelines are covered by the Mutual Acceptance of Data, implying that data generated in the testing of chemicals in an OECD member country, or partner country, in accordance with OECD guidelines be accepted in other OECD countries.[3] A common misconception is that guidances are hard and fast regulations for conduct of nonclinical studies. Guidances are recommendations having the weight of past experience but written to allow for case by case exceptions when scientifically justified.[4,5] Good Laboratory Practices are intended to assure the

[1] https://www.fda.gov:80/FDAgov/Drugs/GuidanceCompliance RegulatoryInformation/Guidances/default.htm

[2] http://www.ema.europa.eu/ema/index.jsp?curl=pages/regulation/general/general_content_000043.jsp

[3] http://www.oecd.org/chemicalsafety/testing/goodlaboratorypracticeglp.htm

[4] http://federalregister.gov/a/2016-19875

[5] https://www.accessdata.fda.gov/scripts/cdrh/cfdocs/cfcfr/CFRSearch.cfm?CFRPart=58

quality and integrity of data submitted to regulatory authorities and are required for all studies intended to support human safety. The GLP specify managerial, organizational, and record-keeping conditions for laboratories in which nonclinical safety studies are planned and conducted. This may also include standard operating procedures for maintenance of laboratory equipment, sample preparation and collection. Compliance with GLP standards does not, however, guarantee a well-designed or scientifically sound study.

9   Whole Animal Safety Assessment

Repeat-dose animal studies are usually conducted in at least two species, one rodent and one nonrodent, and for varying durations of time. Unless there are special considerations due to the proposed indication or patient population, studies of 28 days, 90 days, 6 months (rodent); and 9 months (nonrodent) are normally conducted, usually by the intended route of clinical administration in accordance with ICH M3(R2) timelines. Carcinogenicity studies represent a special case of chronic safety assessment in which animals, usually rats and mice, will receive drug for approximately 2 years. This is accompanied by assessment and incidence of neoplasia in multiple tissues. While carcinogenicity studies focus upon the neoplastic potential of a new drug, gross and microscopic examination allow for the evaluation of chronic effects upon the liver. Carcinogenicity studies are not required for all drugs, but rather depend upon the likely duration or frequency of exposure for the intended patient population. Such studies may be waived if life expectancy of the patient population is less than 3 years.

The general design of rodent safety assessment studies includes a vehicle control group and three groups receiving different doses of drug. Additional groups of rodents may be included for toxicokinetic determination or if there is to be a drug-free recovery period for some animals. The OECD guidelines recommend ten rodents per sex per group as sufficient for most cases of subchronic and chronic toxicity testing (http://www.who.int/tdr/publications/documents/safety_handbook.pdf. Accessed 16 Feb 2017). Nonrodent studies follow the same design of a control/vehicle group and three additional groups receiving different doses of drug. For nonrodents, usually dogs or nonhuman primates (NHP), the numbers per group may be quite low. Neither rodent nor nonrodent study group sizes are based upon statistical power calculations. Sponsors may change the number of animals based upon scientific rationale. However, there is a balance between the desire to reduce, refine, and replace animal testing, and the desire to increase numbers of animals to detect a defined toxicological effect, such as a difference in liver enzymes with a certain statistical power.

The small sample size of both rodent and nonrodent safety assessment is compensated for by study designs that minimize variability (e.g., use of inbred animals) and the use of suprapharmacologic or toxicologic doses. These doses are limited by a number of factors. The concept of the lethal dose for 50% of the population (LD50) was abandoned long ago, both for ethical reasons and as it is a gross assessment of toxicity that does not take into account sublethal toxicities. A maximal tolerated dose is preferred as the highest dose in any safety assessment study. This is a dose that causes definite but subtle toxicity that does not threaten survival, such as limited weight loss, decreased rate of gain, or adverse change in clinical chemistry parameters. Other limitations to the doses that may be used include exaggerated pharmacology (e.g., an anticoagulant or antihypertensive), saturation of absorption (raising the dose does not increase exposure), or feasibility (it is impractical or inhumane to try to administer additional drug). The midrange dose is designed to help delineate a dose-response effect. The lowest dose used is intended to produce an exposure similar to that intended for humans. The use of supratherapeutic doses in general raises the possibility that mechanisms will be called into play that do not exist or are irrelevant at pharmacologic or therapeutic doses.

Safety assessment studies sometimes use animal models of disease to study safety or drug efficacy. In routine safety assessment, the rodents and nonrodents are healthy, usually drug naïve, receive no concurrent medications during the study and live under uniform conditions of housing, diet, and exercise for the duration of the study. Mice tend to be inbred, while rats, dogs and NHP are usually outbred. Even so, the commonly used laboratory species show far greater genetic similarity than does the human population. This is a significant limitation to hazard characterization, particularly in the liver where polymorphisms in enzyme expression exist among the human population. This polymorphism in the livers of humans cannot adequately be captured in one genetically limited strain of one species of animal. The variability of human diet, lifestyle choices, comorbid diseases and concurrent medications is not represented in the use of young, healthy, drug naïve animals living under standardized conditions of diet, light cycle and general husbandry. The likelihood of a single animal model study identifying the true idiosyncratic hepatotoxicity of humans that is attributed to as yet incompletely undefined genetic, disease and medication factors is vanishingly small.

10 Clinical Chemistry in Safety Assessment

Despite the limited genetic diversity of the animals, they usually display a spectrum of sensitivity to the drug being tested. The parameters most often used for evaluating hepatic effects are clinical chemistry and histopathology. The primary serum-derived clinical chemistry indicators are subject to variability from factors that include diurnal rhythms, handling, restraint, anesthesia, and the blood sampling procedure itself [16]. The species specificity, plasma half-lives of each clinical chemistry parameter and interpretation are beyond the scope of this chapter. The reader is referred to detailed recommendations published by the American Society for Veterinary Clinical Pathology (ASCVP) for the application of clinical chemistry parameters in detecting hepatic damage [17]. It should be noted, that some parameters are typically given more weight than others. Alanine aminotransferase (ALT) and aspartate aminotransferase (AST) are recommended for assessing hepatocellular injury in rats, dogs, and nonhuman primates in nonclinical studies. Extrahepatic factors such as muscle injury may affect the circulating levels of ALT and AST. Additional or supplemental indicators of liver injury include serum sorbitol dehydrogenase (SDH) and glutamate dehydrogenase (GLDH). These two dehydrogenases are more specific than the transaminases and may be useful in the species where ALT activity is low or not specific to liver, such as in swine and guinea pigs. Alkaline phosphatase (ALP) and total bilirubin are the primary serum indicators for hepatobiliary effects. Bone and intestinal effects may both increase the levels of ALP. There are several possible causes of increased total bilirubin also, making neither ALP nor total bilirubin specific for hepatotoxicity. Circulating bile acids may be useful as indicators of biliary damage although not specific indicators of the kind of damage. See Fig. 1 for a list of clinical chemistry parameters used for identifying hepatobiliary effects [17].

Another way to evaluate the liver for possible drug-induced effects is by the functional capacity. Circulating levels of proteins, in particular albumin, total cholesterol, triglycerides, glucose, and urea may be indicative of the protein synthetic competence of the liver. It is also possible that prior to hepatic necrosis, the protein synthetic machinery is slowed or disabled, making synthetic function a more sensitive indicator of hepatobiliary effects than the serum transaminases or dehydrogenases. Prothrombin, produced by the liver, has the shortest circulating half-life of the coagulation factors and may be a useful indicator of decreased synthetic capacity. Activated partial thromboplastin time is considered another supplemental parameter for liver function [17].

As previously noted, some parameters are given more weight than others. In particular, AST and ALT may receive more attention both from regulators and from drug developers as these are typically monitored in clinical studies. This may lead to missing more subtle signals, such as decreased synthetic capacity of the liver or alterations in coagulation parameters. Given the complexity and redundancy of hemostasis, such changes may not be obvious. Alterations in specific protein synthesis may also be very difficult to identify in a study unless specifically and deliberately examined.

Primary indicators for liver damage	Primary indicators for biliary damage	Indicators of synthetic (functional) capacity
• Alanine aminotransferase (ALT)	• Alkaline phosphatase (ALP)	• Total protein
• Aspartate aminotransferase (AST)	• γ-glutamyltransferase (GGT)	• Albumin
• Sorbitol dehydrogenase (SDH)	• 5'-nucelotidase (5-NT)	• Triglycerides
• Glutamate dehydrogenase (GDH)	• Total bilirubin	• Cholesterol
		• Glucose
		• Urea nitrogen
		• Serum bile acids
		• Activated partial thromboplastin
		• Prothrombin time

Fig. 1 Clinical chemistry parameters used in nonclinical safety assessment

Results or changes in any of the clinical chemistry parameters are usually compared to the concurrent controls. Concurrent controls are preferable as they are the most accurate comparators of the effect of the contemporary animal husbandry and handling techniques upon clinical chemistry and histopathology. When concurrent controls are unavailable, historical controls may be useful if they are from studies conducted at the same facility within a relatively recent number of years as genetic drift may occur with time and geographic isolation of breeding colonies [18]. Husbandry and facility environmental conditions may change over time, all of which are factors contributing to variability in both clinical chemistry parameters and histopathological background.

A combination of altered clinical chemistry parameters that correlate with a histopathological finding in the liver is generally a strong signal for an adverse liver effect. This kind of correlation with a dose response further strengthens the signal for toxicity. While a dose response in multiple parameters helps to identify hepatic involvement, the small numbers of animals in any study make it easy to miss or miss-classify an effect. A group mean value for any of the hepatic-associated clinical chemistry parameters may be elevated by changes in a single animal. Such changes are frequently dismissed as spurious, due to normal variability, or otherwise irrelevant. Given the small sample size of most nonclinical animal studies, any indications of hepatic damage in single animals per drug treatment should be explored rather than dismissed out of hand.

11   Dose Response

It is also important to remember that while a desired pharmacologic effect may be present with a linear dose response, this is not necessarily true for an adverse effect. Plasma levels do not necessarily reflect tissue levels of drug or reactive intermediate. The biologically effective dose for an adverse event represents the amount of the toxic or culpable entity at the critical tissue location and may be influenced by accumulation of drug or metabolite. In the clinic, genetics, diet, concurrent medications and health conditions also play a role. A variety of terms have been used to describe other phenomena such as paradoxical, preconditioning, or adaptive to name a few. These phenomena are accompanied by a dose response curve that may change shape with time [19].

12   The Overall Interpretation

The overall hazard characterization includes

- Identification of a No Observed Adverse Effect Level
- Are there any clinical pathology findings in the animals?
- Are there any histopathology findings in the animals?
- Metabolites: are the human metabolites represented in the nonclinical species?
  - Are there species specific metabolites?
  - Are there structural alerts in the metabolites?
- Is enterohepatic recirculation apparent?
- Does drug or drug product accumulate in the liver?
- What is the nature and severity of the clinical pathology and histopathology findings?
- Are any effects reversible?
- Can the effects be monitored?

A critical question is whether a no observed adverse effect level (NOAEL) has been identified. If so, what is the apparent safety margin between the exposure or dose at which the no adverse effect occurs, and what is the proposed exposure for the therapeutic effect? If clinical data exists, how does the nonclinical information compare? The disease indication and patient population need to be considered also. An acceptable safety margin will depend upon the combination of the nature of the effects (severity, reversibility, can they be monitored), the indication, and the patient population.

Any sponsor finding a signal for adverse liver effects may conduct nonclinical, hypothesis-driven experiments to try to characterize the findings, mechanism of action or potential contributing factors. This information may be helpful in determining the mechanism or apparent safety margin. It may be possible to identify genetic polymorphisms associated with increased risk, potential for drug-drug   interactions,   or   factors   leading   to   adverse   effects.   If   the efficacy and toxicity of the drug are too closely linked in relation to dose, there may be limitations to a safe path forward for that particular drug.

13   For the Future

There is an ongoing effort to find more sensitive and specific biomarkers of general liver and biliary injury, and indicators of susceptibility to idiosyncratic DILI in particular. Any new animal biomarker should be usable in both animals and humans, or "translatable." The clinical chemistry indicators of hepatic injury are used in both humans and nonhumans. The strengths and weaknesses (nonspecificity, residence time in the blood) are also similar across species. Histopathology as used in nonclinical studies is less than desirable as a translational biomarker as it is invasive. A number of entities are being explored for serum-derived biomarkers of DILI as discussed in detail in several chapters in this book. These proposed biomarkers include, GLDH high-mobility group box-1 protein (HMBG1), keratin-18(K-18), and a number of micro-RNAs, such as miR-122 and miR-192, and others. GLDH, a relatively liver-specific enzyme, is expressed in the mitochondrial matrix of hepatocytes and has been documented as a sensitive and specific biomarker in human liver injury and also as a marker of liver mitochondrial injury in rodents administered with acetaminophen [20–22]. It is a good predictor of hepatic necrosis in rats [21, 22]. High-mobility group box 1 (HMGB1) is a chromatin binding protein passively released from necrotic cells. It is actively secreted in a hyper-acetylated form by immune cells, potentially allowing for discrimination of necrosis and immune activation [23, 24]. Keratin-18 (K-18) is a structural protein that is released full length into the serum during necrosis. In the apoptotic process, this molecule undergoes cleavage by caspase, allowing for differentiation of the cellular processes [25]. Micro RNAs may enter the blood stream passively as a result of cell death or may be actively released via exosomes [20–22]. Numerous -omic methodologies are currently being explored also [20, 22]. An important aspect of the success or failure of these potential biomarkers is the validation of the detection system for each species as well as awareness of species differences in the biology, pathophysiology, or tissue selectivity of the biomarker. Moreover, it is unlikely that a single biomarker will be very useful in predicting DILI; however, their utility as biomarkers could be significantly improved when used in combination with other biomarkers and clinical/nonclinical evaluations.

14   Conclusion

Nonclinical safety assessment offers important information about the inherent pharmacological and toxicological properties of a new drug. Sponsors may use QSAR and SAR at multiple times throughout the safety assessment process, both for the analysis of parent drug for structural alerts and for the analysis of metabolites. From a regulatory perspective, radiolabel distribution studies provide valuable information about persistence of drug-associated radiolabel in different organs, including the liver and may provide indications of enterohepatic recycling. The in vitro metabolite studies in conjunction with in vivo metabolite profiles and pharmacokinetic information provide clues as to the possibility of an active or reactive metabolite with prolonged residence time in the liver. While the in vivo safety assessment studies receive a great amount of attention or are given extra weight in the overall interpretation, they have some inherent limitations and it is highly possible to miss subtle signals such as decreased synthetic capacity, especially if a traditional linear dose response curve is not apparent for the toxicity. The in vivo studies may become more informative if enhanced and based upon the QSAR and metabolic data. That is, if there is an alert for a potential reactive metabolite, the in vivo work could be modified to include examination of adverse effects, such as mitochondrial effects, oxidative stress, or interference with hepatic transport systems and by using appropriate biomarkers. A single animal in a dose group showing some form of hepatobiliary adversity is often dismissed as a spurious finding. Instead, given the small sample sizes and genetic limitations of the nonclinical studies, these single or few animal findings should be further explored to determine if they represent a true safety signal. It may be helpful also if the post-treatment observations can be compared with pretreatment values in the same animal. The ultimate goal is to identify hepatotoxic compounds as early in development as possible, for the safety of clinical trial participants and the general public.

Disclaimer

This book chapter reflects the views of the authors and should not be construed to represent FDA's views or policies.

References

1. Peters TS (2005) Do preclinical testing strategies help predict human hepatotoxic potentials? Toxicol Pathol 33(1):146–154

2. Everitt JI (2015) The future of preclinical animal models in pharmaceutical discovery and development: a need to bring in cerebro to the in vivo discussions. Toxicol Pathol 43(1):70–77

3. Owens AH Jr (1962) Predicting anticancer drug effects in man from laboratory animal studies. J Chronic Dis 15:223–228

4. Schein PS, Davis RD, Carter S, Newman J, Schein DR, Rall DP (1970) The evaluation of anticancer drugs in dogs and monkeys for the prediction of qualitative toxicities in man. Clin Pharmacol Ther 11(1):3–40

5. Hayes AW, Fedorowski T, Balazs T, Carlton WW, Fowler BA, Gilman MR, Heyman I, Jackson BA, Kennedy GL, Shapiro RE, Smith CC, Tardiff RG, Weil CS (1982) Correlation of human hepatotoxicants with hepatic damage in animals. Fundam Appl Toxicol 2(2):55–66

6. Igarashi T, Nakane S, Kitagawa T (1995) Predictability of clinical adverse reactions of drugs by general pharmacology studies. J Toxicol Sci 20(2):77–92

7. Olson H, Betton G, Robinson D, Thomas K, Monro A, Kolaja G, Lilly P, Sanders J, Sipes G, Bracken W, Dorato M, Van Deun K, Smith P, Berger B, Heller A (2000) Concordance of the toxicity of pharmaceuticals in humans and in animals. Regul Toxicol Pharmacol 32(1):56–67

8. Tamaki C, Nagayama T, Hashiba M, Fujiyoshi M, Hizue M, Kodaira H, Nishida M, Suzuki K, Takashima Y, Ogino Y, Yasugi D, Yasuo Yoneta Y, Hisada S, Ohkura T, Nakamura K (2013) Potentials and limitations of nonclinical safety assessment for predicting clinical adverse drug reactions: correlation analysis of 142 approved drugs in Japan (PDF download available). J Toxicol Sci 38(4):581–598

9. Chen M, Suzuki A, Borlak J, Andrade RJ, Lucena MI (2015) Drug-induced liver injury: interactions between drug properties and host factors. J Hepatol 63(2):503–514

10. Obach RS, Kalgutkar AS, Soglia JR, Zhao SX (2008) Can in vitro metabolism-dependent covalent binding data in liver microsomes distinguish hepatotoxic from nonhepatotoxic drugs? An analysis of 18 drugs with consideration of intrinsic clearance and daily dose. Chem Res Toxicol 21(9):1814–1822

11. Papoian T, Chiu HJ, Elayan I, Gowraganahalli J, Khan I, Laniyonu AA, Xinguang CL, Saulnier M, Simpson N, Yang B (2015) Secondary pharmacology data to assess potential off-target activity of new drugs: a regulatory perspective. Nat Rev Drug Discov 14(4):294. Epub 2015 Mar 20

12. Roth AD, Lee, M-Y (2017) Idiosyncratic drug-induced liver injury (IDILI): potential mechanisms and predictive assays. Biomed Res Int. ePub 4 Jan 2017

13. Jan YH, Heck DE, Dragomir AC, Gardner CR, Laskin DL, Laskin JD (2014) Acetaminophen reactive intermediates target hepatic thioredoxin reductase. Chem Res Toxicol 27(5):882–894

14. Kaplowitz N (2004) Drug-induced liver injury. Clin Infect Dis 38(Suppl 2):S44–S48

15. Cho T, Uetrecht J (2017) How reactive metabolites induce an immune response that sometimes leads to an idiosyncratic drug reaction. Chem Res Toxicol 30:295–314

16. Everds NE (2017) Deciphering sources of variability in clinical pathology—it's not just about the numbers. Toxicol Pathol 45(2):275–280

17. Boone L, Meyer D, Cusick P, Ennulat D, Provencher Bolliger A, Everds N, Meador V, Elliott G, Honor D, Bounous D, Jordan H (2005) Selection and interpretation of clinical pathology indicators of hepatic injury in preclinical studies. Vet Clin Pathol 34(3):182–188

18. Fahey JR, Katoh H, Malcolm R, Perez AV (2013) The case for genetic monitoring of mice and rats used in biomedical research. Mamm Genome 24(3–4):89–94

19. Calabrese EJ, Calabrese EJ, Bachmann KA, Bailer AJ, Bolger PM, Borak J, Cai L, Cedergreen N, Cherian MG, Chiueh CC, Clarkson TW, Cook RR, Diamond DM, Doolittle DJ, Dorato MA, Duke SO, Feinendegen L, Gardner DE, Hart RW, Hastings KL, Hayes AW, Hoffmann GR, Ives JA, Jaworowski Z, Johnson TE, Jonas WB, Kaminski NE, Keller JG, Klaunig JE, Knudsen TB, Kozumbo WJ, Lettieri T, Liu SZ, Maisseu A, Maynard KI, Masoro EJ, McClellan RO, Mehendale HM, Mothersill C, Newlin DB, Nigg HN, Oehme FW, Phalen RF, Philbert MA, Rattan SI, Riviere JE, Rodricks J, Sapolsky RM, Scott BR, Seymour C, Sinclair DA, Smith-Sonneborn J, Snow ET, Spear L, Stevenson DE, Thomas Y, Tubiana M, Williams GM, Mattson MP (2007) Biological stress response terminology: integrating the concepts of adaptive response and preconditioning stress within a hormetic dose-response framework. Toxicol Appl Pharmacol 222(1):122–128

20. Robles-Diaz M, Medina-Caliz I, Stephens C, Andrade RJ, Lucena MI (2016) Biomarkers in DILI: one more step forward. Front Pharmacol 7:267

21. Thulin P, Hornby RJ, Auli M, Nordhal G, Antoine DJ, Lewis PS, Goldring CE, Park BK, Prats N, Glinghammar B, Schippe-Koisten I (2017) A longitudinal assessment of miR-122 and GLDH as biomarkers of drug-induced liver injury in the rat. Biomarkers 22(5):461–469

22. Church RJ, Watkin PB (2017) The transformation in biomarker detection and management of drug-induced liver injury. Liver Int 37:1582–1590

23. Scaffidi P, Misteli T, Bianchi ME (2002) Release of chromatin protein HMGB1 by necrotic cells triggers inflammation. Nature 418(6894):191–195

24. Bonaldi T, Talamo F, Scaffidi P, Ferrera D, Porto A, Bachi A, Rubartelli A, Agresti A, Bianchi ME (2003) Monocytic cells hyperacetylate chromatin protein HMGB1 to redirect it towards secretion. EMBO J 22(20):5551–5560

25. Ku NO, Strnad P, Zhong B-H, Tao G-H, Omary MB (2007) Keratins let liver live: mutations predispose to liver disease and crosslinking generates Mallory-Denk bodies. Hepatology 46(5):1639–1649

Chapter 20

Hy's Law and eDISH for Clinical Studies

John Senior and Ted Guo

Abstract

We present in this review a brief background of innovative concepts underlying the expression of Hy's law and the diagnostic eDISH program. The term **Hy's law** is a sobriquet stated by Robert Temple in April 1999, with Dr. Hyman Zimmerman present but modestly objecting. Subsequently John Senior and Ted Guo in the Food and Drug Administration (FDA) Office of Pharmacoepidemiology and Statistical Sciences (OPaSS) together developed in 2003–2004 a graphic program called **eDISH**, acronym for *e*valuation of *D*rug-*I*nduced *S*erious *H*epatotoxicity in clinical trial subjects. It aimed at facilitating diagnosis of the probable cause of significant serum liver test abnormalities. Step one was to look at all values over time of serum alanine aminotransferase (ALT) and total bilirubin (TBL) in *all* subjects in a trial, and display peak values of both ALT and TBL for each subject in an x-y plot to assess incidence by severity. Step two was a time course plot and clinical narrative to diagnose whether subjects of interest with more severe changes of both peak ALT and TBL were *caused by the drug*, at least *probably*, meaning more likely than by all other possible causes combined. The eDISH program was intended for use in clinical trials by FDA medical reviewers, but has been copied and widely misunderstood. The first step ALTxTBL plot does **NOT** define a Hy's law case; to do so requires making a medical differential diagnosis of probable drug cause. The eDISH program is **NOT** simply a graph of serum chemistry elevations.

Key words Serum enzyme activities, Serum bilirubin concentration, Causality diagnosis, Time course, Clinical narrative

Abbreviations

AASLD	American Association for the Study of Liver Diseases
ALT	Alanine aminotransferase = serum glutamic-pyruvic transaminase, SGPT
AST	Aspartate aminotransferase = serum glutamic-oxaloacetic transaminase, SGOT
CDER	Center for Drug Evaluation and Research (FDA)
CIOMS	Council for International Organization of Medical Science
DILI	Drug-induced liver injury
eDISH	evaluation of drug-induced serious hepatotoxicity
FDA	Food and Drug Administration

Minjun Chen and Yvonne Will (eds.), *Drug-Induced Liver Toxicity*, Methods in Pharmacology and Toxicology, https://doi.org/10.1007/978-1-4939-7677-5_20, © Springer Science+Business Media, LLC, part of Springer Nature 2018

NAD+	Oxidized form of nicotinamide adenine dinucleotide = old name DPN, diphosphpyridine nucleotide (oxidized form)
NADH	Reduced nicotinamide adenine dinucleotide = old name DPNH$_2$, diphosphpyridine nucleotide (reduced form)
NE, NW, SE, SW	Quadrants of an eDISH first plot (North = Upper, East = right, South = lower; W = left
NIH	National Institutes of Health
OPaSS	Office of Pharmacoepidemiology and Statistical Science
OTS	Office of Translational Sciences
RUCAM	Roussel-Uclaf Causality Assessment Method
TBL	Serum total bilirubin
ULN	Upper limit of normal

1   The Innovators

The time around 1950 was a watershed, the year of formation of the Association for the Study of Liver Diseases (ASLD), renamed 3 years later the American Association for the Study of Liver Diseases (AASLD). The idea of creating a new subspecialty of hepatology had incubated in the library of the Hektoen Institute at Cook County Hospital in Chicago where Dr. Hans Popper [1] had gathered a group of colleagues to meet and talk about liver problems. It was the year when Dr. Hyman Zimmerman at the Washington Veterans Administration Hospital was writing up his first paper [2] on liver injury caused by a drug. He had observed that high doses of oral and intravenous aureomycin sometimes caused liver toxicity, and wrote about a series of six cases, four fatal, of liver failure in patients he had seen during his medical residency at Ballinger Hospital. It was also the year a young student, Arthur Karmen, started in medical school at New York University. Before graduation in 1954 he had developed a rapid method [3] to measure serum transaminase activity to diagnose myocardial infarction that revolutionized clinical medicine. The ground-breaking new ideas of the three investigators led to development of insights that was at first a tale of three cities: Chicago, Washington, and New York, then spread quickly all over the world.

Hans Popper (Fig. 1) was especially interested in the histologic study of the liver, and in using both light and fluorescence microscopy. After his discharge from military service in 1946, he worked with Murray Franklin to review [4] all cases of fatal hepatitis at Cook County Hospital back to 1929 and contrasted post-mortem histologic appearances of those livers with what he had observed in many military personnel during World War II, mostly due to infectious viral hepatitis. Both Popper and Franklin felt they could differentiate between those cases and the "Cook cases" that were mainly diagnosed "toxic hepatitis." Hans Popper's passionate interest attracted colleagues and they decided [1] in 1949 to start a new medical society of hepatology, called at first the Association

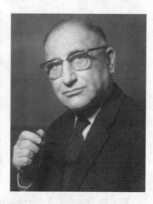

Fig. 1 Hans Popper (24 November, 1903–6 May, 1988), founder of hepatology as a special field

for the Study of Liver Diseases (ASLD). Dr. Leon Schiff of Miami was elected as the first president to serve in 1950 until the following year, with Robert Kark as treasurer, and Popper as secretary (and the driving force behind the scene).

Hyman J. Zimmerman (Hy to his friends) (Fig. 2) also had been an Army doctor in World War II. After discharge he served a medical residency 1946–8 at Ballinger Hospital in Washington (later called DC General Hospital from 1953 until it was closed in 2001). He learned there to do needle biopsy of the liver, and noted a distinction between the very common infectious viral hepatitis that he had seen in World War II and the various liver injuries diagnosed as being caused by drugs at Ballinger. He used liver biopsy to study effects on the liver of many other disease states such as renal, cardiac, malignant, metabolic (diabetes), and pulmonary diseases, as well as in various infections, and to study the diagnosis and management of liver diseases more generally. He published several articles on use of plasma enzymes for disease diagnosis before he focused on toxic hepatopathy, and in 1978 published [5] his monograph "Hepatotoxicity: The Adverse Effects of Drugs and Other Chemical on the Liver."

Arthur Karmen (Fig. 3) was accepted as a medical student at New York University in 1950 and was recruited in 1952 to work with two cardiologists (John S. LaDue and Felix Wroblewski) to search for a new indicator (what we would now term a biomarker) to diagnose myocardial infarction. He worked a year (1952–1953) in the laboratory of Severo Ochoa (who shared with Arthur Kornberg the 1959 Nobel Prize for discoveries of RNA and DNA), learning to measure activity of serum glutamic oxalacetic transaminase (SGOT), first using paper chromatography, required several days, but then by a quick assay needing only 5 min [6].

Coupling the transamination reaction (Fig. 4) to remove the product oxaloacetic acid by reducing it to malic acid by adding

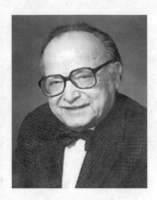

Fig. 2 Hyman J. Zimmerman (19 July, 1914–12 July, 1999), definer of drug-induced liver disease

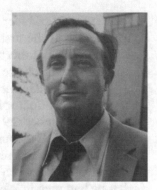

Fig. 3 Arthur Karmen (10 July, 1930–), developer of rapid, simple serum enzyme biomarkers)

malic dehydrogenase and DPNH$_2$ (diphoshopyridine nucleotide, reduced, later called nicotine adenosine dinucleotide, NADH) speeded the reversible transamination reaction, and pulled it more rapidly to completion, as suggested by Ochoa. The second reaction (reduction) rate could be followed by spectrophotometric decrease in absorption peak at wavelength 340 mµ, as NADH was oxidized to NAD$^+$. The new method could also be used to measure glutamic *pyruvic* transaminase activity in serum (SGPT), later renamed alanine aminotransferase (ALT) for the amino acid substrate rather than the product of the reversible reaction. The work of Karmen was immediately confirmed [7] in Italian patients with viral hepatitis by Fernando De Ritis, who had read the preliminary report [3] in Science, published a few months earlier than the full article [6] in the Journal of Clinical Investigation. Another Italian paper [8] considered AST in liver homogenates. While Karmen was busy in 1954–7 with internship and medical residency at NYU, Wrobleski and LaDue pursued study of transaminases, first SGOT in liver disease [9] and then SGPT [10].

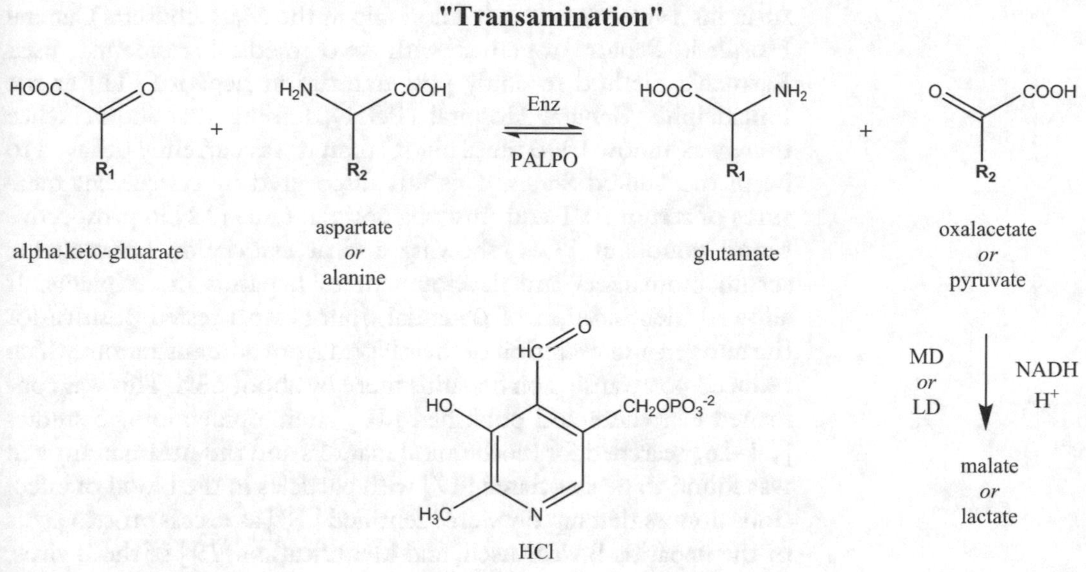

"Transamination"

Fig. 4 Transamination

In medical school at the same time as Karmen, but in Philadelphia at the University of Pennsylvania, one of the coauthors of this chapter (John Senior) was also then an intern who became intrigued by the clever new spectrophotometric assay for serum transaminase activities. He used the paper [6] published by Karmen in January 1955 as a guide to the method and obtained permission to use the equipment of the laboratory at the Hospital of the University of Pennsylvania at night, for helping to diagnose acute myocardial infarction in his patients and those of other interns.

The ideas of Popper, Zimmerman and Karmen stimulated hundreds of other investigators all over the world, and established a basis for the future. Their innovative concepts were:

Hans Popper—development of a new medical subspecialty: **hepatology**;

Hyman Zimmerman—**drug-induced liver injury** distinct from other liver diseases;

Arthur Karmen—evaluating major organ injury by rapid **serum enzyme assay**.

2   Growth and Attempts at Standardization

The discovery of serum enzyme activity as a measure or estimate of liver injury fairly rapidly started a series of short reports from all over the world raising questions on whether elevation of serum enzyme activities such as ALT could be relied upon to diagnose drug causality.

After his 1959–62 research fellowship at the Massachusetts General Hospital, Senior, together with two medical residents, used Karmen's method to study post-transfusion hepatitis [11] at the Philadelphia General Hospital (PGH), finding that its incidence there was almost 1000 times higher than it was currently believed to be in the United States. This was discovered by concurrent measures of serum ALT and Australia antigen (Au) [12] in prospective blood donors at PGH, showing a clear association between the serum biomarkers and development of hepatitis in recipients. It allowed identification of potential donors who tested positive for the antigen and exclusion of their blood from administration, which reduced posttransfusion hepatitis there by about 65%. This was confirmed elsewhere and published [13] later. Epidemiologic studies [14–16] searched for biochemical markers and the Australia antigen was found to be associated [17] with particles in the blood of infectious donors that rapidly were identified [18] as excess protein coats of the hepatitis B virus itself, and identification [19] of the B virus. Hans Popper finally agreed to serve as President of AASLD in 1963, gradually turning its control over to its governing board. He was aware of the PGH work and in 1969 appointed Senior to join the governing board of AASLD. During his 10 years of service there, Senior learned about the seminal ideas [20] of Zimmerman on liver injury caused by drugs, and delved into the first edition of Zimmerman's book. He was the 25th president of AASLD in 1974, and initiated that year a course in the format of a classic clinical-pathological conference (annual courses ever since). With his AASLD vice-president, Bill Summerskill, he also started activities to create a lay organization, the American Liver Foundation in 1976, under Dr. Burt Combes, and in 1981 the journal called Hepatology, first editor Dr. Irwin Arias. By the end of the 1970s, hepatology was well established, and AASLD was attracting hundreds then thousands of registrants to its annual fall meetings. The 1978 monograph by Zimmerman had made drug-induced liver injury increasingly well recognized, although it was still unclear on how to diagnose it. He had repeatedly stated in lectures and writings that "*drug-induced hepatocellular jaundice is a serious lesion*" with substantial mortality. This caught the attention of Dr. Robert Temple at the FDA, who began looking for cases as they came to his attention overseeing reviews of new drugs for approval. In France, interest developed on defining adverse drug reactions [21] and standardizing criteria. They began to appreciate how difficult it was to diagnose [22] drug-induced liver injury (DILI). A very important meeting was called by Benichou and Danan, who were employees of the Roussel Uclaf pharmaceutical company in Paris. They invited leading hepatologists to meet in Paris in June 1989 to discuss drug-induced liver disease, sponsored by the Council for International Organization of Medical Sciences (CIOMS), funded and reported [23] by Roussel Uclaf. Attending were:

France	B. Begaud, Bordeaux
	J. P. Benhamou (chairman), Clichy
	C. Benichou, Paris (Roussel-Uclaf)
	G, Danan, Paris (Roussel-Uclaf)
	G. Lagier, Paris (Ministry of Health)
Denmark	N. Tygstrup, Copenhagen
Germany	J. Bircher, Herdecke
Italy	F. Orlandi. Ancona
Switzerland	Z. Bankowski, Geneva (CIOMS)
	J.F. Dunne, Geneva (World Health Organization)
United Kingdom	J. Neuberger, Birmingham
United States	H. Zimmerman, Washington
	W. Maddrey, Philadelphia

This report was followed in 1993 by the scoring system that has become known as the RUCAM, for *Roussel-Uclaf Causality Assessment Method*, written [21, 25] by Gaby Danan and Christian Benichou, who attempted to simplify and evaluate the conclusions of the Paris meeting 4 years before, especially focusing on the causality problem. They recognized that the experts invited were experts in liver disease but not necessarily in what they called "causality assessment" that required weighting of factors without dependence on their hepatology expertise and could be done by nonhepatologists. Point values from −3 to +3 were somewhat arbitrarily assigned to several factors, namely:

1. time from drug administration to onset of the reaction, 0 to +3;
2. course of the reaction, −2 to +3;
3. risk factors for reactivity, 0 to +2;
4. other drugs administered concomitantly, −3 to 0;
5. other nondrug cause. −3 to +2;
6. previous information on the drug in question, 0 to +2; and finally
7. response to readministration, rechallenge, −2 to +3;

    or plasma concentration known to be toxic, +3;

    or laboratory test with high specificity, sensitivity, and predictive value that has been validated, −3 to +3. (The last presumably referred to some new biomarker that could be relied upon.)

    Despite the attempt to free the scoring system from opinion and experience, the RUCAM still required considerable judgmental skills and was subject to them. Interpretation of final scores as drug-induced was taken as: 0 or less, excluded; 1–2, unlikely; 3–5, possible; 6–8 probable; and >8 highly probable. Assessments were based on narratives or clinical histories of single cases but were proposed for possible use in clinical trials of new drugs. A recapitulation and enthusiastic retrospective endorsement of the RUCAM is included in this volume (Chap. 27 by Rolf Teschke and Gaby Danan).

3   Hy's Law

A second key year was 1999, when several more seminal events took place. Senior had joined the FDA as a medical reviewer for gastrointestinal drugs in June 1995, and became acquainted with reviewers in other divisions. Reports on two new drugs, troglitazone and bromfenac, were disturbing. Both drugs were approved in 1997 despite evidence of liver injury, and after approval patients treated showed serious and sometimes fatal hepatotoxicity. Troglitazone was a promising novel agent for treatment of diabetes. It was an antidiabetic, anti-inflammatory drug of the thiazolidinedione class, developed at first by Daiichi Sankyo in Japan, then by Parke-Davis as REZULIN in the United States for patients with type 2 diabetes mellitus. Although there were signals of liver toxicity, it was approved on 29 January, 1997. Liver dysfunction [26] and deaths were reported [27, 28] soon after. Bromfenac was a nonsteroidal analgesic and anti-inflammatory drug approved for pain relief 15 July, 1997 and marketed by Wyeth-Ayerst as DURACT, with instructions not to use it for more than 10 days. Despite those label warnings, some patients took it for longer, and acute liver failure, liver transplantation, and death occurred in three patients [29–31]. It was withdrawn [30] quickly from the market by the sponsor on 22 June, 1998. Upon learning in the summer of 1998 about the reports of the serious liver toxicity of these new drugs, Senior called Dr. Zimmerman at his home and asked if he thought it might be a good idea to organize a conference of medical and other FDA reviewers to discuss the problem of FDA approval of drugs that caused life-threatening adverse effects. He agreed and offered to participate. We proceeded to plan a conference on serious adverse effects of approved drugs, held 19–20 April 1999 at the University of Maryland Conference Center at Shady Grove (Fig. 5). It attracted about 325 FDA reviewers and had to be repeated in November for 75 more. Hy Zimmerman was present although unable to talk because of progressing lingual carcinoma and had asked Dr. James Lewis [32] to speak for him.

Although other drugs with other toxicities were included, the conference centered on troglitazone and bromfenac. In the discussion period on the first day Robert Temple remarked that he

Food and Drug Administration (FDA)
Center for Drug Evaluation and Research (CDER)
Office of Training and Communication, Division of Training and Development
and the Committee for Advanced Science Education

CDER STAFF COLLEGE COURSE ASE 0202

Drugs and the Liver: What They Do To Each Other
April 19-20, 1999
University of Maryland, Shady Grove Campus Auditorium, Gaithersburg

Monday, 19 April 1999

8:00	Check-in, coffee	
8:30	Welcome, Course Overview	John Senior, HFD-180
8:35	The Problem of Drug-Induced Hepatotoxicity	Mac Lumpkin, HFD-002
8:45	Specific Examples (8-10 minutes each)	
	bromfenac (DURACT)	John Hyde, HFD-550
	tolcapone (TASMAR)	Judy Racoosin, HFD-120
	troglitazone (REZULIN)	Sol Sobel, HFD-510
	tasosartan (VERDIA)	Bob Fenichel, HFD-110
	zileuton (ZYFLO)	Ray Anthracite, HFD-570
	tacrine (COGNEX)	Randy Levin, HFD-120
9:45	FDA Perspective on Drug-Hepatotoxicity	Bob Temple, HFD-004
10:15	Break	
10:45	Drug metabolism and hepatotoxicity in animals; choice of animal species for testing liver effects	Sharon Center, Cornell University School of Veterinary Medicine
11:45	Pharmacology/toxicology preclinical assessments	Andrea Weir, HFD-550
12:15	Lunch	
1:15	Liver function and injury: what the tests mean	John Senior, HFD-180
1:45	What we can learn from hepatic studies in vitro	Jerry Collins, HFD-902
2:15	Human hepatotoxicity of drugs; toxicity or idiosyncracy, cellular or cholestatic?	Jim Lewis, Georgetown University Hy Zimmerman, Armed Forces Institute of Pathology, Walter Reed AMC
3:15	Break	
3:45	Detection of hepatoxicity during NDA review	Tom Laughren, HFD-120
4:15	Clinical panel discussion	Lumpkin, Temple, Senior, Lewis, Zimmerman, Lee, Laughren
5:00	Adjourn	

Fig. 5 First DILI Conference 19 April 1999

CDER STAFF COLLEGE COURSE ASE 0202

Drugs and the Liver: What They Do To Each Other
April 19-20, 1999
University of Maryland, Shady Grove Campus Auditorium, Gaithersburg

Tuesday, 20 April 1999

8:00	Coffee	
8:30	Fialuridine and chronic hepatitis B	David Feigal, HFM-1
8:45	Evaluating drug toxicity in patients with preexisting liver disease	Will Lee, Universityof Texas, Southwestern (Dallas)
9:45	Panel--special problems in treating hepatitis	Zimmerman, Lee, Lewis, Feigal, Senior Graham, Lumpkin, Temple
10:30	Break	
11:00	Post-marketing detection of hepatoxicity	David Graham, HFD-733
11:30	Lessons learned and solutions to be found	Mac Lumpkin, HFD-730
12:00	Lunch	
1:00	Workshop description, questions for breakout groups ...with respect to drug-induced hepatotoxicity, what can be done better to:	Robert Temple; moderator

- detect it in animals and predict it in people?
- use *in vitro* systems to predict it?
- design clinical studies to detect it?
- detect it during NDA review?
- detect and characterize it post-approval?

1:15	Breakout sessions to discuss questions	All Participants
2:45	Reports of breakout groups	Breakout Group Spokespersons
3:30	General discussion in plenary session Consensus & Suggestions: What Might be Done Better	Faculty and Audience
4:00	Adjourn	

Thanks for coming!

Fig. 5 (continued)

had for many years seen cases of liver Injury occurring in patients receiving drugs, and concluded that the Zimmerman statement *"drug-induced hepatocellular jaundice is a serious lesion"* was true, as he reiterated in retrospect in a paper published [33] several years later. Further, Zimmerman had stated [6, page 353] that the mortality rate in patients with jaundice ranged from 10% for isoniazid and alpha-methyldopa to 50% for halothane and cinchophen. James Lewis showed the slide set prepared by Hy Zimmerman and commented [32] on the slides but the major discussion occurred when Hy was able to come to the front and contribute to the discussion, writing notes passed to Senior. The Zimmerman observation was based on his extensive review of thousands of patients with liver dysfunction and failure over four decades of intensive inquiry, where the most important question was whether the abnormal laboratory values indicated by the serum chemical tests were caused by the drug in question or by disease. The next question was whether the characteristic liver changes were due to injury to some underlying hepatocytes or biliary cells; the third question was whether the injury to hepatocytes was extensive enough to cause jaundice because the remaining hepatocytes were unable to carry out whole-liver function of clearing bilirubin from plasma, resulting in visible jaundice. Temple coined the term "Hy's law" as a modification of the Zimmerman term "drug-induced hepatocellular jaundice." Elevation of serum total bilirubin (TBL) above 2× ULN was taken to represent dysfunction of the liver with jaundice (visible possibly in scleral conjunctivae, depending on lighting conditions skin color, and observer experience). Serum transaminase activity of >3× ULN was also used to indicate at least moderate acute hepatocellular injury, as declared by consensus of experts [34] to be "markedly abnormal" at a Fogarty meeting in 1978. (The true complexity of what serum ALT values should be considered normal was discovered [35–37] later.) Both levels were taken arbitrarily at low levels, to increase the sensitivity of detection, with admitted loss of specificity and false positive conclusions. It was emphasized that these measures were not diagnostic for DILI, but required additional clinical determination that the liver injury and dysfunction were caused by the drug and not by some other liver disorder. The Temple definition of the Zimmerman statement that he dubbed "Hy's law" led to modest objection by hy Zimmerman, but since he could not speak he indicated it by shaking his head to signify "no." Temple also indicated that the Hy's law cases (usually just a few) needed to occur in a context where there were more cases of elevated serum ALT without jaundice in more subjects on drug than on control agents as an ancillary finding, which senior then dubbed "Temple's Corollary." Three months later Hy Zimmerman died [38] on 12 July 1999, 1 week before his 85th birthday, but he left autographed copies of his second edition of the monograph for several of his friends and a final review article was published [39] posthumously in early 2000. The meetings of April and November 1999 had included a total of about 400 FDA reviewers, who thereafter began to demand and receive much more detailed data and verbal information about possible liver toxicity of new drugs under development by industry sponsors. This first DILI conference led to another meeting the following year [40] organized by the NIH, and aroused interest by the pharmaceutical industry asking to be included, and a second DILI conference was organized and presented [41] on 12–13 February 2001. That meeting in Chantilly, Virginia brought together speakers and registrants from the FDA, the pharmaceutical industry and academic consultants to both, a pattern that established the format for succeeding DILI conferences.

4   eDISH

Following the first two DILI conferences in 1999 and 2001, Guo and Senior ruminated on how the key ideas expressed by Zimmerman and popularized by Temple as Hy's law might be visualized graphically. To begin, we wanted to apply the concepts developed by Zimmerman in his study of many individual cases to clinical trials in which hundreds of subjects would all be studied in the same way and data recorded. It was felt that it was obviously better to detect serious hepatoxic potential before approval than to find it later. In considering the Zimmerman dictum "drug-induced hepatocellular jaundice" as it might apply to finding cases in clinical trials before approval, it was clear that "jaundice" was easy to detect as elevated serum bilirubin. Hepatocellular injury is nearly always reflected by increased serum ALT, but the hard part was how to determine if those abnormalities were caused by the drug. It looked like the three elements had to be tackled in reverse order: find jaundice, find hepatocellular injury, and consider if it was drug-induced. Just finding the first two was not enough to fulfill the Zimmerman dictum. Very high on the RUCAM list of important factors were time relationships of liver test measures, and a good medical history in narrative form. The latter had been the classic information used for decades to diagnose toxic hepatitis, drug-induced liver injury, toxic hepatopathy, etc. The idea of expressing this graphically came to both Senior and Guo when they were working in the Office of Pharmacoepidemiology and Statistical Sciences (OPaSS) under directorship of Dr. Paul Seligman in 2002–4. Serial data over time would be available for all the subjects in a clinical trial, as required by the protocol, a much more complete data base than ever available in clinical practice for study of isolated single cases. Inclusion of all subjects made possible the estimate of *incidence* of degrees of abnormality of the measures, and of finding serious or severe cases, which were expected to be rare, based on previous clinical experience and the literature. Any such serious cases (disabled, hospitalized, showing liver failure) would then need detailed examination of the time course of changes and clinical history to make possible the difficult *diagnosis* of DILI. Just finding liver trouble was not enough, and fulfilling the Zimmerman dictum or the watered-down Hy's law required that the abnormalities be at least probably drug-induced, not due to some other disease or uncertainty. Uncertainty was 100% when one started with elevated ALT and TBL; the difficult problem was to reduce it. "At least probably" DILI was taken to mean that the combined likelihood of all other possible causes, including uncertainty, were estimated to be less than 50%.

A visualization software tool we named eDISH *(evaluation of Drug-Induced Serious Hepatotoxicity)* was created around year

2002–2003 as a working prototype two-step program with very basic capabilities: to inspect at first the *incidence* of potential liver injury cases in a clinical trial, and secondly try to make a *diagnosis* of their causes. The eDISH tool was created using commercial software named SAS/IntrNet as the platform, designed to mimic the thought process that goes into medical differential diagnosis of probable drug-cause of liver injury. The first key step was to visualize incidence of serious cases of possible concerns by showing all subjects in the study at a glance. That makes some subjects with significantly elevated values "stand out," prominently in the first graph. The second step was aimed at making a medical diagnosis of the most likely cause.

Shown in Fig. 6 is a 2004 example of the first eDISH graph for all-subject visualization. The data used here are based on a real-life new-drug application. To protect the confidentiality of the drug maker, subjects on the active treatment were denoted as "X," and "C" as control arm.

This is a two-dimensional scatter plot by treatment group, based on s subjects' injury-caused ALT measurements and liver-function indicator, TBL. In this scatter plot, the X-axis represents the ALT multiples of the upper limit of normal ranges (ALT × ULN), while the Y-axis, the TBL, displayed on a log 10 scale. The entire plot is divided into four quadrants: SW, NW, NE, and SE quadrants. The dividing lines thus decided were considered reasonable

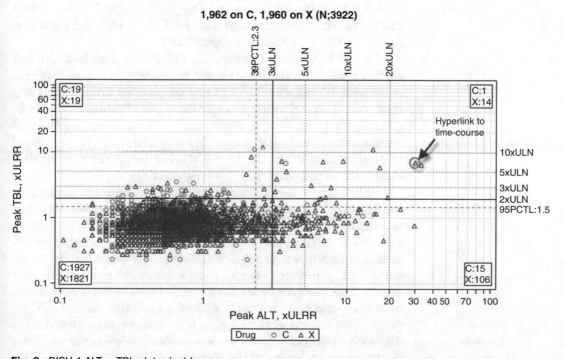

Fig. 6 eDISH 1 ALT × TBL plot—incidence

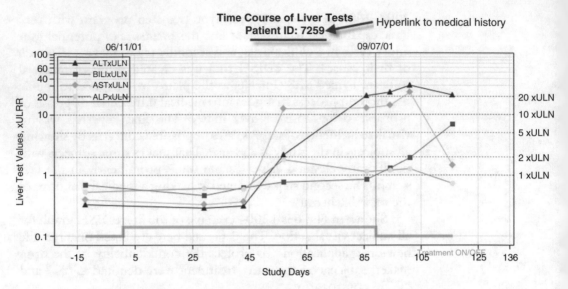

Fig. 7 eDISH 2- time course for diagnosis (with narrative)

at the time, to be inclusive and maximize sensitivity, at the risk of losing specificity. All subjects with peak ALT × ULN >3 and peak TBLxULN > 2 fall into the NE or right upper quadrant. These subjects are potentially Hy's law cases *IF THEY ARE DRUG-INDUCED*, but require further investigation of the time course of liver tests measured over the period subjects were observed and a narrative to make that diagnosis. The graph in Fig. 7 is the second eDISH graph of chemical enzymes (ALT, AST, and ALP) and liver function (TBL) for a single subject 7259.

Here is how eDISH works: After eDISH is launched, the first eDISH graph appears. If we decide to investigate a subject (green circle with ID number 7259 in first graph), we simply point and click on it. This action triggers a SAS program running in the background, resulting in the display of a time-course graph of all enzymes and bilirubin values for that subject during his/her period of obsedrvation in the study, the abscissa being the time in days since starting drug administration (green line).

SAS/IntrNet conveniently provides links between subjects in the first eDISH graph and the second eDISH graph. Among other technical advantages that SAS possesses, such as data processing and a wide range of statistical procedures, we particularly appreciated the drill-down capability SAS/IntrNet provides. In other words, SAS/IntrNet provides such a feature that we can turn a static scatter plot to a dynamic one: each point in the scatter plot is now a hyperlinked to a time-course graph, the second eDISH graph. The second eDISH graph is critical; to help in making a diagnosis of the possible cause, so a medical reviewer can easily see the time-course display of the four chemical measures: ALT, TBL,

AST, and ALP, over the whole period of time the subject was under observation in the study. Subjects located in the right upper or NE quadrant of the first eDISH graph were considered especially worthy of further interrogation as subjects of special interest, but not Hy's law cases until diagnosis of drug-induced cause could be made. Further interrogation augmented the time-course graph through a review of medical history (or clinical narrative), which can be opened easily from within the eDISH program under the second graph.

Cases with elevated serum bilirubin that might be diagnosable as jaundiced are in the upper quadrants (NW and NE), while cases with elevated serum ALT are in the right quadrants NE and SE. Therefore, the subjects in the left lower quadrant (SW) who showed no significant elevations of either biomarker of liver injury or dysfunction were considered "normal" or of low interest. Subjects whose serial clinical trial data placed them in the right upper (NE) quadrant were those who needed the additional information of time course and narrative to diagnose the probable cause of the abnormalities, which possibly could be caused by many different liver disorders. It is incorrect to assume that all subjects whose data put them in the right upper quadrant are Hy's law cases without determining the likely cause of the abnormal findings. The SAS/IntrNet capabilities are especially useful for this 1–2-step process. True Hy's law cases tend to be rare, and it is important to pull these "needles from haystacks" in evaluating new drugs in clinical trials.

Currently, eDISH in SAS/IntrNet is running on the FDA server and can be accessed by the medical reviewers via Intranet behind a security firewall. The security is for the data, not for the eDISH program that processes it. The sponsor-provided data were checked for their conformity to the eDISH Data Specifications. If qualified, they were stored in a centrally located file server for eDISH analyses or future research programs. Currently, Potential users of eDISH will request and receive unique access code in accordance with the FDA's security regulations. Over the decade or more that it has been in use, it has been modified and improved. Errors were fixed; unused functions were removed; new features were added. Therefore, it serves as both review and research tools. The eDISH program was not written overnight, but took many months to develop in the period 2002–2004 when Guo and Senior were working together in the same Office of Pharmacoepidemiology and Statistical Science (OPaSS). An initial presentation [42] of these concepts was made to a small group of investigators at a meeting 28 January, 2005 at a local meeting site in Rockville MD.

5   DILI as an Ongoing Global Problem

The NIH funded a study group of hepatologists in the United States in 2004, calling [43] it the *Drug-Induced Liver Injury Network* (DILIN). They elected first to use both the RUCAM system used widely elsewhere, and the process of DILI diagnosis used by Zimmerman, based on the clinical history and physical findings, symptoms and time course of liver tests. However, in all his hundreds of published papers and two monographs of 1978 and 1999, Zimmerman never defined exactly how he made the diagnosis of "drug-induced." He knew one when he saw it, but like recognizing a face, it is difficult to describe in words and remains a thorny problem. The FDA Guidance to Industry "Drug-Induced Liver Injury: Premarketing Clinical Evaluation" that was published [44] in 2009 specified that "no other reasons could be found to explain the combination of increased AT and TBL, such as viral hepatitis A, B, or C; preexisting or acute liver disease; or another drug capable of causing the observed injury." Finding true Hy's law cases in a clinical trial is a matter of great concern, especially if there is more than one, and may delay or prevent drug approval. The RUCAM program [24] was the first effort to tackle the problem, and is still widely used by its original name despite the sale of the Roussel Uclaf company successively to Hoechst, Aventis, and Sanofi. When the DILIN was formed, the team members used both the RUCAM and overall judgment. The clinical narrative included medical history, physical findings, medications, and laboratory data for each patient, and was used for both methods by three of its members who independently rated each case to develop causality scores. After cases were evaluated by both methods, they found [45–47] RUCAM to be less reproducible. After 12 years of experience with hundreds of cases, the DILIN group recognizes [48] that expert opinions vary, that the process is costly, cumbersome, and time-consuming, and that consensus does not always equal truth. Nevertheless, the expert opinion process, modeled after that used by Zimmerman himself, is the best current method [49, 50] for evaluating the likelihood that an observed predominantly hepatocellular injury sufficiently severe to cause jaundice and probably caused by the drug in question is still the gold standard. The eDISH program has been partially copied by many companies that were not using the SAS/IntrNet program available only within the FDA, considering only the first relative incidence plot of ALT × TBL, and incorrectly calling the right upper quadrant cases as Hy's law cases. They are, however, cases of special interest which require additional examination by time course and narrative to diagnose Hy's law, which primarily requires that the liver test abnormalities be caused by the drug and not by some other liver disease, a determination that is not always easy [51] and may lead to wrong diagnosis in many cases. Beyond that, the right upper quadrant cases sometimes have been wrongly claimed to be diagnostic of HY's law. To misdiagnose Hy's law cases by counting all cases of elevated serum ALT and TBL is incorrect. It is important in review of new drugs for approval to detect true Hy's law cases, which is not easy and requires more information than simple serum chemistry elevations for diagnosis. It is also important in follow-up of approved drugs to diagnose Hy's law correctly, to avoid costly investigation of false positive cases and to begin correct treatment of the real cause. Reviewers should be aware that the cases of combined elevations of ALT and TBL indicate cases of special interest but are not diagnostic of Hy's law, and require study and more work to establish a correct diagnosis of their cause. This is applicable to premarketing studies before approval and also to post-marketing studies in larger numbers of "real-world" patients treated after conditional approval.

Disclaimer

The views expressed are those of the authors and do not necessarily represent the position of nor imply endorsement from the U. S. Food and Drug Administration of the United States' Government.

References

1. Popper H (1982) History of the American Association for the Study of liver diseases. Hepatology 2(6):874–878

2. Lepper MH, Wolfe CK, Zimmerman HJ, Caldwell ER, Spies HW, Dowling HF (1951) Effect of large doses of aureomycin on the human liver. AMA Arch Int Med 88(3):271–283

3. La Due JS, Wroblewski F, Karmen A (1954) Serum glutamic oxalacetic transaminase in human acute transmural myocardial infarction. Science 120(3117):497–499

4. Popper H, Franklin M (1947) Infectious hepatitis contrasted with toxic hepatitis. Proc Inst Med Chic 16(12):353

5. Zimmerman HJ (1978) Hepatotoxicity: the adverse effects of drugs and other chemicals on the liver. Appleton-Century-Crofts, New York

6. Karmen A, Wroblewski F, La Due JS. Transaminase activity in human blood. J Clin Invest 1955:34(1):128–133

7. De Ritis F, Coltorti M, Giusti G Attivita transaminasica del siero umano nell'epatite virale. (Transaminase activity of human serum in viral hepatitis). Minerva Med 46(34):1207–1209

8. Careddu P (1955) Modificazoni di attivita enzymatiche nella nefrosi sperimentale da siero antirene. IV. Attivita dl-aspartico transaminasica negliomogenati di rene e di fegato in ratto nefrosico. [Variations in enzyme activity in experimental nephrosis induced by antirenal serum. IV. dl-aspartic transaminase activity of kidney and liver homogenates of nephrotic rats]. Boll Soc Ital Biol Sper 6:639–641

9. Wroblewski F, La Due JS (1955) Serum glutamic oxalacetic transaminase activity as an index of liver cell injury: a preliminary report. Ann Intern Med 43(2):345–360

10. Wroblewski F, La Due JS (1956) Serum glutamic pyruvic transaminase (SGP-T) in hepatic disease: a preliminary report. Ann Intern Med 45(5):801–811

11. Hampers CL, Prager D, Senior JR (1964) Post-transfusion anicteric hepatitis. N Engl J Med 271(15):747–754

12. Blumberg BS, Alter HJ, Visnich SA (1965) "New" antigen in leukemia serum. JAMA 191(7):841–846

13. Senior JR, Sutnick AI, Goeser E, London WT, Dahlke MB, Blumberg BS (1974) Reduction of post-transfusion hepatitis by exclusion of Australia antigen from donor blood in an urban public hospital. Am J Med Sci 267(3):171–177

14. Rees E (1964) Epidemiology of infectious hepatitis. Brit Med J 2(5401):69–70

15. West ED (1964) Drug and viral hepatitis. Brit Med J 2(5406):445. (reply to 14)

16. De Ritis F, Giusti G, Piccinino F, Cacciatore L (1965) Biochemical laboratory tests in viral hepatitis and other hepatic diseases. Bull World Health Organ 32:59–72

17. Prince AM (1968) Relation of Australia and SH antigens. Lancet 2(7565):462–463

18. Hirschman RJ, Shulman NR, Barker LF, Smith KO (1969) Virus-like particles in sera of patients with infectious and serum hepatitis. JAMA 208(9):1667–1670

19. Dane DS, Cameron CH, Briggs M (1970) Virus-like particles in serum of patients with Australia-antigen-associated hepatitis. Lancet 7649:695–698

20. Zimmerman HJ (1978) Drug-induced liver disease. Drugs 45(5):801–811

21. Benichou C, Danan G (1987) Reunions de consensus sur les definitions en pharmacovigilance. [Consensus conference on definitions in drug monitoring]. Therapie 42(4):347–350

22. Danan G, Benichou C (1987) Criteres d'imputation d'une hepatite aigue a un medicament. Resultats de reunion de consensus. [Criteria of imputation of acute hepatitis to a drug. Results of consensus meetings]. Gastroenterol Clin Biol 11(8–9):581–585

23. Benichou C (1990) Criteria of drug-induced liver disorders. Report of an international consensus meeting. J Hepatol 11(2):272–276

24. Danan G, Benichou C (1993) Causality assessment of adverse reactions to drugs – I. A novel method based on the conclusions of international consensus meetings: application to drug-induced liver injuries. J Clin Epidemiol 46(11):1323–1330

25. Benichou C, Danan G (1993) Causality assessment of adverse reactions to drugs – II. An original model for validation of drug causality assessment methods: case report with positive rechallenge. An application to drug-induced liver injuries. J Clin Epidemiol 46(11):1331–1336

26. Watkins PB, Whitcomb R (1998) Hepatic dysfunction associated with troglitazone. Ann Intern Med 338(13):916–917

27. Neuschwander-Tetri BA, Isley WL, Oki JC (1998) Troglitazone-induced hepatic failure leading to transplantation. A case report. Ann Intern Med 129(1):38–41

28. Misbin RI (1999) Troglitazone-associated hepatic failure. Ann Intern Med 130(4 Pt 1):330

29. Moses PL, Schroeder B, Alkhatib O, Ferrentino N, Suppan T, Lidofsky SD (1999) Severe hepatotoxicity associated with bromfenac sodium. Am J Gastroenterol 94(5):1393–1396

30. Hunter EB, Johnston PE, Tanner G, Pinson CW, Awad JA (1999) Bromfenac (Duract)- associated hepatic failure requiring liver transplantation. Am J Gastroenterol 94(8):2299–2301

31. Rabkin JM, Smith MJ, Orloff SL, Corless CL, Stenzel P, Olyaei AJ (1999) Fatal fulminant hepatitis associated with bromfenac use. Ann Pharmacother 33(9):945–975

32. Lewis JH (2006) Hy's law, the 'Rezulin rule,' and other predictors of severe drug-induced hepatotoxicity: putting risk-benefit into perspective. Pharmacepidemiol. Drug Saf 15(4):221–229

33. Temple R. (2016) Hy's law: predicting serious hepatotoxicity. Pharmacepidemiol Drug Saf 15(4):241–243

34. Davidson CS, Leevy CM, Chamberlayne EC (eds) (1979) Guidelines for detection of hepatotoxicity due to drugs and chemicals. [Fogarty conference, 1978] NIH Publication no. 79–313. US Government Printing Office, Washington, DC, p 109

35. Senior JR (2012) Alanine aminotransferase: a clinical and regulatory tool for detecting liver injury---past, present, and future. Clin Pharmacol Ther 92(3):332–339

36. Dufour DR, Lott JA, Nolte FS, Gretch DR, Koff RS, Seeff LB (2000) Diagnosis and monitoring of hepatic injury. I. Performance characteristics of Laboratory tests. Clin Chem 46(12):2027–2049

37. Dufour DR, Lott JA, Nolte FS, Gretch DR, Koff RS, Seeff LB (2000) Diagnosis and monitoring of hepatic injury. II. Recommendations for use of laboratory tests in detecting, diagnosing, and Monitoring. Clin Chem 46(12):2050–2068

38. Seeff LB, Hyman J, Zimmerman MD (2000) JAMA 283(6):812

39. Zimmerman HJ (2000) Drug-induced liver disease. Clin Liver Dis 4(1):73–96

40. Bissell DM, Gores GJ, Laskin DL, Hoofnagle JH (2000) Drug-induced liver injury: mechanisms and test systems. Hepatology 33(4):1009–1013

41. Second DILI Conference 2001. A national and global problem. Speaker (choose), biosketch, abstract, slides shown. FDA Archive: Drug-Induced Liver Toxicity

42. Senior JR. Fifth DILI conference 2005. Recognizing drug-induced liver injury (DILI)

in exposed populations. FDA Archive: Drug-Induced Liver Toxicity

43. Fontana RJ, Watkins PB, Bonkovsky HL, Chalasani N, Davern T, Serrano J, Rochon J (2009) For the DILIN study group. Drug-induced liver injury network (DILIN) prospective study: rationale, design, and conduct. Drug Saf 32(1):55–68

44. Guidance for Industry 2009. Drug-Induced Liver Injury: premarketing clinical evaluation GuidanceComplianceRegulatoryInformation/Guidances/ucm174090.pdf

45. Rockey DC, Seefe LB, Rochon J, Freston J, Chalasani N, Bonacini M, Fontana RJ, Hayashi PH (2007) Drug-induced liver injury network. Comparison between expert opinion and rucam for assignment of causality in drug-induced liver injury. Gastroenterology 132(4):A-773. (M1777)

46. Rochon J, Protiva P, Seefe LB, Fontana RJ, Liangpunsakul S, Watkins PB, Davern T, McHutchinson JG (2008) Reliability of the Roussel Uclaf causality assessment method for assessing causality in drug-induced liver injury. Hepatology 48(4):1175–1183

47. Rockey DC, Seefe LB, Rochon J, Freston J, Chalasani N, Bonacini M, Fontana RJ, Hayashi PH (2010) For the drug-induced liver injury network. Causality assessment in drug-induced liver injury using a structured expert opinion process: comparison to the Roussel-Uclaf causality assessment method. Hepatology 51(6):2117–2123

48. Hayashi PH (2016) Drug-induced liver injury network causality assessment: criteria and experience in the United States. Int J Mol Sci 17(2):201–210

49. Robles-Diaz M, Lucena MI, Kaplowitz N, Stephens C, Medina-Caliz I, Gonzalez-Jimenez A, Ulzurrun E, Gonzalez AF, Fernandez MC, Romero-Gomez M, Jimenez-Perez M, Bruguera M, Prieto M, Bessone F, Hernandez N, Arrese M, Andrade RJ (2014) Use of Hy's law and a new composite algorithm to predict acute liver failure in patients with drug-induced liver injury. Gastroenterology 147(11):109–118

50. Regev A, Seefe LB, Merz M, Omarsdottir S, Aithal GP, Gallivan J, Watkins PB (2014) Causality assessment for suspected DILI during clinical phases of drug development. Drug Saf 37(Suppl 1):s47–s56

51. Marrone G, Vaccaro FG, Bolato M, Miele L, Liquori A, Araneo C, Onziani FR, Mores N, Gasbarrini A, Grieco A (2017) Drug-induced liver injury 2017: the diagnosis is not easy but always to keep in mind. Eur Rev Med Pharmacol Sci 21(1 Suppl):122–134

Chapter 21

Variability in Baseline Liver Test Values in Clinical Trials: Challenges in Enhancing Drug-Induced Liver Injury Assessment in Subjects with Liver Disease

Bereket Tesfaldet, Gyorgy Csako, Tejas Patel, Md Shamsuzzaman, and Eileen Navarro Almario

Abstract

Baseline liver test (LT: alanine aminotransferase, aspartate aminotransferase, alkaline phosphatase, total bilirubin) values were examined in contemporaneous drug product applications for autoimmune disease (Group A), for diseases that could involve the liver (Group B), for hepatobiliary disease (Group C) and in a reference group with no overt liver disease. The upper limit of normal (ULN) values and hence the classification of an LT as a multiple of ULN varied widely across trials. Most baseline LT values were within the ULN, although the distribution curves of LT values in overt hepatobiliary disease gradually diverged from the other disease groups within the range of values considered to be normal, consistent with the exclusion of subjects with baseline LT 1.5–2 × ULN from most studies. Nonetheless, LT values >3 × ULN occurred in all groups, as in the reference group, suggesting underlying liver disease in the populations studied. Drug-induced liver injury (DILI) is challenging to assess in subjects whose baseline LT values are greater than ULN. Detection of DILI in subjects with liver disease will require an assessment of disease status, liver morphology and function, and LT elevations should be interpreted in light of natural disease variation. Population- and disease-specific thresholds predictive of DILI are needed to guide drug use in subjects with liver disease, given the increasing prevalence of nonalcoholic steatohepatitis (NASH), alcoholic steatohepatitis (ASH) and multidrug and supplement use. Standard definitions of liver cirrhosis and decompensation and standardized data on liver morphology and function can support these assessments.

Key words Liver injury, Adverse reactions, Drug trials, Data standards, Reference standards, Diagnosis, US Food and Drug Administration

1 Introduction

Drug-induced liver injury (DILI) is an uncommon adverse reaction that can result in liver failure and death. Liver injury is possible when values of alanine aminotransferase (ALT), aspartate aminotransferase (AST) and alkaline phosphatase (ALP) are observed above the upper limit of normal (ULN). Low-level elevations of these enzyme test values are common [1], and can be an artifact of

Minjun Chen and Yvonne Will (eds.), *Drug-Induced Liver Toxicity*, Methods in Pharmacology and Toxicology, https://doi.org/10.1007/978-1-4939-7677-5_21, © Springer Science+Business Media, LLC, part of Springer Nature 2018

testing [2] or represent injury from disease [3], environmental toxins [4, 5], and drugs or nutritional supplements [6, 7]. On the other hand, more extensive test elevations (liver test [LT] >3 × ULN) following drug exposure have been shown to predict mortality [8] when accompanied with organ dysfunction as evidenced by visible jaundice equivalent to at least twice the value of direct bilirubin. These LT elevations, unexplained by any other cause, accompanied by an increased incidence in the new drug relative to control is the most specific predictor of a drug's potential for severe hepatotoxicity [2]. The US Food and Drug Administration (FDA) guidance recommends routine monitoring of these LTs for all drugs in development [9, 10] and has instituted hepatic expert consultation as a key element of DILI screening in review of new drug applications (NDA). Review efficiency is enhanced by the use of the e-DISH (evaluation of drug-induced serious hepatotoxicity), a program that computes postbaseline LT elevation as a multiple of the ULN and relies on data adherent to the Clinical Data Interchange Standards Consortium (CDISC) Study Data Tabulation Model (SDTM) format currently required for FDA submissions [11].

The utility of DILI prediction based on comparison to a normal reference has not been evaluated in subjects whose baseline LT values are above the ULN [12], such as in patients with liver disease. In these patients, LT values can be monitored to assess toxicity, but, when the natural history of their variation is well understood (e.g., ALP and bilirubin [BILI] for primary biliary cholangitis [PBC] or ALT for chronic hepatitis C [CHC] [2, 13–38]), also serve as endpoints of successful treatment of liver disease. Any changes in LT values in these patients therefore need interpretation in context of the extent of liver dysfunction, the subject's age, gender, comedications, and other comorbid conditions.

In this chapter, we describe the variability in four LT (ALT, AST, ALP and total BILI) baseline values obtained in registrational trials received at the FDA in subjects with and without liver disease and review the trial protocols to characterize the populations studied and available documentation of liver morphology and function. A description of the variability in baseline LT in these populations could inform design and patient selection in trials of new drugs to treat liver disease and promote submission of clinical trial data in a standard format.

2   Materials and Methods

2.1   Data Source and Trial Selection

New drug applications and biologic licensing applications (BLAs) are currently required to be submitted in electronic format to support computerized data analyses [39]. Applications that enrolled predominantly adult subjects in phase 1–3 trials and that adhered to the standardized study data requirements were selected for inclusion. Trial subjects who received at least one dose of treatment, and had pretreatment results for all four LTs, with specified ULN comprised the analysis population.

2.2   Trial Grouping for Analysis

Eligible studies were classified into three groups of subjects whose baseline LT could be greater than ULN due to previous treatment with drugs known to cause DILI (Group A), or whose underlying disease could involve the liver (Group B) or who had overt liver disease (Group C), whereas subjects with no overt liver disease served as a reference. Group A consisted of subjects with the autoimmune diseases ankylosing spondylitis (AS), multiple sclerosis (MS), psoriasis/psoriatic arthritis (PS) or rheumatoid arthritis (RA). Group B consisted of subjects with cancer with or without liver metastasis, Type 2 diabetes mellitus (T2DM) with potential NASH, community acquired pneumonia (CAP) with or without bacteremia, or tuberculosis (TB). Group C consisted of subjects with known hepatobiliary disease, i.e., chronic hepatitis B (CHB), CHC, NASH, or PBC. To represent the range of LT values in a relatively healthy population, our reference group consisted of community-dwelling subjects with no overt liver disease, including schoolchildren with head lice (HL), enteric disorders (ED) such as intestinal parasites, functional bowel disorders and vacationing travelers who received prophylaxis for diarrhea, and older adults of both sexes (hypogonadal males [HG-M] and postmenopausal osteoporotic females [OP-F]).

2.3   Data Collection and Protocol Review

Protocol specifications for inclusion and exclusion criteria, age, body weight or body mass index (BMI), status of liver function (presence of cirrhosis and decompensation), underlying disease severity, disease activity, co-occurring viral infections, presence of underlying liver disease, drug and alcohol abuse, comorbidities, concomitant medications, dietary restrictions, frequency and extent of monitoring of LTs, and discontinuation criteria are summarized in Tables 1a, and 1b, along with specifications for DILI data and analyses required in the FDA guidance [9, 10]. In addition to demographics, the following patient-level data were extracted from the trial datasets: treatment arm, treatment start date, visit days, values for ALP, ALT, AST, and BILI, and the corresponding ULN value. Pretreatment values represent all measurements of LTs obtained for screening purposes as well as those flagged as baseline in SDTM (or taken at day 1 for non-SDTM data) prior to administration of test drugs.

2.4   Data Analysis

Tabulation data were curated to a uniform format and a common data model to enable integrated analyses using SAS version 9.4 (SAS Institute, Cary, NC). For continuous variables, mean values with standard deviation (SD) and median with first (Q1) and third (Q3) quartiles were calculated, and the minimum and maximum values identified. Categorical variables were expressed in percentages. Box-and-whisker plots were used to describe the variability of LTs along a logarithmic scale to better illustrate outlier values.

Table 1a

Protocol-specified patient selection criteria and data elements collected to assess hepatic safety in representative new drug and biologic applications for the reference group

Protocol element	Data and analyses specified in DILI guidance	Reference group					SDTM domains for collected data
		Enteric disorders	IBS-D+	HL	HG-M	OP-F	
Intervention	Dose/regimen	1–3 days	12 weeks	Single dose (topical)	12–24 months	12–24 months	TA EX
Demographics Age (years), sex	Age, sex, race, ethnicity (other — gene variant, CYP, HLA etc.), individual risk factors	> 6 Males, females	18–65 (some 80 years) Males, females	>6 months	>50 (some >18 years) Males	>50 <80 (some 85 years) Females	DM (PB, PF, PG, SB)
Inclusion: subjects with liver specific inclusion criteria	All subjects must have the liver marker values for aminotransferases, total bilirubin, alkaline phosphatase, GGTP						LB PR for Imaging BR for biopsy SB for viral genotype TU/TR for cancer
Exclusion: based on screening tests	Screening should be conducted every 2–4 weeks for a few months	Investigator defined "clinically significant" abnormalities	AST/ALT >2×ULN BILI >2×ULN		Investigator defined "clinically significant" abnormalities One study "screening AST or ALT > 2.5×ULN"	Investigator defined "clinically significant" or > than normal range or "abnormal" ALP, AST/ALT BILI >1.5×ULN, ALP >2× ULN or >130 U/L**	LB
Exclusion based on BMI (kg/m²) or weight (kg)	BMI	Not specified	Not specified	Not specified	< 25 to > 42 kg/m²	>30 or >25–30% of ideal body weight	VS
Presence of liver disease	Subjects with liver abnormalities can be included, Rule out the following etiology: (1) viral, (2) autoimmune, (3) alcoholic, (4) ischemic hepatitis, (5) biliary tract disease, (6) acute heart failure/shock or hypotension	Investigator defined	Investigator defined liver disease: (1) inflammatory/immune, (2) Gilbert's, (3) unstable hepatic status, (4) biliary		Investigator defined	Investigator defined	LB MH for liver disease MI for histology PF, PG, MH CE QS PR for imaging BR for biopsy (Analysis domains—CPT score, derived data (LB, PE, CE))
Data to test liver function cirrhosis, decompensation	"but not if bilirubin excretory or protein synthesis (albumin, prothrombin) is impaired, unless a strong need for them to be treated"	No	No	No	No	No	MELD – LB, PR AST/platelet ratio

Protocol element	Data and analyses specified in DILI guidance	Reference group					SDTM domains for collected data
		Enteric Disorders	IBS-D+	HL	HG-M	OP-F	
Alcohol and drug abuse history	Alcohol, recreational drug use (special diets)	Not specified	DSM-IV-TR defined, 2 years prior	Not specified	Active use	Active alcohol and/or drug use	SU MH for a DSM IV diagnosis
HIV Hepatitis serologies	HAV, CHC, CHB, HIV Delta Antigen HEV serology HBV DNA viral load	Not specified	CHC, CHB, HIV	Not specified	CHC, CHB, HIV	CHC, CHB, HIV	LB IS
History of recent disease or procedures	"Exposure to environmental chemical agents"	Not specified	Cholecystitis <6 months diverticulitis <3 months gastric banding bariatric surgery	Not specified	Not specified	Not specified	PR
Lipid	Cholesterol, HDL, hypertriglyceridemia (assessed with diabetes, elevated BMI, do liver ultrasound for NASH)	Not specified	Not specified	Not specified	Not specified	Not specified	LB PR
Excluded concomitant medications that could confound hepatic safety	Including nonprescription, herbal, dietary supplements	Not specified	One program excluded probiotics	Not specified	Not specified	Estrogen	CM
AESI Endpoint	ABOVE plus: (1) Reliance on early symptoms, physical examination findings, (2) Unscheduled lab tests, (3) Imaging, (4) Biopsy/autopsy	No	No	No	No	No	LB AE PE VS PR BR/MI

Adapted from information in Drugs@FDA

*Laboratory criteria specified in certain protocols

**Specified in one trial that included women receiving low dose estrogen

+ Trials for IBS-D described separately due to extensive drug exposure and baseline testing

@Data collected when DILI is identified as a serious adverse event of special interest (SASE)

SDTM study data tabulation model, *AESI* adverse event of special interest

Table 1b

Protocol-specified patient selection criteria and data elements collected to assess hepatic safety in representative new drug and biologic applications in groups A, B and C

Protocol element	Group A				Group B					Group C			
	AS	MS	PS	RA	CANCER	T2DM CVOT	T2DM Non CVOT	CAP	TB	CHB	CHC	NASH	PBC
Intervention	16 weeks 12, 24 months	9–12, 24, 48, 84 months	12 weeks to 12 months	12–24 months	4–6 cycles of treatment	36 months	24 weeks	5–7 days	8 weeks to 24 months	48 weeks	12–24 weeks	52–72 weeks	12 months
Age (years) Sex	≥18 Males, females	18–55 Males, females	≥18 Males, females	>18 <65 Males, Females	>18 Males, females	>40 to >50 Males, females	>18 Males, females	>18 Males, females	>18	>12 Males, females	>18 Males, females	18–75 Males, females	18–75 Males, females
Inclusion: subjects with liver specific inclusion criteria					Adequate hepatic function BILI<ULN AST/ALT≤2.5× ULN, with liver metastases, ALT≤10× ULN ALP≤5×ULN					HBV DNA 2×10^4 IU/mL	HCV RNA >10^4 or >10^5 IU/mL plus viral genotype	ALT ≥47 U/L females ≥57 U/L males AST ≥47 U/L females ≥60 U/L males Enlarged liver on imaging Liver biopsy NASH score	ALP >1.67×ULN BILI >1 ×<2 ×ULN Phase 2 allowed AST/ALT <5 ×ULN Liver biopsy + AMA titer or PBC antibodies
Exclusion: based on Screening tests	Investigator identified significant liver disease or injury or ALT/AST >2 × ULN, BILI >1.6 mg/dL	Investigator identified significant hepatic disease	Investigator identified significant laboratory tests or history of liver disease	AST /ALT >1.5 × ULN BILI >1.5 × ULN (AST /ALT >3 × ULN in areas where CHB is prevalent)	AST/ALT >3 × ULN Active inflammation on histopathology	AST/ALT, ALP >3 × ULN BILI 1.5–2 × ULN	AST/ALT, ALP >2 × ULN, BILI >2 mg/dL	Phase 2 studies excluded subjects with AST/ ALT BILI > 3 × ULN No such exclusion for phase 3		AST/ALT <10 × ULN BILI >2.5 × ULN	AST/ALT <5 or <10 × ULN BILI within ULN or <1.5 × ULN	ALT ≥300U/L Or >155 U/L Females ≥185 U/L Males AST ≥155U/L Females ≥185 U/L Males	No aminotransferase thresholds AP >1.67 to <10 × ULN
Exclusion: based on BMI (kg/m²) or Weight (kg)	Not specified	Not specified	Not specified	>50 kg for males or >45 kg for females	Not specified	>40–50	>40	Not specified	<15 or >28	No criteria	<35	Not specified	Not specified
Presence of liver disease	Lab defined inclusion (see above) Chronic infection such as TB	See above Investigator identified exclusionary criteria: Recent infection requiring hospitalization Allergy or hypersensitivity	Investigator identified chronic infection such as TB Immunosuppression	Investigator defined Felty's syndrome Autoimmune disease Chronic infections other than CHC Hypersensitivity reactions Genetic testing for Gilbert's syndrome	See above History of allergy, auto-immune disorder for exclusion	Lab defined Documented or suspected history or evident hepatic decompensation (encephalopathy, ascites, variceal bleeds)			Subjects with known toxicities of ALT or AST grade 2 or greater or >2.5 × ULN ALP ≥grade 2 or >2.5 × ULN, BILI ≥grade 2 or >1.6 × ULN	Serology Histology CPT score Alpha feto protein	Histology Serology	Documented/ suspected hepatic decompensation (encephalopathy, ascites, variceal bleeds) r/o (1) viral, (2) autoimmune, (3) alcoholic, (4) liver cancer	Investigator defined or by history— NASH, alcoholic liver disease, Gilbert's, liver transplant

Protocol element	Group A				Group B					Group C			
	AS	MS	PS	RA	CANCER	T2DM CVOT	T2DM Non CVOT	CAP	TB	CHB	CHC	NASH	PBC
Data to test adequacy of liver function (cirrhosis, decompensation)	No	No	No	No	Prothrombin Platelets	Lab tests: Albumin, INR, prothrombin* Biopsy	Investigator defined cirrhosis	No	No	History, biopsy and lab tests Prothrombin time Albumin <3, alpha feto protein >50 liver imaging	Cirrhosis Definitions specified Platelets, Albumin, INR Biopsy Imaging, fibroscan vs. Metavir, AST/platelet ratio some variation in instrument/ score, HLA typing	Full panel of liver markers include Aminotransferases. BILI, Alkaline phosphatase, GGT, Function tests (albumin, platelets, INR) Bile acids, Imaging and Transient elastography	Decompensation and disease prognostic risk definitions specified histologic (biopsy specific elements and criteria), questionnaire and PRO data, (pruritus VAS), MELD score and clinical findings data (portal hypertension elements) Function tests: Platelets, Albumin, INR, Fibrosis biomarkers— ELF, Transient elastography
Alcohol and drug abuse history	Not specified	Last 2 years	Not specified	Up to 5 years prior		Active to up 12 months	Active to up 12 months		Current or past history of alcohol or substance abuse	Active use		20 g alcohol daily (females) 30 g/day (males) 3 months 1 year pre screening	210 mL of alcohol per week Substance abuse within 12 months
HIV Hepatitis Serologies	CHC, CHB, HIV	CHC, CHB, HIV, Varicella zoster in 6 months, varicella/live virus vaccine	HIV AIDS	CHC, CHB, HIV HBV DNA as indicated		CHC, CHB, Some excluded HIV		HIV with CD4 count <200	HIV with CD4 count <300 or requiring treatment	CHC, CHB, HIV Delta hepatitis	CHC, CHB, HIV	CHC, CHB, HIV	CHC, HBV, HIV
History of Recent Procedures	Not specified	Recent elective surgery	Not specified	Not specified		Bariatric surgery, lap band procedures	Bariatric surgery lap band procedure	Requiring ventilator support	Not specified			Bariatric surgery	Portocaval shunting or TIPS

(continued)

Table 1b (continued)

Protocol element	Group A					Group B				Group C			
	AS	MS	PS	RA	CANCER	T2DM CVOT	T2DM Non CVOT	CAP	TB	CHB	CHC	NASH	PBC
Lipid	Not specified	Not specified	Not specified	hypercholesterolemia (>350 mg/dL, 9.1 mmol/L) or hypertriglyceridemia (>500 mg/dL, 5.6 mmol/L)	Not specified	Not specified	LDL-C > 250 mg/dL Triglycerides >1000 mg/dL HDL-C <25 mg/dL previous 6 months	Not specified	Not specified	Not specified	Not specified	Free fatty acids, LDL, HDL, cholesterol, serum triglycerides,	Not specified
Excluded concomitant medications that could confound hepatic safety	Chronic steroid use	Azathioprine, methotrexate, mitoxantrone, T cell or T cell receptor vaccine, total body irradiation	Not specified	Active treatment for autoimmune disease, or infections (preventive therapy for CHB allowed in endemic sites)	Not specified	Weight loss medications	Weight loss medications				Herbal products, "hepatic protective medication"	Amiodarone, methotrexate, systemic steroids, tetracyclines, tamoxifen, high dose estrogens valproic acid anabolic steroids	Colchicine methotrexate azathioprine fibrates other hepatotoxic drugs
AESI Endpoint	No	No	No	ALT elevation of 3 × ULN w/BILI 2 × ULN	No	No	No					Hepatocellular injury Change in liver function	Hepatocellular injury Change in liver function, including histology

Adapted from information in Drugs@FDA

*Laboratory criteria specified in certain protocols

**Specified in 1 trial that included women receiving low dose estrogen

⁺Trials for IBS-D described separately due to extensive drug exposure and baseline testing

@Data collected when DILI is identified as a serious adverse event of special interest (SASE)

Acronyms: *CVOT* cardiovascular outcome trial, *MELD* model for end stage liver disease, *CPT* child pugh turcotte, *AESI* adverse event of special interest, *PRO* patient reported outcome

Table 2
Aggregated LT database by therapeutic area in various study groups

Group	Therapeutic area	Number of trials	Number of subjects	Number of pretreatment lab values per subject	
				Mean	Median (range)
REF	ED	7	3966	2	2 (1–4)
	HG-M	12	1898	1.2	1 (1–4)
	HL	5	876	1	1 (1–1)
	OP-F	29	30236	1.5	2 (1–5)
	Subtotal	**53**	**36,976**	**1.6**	**2 (1–5)**
A	AS	2	589	2.1	2 (1–4)
	MS	6	6939	1.9	2 (1–5)
	PS	14	5468	2	2 (1–4)
	RA	16	6548	1.8	2 (1–4)
	Subtotal	**38**	**19,544**	**1.9**	**2 (1–5)**
B	CANCER	21	5670	1.7	2 (1–6)
	T2DM	62	40918	3.3	3 (1–12)
	CAP	3	1503	1.2	1 (1–2)
	TB	1	1052	2.4	2 (1–5)
	Subtotal	**87**	**49,143**	**3.1**	**3 (1–12)**
C	CHB	2	1298	2.1	2 (1–4)
	CHC	50	15034	1.9	2 (1–6)
	NASH	1	64	2	2 (2–2)
	PBC	3	440	3.2	3 (1 5)
	Subtotal	**56**	**16,836**	**2**	**2 (1–6)**
	Total	**234**	**122,499**	**2.5**	**2 (1–12)**

Frequency of elevations above the ULN was tabulated and represented in bar charts by disease group.

3   Results

3.1   Demographics   The aggregated dataset consists of 122,499 subjects with screening and baseline LTs from 234 phase 1–3 clinical trials (Table 2). Of these subjects, 40% were in Group B, 16% were in Group A and

Table 3
Demographic characteristics of subjects enrolled by study group

	Reference (*N* = 36,976)	Group A (*N* = 19,544)	Group B (N = 49,143)	Group C (N = 16,836)
Sex, n(%)				
Female	33,534 (90.7)	11,867 (60.7)	21,836 (44.4)	6799 (40.4)
Male	3442 (9.3)	7677 (39.3)	27,307 (55.6)	10,037 (59.6)
Races, n(%)				
Alaskan	33 (0.1)	283 (1.5)	549 (1.1)	51 (0.3)
Asian	2911 (7.9)	2571 (13.2)	7798 (15.9)	1660 (9.9)
Black	2399 (6.5)	359 (1.8)	3190 (6.5)	1430 (8.5)
Hawaiian	8 (<0.01)	12 (0.1)	69 (0.1)	37 (0.2)
Other	771 (2.1)	2135 (10.9)	1114 (2.3)	245 (1.5)
White	30,854 (83.4)	14,184 (72.6)	36,423 (74.1)	13,413 (79.7)
Age (yrs), mean ± SD	60.21 ± 13.1	44.88 ± 13.1	56.93 ± 11.8	50 ± 11.1
Age groups, n(%)				
Not Stated	7 (<0.01)	643 (3.3)	22 (<0.01)	
<18	644 (1.7)			
18–45	2813 (7.6)	9352 (47.9)	7237 (14.7)	4519 (26.8)
45–65	18,187 (49.2)	8092 (41.4)	28,737 (58.5)	11,258 (66.9)
65–75	12,371 (33.5)	1285 (6.6)	10,560 (21.5)	1002 (6)
75+	2954 (8)	172 (0.9)	2587 (5.3)	57 (0.3)
BMI (kg/m^2), mean ± SD	26.87 ± 5.6	27.33 ± 6.5	30.95 ± 8	26.78 ± 5
BMI groups, n(%)				
Not stated	12,139 (32.8)	63 (0.3)	3390 (6.9)	21 (0.1)
<18.5	368 (1)	632 (3.2)	1388 (2.8)	248 (1.5)
18.5–25	2663 (7.2)	7430 (38)	5797 (11.8)	6386 (37.9)
25–30	3126 (8.5)	6019 (30.8)	12,612 (25.7)	6411 (38.1)
30+	18,680 (50.5)	5400 (27.6)	25,956 (52.8)	3770 (22.4)

14% were in Group C. The majority of the trial population consisted of white adult subjects. Asians were the second largest demographic group (Table 3). The reference group, representing a third of the population, enrolled subjects representing the broadest age range, although the majority of individuals were postmenopausal females with osteoporosis. Females in the osteoporosis trials were older (mean age 64.3 ± 7.68 years) and lighter (mean BMI 25.7 ± 4.1 kg/m²) than males with male hypogonadism (mean age 48.7 ± 9.75 years and mean BMI 32.4 ± 4.8). There was a higher proportion of women in trials of autoimmune disorders (Group A) than in trials of systemic disease (Group B), or known hepatobiliary disease (Group C). Subjects with autoimmune disease (Group A) were younger than subjects in the other study groups.

3.2 Variability in ULN Values and Pretreatment LT Results

The ULN value was provided for individual subjects and was age- and gender-specific, based on the respective central laboratory reference interval [25, 40–42]. The exception was a new drug application with multiregional trials that utilized multiple central laboratories and scaled all test values to an ULN value cited in a textbook. The majority of subjects had two sets of LTs collected prior to treatment (one screening and one baseline) and the mean and median number of tests were close; the notable exception was in patients with T2DM, who made up the largest patient group, and for which the mean number was larger than the median, indicating a distribution with a positive skew. Patients with T2DM had more baseline LTs tests conducted, including one subject with an extreme of up to 12 sets of pretreatment LTs performed (Table 2). There were fewer baseline tests conducted in the reference group compared to subjects in other groups.

The median and inter quartile range (IQR) of baseline ALT values divided by the corresponding ULN values were calculated (Fig. 1a). The ULN values ranged from 20 to as high as 80 U/L across various trials and varied by disease group. Subjects enrolled in the trials of Group A had the narrowest range of ULN reference values (20–56 U/L), whereas Group B had the broadest range of ULN (24–80 U/L). The ULN range of the reference group was 20–74 U/L. As expected, for subjects with hepatobiliary disease (Group C) the median (and IQR) in baseline ALT values were generally greater than ULN compared to Groups A and B. Note that for Group C, the median and IQR approached the norm (1 × ULN) in subjects with a reference ULN closer to the maximum value of 67 U/L. For Groups A and B, the median and IQR generally fell below 1× ULN and exceeded this value when the ULN reference was close to the lower end of the range (25–30 U/L).

The ranges and cumulative distributions of the raw baseline ALT values, the normalized baseline ALT values, and the ULN ALT values for Groups A, B, and C and the reference group are shown in Fig. 1b. The cumulative distributions for both the raw and normalized baseline ALT values were similar across groups, however, the distribution curves of ALT values in Group C gradually diverged from the disease groups without overt liver disease within the range of values considered to be normal. The separation

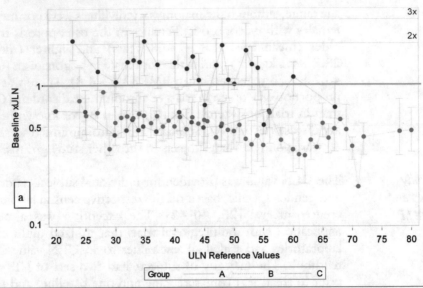

y axis = median and IQR of baseline ALT x ULN   x axis = value of the reference upper limit of normal (U/L)

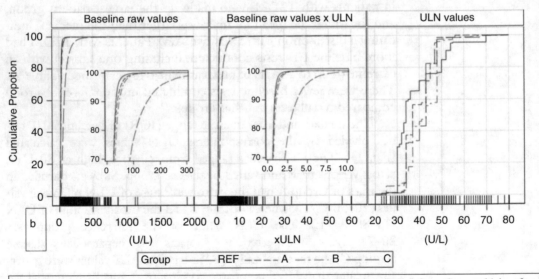

y axis = cumulative frequency of LT values   x axis = raw values of baseline ALT tests (U/L, left panel), as multiples of ULN (x ULN, middle panel) and actual value of the reference ULN (U/L, right panel). Black bars on the x axis represent individual samples. The magnified inset represents the range of values where the widest separation of values occurs between subjects with liver disease (group C) vs the reference and groups A and B.

Fig. 1 Baseline ALT (U/L) Values by Study Group (**a**) Multiples of ULN over the Normal Range, (**b**) Cumulative Distribution of ULN values, raw ALT values and Multiples of ULN

of ALT values for Group C appears to be most evident for raw ALT values at 100–200 IU (magnified inset on the left pane) and for normalized values at 2.5–5 × ULN (inset in the middle pane).

Table 4
Proportion of subjects with elevated baseline ALT compared to reported prevalence of elevated values by study group

Baseline ALT × ULN								
		This Study, n (%)				Reported in Literature		
Group	Disease	>1 × ULN	>2 × ULN	>3 × ULN	>5 × ULN	> ULN or (Actual value)	% > ULN or (U/L, range)	[Reference]
REF	ED	496 (12.5)	59 (1.5)	8 (0.2)	2 (0.1)	(Median)	(15 U/L, 9–44)	[43]
	HL	218 (24.9)	34 (3.9)	16 (1.8)	2 (0.2)			
	HG-M	204 (10.7)	18 (0.9)	1 (0.1)	0 (0)	(Mean)	(26 U/L, 5–46)	[45]
	OP-F	1600 (5.3)	69 (0.2)	24 (0.1)	5 (<0.1)	(Mean)	(20 U/L, 5–190)	[44]
A	AS	35 (5.9)	4 (0.7)	2 (0.3)	0 (0)	> 1 × ULN	0	[24, 51]
	MS	792 (14.5)	62 (0.9)	23 (0.3)	6 (0.1)	> 1 × ULN	6–9.1	[17, 18]
	PS	502 (7.2)	97 (1.8)	24 (0.4)	2 (<0.1)	> 2 × ULN	1-2	[49, 50]
	RA	465 (7.1)	30 (0.5)	6 (0.1)	1 (<0.1)	> 2 × ULN	1-2	[49, 50]
B	CANCER	573 (10.1)	84 (1.5)	25 (0.4)	2 (<0.1)	> 1 × ULN (Mean)	33.8-36 (124 U/L M 58 U/L F)	[53, 54, 80]
	T2DM	5489 (13.4)	490 (1.2)	82 (0.2)	13 (<0.1)	(> 43 U/L)	17	[24]
						> 2 × ULN	23	[81]
	CAP	273 (18.2)	47 (3.1)	12 (0.8)	2 (0.1)	> 1 × ULN	8.3–17	[55, 56]
	TB	223 (21.2)	54 (5.1)	16 (1.5)	3 (0.3)	> 2 × ULN	4	[33]
						>5 × ULN	0.4	
C	CHB	1162 (89.5)	640 (49.3)	345 (26.6)	149 (11.5)	> 1 × ULN	49 (M) 58 (F)	[40][a]
	CHC	11298 (75.1)	4865 (32.4)	2283 (15.2)	581 (3.9)	> 1 × ULN	92	[34]
	NASH	15 (23.4)	3 (4.7)	1 (1.6)	0 (0)	> 1 × ULN	23	[27, 61]
							77	[60]
	PBC	260 (59.1)	123 (28)	55 (12.5)	12 (2.7)	> 1 × ULN	45	[65]
						> 5 × ULN[a]	47–95	[66]

[a] overlap syndrome with autoimmune hepatitis
M males, F females

3.3 Baseline Data, Subject Selection, and Impact on DILI Prediction by Disease Group

The frequency of baseline elevations of ALT relative to ULN by disease group are compared to the prevalence of elevated ALT as reported in the literature (Table 4), whereas the variability of baseline values (mean, median, IQR and outliers) for all four LTs are shown by disease grouping in Figs. 3, 4, 5, and 6. The rate of ALT elevation >1 × ULN was lowest in Group A, followed by Group B, the reference group and Group C, in ascending order. The observed prevalence of tests >1 × ULN was lower in trials of cancer and diabetes (Table 4) in comparison to the reported rates of these ALT abnormalities in the published literature.

3.3.1 Reference Group—LT Values in Subjects with no Overt Liver Disease

This group consisting of a broad age range of ambulant subjects with little comorbidity served as our reference population and made up a third of our total study sample (Tables 2 and 3). The mean and median LTs of most subjects in this group were within reported ULN values (Fig. 3) [43–45]; similarly, the prevalence of values that exceeded 1× ULN is consistent with the reported range of values in a healthy population [1, 29, 32, 42, 46, 47]. The maximum ALT ULN value (75 U/L) exceeds published US ULN reference (33–35 U/L) [1, 48] whereas the minimum value (20 U/L in subjects with HL) is less than the values proposed as discriminatory for liver disease in the US population (29 U/L in females and 22 U/L in males) [47].

As noted, the HL trials had the lowest reference ULN values (Fig. 2) and could account for the falsely elevated normalized ALT values that exceeded the other rates in the group (Table 4, Fig. 3). By comparison, the ULN for hypogonadism (HG) was at the extreme end of the range (55 U/L) (Fig. 2) and the proportion of subjects with ALT >2 × ULN was well within the reported frequency of these values in a US population (Table 4). Subjects with known liver disease were excluded from these trials based on the investigator's definition of clinically significant LT abnormalities or based on the prespecified exclusion criterion of >1.5 × ULN (Table 1a).

3.3.2 Group A—Autoimmune Diseases Treated with Drug Known to Cause DILI

The 38 trials of treatments for autoimmune diseases included a total of 19, 544 subjects, among whom patients with AS were in the minority. Many patients in these trials had previously failed disease-modifying antirheumatic drugs with a known DILI risk (Table 1b). The protocols for this group of disorders generally excluded subjects with elevated baseline tests, chronic viral hepatitis, and investigator-identified "significant underlying liver disease". The LT mean, median and IQR values in this group were generally within the ULN (Fig. 4), with a wide range of outlier values. The finding that 1.8% of PS subjects had ALT values >2 × ULN is consistent with the prevalence of elevated LTs reported in the literature [49, 50]; the observed rates for

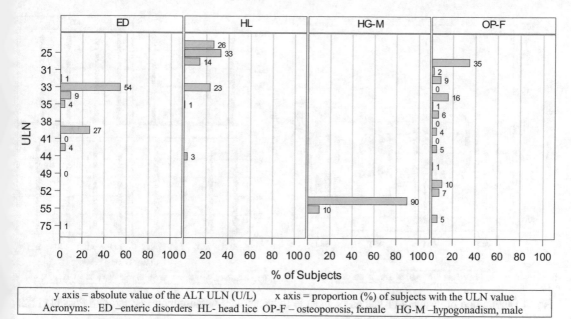

y axis = absolute value of the ALT ULN (U/L)   x axis = proportion (%) of subjects with the ULN value
Acronyms: ED –enteric disorders HL- head lice OP-F – osteoporosis, female   HG-M –hypogonadism, male

Fig. 2 Range and Frequency of ULN Values for ALT in the Reference Group

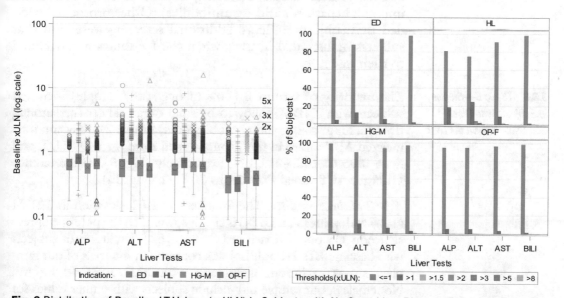

Fig. 3 Distribution of Baseline LT Values (× ULN) in Subjects with No Overt Liver Disease (Reference Group)

AS were higher than reported [51]. Trials conducted in countries where hepatitis B is endemic enrolled subjects with baseline LT values of up to 3 × ULN (Table 1b), with serial monitoring and preemptive treatment of hepatitis B. The occurrence of ALT elevations on treatment prompted collection of additional data to assess causality (e.g., screening panel for

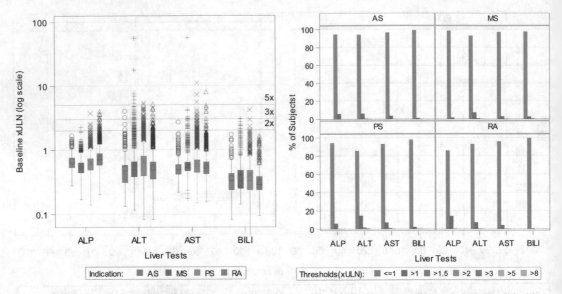

Fig. 4 Distribution of Baseline LT Values (× ULN) in Subjects with Autoimmune Disease and Possible Liver Toxicity from Concurrent Therapy (Group A)

alternative liver disease, including chronic viral infection, autoimmune hepatitis, antidrug antibodies). Other protocols specified that subjects undergo additional screening tests and that subjects be included in trials when the LT values had declined to their nadir.

3.3.3 Group B—Studies in Subjects with Disease that Could Involve the Liver

The majority of Group B (40% of our study sample) included subjects with T2DM, followed by solid organ cancer (melanoma, thyroid, lung, colon, and neuroblastoma) (Table 2). Raw and normalized ALT values in this group ranged from 3 to 499 U/L and from 0.06 to 14.34 × ULN, respectively (Fig. 5). The reference ULN for ALT varied from 24 to 80 U/L (Fig. 1a).

Type 2 diabetes mellitus. The frequency of ALT elevation in T2DM (1.2% with values >2× ULN) is clearly lower than the published prevalence in US population-based surveys [52]. Exclusion of subjects with baseline LTs 2–3 × ULN was common in the trials of our sample, as was exclusion of subjects with BMI > 35-40 kg/m². Nonetheless, our sample did include subjects with outlier values for ALT and AST of up to 10 × ULN, and these values were more extreme than those observed in the other diseases within this study group. Subjects with end-stage liver disease, defined either through laboratory parameters (albumin, prolonged prothrombin time, and a raised INR) or through clinical events (ascites, encephalopathy, variceal bleed, or a prior transplant), were excluded as were subjects on a recent weight loss program, or those who initiated therapy with anti-obesity drugs or had undergone bariatric surgery (Table 1b).

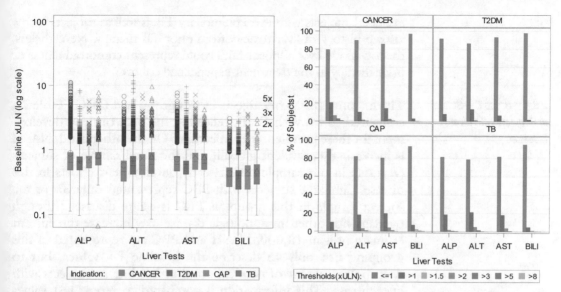

Fig. 5 Distribution of Baseline LT Values (× ULN) in Subjects with Potential Hepatic Involvement due to Underlying Disease (Group B)

Cancer with or without liver metastases. Most cancer protocols excluded subjects with baseline values >3 × ULN, including trial protocols that evaluate DILI as an adverse event of special interest (AESI); consequently, published rates of elevated LT in cancer are higher than those observed in these trials (Table 4). Protocols in metastatic disease, such as metastatic melanoma, however, allowed for the inclusion of subjects with aminotransferase elevations of 5–10 × ULN. In this setting, outlier ALP values up to 10 × ULN (Fig. 5) have been observed, consistent with the published frequency of abnormal LTs in this malignancy [53, 54]. Trials that include patients with liver metastases collect additional tests for ALP fractions to distinguish cancer spread to the bone or liver, data on liver morphology (fibrosis tests) and function (albumin, international normalized ratio [INR], platelets, prothrombin, Model for End Stage Liver Disease (MELD) and Child–Pugh–Turcotte (CTP) scores). To assess immune-mediated liver toxicity for biologic therapeutic classes with a known DILI signal, protocols specified collection of additional tests such as antidrug and other antibody markers and liver biopsy with special staining.

Acute vs. *chronic lung infection: community acquired pneumonia with or without bacteremia and tuberculosis.* ALT elevations are of prognostic significance in CAP [55, 56] and a trial protocol that allowed the inclusion of patients with bacteremic CAP could account for outlier ALT values in this group. Similarly, the frequency of ALT elevations >2 × ULN among the subjects with TB is consistent with the reported prevalence of disseminated military TB or liver injury from anti-TB therapy [33]. The protocols for the trial in this sample, however, excluded subjects with extra pulmonary TB as well as subjects with a known history of liver toxicity from prior TB therapy. Nevertheless, the low grade liver abnormalities could represent comorbid illness or prior therapy in the treatment-experienced cohort.

3.3.4 Group C—Studies in Subjects with Liver Diseases

The majority (89%) of subjects in this group had CHC (Table 2), compared to 8% with CHB, reflecting the pace of drug development for these prevalent liver infections. On the other hand, NASH is increasingly prevalent globally and the small sample of subjects ($n = 64$) in our sample reflects early development efforts in this disease. Similarly, subjects with PBC represented only 3% of the subject sample in this group, as PBC is a rare disease, although overlap with other immunologic disease may increase the current estimate of 4 in 10,000. NASH and PBC are represented in this grouping not only to describe the baseline LT values, but to describe the extent of data collected at baseline in subjects with liver disease. This information is compared to repeat test values obtained on treatment to characterize treatment response as well as retrospectively assess whether liver abnormalities on treatment are attributable to drug or disease. The spread of raw ALT values from subjects in this group was greater than in other groups, ranging from 4 to 1160 U/L, and when normalized to the ULN, varied from 0.1 to 33.12 × ULN (Fig. 1a). The reference ULN value for ALT varied from 23 to 67 U/L. Except for a small number of subjects with NASH, the majority of the population in this group had values that exceed 1 × ULN (Fig. 6) for ALT and AST.

Chronic hepatitis B and C. The populations enrolled in these studies were monoinfected with either hepatitis B or hepatitis C, except for small trials of HIV coinfected subjects. Close to half of subjects with CHB and 30% with CHC had values of ALT >2 × ULN at baseline. Protocols allowed for inclusion of subjects with AST/ALT values <10 × ULN and BILI of <1.5–2 × ULN; studies in CHC specified at least two measures of ALT elevations, with at least 1 elevated value identified within 1–2 months of the first dose of study drug. The mean, IQR and outlier ALT values for CHB were higher than that observed for CHC (Fig. 6). Of the CHC subjects with cirrhosis, 56% had baseline values of both ALT and AST > 2 × ULN [57]; the comparable values in subjects without cirrhosis were 28% for ALT and 18% for AST (data not shown). Patients with chronic hepatitis who have previously failed treatment and have documented cirrhosis have had more extensive data collected at baseline, including tests of hepatic morphology and function, in addition to tests for viral load, viral genotype, and LT values. The test criteria used to establish cirrhosis varied across protocols reviewed (e.g., Knodel vs CPT vs MELD scores) [58, 59].

Nonalcoholic steatohepatitis. A minority (4.7%) of subjects enrolled in this trial had baseline LTs > 2 × ULN, substantially less than the

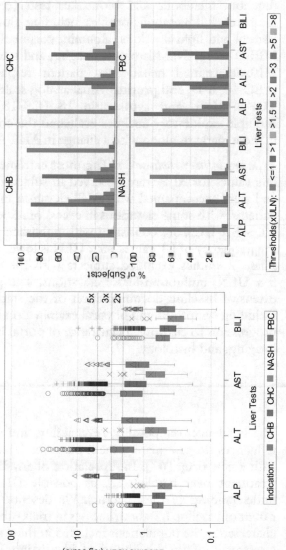

Fig. 6 Distribution of Baseline LT Values (× ULN) in Subjects with Hepatobiliary Disease (Group C)

published prevalence of LT abnormalities in this disease (Table 4) [27, 60, 61]. Compared to the other disease categories in this group, subjects with NASH tended to have a higher proportion of baseline mean and median LT values within the ULN, with a few outlier ALT and AST values >2 × ULN but well within the <5 × ULN limit specified in the protocol exclusion criteria. The database had extensive documentation of liver morphology and function, metabolic and biomarker tests (e.g., anthropometric measures, full metabolic profiles including glucose handling, cholesterol and lipid fractions, albumin, coagulation tests, bile acids, MELD score, liver histology, imaging and transient elastography, MRI-determined hepatic fat, patient response questionnaires (PBC-40, 5-D, and pruritus visual analog scale) [62, 63], TNF-α, TGF-β, IL-6, and cytokeratin 18 (CK-18) fragment assay). Multiple exploratory analyses evaluated the change from baseline in these markers, along with a change in ALT, AST, and BILI [64].

Primary biliary cholangitis. The most extreme elevations in baseline values for ALP were observed in subjects with PBC (Fig. 6) and were accompanied with ALT elevation in close to a third of patients, with some elevations in excess of >5 × ULN. The rates of LT > 1 × ULN are consistent with published estimates [65], but the frequency of LT values >5 × ULN is lower than reported [66]. Phase 2 studies excluded subjects with these more extreme (> 5 × ULN) aminotransferase elevations. The protocols called for extensive baseline documentation of the status of PBC activity, including symptoms and physical examination findings, markers of progression to cirrhosis, occurrence of portal hypertension, lipids, imaging, and histology.

4   Discussion

The incidence, temporality, reversibility, and severity of an event influences the risk management plans for DILI signals that occur with a new drug [67]. Interpretation of any LT changes on drug treatment over baseline LT as possible DILI requires a good understanding of these factors. We describe the frequency and extent of baseline LT abnormalities in trials submitted to FDA, and characterize the populations included in these studies to inform an assessment of the likelihood of identifying DILI using current review practice and to enable consideration of future trial design and patient selection criteria.

In patients without known hepatobiliary disease, (Groups A and B, and the reference group) there was little variability in baseline LT values, as shown by the steep and similar cumulative distribution functions in Fig. 1. The majority of the trial population had homogenous LT values despite the variation in ULN values across studies, differences in laboratories utilized in the individual trials and the fact that trial populations were recruited from multiple regions with genetically different populations [68, 69]. Patients with hepatobiliary disease had higher and more variable LT values, as expected, although ALT values within ULN are common in subjects with CHC [70]. Persistent ALT elevation of 2.25 × ULN in subjects with CHC, for example, results in liver cirrhosis [34], ALT elevations at this level result in a visible separation of subjects with hepatobiliary disease from the groups with no known liver disease, although would still fall within the steep slope of the normalized baseline cumulative distribution curve in our trial sample. An observed decline from this baseline elevation in ALT with effective treatment is expected to be beneficial to patients with CHC. The distributions curve that results in visible separation of subjects with hepatobiliary disease from the rest of the treatment groups could signify the appropriateness of the inclusion criteria selected for these trials.

On the other hand, while the occurrence of outlier ALT values (> 3 × ULN) in all groups could suggest unrecognized liver disease in our study sample, the prevalence of LT values within ULN may not entirely exclude hepatic disease. For example, the difference between ALT values reported for metabolically healthy women (ALT 18.4 ± 6.4 U/L) and their counterparts with metabolic syndrome (ALT 27.4 ± 14.7) [71] is narrow, with potential overlap. These values would similarly fall within the steep slope of the raw baseline ALT values in our cumulative distribution curve and depending on the ULN value, may be considered within the range of normality. We note as well that the prevalence of ALT elevations >2 × ULN in T2DM in our trial sample is lower than reported. The exclusion of subjects with LT abnormalities and significant comorbidity in new drug applications for a broad range of diseases could have contributed to the lack of variability in LT values among patients without hepatobiliary disease, as could the practice of enrolling patients after they reach acceptable nadir values after serial baseline testing.

Conducting a trial in which the majority of subjects have a baseline LT value within 1 × ULN is useful in that on treatment changes can potentially be better discriminated. However, exclusion of subjects with comorbid liver disease and more severe liver dysfunction could limit experience in the safe use of these products, and raise questions about the approach to take (e.g., stopping rules and risk mitigation efforts) when LT elevations progress, because subjects with diminished liver reserve may not recover from DILI.

Our data show that ALT values alone may not discriminate between healthy subjects and those with preexisting liver injury and highlights the need to interpret postbaseline LT elevation along with disease markers and other clinical data. Baseline LT values in populations with liver disease need to be assessed against a subject's age, gender, and BMI, taking into account the individual variability in their test values. Moreover, because low-level LT elevations are common in healthy populations and because significant liver disease can occur with normal or slightly elevated LT values, until a more specific DILI biomarker is identified it seems appropriate to fully characterize the status of the liver disease at baseline along with liver morphology and function, concomitant supplements and medication. Any assessment of LT elevations on treatment needs to take these factors into account before attributing these changes to a new drug. Efficient review of a DILI signal in a new drug application will depend on adequate collection and standardization of these data.

Subjects with baseline LT test values >3 × ULN were present in all disease groups including the reference, and could be explained by factors such as the prevalence of obesity and cardiometabolic disorders leading to NASH, ubiquitous supplement, alcohol or recreational or therapeutic drug use, and even the influence of environmental toxins [4]. While these subjects are proposed for exclusion in first-in-human trials [72], inclusion of patients with baseline LT elevations in trials of diabetes or cardiometabolic disease leading to NASH could lead to an earlier assessment of the impacts of new treatments [73, 74]. The single trial in NASH, for example, excluded subjects with ALT >2 × ULN but completed documentation of a metabolic and endocrine panel, events or imaging consistent with hepatic decompensation, imaging for fibrosis or fat or tumor infiltration, virologic markers, markers of congenital or acquired hepatic disease, and genetic markers of disease. Systematic assessment of this collected data is needed in populations likely to be treated with any new drug to identify valid, reliable and clinically meaningful endpoints in this highly prevalent disease. Further, inclusion of patients with diminished hepatic reserve may affect drug exposure and enable efficient assessment of appropriate dosing. Other trials conducted in a development program for a new drug, such as dose-ranging or placebo-controlled phase 2 monotherapy trials, can be valuable in the assessment of DILI. In these studies it would be appropriate to exclude subjects with any baseline LT abnormality to enhance the detection of a DILI signal.

Given the overlap in values among the disease groups observed in this study, population-specific reference criteria for routine baseline LTs need to be established to enable interpretation of elevations in light of natural disease variation. Standardized definitions of liver cirrhosis and decompensation and standardized data for liver morphology, function and predictive biomarkers can facilitate systematic assessment of DILI in future trials. Terminology for imaging, histology, markers for autoimmunity and immune reconstitution, concomitant medication, and dietary information needs to be consistently represented in the appropriate SDTM domains. Most of the listed concepts can be represented in the Events, Findings, and Interventions domain of the CDISC SDTM, represented in Tables 1a and 1b by their 2-letter variable name. Standard data representation and analyses can be modeled to enable composite visualization of population and individual subject data for systematic regulatory review.

Optimized analyses and displays of trial data, as specified in US FDA Guidance [75, 76], has enabled the early identification of drugs with a potential for DILI [77]. Challenges in identification of DILI in patients with liver disease can be similarly overcome as greater insight is gleaned from the accumulating trial data in these patient populations.

5 Conclusion and Future Directions

Data characterizing liver function and morphology can complement routine LT in assessing treatment efficacy or DILI causality in subjects with overt or unrecognized liver disease. Adoption of population-based reference ranges [8, 78, 79] can improve assessment of LT elevations and enhance understanding of LT values reported from multiregional trials. DILI detection can be optimized with strict LT exclusion criteria in early phase studies; whereas data from later-phase studies that include baseline LT elevations enable generalization of safety findings to populations likely to receive the marketed drug. Collection of blood samples for functional, genomic, and mechanistic biomarker testing [12] can be performed prospectively in high-risk subjects or when DILI is suspected to have occurred in select trial subjects. SDTM adherent data can be shared across trials and mined to assess predictors for DILI risk. Understanding the baseline rates of LT abnormalities in various study populations could help develop population-specific thresholds to validate DILI signals from ongoing clinical trials.

Acknowledgments

This chapter reflects the views of the authors and should not be construed to represent FDA's or NIII's views or policies.

References

1. Ioannou GN, Boyko EJ, Lee SP (2006) The prevalence and predictors of elevated serum aminotransferase activity in the United States in 1999-2002. Am J Gastroenterol 101(1):76–82. https://doi.org/10.1111/j.1572-0241.2005.00341.x

2. Liu Z, Que S, Xu J, Peng T (2014) Alanine aminotransferase-old biomarker and new concept: a review. Int J Med Sci 11(9):925–935. https://doi.org/10.7150/ijms.8951

3. Bell BP, Manos MM, Zaman A, Terrault N, Thomas A, Navarro VJ, Dhotre KB, Murphy RC, Van Ness GR, Stabach N, Robert ME, Bower WA,

Bialek SR, Sofair AN (2008) The epidemiology of newly diagnosed chronic liver disease in gastroenterology practices in the United States: results from population-based surveillance. Am J Gastroenterol 103(11):2727–2736.; quiz 2737. https://doi.org/10.1111/j.1572-0241.2008.02071.x

4. Pan WC, Wu CD, Chen MJ, Huang YT, Chen CJ, Su HJ, Yang HI (2016) Fine particle pollution, alanine transaminase, and liver cancer: a Taiwanese prospective cohort study (REVEAL-HBV). J Natl Cancer Inst 108(3). https://doi.org/10.1093/jnci/djv341

5. Fischbein A (1985) Liver function tests in workers with occupational exposure to polychlorinated biphenyls (PCBs): comparison with yusho and yu-cheng. Environ Health Perspect 60:145–150

6. Chak E, Talal AH, Sherman KE, Schiff ER, Saab S (2011) Hepatitis C virus infection in USA: an estimate of true prevalence. Liver Int 31(8):1090–1101.https://doi.org/10.1111/j.1478-3231.2011.02494.x

7. Younossi ZM, Stepanova M, Afendy M, Fang Y, Younossi Y, Mir H, Srishord M (2011) Changes in the prevalence of the most common causes of chronic liver diseases in the United States from 1988 to 2008. Clin Gastroenterol Hepatol 9(6):524–530. e1.; quiz e60. https://doi.org/10.1016/j.cgh.2011.03.020

8. Seeff LB (2015) Drug-induced liver injury is a major risk for new drugs. Dig Dis 33(4):458–463. https://doi.org/10.1159/000374089

9. U.S. Department of Health and Human Services, Food and Drug Administration, Center for Drug Evaluation and Research (CDER), Center for Biologics Evaluation and Research (CBER) (July 2009) Guidance for industry. Drug induced liver injury: premarketing clinical evaluation. https://www.fda.gov/downloads/Drugs/.../guidances/UCM174090.pdf. Accessed 23 Feb 2017

10. Senior JR (2015) Drug-induced liver injury: clinical and diagnostic aspects. In: Urban L, Patel VF, Vaz RJ (eds) Antitargets and drug safety. Wiley-VCH Verlag GmbH & Co., KGaA, Weinheim, Germany, pp 83–106. https://doi.org/10.1002/9783527673643.ch05

11. Senior JR (2014) Evolution of the Food and Drug Administration approach to liver safety assessment for new drugs: current status and challenges. Drug Saf 37(Suppl 1):S9–17. https://doi.org/10.1007/s40264-014-0182-7

12. Avigan MI, Bjornsson ES, Pasanen M, Cooper C, Andrade RJ, Watkins PB, Lewis JH, Merz M (2014) Liver safety assessment: required data elements and best practices for data collection and standardization in clinical trials. Drug Saf 37(Suppl 1):S19–S31. https://doi.org/10.1007/s40264-014-0183-6

13. Suzuki A, Yuen NA, Ilic K, Miller RT, Reese MJ, Brown HR, Ambroso JI, Falls JG, Hunt CM (2015) Comedications alter drug-induced liver injury reporting frequency: data mining in the WHO VigiBase™. Regul Toxicol Pharmacol 72(3):481–490. https://doi.org/10.1016/j.yrtph.2015.05.004

14. Stine JG, Chalasani N (2015) Chronic liver injury induced by drugs: a systematic review. Liver Int 35(11):2343–2353. https://doi.org/10.1111/liv.12958

15. Kappos L, Wiendl H, Selmaj K, Arnold DL, Havrdova E, Boyko A, Kaufman M, Rose J, Greenberg S, Sweetser M, Riester K, O'Neill G, Elkins J (2015) Daclizumab HYP versus interferon beta-1a in relapsing multiple sclerosis. N Engl J Med 373(15):1418–1428. https://doi.org/10.1056/NEJMoa1501481

16. Marrone A, Signoriello E, Alfieri G, Dalla Mora L, Rinaldi L, Rainone I, Adinolfi LE, Lus G (2014) Epstein Barr virus infection reactivation as a possible trigger of primary biliary cirrhosis-like syndrome in a patient with multiple sclerosis in the course of fingolimod treatment. Infez Med 22(4):331–336

17. Tremlett H, Seemuller S, Zhao Y, Yoshida EM, Oger JD, Petkau J (2006) Liver test abnormalities in multiple sclerosis: findings from placebo-treated patients. Neurology 67(7):1291–1293. https://doi.org/10.1212/01.wnl.0000238515.27055.62

18. Francis GS, Grumser Y, Alteri E, Micaleff A, O'Brien F, Alsop J, Stam Moraga M, Kaplowitz N (2003) Hepatic reactions during treatment of multiple sclerosis with interferon-beta-1a: incidence and clinical significance. Drug Saf 26(11):815–827

19. Villamil A, Mullen E, Casciato P, Gadano A (2015) Interferon beta 1a-induced severe autoimmune hepatitis in patients with multiple sclerosis: report of two cases and review of the literature. Ann Hepatol 14(2):273–280

20. Kremer JM (2002) Not yet time to change the guidelines for monitoring methotrexate liver toxicity: they have served us well. J Rheumatol 29(8):1590–1592

21. Kremer JM, Lee RG, Tolman KG (1989) Liver histology in rheumatoid arthritis patients receiving long-term methotrexate therapy. A prospective study with baseline and sequential biopsy samples. Arthritis Rheum 32(2):121–127

22. Singh JA, Hossain A, Tanjong Ghogomu E, Mudano AS, Tugwell P, Wells GA (2016) Biologic or tofacitinib monotherapy for rheumatoid arthritis in people with traditional disease-modifying anti-rheumatic drug (DMARD) failure: a Cochrane systematic review and network meta-analysis (NMA). Cochrane Database Syst Rev 11:CD012437

23. Ijaz B, Ahmad W, Javed FT, Gull S, Hassan S (2011) Revised cutoff values of ALT and HBV DNA level can better differentiate HBeAg (−) chronic inactive HBV patients from active carriers. Virol J 8:86. https://doi.org/10.1186/1743-422x-8-86

24. Ohira H (2016) The liver in systemic diseases [hardcover and eBook]. Springer International Publ. AG, Cham, Switzerland. 978-4-431-55789-0

25. Clark JM, Brancati FL, Diehl AM (2003) The prevalence and etiology of elevated aminotransferase levels in the United States. Am J Gastroenterol 98(5):960–967

26. Ruhl CE, Everhart JE (2003) Determinants of the association of overweight with elevated serum alanine aminotransferase activity in the United States. Gastroenterology 124(1):71–79. https://doi.org/10.1053/gast.2003.50004

27. Gholam PM, Flancbaum L, Machan JT, Charney DA, Kotler DP (2007) Nonalcoholic fatty liver disease in severely obese subjects. Am J Gastroenterol 102(2):399–408. https://doi.org/10.1111/j.1572-0241.2006.01041.x

28. Pirttiaho HI, Salmela PI, Sotaniemi EA, Pelkonen RO, Pitkanen U, Luoma PV (1984) Drug metabolism in diabetic subjects with fatty livers. Br J Clin Pharmacol 18(6):895–899

29. Dutta A, Saha C, Johnson CS, Chalasani N (2009) Variability in the upper limit of normal for serum alanine aminotransferase levels: a statewide study. Hepatology 50(6):1957–1962. https://doi.org/10.1002/hep.23200

30. Gong Z, Tas E, Yakar S, Muzumdar R (2016) Hepatic lipid metabolism and non-alcoholic fatty liver disease in aging. Mol Cell Endocrinol 455:115–130. pii: S0303-7207(16):30545-30547. https://doi.org/10.1016/j.mce.2016.12.022

31. Kwo PY, Cohen SM, Lim JK (2017) ACG clinical guideline: evaluation of abnormal liver chemistries. Am J Gastroenterol 112(1):18–35. https://doi.org/10.1038/ajg.2016.517

32. Weil JG, Bains C, Linke A, Clark DW, Stirnadel HA, Hunt CM (2008) Background incidence of liver chemistry abnormalities in a clinical trial population without underlying liver disease. Regul Toxicol Pharmacol 52(2):85–88. https://doi.org/10.1016/j.yrtph.2008.06.001

33. Xiang Y, Ma L, Wu W, Liu W, Li Y, Zhu X, Wang Q, Ma J, Cao M, Wang Q, Yao X, Yang L, Wubuli A, Merle C, Milligan P, Mao Y, Gu J, Xin X (2014) The incidence of liver injury in Uyghur patients treated for TB in Xinjiang Uyghur autonomous region, China, and its association with hepatic enzyme polymorphisms nat2, cyp2e1, gstm1 and gstt1. PLoS One 9(1):e85905. https://doi.org/10.1371/journal.pone.0085905

34. Pradat P, Alberti A, Poynard T, Esteban J-I, Weiland O, Marcellin P, Badalamenti S, Trépo C (2002) Predictive value of ALT levels for histologic findings in chronic hepatitis C: a European collaborative study. Hepatology 36(4):973–977. https://doi.org/10.1053/jhep.2002.35530

35. Ekstedt M, Franzén LE, Mathiesen UL, Thorelius L, Holmqvist M, Bodemar G, Kechagias S (2006) Long-term follow-up of patients with NAFLD and elevated liver enzymes. Hepatology 44(4):865–873. https://doi.org/10.1002/hep.21327

36. Hu Y, Snitker S, Ryan KA, Yang R, Mitchell BD, Shuldiner AR, Zhu D, Gong D-W (2012) Serum alanine aminotransferase is correlated with hematocrit in healthy human subjects. Scand J Clin Lab Invest 72(3):258–264. https://doi.org/10.3109/00365513.2012.660536

37. Lee M-H, Yang H-I, Yuan Y, L'Italien G, Chen C-J (2014) Epidemiology and natural history of hepatitis C virus infection. World J Gastroenterol 20(28):9270–9280. https://doi.org/10.3748/wjg.v20.i28.9270

38. Seeff LB, Hoofnagle JH (2003) Appendix: the National Institutes of Health consensus development conference Management of Hepatitis C 2002. Clin Liver Dis 7(1):261–287

39. U.S. Department of Health and Human Services, Food and Drug Administration, Center for Drug Evaluation and Research (CDER), Center for Biologics Evaluation and Research (CBER) (December 2014) Guidance for industry. Providing regulatory submissions in electronic format - standardized study data. https://www.fda.gov/downloads/Drugs/GuidanceComplianceRegulatoryInformation/Guidances/UCM292334.pdf. Accessed 23 Feb 2017

40. Ruhl CE, Everhart JE (2013) Diurnal variation in serum alanine aminotransferase activity in the US population. J Clin Gastroenterol 47(2):165–173. https://doi.org/10.1097/MCG.0b013e31826df40a

41. Neuschwander-Tetri BA, Unalp A, Creer MH (2008) Influence of local reference populations on upper limits of normal for serum alanine aminotransferase levels. Arch Intern Med 168(6):663–666. https://doi.org/10.1001/archinternmed.2007.131

42. Neuschwander-Tetri BA, Ünalp A, Creer MH (2004) The upper limits of normal for serum ALT levels reported by clinical laboratories depend on local reference populations. Arch Intern Med 168(6):663–666. https://doi.org/10.1001/archinternmed.2007.131

43. Cruz AA, Lima F, Sarinho E, Ayre G, Martin C, Fox H, Cooper PJ (2007) Safety of anti-immunoglobulin E therapy with omalizumab in allergic patients at risk of geohelminth infection. Clin Exp Allergy 37(2):197–207. https://doi.org/10.1111/j.1365-2222.2007.02650.x

44. Demirdal US, Ciftci IH, Kavuncu V (2010) Markers of autoimmune liver diseases in postmenopausal women with osteoporosis. Clinics (Sao Paolo) 65(10):971–974. https://doi.org/10.1590/S1807-59322010001000008

45. Wang W-B, She F, Xie L-F, Yan W-H, Ouyang J-Z, Wang B-A, Ma H-Y, Zang L, Mu Y-M

(2016) Evaluation of basal serum adrenocorticotropic hormone and cortisol levels and their relationship with nonalcoholic fatty liver disease in male patients with idiopathic hypogonadotropic hypogonadism. Chin Med J 129(10):1147–1153. https://doi.org/10.4103/0366-6999.181967

46. Artmeier-Brandt U, Boettcher M, Wensing G (2005) Distribution of laboratory values in healthy subjects. [abstract P-56]. Eur J Clin Pharmacol 61(9):701–702

47. Ruhl CE, Everhart JE (2012) Upper limits of normal for alanine aminotransferase activity in the United States population. Hepatology 55(2):447–454. https://doi.org/10.1002/hep.24725

48. Kratz A, Ferraro M, Sluss PM, Lewandrowski KB (2004) Case records of the Massachusetts General Hospital. Weekly clinicopathological exercises. Laboratory reference values. N Engl J Med 351(15):1548–1563. https://doi.org/10.1056/NEJMcpc049016

49. Walker NJ, Zurier RB (2002) Liver abnormalities in rheumatic diseases. Clin Liver Dis 6(4):933–946

50. Curtis JR, Beukelman T, Onofrei A, Cassell S, Greenberg JD, Kavanaugh A, Reed G, Strand V, Kremer JM (2010) Elevated liver enzyme tests among patients with rheumatoid arthritis or psoriatic arthritis treated with methotrexate and/or leflunomide. Ann Rheum Dis 69(1):43–47. https://doi.org/10.1136/ard.2008.101378

51. Sheehan NJ, Slavin BM, Kind PR, Mathews JA (1983) Increased serum alkaline phosphatase activity in ankylosing spondylitis. Ann Rheum Dis 42(5):563–565

52. Jeon CY, Roberts CK, Crespi CM, Zhang Z-F (2013) Elevated liver enzymes in individuals with undiagnosed diabetes in the U.S. J Diabetes Complicat 27(4):333–339. https://doi.org/10.1016/j.jdiacomp.2013.04.005

53. Wyld L, Gutteridge E, Pinder SE, James JJ, Chan SY, Cheung KL, Robertson JF, Evans AJ (2003) Prognostic factors for patients with hepatic metastases from breast cancer. Br J Cancer 89(2):284–290

54. Eskelin S, Pyrhönen S, Hahka-Kemppinen M, Tuomaala S, Kivelä T (2003) A prognostic model and staging for metastatic uveal melanoma. Cancer 97(2):465–475. https://doi.org/10.1002/cncr.11113

55. Jinks MF, Kelly CA (2004) The pattern and significance of abnormal liver function tests in community-acquired pneumonia. Eur J Intern Med 15(7):436–440. https://doi.org/10.1016/j.ejim.2004.06.011

56. Daxboeck F, Gattringer R, Mustafa S, Bauer C, Assadian O (2005) Elevated serum alanine aminotransferase (ALT) levels in patients with serologically verified *Mycoplasma pneumoniae* pneumonia. Clin Microbiol Infect 11(6):507–510. https://doi.org/10.1111/j.1469-0691.2005.01154.x

57. Lens S, Torres F, Puigvehi M, Marino Z, Londono MC, Martinez SM, Garcia-Juarez I, Garcia-Criado A, Gilabert R, Bru C, Sola R, Sanchez-Tapias JM, Carrion JA, Forns X (2016) Predicting the development of liver cirrhosis by simple modelling in patients with chronic hepatitis C. Aliment Pharmacol Ther 43(3):364–374. https://doi.org/10.1111/apt.13472

58. Malinchoc M, Kamath PS, Gordon FD, Peine CJ, Rank J, ter Borg PC (2000) A model to predict poor survival in patients undergoing transjugular intrahepatic portosystemic shunts. Hepatology 31(4):864–871. https://doi.org/10.1053/he.2000.5852

59. Baliga P, Merion RM, Turcotte JG, Ham JM, Henley KS, Lucey MR, Schork A, Shyr Y, Campbell DA Jr (1992) Preoperative risk factor assessment in liver transplantation. Surgery 112(4):704–710. discussion 710-701

60. Verma S, Jensen D, Hart J, Mohanty SR (2013) Predictive value of ALT levels for non-alcoholic steatohepatitis (NASH) and advanced fibrosis in non-alcoholic fatty liver disease (NAFLD). Liver Int 33(9):1398–1405. https://doi.org/10.1111/liv.12226

61. Kunde SS, Lazenby AJ, Clements RH, Abrams GA (2005) Spectrum of NAFLD and diagnostic implications of the proposed new normal range for serum ALT in obese women. Hepatology 42(3):650–656. https://doi.org/10.1002/hep.20818

62. Jacoby A, Rannard A, Buck D, Bhala N, Newton JL, James OF, Jones DE (2005) Development, validation, and evaluation of the PBC-40, a disease specific health related quality of life measure for primary biliary cirrhosis. Gut 54(11):1622–1629. https://doi.org/10.1136/gut.2005.065862

63. Elman S, Hynan LS, Gabriel V, Mayo MJ (2010) The 5-D itch scale: a new measure of pruritus. Br J Dermatology 162(3):587–593. https://doi.org/10.1111/j.1365-2133.2009.09586.x

64. Goessling W, Massaro JM, Vasan RS, D'Agostino RB Sr, Ellison RC, Fox CS (2008) Aminotransferase levels and 20-year risk of metabolic syndrome, diabetes, and cardiovascular disease. Gastroenterology 135(6):1935–1944., 1944.e1931. https://doi.org/10.1053/j.gastro.2008.09.018

65. Triger DR, Berg PA, Rodes J (1984) Epidemiology of primary biliary cirrhosis. Liver 4(3):195–200. https://doi.org/10.1111/j.1600-0676.1984.tb00927.x

66. Chazouillères OWD, Serfaty L, Montembault S, Rosmorduc O, Poupon R (1998) Primary biliary cirrhosis–autoimmune hepatitis overlap syndrome: clinical features and response to therapy. Hepatology 28(2):296–301. https://doi.org/10.1002/hep.510280203

67. U.S. Department of Health and Human Services, Food and Drug Administration, Center for Drug Evaluation and Research (CDER), Center for Biologics Evaluation and Research (CBER) (September 2016) Draft guidance for industry: FDA's application of statutory factors in determining when a REMS is necessary. https://www.fda.gov/downloads/Drugs/GuidanceComplianceRegulatoryInformation/Guidances/UCM521504.pdf. Accessed 23 Feb 2017

68. Mercke Odeberg J, Andrade J, Holmberg K, Hoglund P, Malmqvist U, Odeberg J (2006) UGT1A polymorphisms in a Swedish cohort and a human diversity panel, and the relation to bilirubin plasma levels in males and females. Eur J Clin Pharmacol 62(10):829–837. https://doi.org/10.1007/s00228-006-0166-3

69. Olagnier V, Sibille M, Vital Durand D, Deigat N, Baltassat P, Levrat R (1993) Critical value of bilirubin in the selection of healthy volunteers in for phase I. Therapie 48(6):617–622

70. Prati D, Shiffman ML, Diago M, Gane E, Rajender Reddy K, Pockros P, Farci P, O'Brien CB, Lardelli P, Blotner S, Zeuzem S (2006) Viral and metabolic factors influencing alanine aminotransferase activity in patients with chronic hepatitis C. J Hepatol 44(4):679–685. https://doi.org/10.1016/j.jhep.2006.01.004

71. Messier V, Karelis AD, Robillard ME, Bellefeuille P, Brochu M, Lavoie JM, Rabasa-Lhoret R (2010) Metabolically healthy but obese individuals: relationship with hepatic enzymes. Metabolism 59(1):20–24. https://doi.org/10.1016/j.metabol.2009.06.020

72. Breithaupt-Groegler K, Coch C, Coenen M, Donath F, Erb-Zohar K, Francke K, Goehler K, Iovino M, Kammerer KP, Mikus G, Rengelshausen J, Sourgens H, Schinzel R, Sudhop T, Wensing G (2017) Who is a 'healthy subject'?-consensus results on pivotal eligibility criteria for clinical trials. Eur J Clin Pharmacol 73(4):409–416. https://doi.org/10.1007/s00228-016-2189-8

73. Mavrogiannaki AN, Migdalis IN (2013) Nonalcoholic fatty liver disease, diabetes mellitus and cardiovascular disease: newer data. Int J Endocrinol 2013:450639. https://doi.org/10.1155/2013/450639

74. Williams KH, Shackel NA, Gorrell MD, McLennan SV, Twigg SM (2013) Diabetes and nonalcoholic fatty liver disease: a pathogenic duo. Endocr Rev 34(1):84–129. https://doi.org/10.1210/er.2012-1009

75. Merz M, Lee KR, Kullak-Ublick GA, Brueckner A, Watkins PB (2014) Methodology to assess clinical liver safety data. Drug Saf 37(Suppl 1):33–45. https://doi.org/10.1007/s40264-014-0184-5

76. de Denus S, Spinler SA, Miller K, Peterson AM (2004) Statins and liver toxicity: a meta-analysis. Pharmacotherapy 24(5):584–591

77. Chen M, Borlak J, Tong W (2013) High lipophilicity and high daily dose of oral medications are associated with significant risk for drug-induced liver injury. Hepatology 58(1):388–396. https://doi.org/10.1002/hep.26208

78. Kullak-Ublick GA, Merz M, Griffel L, Kaplowitz N, Watkins PB (2014) Liver safety assessment in special populations (hepatitis B, C, and oncology trials). Drug Saf 37(Suppl 1):S57–S62. https://doi.org/10.1007/s40264-014-0186-3

79. Schadt S, Simon S, Kustermann S, Boess F, McGinnis C, Brink A, Lieven R, Fowler S, Youdim K, Ullah M, Marschmann M, Zihlmann C, Siegrist YM, Cascais AC, Di Lenarda E, Durr E, Schaub N, Ang X, Starke V, Singer T, Alvarez-Sanchez R, Roth AB, Schuler F, Funk C (2015) Minimizing DILI risk in drug discovery - a screening tool for drug candidates. Toxicol In Vitro 30(1 Pt B):429–437. https://doi.org/10.1016/j.tiv.2015.09.019

80. Lopez J, Balasegaram M, Thambyrajah V, Timor J (1996) The value of liver function tests in hepatocellular carcinoma. Malays J Pathol 18(2):95–99

81. Salmela PI, Sotaniemi EA, Niemi M, Maentausta O (1984) Liver function tests in diabetic patients. Diabetes Care 7(3):248–254

Chapter 22

Postmarketing Surveillance of Drug-Induced Liver Injury

S. Christopher Jones, Cindy Kortepeter, and Allen D. Brinker

Abstract

Background Most clinical trials that support approval are not adequately powered to detect rare adverse reactions (e.g., drug-induced liver injury, Stevens–Johnson syndrome, and others) that may emerge under real-world use of a drug. The US Food and Drug Administration (FDA) and other global drug regulatory bodies conduct postmarketing surveillance for these types of adverse events.

FDA Methods FDA's Center for Drug Evaluation and Research (CDER)—Division of Pharmacovigilance (DPV) is devoted to postmarketing adverse event surveillance for drug-induced liver injury (DILI) and other adverse events. DPV predominantly relies on clinical assessment of spontaneous reports submitted to the FDA Adverse Event Reporting System (FAERS) and published case reports to assess for DILI in the postmarketing setting. DPV uses criteria established by the Drug-Induced Liver Injury Network (DILIN), and others, to assess cases for causality and severity. In the past, the FDA has collaborated with professional groups with an interest in DILI to improve the quality of case reports. DPV also uses disproportionality and reporting rate analyses to detect and assess potential safety signals. Additionally, DPV collaborates with CDER epidemiologists who conduct analyses to refine DILI signals that emerge from surveillance.

Conclusion DILI continues to be a significant concern for marketed drugs and a leading cause of drug withdrawal from the worldwide market. Because events such as DILI are rare, systems such as those described in this chapter are important components of postmarketing surveillance, which is designed to recognize liver injury that may have gone undetected in a clinical development program for a drug.

Key words Drug-induced liver injury, Postmarket, Surveillance, Epidemiology, Drug safety, Causality assessment, Hepatotoxicity, Drug toxicity, Adverse event

1 Introduction and Background

The World Health Organization defines pharmacovigilance as the science and activities relating to the detection, assessment, understanding, and prevention of adverse effects or any other drug-related problem [1]. Surveillance is an important component of pharmacovigilance and this allows a drug regulatory body to detect and assess a new drug related safety signal. Although there are several definitions for the term "signal," simply put, a signal is a report or reports of an event with an unknown causal relationship to treatment that is recognized as worthy of further exploration and

Minjun Chen and Yvonne Will (eds.), *Drug-Induced Liver Toxicity*, Methods in Pharmacology and Toxicology, https://doi.org/10.1007/978-1-4939-7677-5_22, © Springer Science+Business Media, LLC, part of Springer Nature 2018

continued surveillance [2]. The US Food and Drug Administration (FDA) and other global regulatory bodies conduct surveillance for adverse events after a drug is approved for marketing in order to identify safety signals. In the USA, this activity is mandated in the US Code of Federal Regulations (21CFR §314.80 and §600.80 for approved new drugs and biologics, respectively). Surveillance activities in the USA can also capture events linked to products that fall into "grey-areas," such as dietary supplements or nutraceuticals [3]. Drug-induced liver injury is a possible complication of medication use, and one that the FDA closely monitors once a drug is marketed. In fact, DILI has been one of the most frequent reasons for market withdrawal in the United States [4]. There are at least 60 known drugs that have either been withdrawn or discontinued worldwide over concerns of liver toxicity [5, 6]. Bell and Chalasani have estimated that drug-induced liver injury has an annual incidence of 44,000 cases in the USA, and a subset of these will die (10%) as result of DILI or require a liver transplant to avert death [7]. DILI is a relatively rare adverse reaction, and has been estimated to occur at a rate of one case per 10,000 to 100,000 treated patients [8].

Because events such as DILI are expected to be rare, postmarketing surveillance for emerging safety signals is an important activity in the life cycle of FDA approved drugs. While premarketing clinical trials provide important information regarding the efficacy and safety of a drug, most are powered to test an efficacy endpoint, but are underpowered to detect rare adverse drug events. For instance, let us assume that Drug X is a newly approved antibiotic used to treat community acquired pneumonia. However, before approval, there was a preclinical hepatotoxicity concern. In addition, several patients in the clinical trials developed greater than twofold elevation in alanine aminotransferase (ALT), a biomarker for liver injury. The total number of patients who received one or more doses of Drug X is 200. In all patients who experienced elevations in ALT, it returned to normal after the drug was discontinued. There were no cases of clinically meaningful hepatitis or Hy's law cases, defined as transaminitis with elevated bilirubin, observed during the clinical trial, and possible alternative causes of elevated ALT were excluded [4]. Can we conclude that the drug is not a hepatotoxin? The answer is no, because there was insufficient enrollment in the trial to detect an event such as DILI that has a low background incidence rate among the general population of medication users.

Using the concept of the rule of three (application of three events in the numerator when zero events were observed to result in the upper bound of a confidence interval [9]) if a total of 200 patients received the treatment and none experienced significant liver injury, then we could conclude with 95% confidence that no more than 1.5% (3/200) would experience significant liver injury if given the drug. However, once the drug is administered to a much larger population of patients who have a wide range of comorbidities, are different ages, use various concomitant medications, or have differing pharmacogenetics that can alter drug metabolism, we may see clinically significant cases of liver injury that were not apparent in the clinical development program. The inability to detect rare events in small clinical trials is a known limitation of modern drug development and is one basis for pharmacovigilance after a drug is approved. Pharmacovigilance, operationalized, is the surveillance of marketed drug products for adverse events under real-world conditions. This surveillance is important because we cannot be fully aware of the complete spectrum of toxicities, including liver injury, at the time a new drug is approved and introduced into the market.

The purpose of this chapter is to provide an overview of the FDA's Center for Drug Evaluation and Research (CDER) approach to surveillance of approved drugs for potential liver injury in the postmarketing setting.

2   Data Sources for Detecting DILI in the Postmarketing Setting

DPV uses a variety of data sources to detect and assess DILI for marketed drugs. In addition to drug-approving divisions, the agency has a Division of Pharmacovigilance (DPV) that conducts postapproval safety surveillance for CDER approved drugs. This group is divided into teams of safety reviewers, typically comprised of pharmacists and physicians, who focus on specific therapeutic classifications of drugs. For instance, DPV will have a team devoted to the pharmacovigilance of oncology drugs with several pharmacists having specialty residency training and experience in hematology/oncology and a specialty trained physician as a medical advisor. The team will assess currently available data, which are typically literature or spontaneous case reports submitted to the agency, to determine if an administered drug or a manifestation of disease or some other cause is responsible for an adverse event being reported to FDA. For reports of hepatotoxicity, this group may reach out to FDA employed hepatologists for advice and assessment of cases that are particularly challenging to discern whether a drug could have caused the event. The agency may occasionally seek the advice of outside practicing hepatologists as Special Government Employees (SGEs) to aid in case adjudication. FDA-CDER also has teams of epidemiologists who aid in refining hepatotoxicity signals and others once these emerge. This section of the chapter reviews some of the data sources that DPV staff may consult to assess DILI in the postmarketing setting.

2.1 FAERS Case Assessment

Since 1969, CDER has maintained a database of case reports received by the FDA that reports an adverse event to some drug. The database is known as the FDA Adverse Event Reporting System (FAERS), and it is an important component of FDA's post-marketing surveillance strategy. FAERS is the repository for spontaneous adverse event reports submitted from drug sponsors and the general public under real use conditions. Importantly, healthcare professionals and the public at large can report DILI and other adverse events directly to FDA via the MedWatch program using the online portal, mailing a paper form, or sharing information by phone or facsimile with the agency [10]. It is important to note that any observed or suspected adverse event can be reported and there is no requirement for the reporter to prove that the adverse event was caused by the drug.

The FAERS database currently houses over 13 million reports describing 9.9 million distinct cases of adverse events to approved drugs (Fig. 1). The majority of reports in the FAERS database are spontaneously reported, meaning these reports are passively reported to manufacturers or directly to the FDA. The FDA does not solicit these reports. This type of system has several advantages in surveillance, with its predominant advantage being its ability to detect rare and serious adverse events. Recall the example provided in Sect. 1 of the chapter (Introduction and background) using Drug X. There was some preapproval evidence, albeit not conclusive, that Drug X may be associated with liver toxicity after

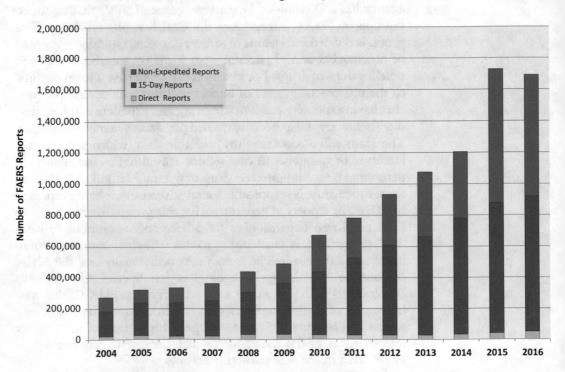

Fig. 1 FAERS Reports by year and type

being administered to 200 patients. After the drug is approved and used in a variety of clinical settings and in patients with different health statuses, clinicians may occasionally observe patients with unexplained transaminase elevation concurrent with bilirubin elevation, which could indicate serious liver injury. Pharmacovigilance staff at CDER look closely for cases such as these and will review them for the role of the drug in the event. A spontaneous reporting system such as FAERS is a comprehensive surveillance system for all FDA-approved drugs.

FAERS, however, has weaknesses that are important to understand. The data are passively reported to manufacturers or directly to the FDA. The manufacturers, in turn, submit reports of adverse events that they have received to the FDA. Since the data are not acquired through an active process, it is assumed that not all incident cases will be reported to the FDA. This concept is termed underreporting. Without full enumeration of all cases, it is therefore not possible to use spontaneous cases to estimate the actual incidence of an adverse event in association with a product. Although estimates of the magnitude of underreporting have been made at 1–10 percent of all adverse reactions, [11] the true size remains unknown and is likely variable by drug and event [12]. Data quality is also highly variable in spontaneous reports and poorly documented submissions can significantly hamper FDA's ability to conduct an adequate assessment of the case. Despite these limitations, spontaneous case reports in the FAERS database remain an important and primary tool that DPV uses to conduct surveillance for rare and serious adverse events for currently marketed drugs.

Once FDA identifies new cases of liver injury from FAERS or other data sources, DPV staff will conduct a causality assessment to better understand if a drug could be the cause. The diagnosis of DILI is based on excluding more common causes of liver injury, such as viral hepatitis. Causality assessment scales that are specific to DILI, such as the Roussel Uclaf Causality Assessment Method (RUCAM), or the Drug-Induced Liver Injury Network (DILIN), [13] are particularly useful to assess a drug as a potential cause. The causality assessment methods are detailed in other chapters in this book. These scales consider temporality, time to onset after a drug exposure, evidence of positive dechallenge, positive rechallenge, exclusion of other probable causes (e.g., viral hepatitis, chronic alcohol intake), and known hepatotoxicity of the drug or other drugs that are chemically similar to the suspect drug, as factors to consider in the causality assessment. DPV staff will gather case details, such as results from a liver biopsy, laboratory tests results, and the clinical description of the liver injury, to better understand if the injury pattern is hepatocellular, cholestatic, or mixed. DPV will also use a severity scale, typically the scale developed by the DILIN [13], to further grade possible cases as mild, moderate, moderate to severe, or severe.

The FDA recently used FAERS to identify liver injury associated with dimethyl fumarate (DMF) in multiple sclerosis patients [14]. Much like the example of Drug X, the incidence of elevation of liver aminotransferases was higher for DMF users compared to study comparators. However, there were no apparent cases of serious liver injury identified preapproval. After approval, CDER/DPV became aware of a report in the literature where severe DILI was linked to DMF. CDER/DPV also reviewed FAERS cases for DILI, and found that many reports either described nonclinically significant elevations in liver aminotransferases, lacked details to make causal inference, or were too poorly documented to adequately assess. However, 14 cases of clinically significant DILI were identified, and all were considered possible or probable on a causality scale. Ten of these cases resulted in hospitalization for DILI. CDER/DPV assessed each case for biopsy results, hepatic enzymes, and other causes for the liver injury. Using information from this postmarket surveillance, FDA was able to identify and characterize DMF-associated DILI and update the DMF labeling to include a new warning that liver injury requiring hospitalization could occur [15].

2.2 FAERS Disproportionality Assessment and Reporting Rates

FDA also conducts hypothesis generating disproportionality analyses using FAERS data (also referred to as data-mining). The growth of spontaneous adverse event reports submitted to the FDA and entered into the FAERS database is exponential (see Fig. 1). With a growing number of reports, FDA increasingly relies on strategies to review these data systematically. One strategy is disproportionality analysis. If we revisit our example of Drug X, we can illustrate how DPV could use disproportionality to detect DILI. Suppose we have observed a few cases of varying degrees of liver injury with Drug X. How many cases should we observe before we become concerned and take regulatory action? This relies on a number of factors that could include the severity of the cases, the benefits of the drug, and the unmet medical need the drug fulfills. We could also consider the proportion of cases of liver injury for Drug X compared to the proportion of cases of liver injury for all other drugs in the database. If a larger proportion of cases than expected are seen with Drug X, then this may indicate a new signal specific to that drug. Although there are a number of disproportionality test statistics available for use, we will describe the proportional reporting ratio (PRR) in an example for its ease of comprehension and calculation.

Suppose we observe the following for Drug X in the FAERS database (Table 1). The PRR is calculated by taking the proportion of DILI reports for Drug X and dividing it by the proportion of DILI reports for all other drugs in the database. Each cell in Table 1 contains both a value and a label (A,B,C,D) with the PRR = [(A/A + B)/(C/C + D)]. In the case of Drug X and DILI,

Table 1
FAERS DILI reporting with Drug X and all other drugs in the database

	DILI	All other events in FAERS
Reports for drug X	10 (A)	500 (B)
Reports for all other drugs	50 (C)	15,000 (D)

Not actual data from FAERS, these data are used for illustrative purposes only

the PRR is $[(10/(10 + 500))/(50/(50 + 15,000)]$, which is 5.9. CDER/DPV would interpret this as FAERS reporting for Drug X and DILI to be 5.9 times more frequent than what we observe for all other drugs and DILI in FAERS. This is suggestive, not confirmatory, for a possible signal that would require further investigation by a thorough review of existing DILI data for Drug X. If the PRR had been computed as one or a number less than one, we would interpret this as the number of reports of DILI for Drug X to not be disproportional to all other drugs in FAERS. The PRR can be large when events are reported in low frequency to FAERS. There are other measures of disproportionality such as the reporting odds ratio (ROR) and the Empirical Bayes Geometric Mean (EBGM) that are used in pharmacovigilance. FDA primarily relies on the EBGM as a measure of disproportionality because the statistic adjusts for low report counts. Regardless of the type of measure of disproportionality used, any data mining of FAERS data is subject to the same limitations and considerations of spontaneous reporting (duplicate reports, stimulated reporting, etc.) and interpretation of the numeric results is done judiciously, often involving a hands-on analysis of the cases.

Reporting rates can be used to help assess and provide context to new DILI safety signals. A reporting rate is calculated by dividing the number of US FAERS reports of a particular adverse event for a given drug (numerator) by a US use estimate of that drug (denominator) in a specified time period. The use estimate is frequently the projected number of prescriptions dispensed or the projected number of unique patients who received a prescription for a drug. Ideally, however, the numerator and denominator should represent the same populations (i.e., from the same data source), but because this is not possible using FAERS data, the reporting rates are therefore hypothesis generating exercises, not confirmatory of a new signal. Accordingly, reporting rates, when calculated, must be interpreted with caution when attempting to glean insight into the size of the at-risk population when considering other drugs in the class or background rate of the adverse event. As an example, if we assume that Drug X is one of three drugs in a therapeutic class, and there was some concern of hepa-

Table 2
Spontaneous report counts and number of prescriptions dispensed for Drug X and others in the therapeutic class

Drug	US spontaneous report count of suspected DILI	US number of prescriptions dispensed	Reporting rate (per 10,000)
Drug X	17	15,200	11.2/10,000
Drug Y	30	330,000	0.91/10,000
Drug Z	60	700,000	0.85/10,000

Not actual data from FAERS, these data are used for illustrative purposes only

totoxicity at approval for Drug X, then we could use reporting rates to better understand the reporting observed in FAERS. If we observe three times the number of reports for Drug X compared to others in the class, does this mean this is a new signal? If we apply reporting rates, it could help us interpret the number reports that we have observed. In Table 2, if we only consider the number of reports (numerator) and not make an adjustment for the likely exposure to the drug, then we may conclude that since the reporting volume for Drug X is much less than others in the drug class, there is no safety concern with the drug. However, if we adjust the reporting volume using the number of prescriptions dispensed, then we learn that the reporting rate for Drug X is a little over ten times higher than for other drugs. We also know that the expected rate of DILI among medication users approximates 1 case per 10,000–100,000 users, so a rate of 11.2/10,000, would be considered an unusual observation. This does not prove that Drug X is causing DILI but it is suggestive of a signal identified in the surveillance of Drug X, and warrants further evaluation. The same limitations that are found when using the FAERS database are applicable when FAERS data are used to compute a reporting rate (duplicate reports, uncertain causality, stimulated reporting, different marketing periods for different products etc.). Furthermore, there is additional uncertainty in estimates of the exposure. For pragmatic purposes, reporting rates are likely most useful when there is at least an order of magnitude difference between the drug of interest and the comparator rate.

2.3 Literature Monitoring

The published biomedical literature is a rich source of drug safety signals used in the surveillance of DILI. Compared to FAERS cases, literature cases are much fewer, but they are often better documented cases with relevant clinical details of a liver adverse event thereby allowing one to conduct a more rigorous causality assessment. Unlike FAERS cases, which have highly variable data quality, literature cases have typically undergone peer review to meet acceptable quality prior to publication. DPV leverages automated alerts that may be established in PubMed, Embase, or other literature monitoring tools, which can notify a safety reviewer of a new published case report or observational studies of DILI for a drug. For example, the FDA recently reassessed the risks of liver injury of ketoconazole [16]. At that time, a number of published case reports and some observational data, which had evaluated the risk of liver injury attributed to ketoconazole, were reviewed. One particular study, by Garcia Rodriguez [17], assessed the risk of acute liver injury for ketoconazole users compared to nonusers and to other antifungals used in the treatment of dermatophyte infections. The relative risk of acute liver injury for ketoconazole users was 228 (95% CI 33.9–933.0) compared to nonusers. While this study has limitations, such as the few observed instances of acute liver injury, and the sensitivity of the relative risks to small changes in the number of cases observed, it nonetheless, served as an important information source for CDER to further investigate ketoconazole-associated liver injury. Published investigations from large administrative databases, pharmacoepidemiology studies, can also be very useful for assessing rare adverse events that were not apparent at approval, and can serve as sources of signals in adverse event detection.

2.4 Clinical Specialty Networks

Clinical specialty networks are an important source of information when assessing a DILI signal. One example of a clinical specialty network is the United Network for Organ Sharing (UNOS). UNOS exists to make organs available for transplant by matching patients to available organs. This organization is able to track the number of transplants (e.g., liver and others) with details on the reason for transplant (liver failure from hepatitis, DILI, etc.). Since liver transplant is a severe outcome of DILI, this specialty network could prove useful to assess liver injury that has resulted in transplant that is attributed to a drug.

FDA has also partnered with the Drug-Induced Liver Injury Network (DILIN) established by the National Institute of Diabetes and Digestive Kidney Disease (NIDDK) in collaboration with select clinical centers across the USA to collect details of cases of DILI linked to marketed prescription and over-the-counter drugs and dietary supplements. In the past, DILIN has collected and submitted high quality case reports of DILI to FAERS via the MedWatch program. These cases then become available to our pharmacovigilance teams who assess each report when evaluating a new DILI signal. FDA has also established similar collaborative efforts with the Acute Liver Failure Study Group (ALFSG) and the Pediatric Acute Liver Failure (PALF) Registry Study Group. These partnerships are greatly valued, as it enriches the quality of DILI reports.

2.5   Sentinel

Sentinel is a national electronic system designed to conduct active safety surveillance for FDA approved medical products. The impetus for the system was the Food and Drug Administration Amendments Act (FDAAA) of 2007, which required that the FDA develop a tool for the active safety monitoring of medical products. The system has been implemented using a phased approach, with the launch of Mini-Sentinel in May 2008, followed by a transition to the Sentinel System in September, 2014 [18]. The full Sentinel system launched in February 2016, and is comprised of data from multiple partner institutions that provide health insurance coverage to well over 100 million members [19]. Because the data partners are health insurers, each will have administrative data for diagnoses using ICD (International Classification of Diseases) codes from physicians as well as dispensing codes from pharmacies. These codes can be used to identify outcomes of interest in drug safety research.

Sentinel is intended to be a complementary analytical tool to FAERS and other databases that are used to conduct postmarketing drug safety surveillance. For instance, Sentinel has been successfully used to assess the bleeding rates of dabigatran and warfarin [20]. In early 2011, the FDA identified an unusually large number of FAERS reports of clinically significant bleeding with dabigatran compared to warfarin, shortly after dabigatran was approved. Although the rates of bleeding were similar among dabigatran and warfarin users in the Randomized Evaluation of Long Term Anticoagulation Therapy (RE-LY) trial, there was concern that the risk of bleeding could be significantly higher in dabigatran users if the drug was being used in settings that were not represented in the clinical development program. Ultimately, Sentinel was used to provide context to the spontaneous reporting seen with dabigatran, and FDA concluded that bleeding rates associated with dabigatran did not appear to be higher than those with warfarin.

The use of Sentinel to study different outcomes, including DILI, is still being explored. One group has investigated the validity of diagnostic codes and laboratory tests to identify severe cases of liver injury [21, 22]. Thus far, Sentinel has not been a reliable tool for detecting severe liver injury as an outcome using administrative billing codes. The positive predictive value for identifying cases of acute liver injury has been generally low at 5–15%. Studies of acute liver injury in Sentinel will likely need medical chart review to confirm the outcome. Sentinel is a new tool and the FDA is still exploring how to better integrate it into regulatory decision-making for DILI.

2.6   Select Other Pharmacovigilance Surveillance Data Sources

In addition to data sources cited above and as needed, CDER/FDA will consult other data sources to assess liver injury attributed to a drug. One drug that is regarded as a leading cause of liver injury is acetaminophen. FDA researchers have evaluated US rates of acetaminophen related adverse events, including hepatotoxicity, using a variety of data sources such as the National Inpatient Sample (NIS), National Electronic Injury Surveillance System-Cooperative Adverse Drug Event Surveillance (NEISS-CADES), and data from the American Association of Poison Control Centers (AAPCC) [23]. Additionally, a British-based primary care database such as the Clinical Practice Research Datalink (CPRD) has been used to assess acute liver injury in the post-market setting for keto-conazole and antibiotics [17, 24]. Occasionally, DPV will also search the Uppsala Monitoring Center's VigiBase® for additional evidence of a drug-induced event. VigiBase®, like FAERS, is another spontaneous reporting system that contains reports from over 110 countries [25]. CDER also frequently meets with drug regulators from other countries to share information related to new safety signals, including liver injury for drugs. This open communication is an important tool to corroborate signals that one or more groups may find during postmarketing surveillance of the new drug.

3 Telithromycin and DILI—A Postmarketing Case Study

Telithromycin, a semisynthetic erythromycin derivative, was the first of a new class of antimicrobials called ketolides that were introduced to the US market in 2004 [26]. Similar to the macrolide antibiotics, telithromycin prevents bacterial growth by interfering with bacterial protein synthesis. The French pharmaceutical company Hoechst Marion Roussel (now Sanofi) began clinical trials of telithromycin for the treatment of common upper respiratory infections in 1998 [26]. Telithromycin was approved by the European Commission in July 2001 and was subsequently marketed in Europe in October 2001 [27]. The original NDA for telithromycin was submitted to FDA/CDER in February 2000 with clinical trial experience for acute bacterial sinusitis (ABS), acute exacerbation of chronic bronchitis (AECB), and community–acquired pneumonia (CAP).

The initial CDER review of telithromycin identified multiple issues of concern including, cardiac, hepatic, visual, and vascular safety [28]. With specific interest in hepatic events, some differential hepatotoxicity was identified in animals. In addition, two patients in a Phase 3 CAP trial experienced hepatitis versus no (zero) patients randomized to active control. CAP patients treated with telithromycin also experienced more ALT and aspartate aminotransferase (AST) elevations than control patients. No differential in transaminase elevations was observed in patients treated for AECB or ABS. Like many new agents, telithromycin was discussed at the public FDA Advisory Committee meetings. These meetings permit outside experts to offer opinions to the FDA on regulatory actions, such as new drug approvals. Telithromycin was first presented before the Anti-Infective Drug Advisory Committee in April 2001. This committee generally concurred with CDER's assessment that significant safety concerns precluded US approval [29]. To address these concerns, the sponsor conducted a large safety study (termed "Study 3014"). This study, started in 2001, was a randomized, open-label, comparative study designed to characterize the safety and effectiveness of telithromycin vs. amoxicillin-clavulanic acid when used for the treatment of community-acquired respiratory tract infections in a large population of subjects. Adverse events of special interest (hepatic, cardiac, vascular, and visual) were to be adjudicated by a blinded independent panel of external experts. When completed, Study 3014 included 24,140 subjects, including 12,161 subjects in the telithromycin arm. Although Study 3014 reported no difference in hepatic events between telithromycin and amoxicillin-clavulanic acid, the study suffered many integrity problems which did not allow for a meaningful assessment of the hepatic safety concerns for which the study was designed [30]. However, the full extent of the problems were not presented to the second Advisory Committee (January 2003) [30]. Without a liver signal from Study 3014 and with a supporting analysis based on spontaneous adverse event reporting from Europe, the Advisory Committee voted for approval. Telithromycin (as Ketek) was approved by the FDA in April 2004 and entered the US market in fall of 2004. Ketek was approved for the oral treatment of ABS, AECB, and CAP.

Following marketing of Ketek in the USA, the FDA/CDER—including both premarketing and postmarketing (pharmacovigilance) groups—began to monitor spontaneous adverse event reports. Such reports are required for submission by a drug sponsor but also include reports sent in directly to FDA by the public via the FDA MedWatch system for inclusion in the FAERS database. Given lingering concern for liver injury, reports of hepatitis or liver injury were considered a focus for ongoing review. The first analysis of such reports (completed in June 2005 and thus restricted to the first 6 months of marketing) identified cases of liver injury generally consistent with the approved label. This included cases of isolated ALT/AST elevation and cholestatic jaundice that resolved with discontinuation of Ketek. Importantly, there was one case consistent with Hy's law [31]. This case described fulminant hepatic failure with an outcome of death and with limited alternative possible etiologies. This case, which would be identified later as "Case 3" in the sentinel publication [32], was not—in itself—enough for the FDA review team to advance a "signal" for risk of hepatocellular injury with telithromycin as there is a background rate of acute liver failure in the population at large. However, when "Case 3" was published alongside two additional cases in January

2006, the Agency published a public health advisory for serious liver toxicity in association with telithromycin [32, 33]. These cases and an analysis of all available data led to the addition of a Warning for serious liver toxicity to approved labeling for telithromycin in June 2006 [34].

In time, additional cases of acute liver failure in association with telithromycin were submitted to the Agency (Fig. 2) and this prompted an additional review by the pharmacovigilance group at CDER [35]. While this second review was ongoing, the Agency prepared to discuss the risk of liver injury caused by telithromycin at a third public FDA Advisory Committee. This FDA Advisory Committee meeting took place on December 14 and 15, 2006 and included the review of a total of 12 cases of acute liver failure associated with telithromycin through April 2006. [The existence of a 13th case received after April 2006 was also mentioned.] The review of cases was supported by the participation of outside expert hepatologists (as Special Government Employees) to aid in the case adjudication process [36]. The case series was remarkable for the short time-to-onset (median 4 days) and severity of outcome (4 deaths, 1 transplant). At baseline, before exposure to telithromycin, the cases appeared healthy and reported few confounding drugs or conditions. The most common condition for which telithromycin was used was sinusitis ($n = 5$).

In order to put these cases in context of utilization, and in context of similar agents, a reporting rate analysis was conducted to compare reporting rates of acute liver failure with telithromycin during early marketing to similar rates for fluoroquinolones. The fluoroquinolones all carried a Warning for hepatotoxicity in the approved labeling [37]. Importantly, there are numerous limitations of such analyses and the results should be interpreted with caution [38]. On the surface, however, it should be of interest to question how, for example, two antimicrobials could have reporting rates that differ by tenfold (for example) unless the risk for the event was different between them. As presented at the Advisory Committee meeting, the reporting rate analysis showed a reporting rate for telithromycin some fourfold higher than for recently approved fluoroquinolones [35]. This was deemed not robust enough to suggest that the risk of serious drug-induced liver injury was higher for telithromycin than comparator agents that carried a hepatotoxicity Warning. Following the Advisory Committee meeting, which included numerous other data streams than spontaneous reports for assessment of liver toxicity and other safety issues, the FDA and the drug sponsor agreed to additional labeling changes for Ketek including removal of certain indications (ABS and AECB). As of December 2016, telithromycin was not marketed in the USA.

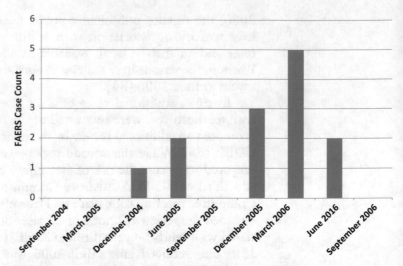

Fig. 2 Telithromycin spontaneously reported acute liver failure cases (*n* = 13) as adjudicated by FDA through September 2006

4   Conclusion

Drug-induced liver injury continues to be a significant concern for marketed drugs and other consumable products, such as dietary supplements and nutraceuticals. Because events such as DILI are rare, surveillance systems and methods such as those described in this chapter are important components of the safety net, which is designed to recognize liver injury that may have gone undetected in a clinical development program for a drug. FDA predominantly relies on clinical assessment of spontaneous reports submitted to FAERS and published case reports to assess DILI in the postmarketing setting.

Acknowledgments

The views expressed are those of the authors and do not necessarily represent the position of, nor imply endorsement from, the US Food and Drug Administration or the US Government.

References

1. World Health Organization. Available via http://www.who.int/medicines/areas/quality_safety/safety_efficacy/pharmvigi/en/. Accessed 22 Jan 2017

2. Council for International Organization of Medical Sciences (CIOMS) Report of Working Group VIII (2010). Practical aspects of signal detection in Pharmacovigilance. Geneva, Switzerland, 14

3. Avigan MI, Mozersky RP, Seeff LB (2016) Scientific and regulatory perspectives in herbal and dietary supplement associated hepatotoxicity in the United States. Int J Mol Sci 17(3):331

4. United States Food and Drug Administration (2009) .Guidance for industry drug-induced liver injury: premarketing clinical evaluation. http://www.fda.gov/downloads/Drugs/Guidances/UCM174090.pdf. Accessed 11 Jan 2017

5. WITHDRAWN: a resource for withdrawn and discontinued drugs. http://cheminfo.charite. de/withdrawn/index.html. Accessed 9 Feb 2017

6. Siramshetty VB, Nickel J, Omieczynski C, Gohlke B-O, Drwal MN (2015) Robert Preissner; WITHDRAWN—a resource for withdrawn and discontinued drugs. Nucleic Acids Res 44(D1):D1080–D1086. https:// doi.org/10.1093/nar/gkv1192

7. Bell LN, Chalasani N (2009) Epidemiology of idiosyncratic drug-induced liver injury. Semin Liver Dis 29(4):337–347

8. Navarro VJ, Senior JR (2006) Drug-related hepatotoxicity. N Engl J Med 354(7):731–739

9. Philips B (2005) Towards evidence based medicine for paediatricians. Arch Dis Child 90:642–650

10. US Food and Drug Administration-MedWatch Program. Available at http://www.fda.gov/ Safety/MedWatch/HowToReport/. Accessed 13 Feb 2017

11. US Government General Accounting Office. General Accounting Office Report on Adverse Drug Events Substantial Problem but Magnitude Uncertain, 1 Feb 1 2000. http:// www.gao.gov/new.items/he00053t.pdf. Accessed 22 Jan 2017

12. McAdams M, Staffa J, Dal Pan G (2008) Estimating the extent of reporting to FDA: a case study of statin-associated rhabdomyolysis. Pharmacoepidemiol Drug Saf 17:229–239

13. LiverTox. https://livertox.nih.gov/index. html. Accessed 09 Feb 2017

14. Munoz MA, Kulick CG, Kortepeter CM, Levin RL, Avigan MI (2017) Liver injury associated with dimethyl fumarate in multiple sclerosis patients. Mult Scler J. https://doi. org/10.1177/1352458516688351

15. Drugs@FDA updated prescribing information for Tecfidera. https://www.accessdata.fda.gov/ drugsatfda_docs/label/2017/204063s017lbl. pdf. Accessed 30 Mar 2017

16. US Food and Drug Administration. Drug safety communication, July 26, 2013. http://www.fda. gov/Safety/MedWatch/SafetyInformation/ SafetyAlertsforHumanMedicalProducts/ ucm362672.htm. Accessed 22 Jan 2017

17. Garcia Rodriguez LA, Duque A, Castellsague J, Perez-Gutthann S, Stricker BH (1999) A cohort study on the risk of acute liver injury among users of ketoconazole and other antifungal drugs. Br J Clin Pharmacol 48:847–852

18. Ball R, Robb M, Anderson SA, Dal Pan G (2016) The FDA's sentinel initiative-a comprehensive approach to medical product surveillance. Clin Pharmacol Ther 99(3):265–267

19. US Food and Drug Administration-Sentinel Initiative. http://www.fda.gov/Safety/ FDAsSentinelInitiative/default.htm. Accessed 13 Feb 2017

20. Southworth MR, Reichman ME, Unger EF (2013) Dabigatran and postmarketing reports of bleeding. N Engl J Med 368(14):1272–1274

21. Lo Re V III, Haynes K, Goldberg D, Forde KA, Carbonari DM, Leidl KB, Hennessy S, Reddy KR, Pawloski PA, Daniel GW, Cheetham TC, Iyer A, Coughlin KO, Toh S, Boudreau DM, Selvam N, Cooper WO, Selvan MS, VanWormer JJ, Avigan MI, Houstoun M, Zornberg GL, Racoosin JA, Shoaibi A (2013) Validity of diagnostic codes to identify cases of severe acute liver injury in the US Food and Drug Administration's mini-sentinel distributed database. Pharmacoepidemiol Drug Saf 22(8):861–872

22. Lo Re V III, Carbonari DM, Forde KA, Goldberg D, Lewis JD, Haynes K, Leidl KB, Reddy RK, Roy J, Sha D, Marks AR, Schneider JL, Strom BL, Corley DA (2015) Validity of diagnostic codes and laboratory tests of liver dysfunction to identify acute liver failure events. Pharmacoepidemiol Drug Saf 24(7):676–683

23. Major JM, Zhou EH, Wong HL, Trinidad JP, Pham TM, Mehta H, Ding Y, Staff JA, Iyasu S, Wang C, Willy MF (2016) Trends in rates of acetaminophen-related adverse events in the United States. Pharmacoepidemiol Drug Saf 25:590–598

24. Brauer R, Douglas I, Garcia Rodriguez LA, Downey G, Huerta C, de Abajo F, Bate A, Tepie MF, de Groot MCH, Schlienger R, Reynolds R, Smeeth L, Klungel O, Ruigomez A (2016) Risk of acute liver injury associated the use of antibiotics. Comparative cohort and nested case-control studies using two primary care databases in Europe. Pharmacoepidemiology. Drug Saf 25(suppl 1):29–38

25. World Health Organization-Uppsala Monitoring Centre. https://www.who-umc. org/vigibase/vigibase/. Accessed 13 Feb 2017

26. Bearden DT, Neuhauser MM, Garey KW (2001) Telithromycin: an oral ketolide for respiratory infections. Pharmacotherapy 21(10):1204–1222

27. Aventis. Ketek (telithromycin): Briefing document for the FDA Anti-Infective Drug Products Advisory Committee Meeting. January 2003. Accessed 3 Feb 2017 at http:// www.fda.gov/ohrms/dockets/ac/03/ briefing/3919B1_01_Aventis-KETEK.pdf

28. Soreth J. Ketek (telithromycin) NDA background for the FDA anti-infective drug products advisory committee meeting (2003). Accessed 3 Feb 2017 at http://www.fda.gov/

ohrms/dockets/ac/03/slides/3919S1_01_FDA-Soreth.ppt

29. Cooper C. Medical officer safety review of NDA 21–144: telithromycin (Ketek), 31 Mar 2004. Accessed 3 Feb 2017 at http://www.fda.gov/cder/foi/nda/2004/21-144_Ketek.htm

30. Ross DB (2007) The FDA and the case of Ketek. N Engl J Med 356(16):1601–1604

31. Senior JR (2009) Monitoring for hepatotoxicity: what is the predictive value of liver "function" tests? Clin Pharmacol Ther 85(3):331–334

32. FDA Public Health Advisory for Ketek (telithromycin). 20 Jan 2006. Accessed 3 Feb 2017 at http://www.fda.gov/Drugs/DrugSafety/PostmarketDrugSafetyInformationforPatientsandProviders/ucm051301.htm

33. Clay KD, Hanson JS, Pope SD, Rissmiller RW, Purdum PP III, Banks PM (2006) Brief communication: severe hepatotoxicity of telithromycin: three case reports and literature review. Ann Intern Med 144:415–420

34. Soreth J, Cox E, Kweder S, Jenkins J, Galson S (2007) Ketek - the FDA perspective. N Engl J Med 356(16):1675–1676

35. Brinker A, Wassel R. Telithromycin-associated hepatotoxicity. 14 Dec 2006. Accessed 3 Feb 2017 at http://www.fda.gov/ohrms/DOCKETS/ac/06/slides/2006-4266s1-01-07-FDA-Brinker.ppt

36. Brinker AD, Wassel RT, Lyndly J, Serrano J, Avigan M, Lee WM, Seeff LB (2009) Telithromycin-associated hepatotoxicity: clinical spectrum and causality assessment of 42 cases. Hepatology 49(1):250–257

37. Orman ES, Conjeevaram HS, Vuppalanchi R, Freston JW, Rochon J, Kleiner DE, Hayashi PH, DILIN Research Group (2011) Clinical and histopathologic features of fluoroquinolone-induced liver injury. Clin Gastroenterol Hepatol 9(6):517–523

38. Brinker A, Goldkind L, Bonnel R, Beitz J (2004) Spontaneous reports of hypertension leading to hospitalisation in association with rofecoxib, celecoxib, nabumetone and oxaprozin. Drugs Aging 21(7):479–484

Part V

Methodologies for Clinical Studies

Chapter 23

Host Risk Modifiers in Idiosyncratic Drug-Induced Liver Injury (DILI) and Its Interplay with Drug Properties

Camilla Stephens, M. Isabel Lucena, and Raúl J. Andrade

Abstract

Idiosyncratic drug-induced liver injury (DILI) occurs in a small proportion of individuals exposed to a drug and is unpredictable based on the drug's pharmacological action and ingested dose. Due to the multifactorial pathology of this condition various factors associated with both the drug and the patient can affect DILI susceptibility and clinical presentation. A major challenge in the area of DILI is therefore to determine these risk factors and their interactions in order to predict individuals at risk of developing DILI. This would enable patients without significant DILI risk to securely benefit from an effective treatment (including medications with black box warnings for hepatotoxicity), while ensuring patient safety to those at increased risk by providing an alternative medication. Host-related DILI modifiers proposed to date include age, sex, genetic variations, associated conditions, concomitant medications and lifestyle. In addition, physicochemical and toxicological drug properties such as dose, lipophilicity, reactive metabolite formation, mitochondrial liability, and transporter inhibition are likewise assumed to have a potential modulating effect on DILI. Individually none of these host and drug-related features are likely to be sufficient to induce liver injury, but when combined could lead to DILI development. Hence, considering interactions between DILI host and drug factors could be more useful in predicting individuals at increased risk of developing DILI. In this chapter we provide an overview of the current understanding of risk factors for idiosyncratic DILI.

Key words Genetic variations, Age and gender, Lifestyle, Comorbidities and concomitant medications, Physicochemical drug properties

1 Introduction

Idiosyncratic drug-induced liver injury (DILI) occurs in a small proportion of individuals exposed to a drug and is unpredictable based on the drug's pharmacological action and ingested dose. Despite advances in the mechanistic understanding of dose-dependent (intrinsic) acetaminophen hepatotoxicity, the cellular processes behind idiosyncratic DILI are not yet fully understood. Nevertheless it is generally believed that DILI is a multifactorial process that involves cellular stress and immune responses [1–3]. The development of DILI is subsequently affected by various

Minjun Chen and Yvonne Will (eds.), *Drug-Induced Liver Toxicity*, Methods in Pharmacology and Toxicology,
https://doi.org/10.1007/978-1-4939-7677-5_23, © Springer Science+Business Media, LLC, part of Springer Nature 2018

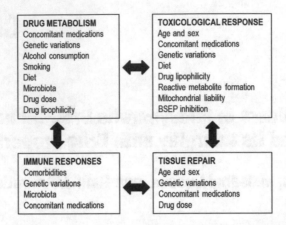

Fig. 1 Idiosyncratic drug-induced liver injury risk factors. Idiosyncratic DILI is assumed to be a multifactorial process and the consequence of simultaneous occurrence of several interacting elements, constituted by drug properties and host factors. These interactions can affect cellular processes such as drug metabolism, toxicological responses, immune responses, and tissue repair

factors associated with both the drug and the patient (Fig. 1). This combination of drug and host factors required to induce idiosyncratic DILI is a main reason for the lack of fully functional animal models for idiosyncratic DILI, while well-established murine models currently exist for acetaminophen hepatotoxicity.

A major challenge in the area of DILI is therefore to determine these risk factors and their interactions in order to predict individuals at risk of developing idiosyncratic DILI. This would enable patients without significant DILI risk to securely benefit from an effective treatment (including medications with black box warnings for hepatotoxicity), while ensuring patient safety to those at increased risk by providing an alternative medication. In this chapter we present an overview of the current understanding of physicochemical and toxicological drug properties and host factors as potential DILI susceptibility and phenotype modifiers.

2 Host Factors

Many drugs have the capacity to induce cellular stress, however the outcome is dependent on the patient's cellular ability to counteract this feature and consequently control potential cell damage. Specific host factors may also potentiate drug properties that on their own are not sufficient to produce liver injury. Hence, host factors can contribute to individual susceptibility and clinical phenotypes by influencing drug metabolism, toxicological responses, immune responses and tissue repair processes [4] (Table 1). The difficulty to reproduce multiple host factor contributions in animal models can explain why idiosyncratic hepatotoxicity is seldom detected in animal models, which often involve young healthy animals.

Table 1
Potential risk modifiers of idiosyncratic drug-induced liver injury and their effects

Risk modifiers	Effects
Host factors	
Age	Pharmacokinetic variations (e.g., ↑ age → ↓ drug clearance, ↓ liver mass, ↓ hepatic blood flow, ↓ protein synthesis
Sex	Hormone-related pharmacokinetic and pharmacodynamic variations
Comorbidities	↑ oxidative stress level Heightened inflammatory state
Concomitant medications	Variations in drug metabolism of the causative drug due to induction, inhibition or competition Positive or negative effect on tissue repair → variations in clinical outcome
Genetic variations	Variations in gene expression leading to suboptimal drug metabolism, detoxification and immune responses
Alcohol and tobacco	Potential variations in drug metabolism, such as induction of CYP2E1 → ↑ ROS formation
Diet	Malnutrition: ↓ drug and xenobiotic clearance Obesity: ↑ CYP2E1 → ↑ ROS formation
Microbiota	Variations in drug metabolism Bacterial translocation to the liver
Drug properties	
Dose	Overcome threshold for cellular damage Tissue repair response regulation
Lipophilicity	↑ lipophilicity → ↑ off-target binding ↑ lipophilicity → extensive metabolism
Reactive metabolite formation	ROS formation → oxidative stress → initiation of signaling pathways Binding to cellular macromolecules → ↓ function Haptenization → immune response
Mitochondrial liability	↓ ATP formation ↑ ROS formation ↑ mtDNA mutations
Hepatic transporter inhibition	BSEP inhibition → ↑ hepatocyte bile salt accumulation ↓ drug elimination

Abbreviations: ↑ increased, ↓ decreased, *CYP2E1* cytochrome P450 2E1, *ROS* reactive oxygen species, *ATP* adenosine triphosphate, *mtDNA* mitochondrial DNA, *BSEP* bile salt export pump

2.1 Age and Sex   Aging is well known to produce pharmacokinetic changes, although this has not been demonstrated to increase the risk of DILI. In fact, data from large prospective DILI registries do not support old age as a general risk factor, with 46% of Spanish DILI patients being ≥60 years and 16.6% of North American DILI patients being ≥65 years [5, 6].

Older age has, however, been associated with increased risk of DILI with persistent/chronic liver profile abnormalities [7, 8]. This could potentially result from a decline in tissue repair function occurring with age. While not a general susceptibility risk factor, age appears to be important for hepatotoxicity induced by specific medications. Valproic acid, for example, is more likely to produce DILI in young children, with children under the age of two being particularly prone to severe forms of valproic acid hepatotoxicity [9]. It has been suggested that this age-related risk is due to differences in drug metabolism and reduced plasma protein binding [10]. In contrast, the risk of DILI due to isoniazid appears to increase with age, with speculation of altered pharmacokinetics and/or cumulative mitochondrial functional impairment being responsible for this occurrence [11, 12].

In addition, age appears to affect the clinical presentation of DILI. A study of 603 Spanish DILI cases found that older DILI patients are more prone to develop cholestatic liver injury, particularly males, while younger patients, particularly females, more frequently present with hepatocellular damage [5]. Age differences in reporting frequency of liver events in the WHO Safety Report Database, VigiBase, support these findings, with the highest incidence of hepatocellular injury found in younger patients and cholestatic injury in elderly ($\geq$65 years) patients [13]. Interestingly, this relationship contradicts old age as a risk factor for isoniazid as it predominantly produces a hepatocellular pattern. This highlights the intricate interplay between DILI risk factors, in which the effect of a single risk factor may vary depending on the presence or absence of additional modulating factors.

Differences in incidence rates between males and females are known for various hepatic conditions. For example, women are more prone to develop primary biliary cirrhosis and autoimmune hepatitis, while men predominate among patients with sclerosing cholangitis and hepatocellular carcinoma [14]. Patient sex as a predisposing risk factor in DILI is less clear-cut. Results from large DILI cohorts demonstrate a relatively equal distribution, with 49%, 59%, and 56% female DILI patients in Spain, the USA, and Iceland, respectively [5, 6, 15]. Nevertheless, increased female susceptibility for specific drugs has been noted, such as minocycline and nitrofurantoin [6, 16]. These medications, however, often produce hepatotoxicity with autoimmune features, which may be why women appear to be more susceptible to these forms of DILI. While the role of patient sex in DILI susceptibility is disputable, strong evidence has been presented from several studies that female DILI patients are significantly more likely to progress to acute liver failure [17, 18].

2.2 Comorbidities and Concomitant Medications

Controversy exists as to whether preexisting conditions, particularly liver diseases, is a hepatotoxicity susceptibility factor. A comparison of American DILI patients with and without known preexisting liver diseases suggests that the former group has a higher risk of mortality, although the rate of liver-related mortality did not differ significantly between the two groups [6]. Nevertheless, HIV patients on antiretroviral therapy containing protease inhibitors have been demonstrated to be more susceptible to DILI when having viral hepatitis B and C coinfections [19]. Similar results have been reported for DILI induced by nonnucleoside reverse transcriptase inhibitors and antituberculosis treatments [20, 21]. In terms of nonhepatic conditions, the effect of diabetes mellitus on DILI susceptibility is unknown. However, a study of 300 North American DILI cases found that having diabetes mellitus more than doubled the risk of developing severe DILI [22]. As comorbidities often entail additional drug treatments it can be difficult to determine if any apparent increase in DILI risk is due to the underlying condition or to concomitant treatments. Concomitant drugs should not be overlooked as many drugs have the capacity to modulate the metabolism of additional drugs through induction, inhibition or competition for CYP450 reactions and hepatic transporter systems and consequently affect the hepatotoxicity potential of other drugs. Concomitant drugs have also been reported to affect hepatotoxicity risk and clinical outcome based on retrospective database analyses of liver event reporting frequency of acetaminophen, isoniazid, valproic acid and amoxicillin-clavulanate in the presence of coreported medications [23, 24].

2.3 Genetic Variations

Genetic variations are assumed to play a major role in the idiosyncratic nature of DILI and various studies have explored this area. Genetic DILI studies have to a large extent focused on genes involved in drug metabolism, as polymorphisms in such genes can potentially generate increased drug plasma concentrations and/or decreased clearance rates in patients treated with standard medication doses. In fact, drug metabolizing gene polymorphisms are estimated to influence the clinical outcome in 20–25% of all drug therapies [25]. Associations between increased risk of DILI development and various specific genotypes have been detected [26]. For example, N-acetyltransferase 2 slow acetylator genotype carriers appear more susceptible to isoniazid-related liver injury [27, 28], while the glutathione S-transferase M1 and T1 double null genotype appears to increase DILI susceptibility nonspecifically to a large variety of causative agents [29]. All individual risk genotypes identified to date coincide in having modest effect sizes. The effect of a specific genetic variation is, however, dependent on the genomic setting of each individual and discrete genotypes with seemingly low impacts may collectively play a substantial role in disease development in conjunction with supplementary drug properties. In addition, variations in different genes in the same or related pathways may lead to the same cellular phenotype and consequently promote the same disorder, which complicates the identification of genetic risk factors. Genetic heterogeneity is common in complex diseases [30], and this is unlikely to differ in idiosyncratic DILI.

Surprisingly, few of the earlier results in drug metabolizing genes have been reproduced in later genome-wide association (GWA) studies using single nucleotide polymorphism (SNP) array technology. Most DILI GWA studies have in fact detected specific human leukocyte antigen (HLA) alleles as potential DILI risk factors [31–34]. Considering the strong linkage disequilibrium that exists in the HLA region on chromosome 6, it is possible that other alleles rather than HLA alleles are the true risk factors. Nevertheless, a large proportion of the genes situated in the HLA region are involved in the immune system, which reinforces the assumed importance of immune responses in DILI development. Most identified HLA risk alleles have low predictive value but relatively high negative predictive value, and subsequently are of limited use for genetic screening prior to drug prescription in order to prevent liver injury. However, they could aid clinical diagnosis by enabling DILI due to a specific agent to be ruled out in the absence of the corresponding HLA allele(s) and to identify the correct causative agent in DILI cases where the patient has taken multiple drugs with hepatotoxicity potential prior to DILI onset, providing the suspected drug has been previously linked to a given allele in terms of hepatotoxicity risk [35]. As the presence of specific alleles tend to vary depending on ethnicity and geographic regions it is important to keep in mind that identified risk alleles or genotypes may not be applicable to all populations. For example, Spanish carriers of the HLA class I allele B*18:01 have been found to have increased risk of developing hepatotoxicity due to amoxicillin-clavulanate, particularly hepatocellular type of liver injury, while no such association was detected for patients with Northwestern European heritage [36, 37].

2.4 Lifestyle

It is feasible to assume that exposure to conditions that have a biological effect on the body may alter the risk of DILI development and presentation. Hence, variations in patient lifestyle should also be considered as potential DILI moderators, although limited evidence is currently available to confirm this theory. Alcohol abuse is frequently considered to be a DILI risk factor in the literature. In fact, alcohol consumption is included as a risk factor in the Council for International Organizations of Medical Sciences (CIOMS) causality assessment scale and gives an extra point when the scale is applied to a case with known alcohol history [38]. Alcohol induces CYP2E1 activity, which can lead to changes in drug metabolism. This is of particular interest for acetaminophen hepatotoxicity as CYP2E1 catalyzes the formation of the reactive metabolite N-acetyl-p-benzoquinone imine (NAPQI), which if present at high concentrations rapidly depletes cytosolic and mitochondrial glutathione stores. In terms of idiosyncratic hepatotoxicity, studies supporting alcohol as a risk factor are limited to isoniazid, methotrexate, halothane and vitamin A as causative agents [39]. Nevertheless, the recovery of idiosyncratic DILI induced by any causative agent in patients with an underlying alcohol-induced liver condition may be hampered by the latter condition. Cigarette smoking is also believed to induce CYP2E1 activity [40]. In addition, it has been shown to be an independent risk factor for severe hepatotoxicity, acute liver failure and death following acetaminophen overdose, although its effect on idiosyncratic DILI is currently unknown [41].

Diet affects the development of many diseases, including liver conditions. High caloric diets and obesity are now generally assumed to be associated with increased risk of nonalcoholic fatty liver disease (NAFLD). However, the effect on DILI is less studied. Data from large national DILI registries do not support that DILI patients have a higher body mass index than the general population [5, 6]. Nevertheless, high fat diets have been shown to increase CYP2E1 expression in murine models, which can lead to increased reactive oxygen species (ROS) formation [42]. On the one hand, it is tempting to hypothesize that in conjunction with drug-induced hepatocyte stress this could favor hepatotoxicity development. On the other hand, it has been suggested that CYP2E1-derived ROS may induce activation of antioxidant genes and subsequently be protective in eliminating harmful substances [43]. It is important to note that deficiency or excess of most dietary nutrients can impair the balance between antioxidant and pro-oxidant agents and subsequently lead to complications [44]. Hence, nutritional components apart from dietary fat intake could potentially be involved in regulating DILI susceptibility. Furthermore, malnutrition can result in decreased xenobiotic clearance, and could subsequently influence toxicity as seen with acetaminophen [45]. Malnutrition or weight loss (potentially resulting from inadequate food intake due to persistent gastrointestinal symptoms brought on by the treatment) has also been indicated to increase the risk of hepatotoxicity induced by antituberculosis treatments [46, 47].

Dietary intake not only affects body weight but can also have a profound impact on the gut flora with changes in the intestinal microbiota composition [48, 49]. Recent findings suggest that gut dysbiosis plays a role in various liver conditions, such as NAFLD, primary sclerosing cholangitis and primary biliary cirrhosis [50, 51]. The role of the intestinal microbiota in idiosyncratic DILI is currently unknown, but it has been suggested that it could be a potential risk factor influencing DILI susceptibility and outcome [52]. Gut dysbiosis can disrupt the integrity of the intestinal barrier allowing leakage of bacterial components, which can travel to the liver via the portal vein. Such bacterial translocation could produce a heightened inflammatory environment in the liver through Toll-like receptor stimulation, and potentially lead to alterations in immune tolerance. It has been hypothesized that the ability of antibiotics to cause temporal alteration in the microbiota and consequent changes in bacterial exposure, could sensitize the liver to drug-induced injury, and be a reason for antibiotics being a leading cause of hepatotoxicity [3]. Furthermore, evidence that microbiota variations can modulate drug metabolism are also available [53, 54]. In fact, hepatic mRNA levels of more than 50 drug-processing genes have been found to vary between conventional and germ-free mice [55]. Drugs such as salicylazosulfapyridine, digoxin and acetaminophen have all been demonstrated to undergo some form of microbiota-mediated metabolic processes [56–58]. Hence, variations in gut microbiota composition could potentially affect a drugs hepatotoxicity potential and merits further investigations with respect to idiosyncratic DILI.

3 Drug Properties

The hepatotoxicity potential varies between drugs, with some compounds being more prone to induce DILI than others. Such differences occur even within the same therapeutic class. For example the fluoroquinolone trovafloxacin has been withdrawn from the market due to hepatotoxicity, while levofloxacin, similarly a fluoroquinolone, is associated with a minor risk of idiosyncratic DILI. Hence, while defining the pharmacological effect and potency, physicochemical drug properties also play an important role in initiating DILI development, which is either augmented or diminished by host factors (Table 1). Extensive studies have been undertaken to enhance the understanding of drug physicochemical properties with regard to balancing enhanced drug qualities and reduced likelihood of toxicity, an ongoing challenge in the pharmaceutical industry [59, 60].

3.1 Dose

Idiosyncratic DILI was initially believed to be a dose-independent reaction due to the occurrence after drug treatments at recommended daily doses. However, it is now assumed that dose in fact does play a role, as drugs given at a daily dose of 10 mg or less are rarely, if ever, associated with a high incidence of idiosyncratic DILI [61]. It has been suggested that in DILI due to nonoverdose treatments the dose–response curve is shifted to the left causing a hepatotoxic response at a therapeutic dose due to host-related circumstances [62]. Hence, some kind of threshold dose needs to be exceeded even for idiosyncratic DILI to occur, but this threshold may vary among individuals [1]. This is exemplified in DILI cases were a patient tolerate a drug at an initial lower concentration but develops DILI when a dose increase (still within the recommended daily dose range) is required for better pharmacological effect [63]. Furthermore, a study comparing 377 idiosyncratic DILI cases induced by drugs classified by dosage found that drugs with a daily dose of ≥50 mg were associated with a significantly shorter latency period than drugs with a lower daily dose [64].

3.2 Lipophilicity

Lipophilicity (often measured as the log of octanol–water partition coefficient, logP) is known to influence drug potency, pharmacokinetics and toxicity [65, 66]. The effect of lipophilicity on toxicity has been demonstrated using data from animal in vivo toleration studies of 245 preclinical compounds, in which more lipophilic compounds were associated with increased likelihood of toxic events potentially due to increased off-target binding [67]. High lipophilicity in conjunction with high daily dose has been associated with risk of idiosyncratic DILI development. In an analysis of 164 approved medications in the USA, Chen et al. observed that drugs with a recommended daily dose ≥100 mg and a logP value ≥3 had a higher risk of inducing hepatotoxicity. This relationship was defined as the "rule-of-two" [68]. It has been speculated that higher lipophilicity could facilitate drug uptake into hepatocytes and subsequent hepatic metabolism that may result in increased amount of reactive metabolites and thereby a potentially higher risk of DILI [4]. The potential use of the rule-of-two in supporting research and drug development as a predictive tool for hepatotoxicity has recently been demonstrated on direct-acting antiviral medications for chronic viral hepatitis C [69]. An independent study analyzing 975 oral drugs did, however, not confirm the rule-of-two, but found defined daily dose ≥100 mg and extensive liver metabolism (≥50%), but not lipophilicity, to be independent, but not synergistic, risk factors for increased hepatotoxicity potential [70]. An attempt to improve the rule-of-two was recently published in the form of a DILI score algorithm that takes into consideration daily dose, logP and formation of reactive metabolites of the drug in question. In contrast to the rule-of-two, the DILI score algorithm provides a numerical value that gives a better indication of potential DILI severity risk [71].

3.3 Reactive Metabolite Formation

Unbalanced concentrations of reactive drug metabolites can bind to cellular macromolecules and produce cellular stress, an event widely accepted to play a major role in DILI development. The type of reactive metabolites formed by individual drugs is mostly dependent on the drug's chemical structure. Certain structural motifs (referred to as structural alerts) known to be intrinsically electrophilic or have a propensity to form reactive metabolites are therefore avoided in drug design in order to reduce the risk of toxicity [60, 72–74]. However, not all drugs containing structural alerts produce reactive metabolites or have increased hepatotoxicity potential. For example, sudoxicam and meloxicam both contain the 2-aminothiazole structural alert, but reactive acylthiourea is only formed from sudoxicam, and may be responsible for the difference in hepatotoxicity potential between the two drugs [75]. The clinical development of sudoxicam was discontinued due to incidences of severe hepatotoxicity, while meloxicam is associated with low hepatotoxicity potential. It is important to note that while being a prominent risk factor, reactive metabolite formation is not a prerequisite for idiosyncratic DILI development. For example, pemoline (withdrawn from the market due to hepatotoxicity), ambrisentan and flecainide (both with black box warnings for hepatotoxicity) do not appear to produce reactive metabolites [74].

3.4 Mitochondrial Liability and Hepatic Transporter Inhibition

Many drugs known to induce idiosyncratic DILI are hazardous to mitochondria in vitro [76, 77]. Although, drug concentrations in experimental studies often exceed those attained in patients, the ability to cause mitochondrial liability is considered a potential DILI risk. Perturbation of mitochondrial functions can occur through various mechanisms altering different pathways and mitochondrial components. For example, drugs can directly affect energy homeostasis by impairing mitochondrial fatty acid oxidation (amiodarone, valproic acid, glucocorticoids), interfere with electron transfer in the mitochondrial respiratory chain (paroxetine, simvastatin, tamoxifen, efavirenz), the oxidative phosphorylation process (tamoxifen) or interfere with mitochondrial DNA (mtDNA) (tacrine, tamoxifen, ciprofloxacin) [78]. It can be difficult to pinpoint the primary effect of a drug on the mitochondria as the effect of one mechanism often lead to secondary effects. Electron transfer impairment in the respiratory chain will indirectly have a negative effect on fatty acid oxidation as well as lead to increased ROS production that may cause mtDNA damage. Similarly, drugs directly interfering with mtDNA replication or gene expression can impair the electron transfer process by inhibiting or reducing the production of protein complexes constituting the respiratory chain, of which a large proportion are encoded by mtDNA. Accumulated mitochondrial damage can induce signaling transduction pathways and potentially cell death [1].

Cellular stress can also be a consequence of drugs interfering with hepatic transporters. The bile salt export pump (BSEP) is located in the hepatocyte canalicular membrane and is responsible for transporting bile salts into the bile. Information on BESP-mediated transport of pravastatin has also emerged, challenging, the belief of BSEP being a bile salt-specific transporter [79]. BSEP inhibition can lead to impaired bile flow and cholestasis, as seen in patients with *ABCB11* mutations and familial intrahepatic cholestasis [80]. Drugs are known to inhibit BSEP activity and hepatocyte accumulation of toxic bile salts producing cellular stress could subsequently be a contributing factor to hepatotoxicity. In fact, drug-induced BSEP inhibition has been linked to hepatotoxicity with studies demonstrating correlations between a drug's ability to inhibit BSEP in vitro and its known hepatotoxicity potential [81, 82]. Furthermore, BSEP inhibition has been reported to be associated with physicochemical drug properties, such that drugs with higher molecular weight and higher calculated logP value are positively correlated with BSEP inhibition potency [82, 83]. Nevertheless, bile acid homeostasis is an intricately regulated process and a temporary reduction in BSEP activity could potentially be compensated for by increased activity of other transporters to limit intracellular bile salts accumulation. Multidrug resistance-associated protein 3 (MRP3) and 4 (MRP4), for example, play important compensatory roles during cholestasis [84].

Considering BSEP inhibition in conjunction with MRP transporter activities has therefore been suggested to provide a better estimation of idiosyncratic DILI risk [85].

4   Host Factor-Drug Property Interactions as DILI Modulators

Individual DILI susceptibility is affected by risk factors derived from both the host and the drug. Hence, individual risk factors are generally poor predictors of hepatotoxicity as their effect is dependent on the presence or absence of additional DILI modulators. The presence of the "correct" combination of risk factors is what will determine if a patient will or will not develop DILI and may explain clinical observations. DILI risk factors should therefore be considered collectively based on their interactions in order to be most informative [4]. Here we will discuss interactions between host factors and drug properties in different processes potentially involved in DILI development (Table 2).

4.1   Cellular Injury/
Stress Initiation and
Toxicological
Responses

Drugs that undergo extensive hepatic metabolism are more prone to form reactive metabolites, which can bind covalently to proteins resulting in functional changes and cellular stress. The cell is, however, equipped with defense mechanisms to combat such threats, and any direct link between drugs forming reactive metabolites, as a natural consequence of drug metabolism, and idiosyncratic hepatotoxicity development is circumstantial at best. For cell damage to occur the cell's defense mechanism must be overcome. Genetic variations leading to increased reactive metabolite formation or reduced detoxification processes could push the scale in favor of cellular injury. Diclofenac is bioactivated via glucuronidation by UGT2B7 and via oxidative metabolism by cytochrome P450 (including CYP2C8) that result in diclofenac acyl glucuronide and benzoquinone imines that can cause covalent modification of cellular proteins. Carriers of specific UGT2B7 and CYP2C8 genotypes, which could increase the production of reactive metabolites, have been found to be more susceptible to DILI induced by diclofenac [86]. Furthermore, interindividual differences in glutathione S-transferase activities have been demonstrated in vitro to affect inactivation of reactive para-benzoquinone imine metabolites of diclofenac, and could likewise modulate susceptibility risk [87]. Concomitant medications could similarly increase cellular stress formation by modulating the metabolism of the causative agent or compete with the causative agent for a specific enzyme and consequently alter the drug proportion metabolized by otherwise minor pathways. Polypharmacy with valproic acid in conjunction with CYP 450-enzyme inducing anticonvulsant drugs, such as carbamazepine or phenytoin, increases

Table 2
Overview of selected idiosyncratic drug-induced liver injury causative agents, their drug properties and potentially associated host factors

Drug	Drug properties	Host risk factors
Amoxicillin-clavulanate	Amoxicillin: LogP: 0.87 HM: <30%, RM → haptenization RDD >100 mg Clavulanic acid: LogP: −1.5 HM: yes RM: unknown RDD >100 mg	HLA risk alleles: A*02:01, A*30:02 (Hep[§]), B*18:01 (Hep[§]) and DRB1*15:01-DQB1*06:02 (Chol/Mix[§])
Isoniazid	LogP: −0.70 HM: yes , RM: yes Mitochondrial liability RDD: >100 mg	Older age Alcohol consumption Malnutrition *NAT2* slow acetylators Viral hepatitis C infection
Diclofenac	LogP: 4.51 HM: yes, RM: yes Chemical structure with structural alert RDD: >100 mg Can cause lower gastrointestinal complications and increase permeability	Genetic variations in *UGT2B7* and *CYP2C8* Underlying chronic inflammatory conditions Concomitant medications, such as gastroduodenal protective treatments can cause microbiota changes
Valproic acid	LogP: 2.75 HM: yes, RM: yes Metabolism involving beta oxidation Mitochondrial hazardous RDD: >100 mg	Age: young children are at higher risk of severe DILI Genetic variations in *polγ*
Nitrofurantoin	LogP: −0.47 HM: partially metabolized to aminofurantoin RM: unknown RDD: >100 mg	Female sex
Minocycline	LogP: 0.05 HM: yes, RM: yes RDD: ≥100 mg	HLA risk allele: B*35:02 Female sex
Atorvastatin	LogP: 5.7 HM: yes, RM: yes RDD: <100 mg	Older age; concomitant medications
Phenytoin	LogP: 2.47 HM: yes, RM; unknown RDD: >100 mg	Genetic variations leading to epoxide hydrolase deficiency

[§]HLA-A*30:02 and B*18:01 have been found to be risk factors for hepatocellular (Hep) type of DILI, while DRB1*15:01-DQB1*06:02 appears to be risk factors for cholestatic (Chol)/mixed (Mix) type of DILI, *see* ref. 36. Abbreviations: *HM* hepatic metabolism, *RM* reactive metabolite formation, *RDD* recommended daily dose, *HLA* human leukocyte antigen, *NAT2* N-acetyltransferase 2, *UGT2B7* UDP-glucuronosyltransferase 2B7, *CYP2C8* Cytochrome P450 2CB, *polγ*, polymerase gamma

the metabolism of valproic acid to 4-ene valproic acid and (E)-2,4-diene valproic acid [88]. Although not confirmed, many findings speak in favor of these metabolites or derivatives thereof as implicated in valproic acid hepatotoxicity [10].

As the burden of reactive metabolites is related to the amount the cell is exposed to, a higher drug dose is more likely to lead to hepatotoxicity. It is tempting to hypothesize that although idiosyncratic DILI occur during intake of recommended daily doses, in polymedicated patients the various medications might have an accumulative effect with regard to reactive metabolite formation and detoxification leading to cellular stress, in particular in patients with a compromised cellular defense mechanism. Hence, the causative agent might be "the straw that breaks the camel's back."

Drug–host interactions involving genetic variations and drug properties have also been noted. For example, it has been suggested that chemical drug structure and BSEP inhibition potency could influence the effect of the *ABCB11* c.1331T>C risk allele [89]. Furthermore, the risk of developing cholestatic/mixed type of DILI was found to be greater in *SOD2* CC (c.47T>C) carriers taking drugs known to produce highly reactive metabolites, such as quinone imines or epoxides [90].

4.2 Immune Responses and Tissue Repair

It is unlikely that cellular stress induced by the parent drug or metabolites thereof, will be sufficient to induce idiosyncratic DILI. Hence, additional processes are likely to be involved, such as immune responses. This hypothesis is further strengthened by the identification of HLA risk alleles (*see* Sect. 2.3). The liver has a strong natural predisposition toward immune tolerance as it is constantly exposed to foreign antigens. The occurrence of an adaptive immune response therefore needs an interruption of the liver's general immune tolerance. This has been highlighted in recent animal studies targeting immunological checkpoints [91, 92]. Infectious diseases or concomitant illnesses in the host could favor an immune response. Pathogen-associated molecular pattern (PAMP) molecules, such as lipopolysaccharides (LPS) can prompt inflammatory stress and alter immune tolerance. Coexposure to LPS and medications such as trovafloxacin, diclofenac, and chlorpromazine, but not the medications alone, has been found to induce idiosyncrasy-like liver injury in murine models [93–95]. Changes in the host microbiota can similarly lead to hepatic LPS exposure due to increased gut permeability. Certain nonsteroidal antiinflammatry drugs (NSAIDs), such as diclofenac, can cause lower gastrointestinal complications, with inflammation and/or increased permeability recorded in up to 70% of long-term NSAID users [96]. Furthermore, protein pump inhibitors are commonly taken in conjunction with NSAIDs as protection toward upper gastrointestinal tract adverse events. While being effective in preventing gastroduodenal damage, protein pump inhibitors can alter the microbiota composition, which could potentially lead to increased permeability [97].

It has been suggested that severe idiosyncratic DILI could be the result of *defective clinical adaptation* or failure to dampen the initiating mechanisms or injury due to diminished adaptive responses [3, 98]. Tissue repair is an important determinant in DILI outcome. Tissue repair as a response to drug-induced cell damage increases with drug dose until a threshold dose is reached, beyond which cellular signaling inhibition impairs the tissue repair process favoring accelerated tissue injury [99]. In addition to drug dose, animal models have demonstrated that age, nutritional status and comorbidities can affect the tissue repair process. Young age and caloric restrictions appear to affect tissue repair favorably, while the presence of diabetes mellitus has an adverse effect [100–102]. Furthermore, concomitant medications may influence idiosyncratic DILI development based on their effect on tissue repair. For example, several cardiovascular system drug classes such as statins, angiotensin converting enzyme inhibitors, adrenergic blockers and fibrates can reduce liver injury and/or enhance liver repair, [103–106]. This assumption was supported by findings in a retrospective database study in which reported acetaminophen-associated liver injury cases with concomitant use of statins and fibrates were less likely to have a fatal outcome [24]. The presence of dyslipidemia and subsequent stain use has similarly been found to have a protective effect against progression to acute liver failure in an analysis of 771 Spanish DILI patients [17].

5 Conclusion and Future Direction

Idiosyncratic DILI is considered as a multifactorial condition determined by both drug properties and host factors. Hence, individual risk factors have limited capacity to predict DILI susceptibility and clinical phenotypes as patient outcome is determined by the interaction between individual risk modulators. In fact, none of the presented risk factors are likely to have detrimental effects on their own, but when combined could culminate in liver injury. Despite advances in the area, it is not yet possible to predict patient susceptibility, and further studies are needed to elucidate the intricate pathological mechanism behind idiosyncratic DILI. Computational systems biology offers a new direction for hepatotoxicity studies that could shed light on mechanistic aspects of this condition. Here in silico modeling based on physiological understanding and in vitro experiments can be used to predict drug-induced effects on biological processes. This approach also presents the ability to examine the interaction of multiple drug properties and host factors in integrative system analyses [107, 108]. Promising results from hepatotoxicity-directed computational systems biology are emerging. For example, DILIsym, a quantitative systems pharmacology platform for drug-induced liver injury, has unraveled mechanistic aspects of DILI induced by troglitazone and tolvaptan [109, 110]. It has been suggested that incorporating information on the growing understanding of adaptive immune responses into established system biology platforms hold promising potential for future hepatotoxicity studies [108]. On the experimental side, the use of induced pluripotent stem cell-derived hepatocytes (iPSC-HCs) is a promising alternative to animal models and established cell lines to study hepatotoxicity both in search for a better mechanistic understanding as well as for early toxicity evaluations during drug development. The ability to generate PSC-HCs from diverse patient populations enables wider exploration of genetically different backgrounds [111]. In conclusion, a shift in paradigm toward an integrative approach considering drug–host interactions could enhance the mechanistic comprehension of idiosyncratic DILI and identification of determinant risk factors, paving the way for personalized therapy and safer treatment strategies.

References

1. Han D, Dara L, Win S, Than TA, Yuan L, Abbasi SQ, Liu ZX, Kaplowitz N (2013) Regulation of drug-induced liver injury by signal transduction pathways: critical role of mitochondria. Trends Pharmacol Sci 34:243–253

2. Stephens C, Andrade RJ, Lucena MI (2014) Mechanisms of drug-induced liver injury. Curr Opin Allergy Clin Immunol 14:286–292

3. Dara L, Liu ZX, Kaplowitz N (2016) Mechanisms of adaptation and progression in idiosyncratic drug induced liver injury, clinical implications. Liver Int 36:158–165

4. Chen M, Suzuki A, Borlak J, Andrade RJ, Lucena MI (2015) Drug-induced liver injury: interactions between drug properties and host factors. J Hepatol 63:503–514

5. Lucena MI, Andrade RJ, Kaplowitz N, García-Cortes M, Fernández MC, Romero-Gomez M, Bruguera M, Hallal H, Robles-Diaz M, Rodriguez-González JF, Navarro JM, Salmeron J, Martinez-Odriozola P, Perez-Alvarez R, Borraz Y, Hidalgo R, Spanish Group for the Study of Drug-Induced Liver Disease (2009) Phenotypic characterization of idiosyncratic drug-induced liver injury: the influence of age and sex. Hepatology 49:2001–2009

6. Chalasani N, Bonkovsky HL, Fontana R, Lee W, Stolz A, Talwalkar J, Reddy KR, Watkins PB, Navarro V, Barnhart H, Gu J, Serrano J, United States Drug Induced Liver Injury Network (2015) Features and outcome of 899 patients with drug-induced liver injury: the DILIN prospective study. Gastroenterology 148:1340–1352

7. Fontana RJ, Hayashi PH, Barnhart H, Kleiner DE, Reddy KR, Chalasani N, Lee WM, Stolz A, Phillips T, Serrano J, Watkins PB, DILIN Investigators (2015) Persistent liver biochemistry abnormalities are more common in older patients and those with cholestatic drug induced liver injury Am J Gastroenterol 110:1450–1459

8. Medina-Caliz I, Robles-Díaz M, Garcia-Muñoz B, Stephens C, Ortega-Alonso A, Garcia-Cortes M, González-Jimenez A, Sanabria-Cabrera JA, Moreno I, Fernandez MC, Romero-Gomes M, Navarro JM, Barriocanal AM, Montane E, Hallal H, Blanco S, Soriano G, Roman EM, Gómez-Dominguez E, Castiella A, Zapata EM, Jimenez-Perez M, Moreno JM, Aldea-Perona A, Hernández-Guerra M et al (2016) Definition and risk factors for chronicity following acute idiosyncratic drug-induced liver injury. J Hepatol 65:532–542

9. Bryant AE 3rd, Dreifuss FE (1996) Valproic acid hepatic fatalities. III. U.S. experience since 1986. Neurology 46:465–469

10. Felker D, Lynn A, Wang S, Johnson DE (2014) Evidence for a potential protective effect of carnitine-pantothenic acid co-treatment on valproic acid-induced hepatotoxicity. Expert Rev Clin Pharmacol 7:211–218

11. Fountain FF, Tolley E, Chrisman CR, Self TH (2005) Isoniazid hepatotoxicity associated with treatment of latent tuberculosis infection: a 7-year evaluation from a public health tuberculosis clinic. Chest 128:116–123

12. Boelsterli UA, Lee KK (2014) Mechanisms of isoniazid-induced idiosyncratic liver injury: emerging role of mitochondrial stress. J Gastroenterol Hepatol 29:678–687

13. Hunt CM, Yuen NA, Stirnadel-Farrant HA, Suzuki A (2014) Age-related differences in reporting of drug-associated liver injury: data-mining of WHO safety report database. Regul Toxicol Pharmacol 70:519–526

14. Guy J, Peters MG (2013) Liver disease in women: the influence of gender on epidemiology, natural history, and patient outcomes. Gastroenterol Hepatol (N Y) 9:633–639

15. Björnsson ES, Bergmann OM, Björnsson HK, Kvaran RB, Olafsson S (2013) Incidence, presentation, and outcomes in patients with drug-induced liver injury in the general population of Iceland. Gastroenterology 144:1419–1425

16. deLemos AS, Foureau DM, Jacobs C, Ahrens W, Russo MW, Bonkovsky HL (2014) Drug-induced liver injury with autoimmune features. Semin Liver Dis 34:194–204

17. Robles-Díaz M, Lucena MI, Kaplowitz N, Stephens C, Medina-Cáliz I, González-Jimenez A, Ulzurrun E, Gonzalez AF, Fernandez MC, Romero-Gómez M, Jimenez-Perez M, Bruguera M, Prieto M, Bessone F, Hernandez N, Arrese M, Andrade RJ, Spanish DILI Registry, SLatinDILI Network, Safer and Faster Evidence-based Translation Consortium (2014) Use of Hy's law and a new composite algorithm to predict acute liver failure in patients with drug-induced liver injury. Gastroenterology 147:109–118

18. Reuben A, Koch DG, Lee WM, Acute Liver Failure Study Group (2010) Drug-induced acute liver failure: results of a U.S. multicenter, prospective study. Hepatology 52:2065–2076

19. Aceti A, Pasquazzi C, Zechini B, De Bac C, LIVERHAART Group (2002) Hepatotoxicity development during antiretroviral therapy containing protease inhibitors in patients with HIV: the role of hepatitis B and C virus infection. J Acquir Immune Defic Syndr 29:41–48

20. Sulkowski MS, Thomas DL, Mehta SH, Chaisson RE, Moore RD (2002) Hepatotoxicity associated with nevirapine or efavirenz-containing antiretroviral therapy: role of hepatitis C and B infections. Hepatology 35:182–189

21. Lomtadze N, Kupreishvili L, Salakaia A, Vashakidze S, Sharvadze L, Kempker RR, Magee MJ, del Rio C, Blumberg HM (2013) Hepatitis C virus co-infection increases the risk of anti-tuberculosis drug-induced hepatotoxicity among patients with pulmonary tuberculosis. PLoS One 8:e83892. https://doi.org/10.1371/journal.pone.0083892

22. Chalasani N, Fontana RJ, Bonkovsky HL, Watkins PB, Davern T, Serrano J, Yang H, Rochon J, Drug Induced Liver Injury Network (DILIN) (2008) Causes, clinical features, and outcomes from a prospective study of drug-induced liver injury in the United States. Gastroenterology 135:1924–1934

23. Suzuki A, Yuen NA, Ilic K, Miller RT, Reese MJ, Brown HR, Ambroso JI, Falls JG, Hunt CM (2015) Comedications alter drug-induced liver injury reporting frequency: data mining in the WHO VigiBase. Regul Toxicol Pharmacol 72:481–490

24. Suzuki A, Yuen N, Walsh J, Papay J, Hunt CM, Diehl AM (2009) Co-medications that modulate liver injury and repair influence clinical outcome of acetaminophen-associated liver injury. Clin Gastroenterol Hepatol 7:882–888

25. Ingelman-Sundberg M, Sim SC, Gomez A, Rodriguez-Antona C (2007) Influence of cytochrome P450 polymorphisms on drug therapies: pharmacogenetic, pharmacoepigenetic and clinical aspects. Pharmacol Ther 116:496–526

26. Andrade RJ, Robles M, Ulzurrun E, Lucena MI (2009) Drug-induced liver injury: insight from genetic studies. Pharmacogenomics 10:1467–1487

27. Ng CS, Hasnat A, Al Maruf A, Ahmed MU, Pirmohamed M, Day CP, Aithal GP, Daly AK (2014) N-acetyltransferase 2 (NAT2) genotype as a risk factor for development of drug-induced liver injury relating to antituberculosis drug treatment in a mixed-ethnicity patient group. Eur J Clin Pharmacol 70:1079–1086

28. Du H, Chen X, Fang Y, Yan O, Xu H, Li L, Li W, Huang W (2013) Slow N-acetyltransferase 2 genotype contributes to anti-tuberculosis drug-induced hepatotoxicity: a meta-analysis. Mol Biol Rep 40:3591–3596

29. Lucena MI, Andrade RJ, Martínez C, Ulzurrun E, García-Martín E, Borraz Y, Fernández MC, Romero-Gomes M, Castiella A, Planas R, Costa J, Anzola S, Agúndez JA, Spanish Group for the Study of Drug-Induced Liver Disease (2008) Glutathione S-transferase m1 and t1 null genotypes increase susceptibility to idiosyncratic drug-induced liver injury. Hepatology 48:588–596

30. McClellan J, King MC (2010) Genetic heterogeneity in human disease. Cell 141:210–217

31. Grove JI, Aithal GP (2015) Human leukocyte antigen genetic risk factors of drug-induced liver toxicology. Expert Opin Drug Metab Toxicol 11:395–409

32. Petros Z, Makonnen E, Aklillu E (2017) Genome-wide association studies for idiosyncratic drug-induced hepatotoxicity: looking back–looking forward to next-generation innovation. OMICS 21:123–131

33. Urban TJ, Nicoletti P, Chalasani N, Serrano J, Stolz A, Daly AK, Aithal GP, Dillon JF, Barnhart HX, Watkins PB, Fontana RJ (2015) Minocycline hepatotoxicity: clinical characterization and identification of HLA-B*35:02 as a risk factor. Hepatology 62(S1):1149A

34. Nicoletti P, Aithal GP, Björnsson ES, Adrade RJ, Sawle A, Arrese M, Barnhart HX, Bondon-Guitton E, Hayashi PH, Bessone F, Carvajal A, Cascorbi I, Chalasani N, Conforti A, Coulthard SA, Daly MJ, Day CP, Dillon JF, Fontana RJ, Grove JI, Hallberg P, Hernández N, Ibáñez L, Kullak-Ublick GA, Laitinene T et al (2017) Association of liver injury from specific drugs, or groups of drugs, with polymorphisms in HLA and other genes in a genome-wide association study. Gastroenterology 152:1078–1089

35. Aithal GP (2015) Pharmacogenetic testing in idiosyncratic drug-induced liver injury: current role in clinical practice. Liver Int 35:1801–1808

36. Stephens C, López-Nevot MÁ, Ruiz-Cabello R, Ulzurrun E, Soriano G, Romero-Gómez M, Moreno-Casares A, Lucena MI, Andrade RJ (2013) HLA alleles influence the clinical signature of amoxicillin-clavulanate hepatotoxicity. PLoS One 8:e6811. https://doi.org/10.1371/journal.ponc.0068111

37. Lucena MI, Molokhia M, Shen Y, Urban TJ, Aithal GP, Andrade RJ, Day CP, Ruiz-Cabello F, Donaldson PT, Stephens C, Pirmohamed M, Romero-Gomez M, Navarro JM, Fontana RJ, Miller M, Groome M, Bondon-Guitton E, Conforti A, Stricker BH, Carvajal A, Ibanez L, Yue QY, Eichelbaum M, Floratos A, Pe'er I et al (2011) Susceptibility to amoxicillin-clavulanate-induced liver injury is influenced by multiple HLA class I and II alleles. Gastroenterology 141:338–347

38. Danan G, Benichou C (1993) Causality assessment of adverse reactions to drugs-1. A novel method based on the conclusions of international consensus meetings: application to drug-induced liver injuries. J Clin Epidemiol 46:1323–1330

39. Zimmerman HJ (1986) Effects of alcohol on other hepatotoxins. Alcohol Clin Exp Res 10:3–15

40. Benowitz NL, Peng M, Jacob P 3rd (2003) Effects of cigarette smoking and carbon monoxide on chlorzoxazone and caffeine metabolism. Clin Pharmacol Ther 74:468–474

41. Schmidt LE, Dalhoff K (2003) The impact of current tobacco use in the outcome of paracetamol poisoning. Aliment Pharmacol Ther 18:979–985

42. Abdelmegeed MA, Banerjee A, Yoo SH, Jang S, Gonzalez FJ, Song BJ (2012) Critical role of cytochrome P450 2E1 (CYP2E1) in the development of high fat-induced non-alcoholic steatohepatitis. J Hepatol 57:860–866

43. Nieto N, Marí M, Cederbaum AI (2003) Cytochrome P450 2E1 responsiveness in the promoter of glutamate-cysteine ligase catalytic subunit. Hepatology 37:96–106

44. Arrigo T, Leonardi S, Cuppari C, Manti S, Lanzafame A, D'Angelo G, Gitto E, Marseglia L, Salpietro C (2015) Role of th diet as a link between oxidative stress and liver diseases. World J Gastroenterol 21:384–395

45. Nguyen GC, Sam J, Thuluvath PJ (2008) Hepatitis C is a predictor of acute liver injury among hospitalizations for acetaminophen overdose in the United States: a nationwide analysis. Hepatology 48:1336–1341

46. Fernánez-Villar A, Sopeña B, Fernánez-Villar J, Vázquez-Gallardo R, Ulloa F, Leiro V, Mosteiro M, Piñeiro L (2004) The influence of risk factors on the severity of anti-tuberculosis drug-induced hepatotoxicity. Int J Tuberc Lung Dis 8:1499–1505

47. Warmelink I, ten Hacken NH, van der Werf TS, van Altena R (2011) Weight loss during tuberculosis treatment is an important risk factor for drug-induced hepatotoxicity. Br J Nutr 105:400–408

48. Bibbò S, Ianiro G, Giorgio V, Scaldaferri F, Masucci L, Gasbarrini A, Cammarota G (2016) The role of diet on gut microbiota composition. Eur Rev Med Pharmacol Sci 20:4742–4749

49. David LA, Maurice CF, Carmody RN, Gootenberg DB, Button JE, Wolfe BE, Ling AV, Devlin AS, Varma Y, Fischbach MA, Biddinger SB, Dutton RJ, Turnbaugh PJ (2014) Diet rapidly and reproducibly alters the human gut microbiome. Nature 505:559–563

50. Schnabl B, Brenner DA (2014) Interactions between the intestinal microbiome and liver diseases. Gastroenterology 146:1513–1524

51. Ma HD, Wang YH, Chang C, Gershwin ME, Lian ZX (2015) The intestinal microbiota and microenvironment in liver. Autoimmun Rev 14:183–191

52. Fontana RJ (2014) Pathogenesis of idiosyncratic drug-induced liver injury and clinical perspectives. Gastroenterology 46:914–928

53. Swanson HI (2015) Drug metabolism by the host and gut microbiota: a partnership or rivalry? Drug Metab Dispos 43:1499–1504

54. Klaassen CD, Cui JY (2015) Review: mechanism of how intestinal microbiota alters the effects of drugs and bile acids. Drug Metab Dispos 43:1505–1521

55. Selwyn FP, Cui JY, Klaassen CD (2015) RNA-seq quantification of hepatic drug processing genes in germ-free mice. Drug Metab Dispos 43:1572–1580

56. Peppercorn MA, Goldman P (1972) The role of intestinal bacteria in the metabolism of salicylazosulfapyridine. J Pharmacol Exp Ther 181:555–562

57. Haiser HJ, Gootenberg DB, Chatman K, Sirasani G, Balskus EP, Turnbaugh PJ (2013) Predicting and manipulating cardiac drug inactivation by the human gut bacterium *Eggerthella lenta*. Science 341:295–298

58. Clayton TA, Baker D, Lindon JC, Everett JR, Nicholson JK (2009) Pharmacometabonomic identification of a significant host-microbiome metabolic interaction affecting human drug metabolism. Proc Natl Acad Sci U S A 106:14728–14733

59. Meanwell NA (2011) Improving drug candidates by design: a focus on physicochemical properties as a means of improving compound disposition and safety. Chem Res Toxicol 24:1420–1456

60. Kalgutkar AS, Dalvie D (2015) Predicting toxicities of reactive metabolite-positive drug candidates. Annu Rev Pharmacol Toxicol 55:35–54

61. Uetrecht JP (1999) New concepts in immunology relevant to idiosyncratic drug reactions: the "danger hypothesis" and innate immune system. Chem Res Toxicol 12:387–395

62. Roth RA, Ganey PE (2010) Intrinsic versus idiosyncratic drug-induced hepatotoxicity–two villains or one? J Pharmacol Exp Ther 332:692–697

63. Carrascosa MF, Salcines-Caviedes JR, Lucena MI, Andrade RJ (2015) Acute liver failure following atorvastatin dose escalation: is there a threshold dose for idiosyncratic hepatotoxicity? J Hepatol 62:751–752

64. Vuppalanchi R, Gotur R, Reddy KR, Fontana RJ, Ghabril M, Kosinski AS, Gu J, Serrano J, Chalasani N (2014) Relationship between characteristics of medications and drug-induced liver disease phenotype and outcome. Clin Gastroenterol Hepatol 12:1550–1555

65. van de Waterbeemd H, Smith DA, Beaumont K, Walker DK (2001) Property-based design: optimization of drug absorption and pharmacokinetics. J Med Chem 44:1313–1333

66. Leeson PD, Springthorpe B (2007) The influence of drug-like concepts on decision-making in medicinal chemistry. Nat Rev Drug Discov 6:881–890

67. Hughes JD, Blagg J, Price DA, Bailey S, Decrescenzo GA, Devraj RV, Ellsworth E, Fobian YM, Gibbs ME, Gilles RW, Greene N, Huang E, Krieger-Burke T, Loesel J, Wager T, Whiteley L, Zhang Y (2008) Physiochemical drug properties associated with in vivo toxicological outcomes. Bioorg Med Chem Lett 18:4872–4875

68. Chen M, Borlak J, Tong W (2013) High lipophilicity and high daily dose of oral medications are associated with significant risk for drug-induced liver injury. Hepatology 58:388–396

69. Mishra P, Chen M (2017) Direct-acting antivirals for chronic hepatitis C: can drug properties signal potential for liver injury? Gastroenterology 152:1270–1274

70. Weng Z, Wang K, Li H, Shi Q (2015) A comprehensive study of the association between drug hepatotoxicity and daily dose, liver metabolism, and lipophilicity using 975 oral medications. Oncotarget 10:17031–17038

71. Chen M, Borlak J, Tong W (2016) A model to predict severity of drug-induced liver injury in humans. Hepatology 64:931–940

72. Dalvie D, Kalgutkar AS, Chen W (2015) Practical approaches to resolving reactive metabolite liabilities in early discovery. Drug Metab Rev 47:56–70

73. Thompson RA, Isin EM, Ogese MO, Mettetal JT, Williams DP (2016) Reactive metabolites: current and emerging risk and hazard assessments. Chem Res Toxicol 29:505–533

74. Stepan AF, Walker DP, Bauman J, Price DA, Baillie TA, Kalgutkar AS, Aleo MD (2011) Structural alert/reactive metabolite concept as applied in medicinal chemistry to mitigate the risk of idiosyncratic drug toxicity: a perspective based on the critical examination of trends in the top 200 drugs marketed in the United States. Chem Res Toxicol 24:1345–1410

75. Orbach RS, Kalgutkar AS, Ryder TF, Walker GS (2008) In vitro metabolism and covalent binding of enol-carboxamide derivatives and anti-inflammatory agents sudoxicam and meloxicam: insights into the hepatotoxicity of sudoxicam. Chem Res Toxicol 21:1890–1899

76. Boelsterli UA, Lim PL (2007) Mitochondrial abnormalities–a link to idiosyncratic drug hepatotoxicity? Toxicol Appl Pharmacol 220:92–107

77. Porceddu M, Buron N, Roussel C, Labbe G, Fromenty B, Borgne-Sanchez A (2012) Prediction of liver injury induced by chemicals in human with a multiparametric assay on isolated mouse liver mitochondria. Toxicol Sci 129:332–345

78. Pessayre D, Fromenty B, Berson A, Robin MA, Lettéron P, Moreau R, Mansouri A (2012) Central role of mitochondria in drug-

induced liver injury. Drug Metab Rev 44:34–87

79. Hirano M, Maeda K, Hayashi H, Kusuhara H, Sugiyama Y (2005) Bile salt export pump (BSEP/ABCB11) can transport a nonbile acid substrate, pravastatin. J Pharmacol Exp Ther 314:876–882

80. Noe J, Kullak-Ublick GA, Jochum W, Stieger B, Kerb R, Haberl M, Müllhaupt B, Meier PJ, Pauli-Magnus C (2005) Impaired expression and function of the bile salt export pump due to three novel ABCB11 mutations in intrahepatic cholestasis. J Hepatol 43:536–543

81. Morgan RE, Trauner M, van Staden CJ, Lee PH, Ramachandran B, Eschenberg M, Afshari CA, Qualls CW Jr, Lightfoot-Dunn R, Hamadeh HK (2010) Interference with bile salt export pump function is a susceptibility factor for human liver injury in drug development. Toxicol Sci 118:485–500

82. Pedersen JM, Matsson P, Bergström CA, Hoogstraate J, Norén A, LeCluyse EL, Artursson P (2013) Early identification of clinically relevant drug interactions with the human bile salt export pump (BSEP/ABCB11). Toxicol Sci 136:328–343

83. Warner DJ, Chen H, Cantin LD, Kenna JG, Stahl S, Walker CL, Noeske T (2012) Mitigating the inhibition of human bile salt export pump by drugs: opportunities provided by physicochemical property modulation, in silico modelling, and structural modifications. Drug Metab Dispos 40:2332–2341

84. Geier A, Wagner M, Dietrich CG, Trauner M (2007) Principles of hepatic anion transporter regulation during cholestasis, inflammation and liver regeneration. Biochim Biophys Acta 1773:283–308

85. Morgan RE, van Staden CJ, Chen Y, Kalyanaraman N, Kalanzi J, Dunn RT 2nd, Afshari CA, Hamadeh HK (2013) A multifactorial approach to hepatobiliary transporter assessment enables improved therapeutic compound development. Toxicol Sci 136:216–241

86. Daly AK, Aithal GP, Leathart JB, Swainsbury RA, Dang TS, Day CP (2007) Genetic susceptibility to diclofenac-induced hepatotoxicity: contribution of UGT2B7, CYP2C8, and ABCC2 genotypes. Gastroenterology 132:272–281

87. den Braver MW, Zhang Y, Venkataraman H, Vermeulen NP, Commadeur JN (2016) Simulation of interindividual differences in inactivation of reactive para-benzoquinone imine metabolites of diclofenac by glutathione S-transferases in human liver cytosol. Toxicol Lett 255:52–62

88. Gopaul S, Farrell K, Abbott F (2003) Effects of age and polytherapy, risk factors of valproic acid (VPA) hepatotoxicity, on the excretion of thiol conjugates of (E)-2,4-diene VPA in people with epilepsy taking VPA. Epilepsia 44:322–328

89. Ulzurrun E, Stephens C, Crespo E, Ruiz-Cabello F, Ruiz-Nuñez J, Saenz-López P, Moreno-Herrera I, Robles-Díaz M, Hallal H, Moreno-Planas JM, Cabello MR, Lucena MI, Andrade RJ (2013) Role of chemical structures and the 1331T>C bile salt export pump polymorphism in idiosyncratic drug-induced liver injury. Liver Int 33:1378–1385

90. Lucena MI, García-Martín E, Andrade RJ, Martínez C, Stephens C, Ruiz JD, Ulzurrun E, Fernandez MC, Romero-Gomez M, Castiella A, Planas R, Durán JA, de Dios AM, Guarner C, Soriano G, Borraz Y, Agundez JA (2010) Mitochondrial superoxide dismutase and glutathione peroxidase in idiosyncratic drug-induced liver injury. Hepatology 52:303–312

91. Metushi IG, Hayes MA, Uetrecht J (2014) Treatment of PD-1(−/−) mice with amodiaquine and anti-CTLA4 leads to liver injury similar to idiosyncratic liver injury in patients. Hepatology 61:1332–1342

92. Chakraborty M, Fullerton AM, Semple K, Chea LS, Proctor WR, Bourdi M, Kleiner DE, Zeng X, Ryan PM, Dagur PK, Berkson JD, Reilly TP, Pohl LR (2015) Drug-induced allergic hepatitis develops in mice when myeloid-derived suppressor cells are depleted prior to halothane treatment. Hepatology 62:546–557

93. Shaw PJ, Hopfensperger MJ, Ganey PE, Roth RA (2007) Lipopolysaccharide and trovafloxacin coexposure in mice causes idiosyncrasy-like liver injury dependent on tumor necrosis factor-alpha. Toxicol Sci 100:259–266

94. Deng X, Stachlewitz RF, Liguori MJ, Blomme EA, Waring JF, Luyendyk JP, Maddox JF, Ganey PE, Roth RA (2006) Modest inflammation enhances diclofenac hepatotoxicity in rats: role of neutrophils and bacterial translocation. J Pharmacol Exp Ther 319:1191–1199

95. Buchweitz JP, Ganey PE, Bursian SJ, Roth RA (2002) Underlying endotoxemia augments responses to chlorpromazine: is there a relationship to drug idiosyncrasy? J Pharmacol Exp Ther 300:460–467

96. Lanas A, Sopeña F (2009) Nonsteroidal anti-inflammatory drugs and lower gastrointestinal complications. Gastroenterol Clin North Am 38:333–352

97. Jackson MA, Goodrich JK, Maxan ME, Freedberg DE, Abrams JA, Poole AC, Sutter JL, Welter D, Ley RE, Bell JT, Spector TD,

Steves CJ (2016) Proton pump inhibitors alter the composition of the gut microbiota. Gut 65:749–756

98. Watkins PB (2005) Idiosyncratic liver injury: challenges and approaches. Toxicol Pathol 33:1–5

99. Mehendale HM (2005) Tissue repair: an important determinant of final outcome of toxicant-induced injury. Toxicol Pathol 33:41–51

100. Murali B, Korrapati MC, Warbritton A, Latendresse JR, Mehendale HM (2004) Tolerance of aged Fischer 344 rats against chlordecone-amplified carbon tetrachloride toxicity. Mech Ageing Dev 125:421–435

101. Apte UM, Limaye PB, Desaiah D, Bucci TJ, Warbritton A, Mehendale HM (2003) Mechanisms of increased liver tissue repair and survival in diet-restricted rats treated with equitoxic doses of thioacetamide. Toxicol Sci 72:272–282

102. Sawant SP, Dnyanmote AV, Warbritton A, Latendresse JR, Mehendale HM (2006) Type 2 diabetic rats are sensitive to thioacetamide hepatotoxicity. Toxicol Appl Pharmacol 211:221–232

103. Cai SR, Motoyama K, Shen KJ, Kennedy SC, Flye MW, Ponder KP (2000) Lovastatin decreases mortality and improves liver functions in fulminant hepatic failure from 90% partial hepatectomy in rats. J Hepatol 32:67–77

104. Yayama K, Sugiyama K, Miyagi R, Okamoto H (2007) Angiotensin-converting enzyme inhibitor enhances liver regeneration following partial hepatectomy: involvement of bradykinin B2 and angiotensin AT1 receptors. Biol Pharm Bull 30:591–594

105. Oben JA, Roskams T, Yang S, Lin H, Sinelli N, Li Z, Torbenson M, Huang J, Guarino P, Kafrouni M, Diehl AM (2003) Sympathetic nervous system inhibition increases hepatic progenitors and reduces liver injury. Hepatology 38:664–673

106. Donthamsetty S, Bhave VS, Mitra MS, Latendresse JR, Mehendale HM (2008) Nonalcoholic steatohepatitic (NASH) mice are protected from higher hepatotoxicity of acetaminophen upon induction of PPARalpha with clofibrate. Toxicol Appl Pharmacol 230:327–337

107. Bhattacharya S, Shoda LK, Zhang Q, Woods CG, Howell BA, Siler SQ, Woodhead JL, Yang Y, McMullen P, Watkins PB, Andersen ME (2012) Modeling drug- and chemical-induced hepatotoxicity with systems biology approaches. Front Physiol 3:462. https://doi.org/10.3389/fphys.2012.00462

108. Woodhead JL, Watkins PB, Howell BA, Siler SQ, Shoda LK (2017) The role of quantitative systems pharmacology modeling in the prediction and explanation of idiosyncratic drug-induced liver injury. Drug Metab Pharmacokinet 32:40–45

109. Yang K, Woodhead JL, Watkins PB, Howell BA, Brouwer KLR (2014) Systems pharmacology modeling predicts delayed presentation and species differences in bile acid-mediated troglitazone hepatotoxicity. Clin Pharmacol Ther 96:589–598

110. Woodhead JL, Brock WJ, Roth SE, Shoaf SE, Brouwer KL, Church R, Grammatopoulos TN, Stiles L, Siler SQ, Howell BA, Mosedale M, Watkins PB, Shoda LK (2017) Application of a mechanistic model to evaluate putative mechanisms of tolvaptan drug-induced liver injury and identify patient susceptibility factors. Toxicol Sci 155:61–74

111. Mann DA (2015) Human induced pluripotent stem cell-derived hepatocytes for toxicology testing. Expert Opin Drug Metab Toxicol 11:1–5

Chapter 24

Human Leukocyte Antigen (HLA) and Other Genetic Risk Factors in Drug-Induced Liver Injury (DILI)

Ann K. Daly

Abstract

Genetic risk factors, especially HLA alleles, have been investigated widely as risk factors for DILI development. The earlier studies prior to approx. the year of 2000 suffered from a number of problems including small numbers, imprecise phenotype and limited approaches to genotype or phenotype determination. Development of national and international networks to study DILI has resulted in larger numbers of cases being recruited. In combination with development of standardized methods for causality assessment and the introduction of genome-wide association studies (GWAS) in place of the earlier candidate gene approaches, this has resulted in more consistent findings on genetic risk factors. The newer studies using GWAS have confirmed the importance of HLA alleles as risk factors for DILI and have demonstrated that while particular HLA alleles are specific to individual drug causes of DILI, some unrelated drugs show similar HLA associations. Importantly, not all forms of DILI show HLA associations, and polymorphisms in other genes, especially those relevant to drug disposition, protection against oxidative stress and the innate immune system may also be relevant to risk of DILI. Identification of additional genetic risk factors may be feasible but will require larger case numbers than those currently available. The positive predictive value of all genetic risk factors discovered to date is low, but there is potential to combine genetic data with additional patient data such as age and gender to assess the risk of developing DILI with certain drugs.

Key words Human leukocyte antigen, Drug-induced liver injury, Genome-wide association study, Single nucleotide polymorphism

1 Introduction

The last 10 years has seen a considerable number of studies concerned with identifying genetic risk factors for DILI. Many of these involved genome-wide association studies (GWAS) which are increasingly feasible and have a number of advantages over more traditional candidate gene case–control studies. This chapter will consider both these approaches with particular emphasis on the relevance of HLA genes which have emerged as an important determinant of DILI risk in humans. Only idiosyncratic DILI, which includes most cases of DILI with the exception of those due to acetaminophen overdose, will be considered here. Studies on

Minjun Chen and Yvonne Will (eds.), *Drug-Induced Liver Toxicity*, Methods in Pharmacology and Toxicology,
https://doi.org/10.1007/978-1-4939-7677-5_24, © Springer Science+Business Media, LLC, part of Springer Nature 2018

idiosyncratic DILI sometimes divide toxicity into immune-mediated and non-immune-mediated reactions but there is considerable overlap between these categories; in particular, some types of DILI linked to particular HLA genotypes do not exhibit classic "immune" symptoms such as fever and rash so this division will not be considered further here.

2   Approaches to Genetic Studies on DILI

2.1   Early Studies Involving Candidate Gene Approaches

The original approach to genetic studies on DILI generally involved candidate gene case–control studies where the frequency of one or more genetic polymorphisms in biologically plausible genes was compared between cases of the disease and ethnically matched controls, who had either been exposed to the drug without toxicity or were simply healthy volunteers. In general, candidate gene association studies had limited success in finding genetic risk factors which could be replicated independently though some associations discussed in detail in Sects. 3 and 4, particularly HLA associations, were detected originally using a candidate gene approach. There are a number of reasons for the poor success with candidate gene studies on DILI including selection of inappropriate candidate genes, selection of polymorphisms that are not functionally important, use of small sample sizes due to the studies being based at single centers and heterogeneity in phenotype. These problems are not unique to DILI and also arose with many early genetic studies on complex polygenic diseases where family studies are not feasible. Problems with gene and polymorphism selection have been increasingly overcome by use of GWAS approaches as discussed in Sect. 2.2. Issues with sample size still arise but, as discussed in Sect. 2.3. below, have been overcome in part by the development of national and international networks for case recruitment. There are also improved guidelines available to help ensure uniformity in phenotype, as discussed in Sect. 2.4. below.

2.2   Genome-Wide Association Studies (GWAS)

In 2007, the Wellcome Trust Case Control Consortium published the first GWAS of selected human diseases [1]. A GWAS involves simultaneously genotyping approx. 300,000–1 million single nucleotide polymorphisms (SNPs) by microarray technology. Because of the existence of linkage disequilibrium in the human genome where several SNPs will be inherited together, the SNPs genotyped on a GWAS chip can cover all the common genetic variation in the human genome. Genotype for each SNP is tested for association with the disease of interest usually by comparing genotype frequency in the disease group with an ethnically matched healthy control group. Because of the large number of genotyping tests being performed, the *p*-value threshold for statistical significance needs to be set at a lower than normal level to correct for multiple testing. Replication of significant findings in a second set of disease cases is an important feature of the GWAS approach. The technique has now been applied to the study of a diverse range of diseases, including rare adverse drug reactions such as DILI (https://www.ebi.ac.uk/gwas/). A detailed description of methods used for GWAS is outside the scope on this chapter, mainly because generally only DNA preparation from blood samples using straightforward methodology or commercial kits is performed at the investigators' laboratories. Genotyping for GWAS using microarrays is normally performed by specialist academic or commercial providers. Data analysis for GWAS is complex and also outside the scope of this chapter but a detailed account of all aspects of this area is available elsewhere [2]. Specific findings on DILI obtained by GWAS are discussed in detail in Sects. 3 and 4.

2.3 Networks to Study DILI Genetics

A particular problem with genetic studies on DILI is obtaining adequate numbers of cases to discover genetic associations and then replicate them. Due to its relative rarity, case finding for genetic studies on DILI is challenging. Good progress has been made toward understanding the epidemiology of DILI by use of adverse drug reaction reports to national registries [3] and by searching medical records [4, 5] but the need to also obtain DNA samples for genetic studies poses additional challenges. The main success in detection of genetic risk factors for DILI has been achieved by development of national and international networks based on specialist hepatology centers and, to a more limited extent, national registries. Examples of national networks developed to study DILI generally and which continue to recruit include the Spanish Hepatotoxicity Group which has collected cases of DILI prospectively from all regions of Spain since 1994 [6] and now extends to Latin America [7], together with the US DILIN network established in 2004 [8], which collects cases both prospectively and retrospectively. Both networks have also collected material for DNA preparation from all or some of the cases enrolled and have performed genetic analysis on these samples. Networks concerned more specifically with genetic studies on DILI include DILIGEN based in the UK [9] and iDILIC [10], an international network involving Europe, South America, Canada, and Australasia. There are also networks which focus on genetic studies on a range of different types of adverse drug reaction including DILI such as Swedegene based in Sweden [11] and EUDRAGENE which was Europe-wide [12]. The recently established PRO-EURO-DILI registry is biobanking a wide range of biological samples from DILI cases collected prospectively which may facilitate further genetic studies [13].

Idiosyncratic DILI shows considerable heterogeneity with a range of different phenotypes and therefore obtaining an accurate diagnosis is not a simple task. A UK-based study where adverse drug reaction reports were searched retrospectively for cases of DILI and expert hepatology review was performed revealed that approximately half of the cases were not genuinely DILI [3]. Consistent case definition and phenotypic characterization are of paramount importance in investigations designed to identify genetic determinants of DILI susceptibility and this recently prompted the development of consensus criteria which could be applied readily to international studies. Recommendations from an international group of investigators based mainly in Europe and the USA have been developed [14]. Essentially there is a need to collect precise clinical data on suspected cases including details of recently prescribed drugs. Once these data are available, a causality score for the likelihood that this is a DILI case is calculated and ideally the case is then reviewed by a panel of expert hepatologists. The basis for the causality score is use of a scoring system usually referred to as RUCAM which was first described in the 1990s [15].

The recent international guidelines related mainly to DILI resulting from use of prescribed drugs [14]. Some independent guidelines on causality assessment covering herbal medicines, which are an important cause of DILI in a number of countries in addition to pharmaceuticals, have been developed recently [16]. There are also new guidelines regarding phenotype and causality assessment from the Chinese Society of Hepatology which seem valuable for studies in China where natural medicines are a particularly common cause of DILI [17].

3   HLA Genes as Risk Factors for DILI

HLA genes are located on chromosome 6 in the major histocompatibility complex (MHC) region and code for proteins that present foreign peptides, usually derived from pathogens, to T lymphocytes [18]. These genes are divided into two groups, class I and II. Class I genes are expressed on most cells in the body and present peptides to cytotoxic T-cells which may result in local tissue damage. Class II genes are expressed mainly on immune cells and have a key role in stimulating T-helper cells to produce inflammatory mediators. HLA genes show a large amount of genetic polymorphism. This diversity probably arose originally to help protect the body from pathogens but particular HLA alleles have also been shown to be risk factors for adverse drug reactions such as DILI. Some types of DILI may involve an inappropriate T-cell response to a drug, following covalent binding of the drug to cellular proteins.

The first studies on a possible genetic component in DILI susceptibility date from the 1980s and one of the earliest studies concerned a HLA association which was suggested between the HLA serotype DR2 and halothane-related DILI [19]. Following this initial study, other reports of associations between HLA serotypes and DILI induced by specific drugs emerged. These include a study of cases of DILI associated with several different drugs including nitrofurantoin [20] which found an apparent increased incidence in frequency of certain HLA class II serotypes (HLA-DR2 and HLA-DR6) among cases compared with controls. These increased frequencies were not statistically significant, probably due to small numbers. A subsequent larger study also involving a number of different causative drugs found a trend toward significance for the class I serotype HLA-A11 in DILI induced by tricyclic antidepressants and diclofenac and for the class II serotype HLA-DR6 in DILI due to chlorpromazine [21].

More recently, HLA associations with DILI have been studied directly by genotyping slightly larger numbers of DILI cases. The first studies of this nature were on amoxicillin-clavulanate-related DILI. Two independent candidate gene association studies reported an identical association with the *HLA-DRB1*15:01* allele [22, 23], which corresponds to the DR2 serotype already observed as a risk factor for halothane DILI [19].

Subsequent reports on HLA associations have usually involved GWAS, often combined with direct HLA typing if associations in the MHC region are detected. HLA typing is increasingly performed by DNA sequencing but, though this approach provides a large amount of data, it is labor-intensive and expensive. As an alternative, it is now possible to reliably predict HLA genotypes from GWAS data by imputation of SNP data using computer programs. A recent survey of several programs used for this purpose found a high level of accuracy could be achieved with several imputation programs using GWAS chip data, particularly for a European American population [24].

Table 1 provides a summary of HLA associations with DILI reported to date where the association appears robust on the basis of relatively large number of cases and/or replication in a second cohort. Effect sizes vary considerably depending on the drug with odds ratios for risk of DILI of between 2 and 80 reported. The strongest HLA association reported to date for DILI is for reactions due to the antimicrobial flucloxacillin, which is used in some countries to treat gram-positive bacterial infections. This was detected in the first GWAS performed for any type of DILI which reported a very strong association (odds ratio 80) for development of flucloxacillin DILI with the HLA class I allele *B*57:01* [9]. This allele had been shown previously to be a strong risk factor for hypersensitivity reactions to the drug abacavir, but these reactions generally do not involve the liver. *HLA-B*57:01* and some related

Table 1
HLA associations in DILI

Gene	Allele	Drug	Reference
HLA-A	*02:01	Amoxicillin-clavulanate	[25]
HLA-A	*33:01	Terbinafine, Fenofibrate, Ticlopidine	[10]
HLA-A	*33:03	Ticlopidine	[26]
HLA-B	*18:01	Amoxicillin-clavulanate	[25]
HLA-B	*35:02	Minocycline	[27]
HLA-B	*57:01	Flucloxacillin	[9]
	*57:01	Pazopanib	[28]
	*57:02, *57:03	Anti-TB drugs combined with antiretroviral agents	[29]
HLA-DRB1	*07:01	Ximelagatran	[30]
HLA-DRB1	*07:01	Lapatinib	[31]
HLA-DRB1	*15:01	Amoxicillin-clavulanate	[22, 23, 25, 32]
HLA-DRB1	*15:01	Lumiracoxib	[33]
HLA-DRB1	*16:01	Flupirtine	[34]

alleles may also contribute to DILI induced by other drugs. In particular, $B*57:01$ carriage appears to be a risk factor for DILI due to pazopanib though the effect size is much lower than that observed for flucloxacillin [28]. Additional alleles with strong homology to $HLA-B*57:01$ also appear to be risk factors for DILI; a recent report found that both $B*57:02$ and $B*57:03$ which are rare in Europe but more common in Africa were risk factors for DILI in patients treated with both anti-HIV drugs and anti-TB drugs concomitantly [29].

The early studies suggesting an association between $HLA-DRB1*15:01$ and amoxicillin-clavulanate DILI have been confirmed by use of GWAS, with these further studies showing two other HLA associations for amoxicillin-clavulanate-related toxicity involving HLA class I. Some of the reported HLA associations involve two or more different chemically unrelated drugs; for example, the HLA class II allele $DRB1*15:01$ is a risk factor for DILI related to both amoxicillin-clavulanate and lumiracoxib and the class I allele $A*33:01$ is a risk factor for DILI due to terbinafine, fenofibrate, and ticlopidine (Table 1).

The observed HLA associations are interesting but even for flucloxacillin DILI, only 1 in every 500–1000 patients carrying the risk allele *B*57:01* develop the reaction when given the drug. This means that genotyping for *B*57:01* shows a low positive predictive value and knowledge of genotype is unlikely to be a useful predictor of whether a patient treated with flucloxacillin will develop DILI. However, genotyping for *B*57:01* may be useful in confirming that flucloxacillin is the cause of liver injury in patients presenting with symptoms of DILI and help ensure the patient is not treated with this drug in the future.

Understanding the mechanism by which particular HLA alleles are associated with increased risk of DILI is an important issue that could lead to an improved understanding of the underlying biological mechanism and new approaches to identifying drugs that cause idiosyncratic DILI early in development. The mechanism underlying the flucloxacillin association with *HLA-B*57:01* has been the best studied to date. Overall, the underlying mechanism involved in the flucloxacillin DILI reaction appears to be different to the mechanism reported for abacavir [35, 36]. There is some evidence that flucloxacillin binds covalently to proteins prior to triggering a T cell response [35], though a second study using a different approach suggests that covalent binding is not essential [36]. For DILI due to amoxicillin-clavulanate, evidence for T cell responses involving both drugs has been obtained, with several pieces of evidence suggesting a hapten mechanism involving covalent binding of the drugs to proteins [37]. Detailed mechanistic studies relating to other causes of DILI where a HLA association occurs have generally not yet been performed but a very recent report on minocycline DILI suggests that direct binding of minocycline to the *HLA-B*35:02* protein may occur in a mechanism more similar to that reported for abacavir hypersensitivity [27].

4 Non-HLA Genes and DILI

While HLA genes are important genetic risk factors in idiosyncratic DILI, it is clear that HLA genotype only predicts a small proportion of DILI risk. In particular, there are examples of drugs that are common causes of DILI such as diclofenac and isoniazid where data from GWAS analysis suggests HLA genotype is not a predictor of risk [38]. Progress to date in identifying non-HLA genetic risk factors for DILI has been limited but a summary of the main findings is provided in Table 2.

With respect to genes relevant to drug disposition, a recent review has considered their relevance as DILI risk factors in detail [59] but concluded that only a small number of the associations reported appear likely to be genuine and that almost all still require replication in larger numbers of cases, ideally using approaches such as GWAS. The most widely studied association with a non-HLA gene to date for DILI is N-acetyltransferase 2 (*NAT2*) for isoniazid-related DILI but, as discussed recently [59], this association remains somewhat problematic due to most studies being on relatively mild DILI, the complexity of treatment regimens involving isoniazid for tuberculosis treatment with several potentially hepatotoxic drugs used and the failure to date to confirm the association using a GWAS [38].

It remains possible that genes relevant to hepatic function and, more generally, to protection against oxidative stress or the innate immune response could be risk factors for DILI. Examples are shown in Table 2. In general, oxidative stress genes in DILI, especially those affecting mitochondrial function, have been the most investigated [60] of these three gene classes with some borderline significant findings reported [56, 58]. In addition, polymorphisms in the immune-related genes STAT4 and PTPN22 may be risk factors for particular DILI phenotypes but this needs follow-up in larger numbers of cases [38].

Finding additional non-HLA genetic risk factors may best be achieved by larger studies. Much of the success so far in finding HLA risk factors has been due to large effect sizes and the highly polymorphic nature of HLA genes. In line with a range of common diseases, odds ratios for genetic risk factors could be in the range 1–2 and require sample sizes of several thousand cases for detection [61].

5   Conclusions and Future Directions

The development of international networks and clear phenotype guidelines has resulted in a relatively large number of studies on DILI genetics in the last 8 years approximately. Many of these have yielded findings that replicate in additional cohorts and the importance of HLA genes in susceptibility to this adverse drug reaction has become clear. It may be possible to identify additional genetic risk factors but this is likely to require considerably larger numbers of cases, as discussed in Sect. 4.

It has been suggested that genetic studies using alternative approaches such as whole genome sequencing or studies on epigenomics where DNA modification is analyzed may increase understanding of risk for DILI. These approaches remain promising and appear to have not yet been applied to DILI but, unlike GWAS, have generally not proved particularly useful to date in studies on more common polygenic diseases. In the case of whole genome sequencing, this is probably because GWAS combined with imputation of additional genotypes provides adequate coverage of the genome when performing case–control studies on polygenic disease risk, so genome sequencing does not generally provide addi-

Table 2
Selected non-HLA risk factors for DILI

Gene	Drug	Summary findings	References
CYP2B6	Efavirenz Ticlopidine	For DILI due to ticlopidine, upstream CYP2B6 SNP (rs7254579; −2320T>C) (possible high activity variant) was more common among cases. For DILI due to efavirenz, the CYP2B6*6 allele (rs3745274) (low activity variant) appears more common.	[39, 40]
CYP2C9	Bosentan	A possible association with CYP2C9 variant alleles, especially CYP2C9*2.	[41, 42]
CYP2E1	Isoniazid	Inconsistent data. Most studies concern CYP2E1*5 (rs2031920) (detectable using the restriction enzyme RsaI) which may be protective.	[43–45]
NAT2	Isoniazid	Many studies suggest that those homozygous for NAT2 variant alleles (NAT2 slow acetylators) are more susceptible to isoniazid-related DILI. Not all studies, including one GWAS, find this association.	[38, 46, 47]
UGT1A6	Tolcapone	Several polymorphisms in the UGT1A6 promoter region were found to be significantly associated with elevated transaminase levels.	[48]
UGT2B7	Diclofenac	Possession of UGT2B7*2 (rs7439366) was associated with an increased risk of toxicity. In a GWAS substudy of genes relevant to drug disposition only, SNPs in the UGT2B region which were in linkage disequilibrium with the UGT2B7*2-related SNPs were more common.	[38, 49]
GSTM1 and GSTT1	Troglitazone	Individuals homozygous null for both GSTM1 and GSTT1 are at increased risk of DILI due to troglitazone.	[50]
ABCB1	Nevirapine	In African DILI cases, decreased frequency of 3435C>T (rs1045642) seen. This was also reported for a US patient group. A study on a group of European nevirapine DILI patients failed to confirm this association.	[51–53]
ABCB11	Various	Association between cholestatic injury due to various drugs and a polymorphism (rs2287622) in exon 13 of ABCB11 reported.	[54]
ABCC2	Diclofenac	Carriage of an upstream polymorphism in ABCC2 (rs717620; −24C>T) was found to be significantly more common among DILI cases.	[49]
ABCC2	Various	Polymorphism in linkage disequilibrium with rs717620 was a risk factor for hepatocellular DILI; another promoter region polymorphism was a risk factor for cholestatic/mixed DILI.	[55]

(continued)

Table 2
(continued)

Gene	Drug	Summary findings	References
SOD2	Various	Common SOD2 polymorphism (rs4880) was found to be a predictor of hepatocellular DILI, particularly relating to antituberculosis drugs the same genotype was found to be a significant risk factor for cholestatic/mixed DILI due to a range of drugs.	[56, 57]
STAT4	Various	Variant in *STAT4* (rs7574865) which regulates cytokine production and T cell responses increases risk of hepatocellular DILI.	[38]
PTPN22	Various	Variant in PTPN22 (rs2476601) which contributes to T cell responses increases risk of cholestatic DILI.	[38]
NOS2A, BACH1, MAFK	Isoniazid	Particular SNPs in these oxidative stress-related genes increase risk of DILI.	[58]

Studies listed involve a candidate gene approach either by genotyping only for the polymorphism of interest or by extraction of relevant data from a GWAS

tional novel findings, despite being extremely valuable in rare monogenic diseases [62]. Though rare, DILI is generally considered to be a polygenic rather than monogenic disease. With epigenomics, study design remains very challenging and findings subject to multiple issues that make interpretation difficult [63]. Performing such studies on DILI in the future could yield useful data if the study design can be optimized appropriately.

In spite of recent advances in DILI genetics, it is becoming clear that knowledge of patient genotype prior to drug prescription is unlikely to be a useful means of preventing DILI reactions due to low positive predictive value. In parallel with the genetic studies, it has been recognized that patient age and gender are also important factors in DILI. Assessment of risk with these additional factors considered as well as genotype for HLA and other genes may result in improved positive predictive values.

References

1. Wellcome Trust Case Control C (2007) Genome-wide association study of 14,000 cases of seven common diseases and 3,000 shared controls. Nature 447(7145):661–678

2. Gondro C, van der Werf J, Hayes B (2013) Genome-wide association studies and genomic prediction, Methods in molecular biology, vol 1019. Springer, NY

3. Aithal GP, Rawlins MD, Day CP (1999) Accuracy of hepatic adverse drug reaction reporting in one English health region. Br Med J 319(7224):1541–1541

4. Sgro C, Clinard F, Ouazir K et al (2002) Incidence of drug-induced hepatic injuries: a French population-based study. Hepatology 36(2):451–455

5. Russmann S, Kaye JA, Jick SS, Jick H (2005) Risk of cholestatic liver disease associated with flucloxacillin and flucloxacillin prescribing habits in the UK: cohort study using data from the

UK general practice research database. Br J Clin Pharmacol 60(1):76–82

6. Lucena MI, Camargo R, Andrade RJ et al (2001) Comparison of two clinical scales for causality assessment in hepatotoxicity. Hepatology 33(1):123–130

7. Bessone F, Hernandez N, Lucena MI, Andrade RJ (2016) The Latin American DILI registry experience: a successful ongoing collaborative strategic initiative. Int J Mol Sci 17(3):313

8. Chalasani N, Fontana RJ, Bonkovsky HL et al (2008) Causes, clinical features, and outcomes from a prospective study of drug-induced liver injury in the United States. Gastroenterology 135(6):1924–1934. 1934 e1921-1924

9. Daly AK, Donaldson PT, Bhatnagar P et al (2009) HLA-B*5701 genotype is a major determinant of drug-induced liver injury due to flucloxacillin. Nat Genet 41:816–819

10. Nicoletti P, Aithal GP, Bjornsson ES et al (2017) Association of liver injury from specific drugs, or groups of drugs, with polymorphisms in HLA and other genes in a genome-wide association study. Gastroenterology 152(5):1078–1089

11. Wadelius M, Eriksson N, Ying-Yue Q et al (2013) Swedegene: genome-wide association studies of adverse drug reactions. In: 63rd Meeting of the American Society of Human Genetics, Boston, MA. http://www.ashg.org/2013meeting/abstracts/fulltext/f130122057.htm

12. Molokhia M, McKeigue P (2006) EUDRAGENE: European collaboration to establish a case-control DNA collection for studying the genetic basis of adverse drug reactions. Pharmacogenomics 7(4):633–638

13. Slim M, Stephens C, Robles-Diaz M et al (2016) PRO-EURO-DILI registry: a collaborative effort to enhance the understanding of DILI. J Hepatol 64(2 (Supplement)):S293–S294

14. Aithal GP, Watkins PB, Andrade RJ et al (2011) Case definition and phenotype standardization in drug-induced liver injury. Clin Pharmacol Ther 89(6):806–815

15. Danan G, Benichou C (1993) Causality assessment of adverse reactions to drugs--I. A novel method based on the conclusions of international consensus meetings: application to drug-induced liver injuries. J Clin Epidemiol 46(11):1323–1330

16. Danan G, Teschke R (2015) RUCAM in drug and herb induced liver injury: the update. Int J Mol Sci 17(1):E14

17. Yu YC, Mao YM, Chen CW et al (2017) CSH guidelines for the diagnosis and treatment of drug-induced liver injury. Hepatol Int 11(3):221–241

18. Mehta NK (2010) The HLA complex in biology and medicine: a resource book, 1st edn. Jaypee Brothers Medical Publishers Ltd, New Delhi, India

19. Otsuka S, Yamamoto M, Kasuya S et al (1985) HLA antigens in patients with unexplained hepatitis following halothane anesthesia. Acta Anaesthesiol Scand 29(5):497–501

20. Stricker BH, Blok AP, Claas FH et al (1988) Hepatic injury associated with the use of nitrofurans: a clinicopathological study of 52 reported cases. Hepatology 8(3):599–606

21. Berson A, Freneaux E, Larrey D et al (1994) Possible role of Hla in hepatotoxicity–an exploratory-study in 71 patients with drug-induced idiosyncratic hepatitis. J Hepatol 20(3):336–342

22. Hautekeete ML, Horsmans Y, van Waeyenberge C et al (1999) HLA association of amoxicillin-clavulanate-induced hepatitis. Gastroenterology 117(5):1181–1186

23. O'Donohue J, Oien KA, Donaldson P et al (2000) Co-amoxiclav jaundice: clinical and histological features and HLA class II association. Gut 47(5):717–720

24. Karnes JH, Shaffer CM, Bastarache L et al (2017) Comparison of HLA allelic imputation programs. PLoS One 12(2):e0172444

25. Lucena MI, Molokhia M, Shen Y et al (2011) Susceptibility to amoxicillin-clavulanate-induced liver injury is influenced by multiple HLA class I and II alleles. Gastroenterology 141(1):338–347

26. Hirata K, Takagi H, Yamamoto M et al (2008) Ticlopidine-induced hepatotoxicity is associated with specific human leukocyte antigen genomic subtypes in Japanese patients: a preliminary case-control study. Pharmacogenomics J 8(1):29–33

27. Urban TJ, Nicoletti P, Chalasani N et al (2017) Minocycline hepatotoxicity: clinical characterization and identification of HLA-B * 35:02 as a risk factor. J Hepatol 67(1):137–144

28. Xu CF, Johnson T, Wang X et al (2016) HLA-B*57:01 confers susceptibility to pazopanib-associated liver injury in patients with cancer. Clin Cancer Res 22(6):1371–1377

29. Petros Z, Kishikawa J, Makonnen E et al (2017) HLA-B*57 allele is associated with concomitant anti-tuberculosis and antiretroviral drugs induced liver toxicity in ethiopians. Front Pharmacol 8:90

30. Kindmark A, Jawaid A, Harbron CG et al (2008) Genome-wide pharmacogenetic investigation of a hepatic adverse event without

clinical signs of immunopathology suggests an underlying immune pathogenesis. Pharmacogenomics J 8:186–195

31. Spraggs CF, Budde LR, Briley LP et al (2011) HLA-DQA1*02:01 is a major risk factor for lapatinib-induced hepatotoxicity in women with advanced breast cancer. J Clin Oncol 29(6):667–673

32. Donaldson PT, Daly AK, Henderson J et al (2010) Human leucocyte antigen class II genotype in susceptibility and resistance to co-amoxiclav-induced liver injury. J Hepatol 53(6):1049–1053

33. Singer JB, Lewitzky S, Leroy E et al (2010) A genome-wide study identifies HLA alleles associated with lumiracoxib-related liver injury. Nat Genet 42:711–714

34. Nicoletti P, Werk AN, Sawle A et al (2016) HLA-DRB1*16:01-DQB1*05:02 is a novel genetic risk factor for flupirtine-induced liver injury. Pharmacogenet Genomics 26(5):218–224

35. Monshi MM, Faulkner L, Gibson A et al (2013) Human leukocyte antigen (HLA)-B*57:01-restricted activation of drug-specific T cells provides the immunological basis for flucloxacillin-induced liver injury. Hepatology 57(2):727–739

36. Wuillemin N, Adam J, Fontana S et al (2013) HLA haplotype determines hapten or p-i T cell reactivity to flucloxacillin. J Immunol 190(10):4956–4964

37. Kim SH, Saide K, Farrell J et al (2015) Characterization of amoxicillin- and clavulanic acid-specific T cells in patients with amoxicillin-clavulanate-induced liver injury. Hepatology 62(3):887–899

38. Urban TJ, Shen Y, Stolz A et al (2012) Limited contribution of common genetic variants to risk for liver injury due to a variety of drugs. Pharmacogenet Genomics 22(11):784–795

39. Ariyoshi N, Iga Y, Hirata K et al (2010) Enhanced susceptibility of HLA-mediated ticlopidine-induced idiosyncratic hepatotoxicity by CYP2B6 polymorphism in Japanese. Drug Metab Pharmacokinet 25(3):298–306

40. Yimer G, Amogne W, Habtewold A et al (2011) High plasma efavirenz level and CYP2B6*6 are associated with efavirenz-based HAART-induced liver injury in the treatment of naive HIV patients from Ethiopia: a prospective cohort study. Pharmacogenomics J 12(6):499–506

41. Markova SM, De Marco T, Bendjilali N et al (2013) Association of CYP2C9*2 with bosentan-induced liver injury. Clin Pharmacol Ther 94(6):678–686

42. Seyfarth HJ, Favreau N, Tennert C et al (2014) Genetic susceptibility to hepatotoxicity due to bosentan treatment in pulmonary hypertension. Ann Hepatol 13(6):803–809

43. Vuilleumier N, Rossier MF, Chiappe A et al (2006) CYP2E1 genotype and isoniazid-induced hepatotoxicity in patients treated for latent tuberculosis. Eur J Clin Pharmacol 62(6):423–429

44. Cho HJ, Koh WJ, Ryu YJ et al (2007) Genetic polymorphisms of NAT2 and CYP2E1 associated with antituberculosis drug-induced hepatotoxicity in Korean patients with pulmonary tuberculosis. Tuberculosis (Edinb) 87(6):551–556

45. Lee SW, Chung LS, Huang HH et al (2010) NAT2 and CYP2E1 polymorphisms and susceptibility to first-line anti-tuberculosis drug-induced hepatitis. Int J Tuberc Lung Dis 14(5):622–626

46. Daly AK, Day CP (2012) Genetic association studies in drug-induced liver injury. Drug Metab Rev 44(1):116–126

47. Ng CS, Hasnat A, Al Maruf A et al (2014) N-acetyltransferase 2 (NAT2) genotype as a risk factor for development of drug-induced liver injury relating to antituberculosis drug treatment in a mixed-ethnicity patient group. Eur J Clin Pharmacol 70(9):1079–1086

48. Acuna G, Foernzler D, Leong D et al (2002) Pharmacogenetic analysis of adverse drug effect reveals genetic variant for susceptibility to liver toxicity. Pharmacogenomics J 2(5):327–334

49. Daly AK, Aithal GP, Leathart JB et al (2007) Genetic susceptibility to diclofenac-induced hepatotoxicity: contribution of UGT2B7, CYP2C8, and ABCC2 genotypes. Gastroenterology 132(1):272–281

50. Watanabe I, Tomita A, Shimizu M et al (2003) A study to survey susceptible genetic factors responsible for troglitazone-associated hepatotoxicity in Japanese patients with type 2 diabetes mellitus. Clin Pharmacol Ther 73(5):435–455

51. Haas DW, Bartlett JA, Andersen JW et al (2006) Pharmacogenetics of nevirapine-associated hepatotoxicity: an adult AIDS clinical trials group collaboration. Clin Infect Dis 43(6):783–786

52. Ritchie MD, Haas DW, Motsinger AA et al (2006) Drug transporter and metabolizing enzyme gene variants and nonnucleoside reverse-transcriptase inhibitor hepatotoxicity. Clin Infect Dis 43(6):779–782

53. Yuan J, Guo S, Hall D et al (2011) Toxicogenomics of nevirapine-associated cutaneous and hepatic adverse events among populations of African, Asian, and European descent. AIDS 25(10):1271–1280

54. Noe J, Kullak-Ublick GA, Jochum W et al (2005) Impaired expression and function of

the bile salt export pump due to three novel ABCB11 mutations in intrahepatic cholestasis. J Hepatol 43(3):536–543

55. Choi JH, Ahn BM, Yi J et al (2007) MRP2 haplotypes confer differential susceptibility to toxic liver injury. Pharmacogenet Genomics 17(6):403–415

56. Lucena MI, Garcia-Martin E, Andrade RJ et al (2010) Mitochondrial superoxide dismutase and glutathione peroxidase in idiosyncratic drug-induced liver injury. Hepatology 52(1):303–312

57. Huang YS, Su WJ, Huang YH et al (2007) Genetic polymorphisms of manganese superoxide dismutase, NAD(P)H:quinone oxidoreductase, glutathione S-transferase M1 and T1, and the susceptibility to drug-induced liver injury. J Hepatol 47(1):128–134

58. Nanashima K, Mawatari T, Tahara N et al (2012) Genetic variants in antioxidant pathway: risk factors for hepatotoxicity in tuberculosis patients. Tuberculosis (Edinb) 92(3):253–259

59. Daly AK (2016) Are polymorphisms in genes relevant to drug disposition predictors of susceptibility to drug-induced liver injury? Pharm Res 34(8):1564–1569

60. Boelsterli UA, Lee KK (2014) Mechanisms of isoniazid-induced idiosyncratic liver injury: emerging role of mitochondrial stress. J Gastroenterol Hepatol 29(4):678–687

61. Pranavchand R, Reddy BM (2016) Genomics era and complex disorders: implications of GWAS with special reference to coronary artery disease, type 2 diabetes mellitus, and cancers. J Postgrad Med 62(3):188–198

62. Ngeow J, Eng C (2015) New genetic and genomic approaches after the genome-wide association study era--back to the future. Gastroenterology 149(5):1138–1141

63. Birney E, Smith GD, Greally JM (2016) Epigenome-wide association studies and the interpretation of disease -omics. PLoS Genet 12(6):e1006105

Chapter 25

Immune Mechanisms in Drug-Induced Liver Injury

Hartmut Jaeschke and Dean J. Naisbitt

Abstract

Drug-induced liver injury is a serious clinical problem and a challenge for drug development. Although intracellular events including formation of reactive metabolites and oxidant stress are well-established causes of cell injury, immune mechanisms of liver injury are coming more into focus recently. Acute liver injury as observed after acetaminophen overdose leads to release of damage-associated molecular patterns (DAMPs), which triggers formation of cytokines and chemokines through activation of toll like receptors and other pattern recognition receptors causing the activation of innate immune cells including neutrophils, Kupffer cells, and monocytes. The general purpose of this innate immune response is to recruit phagocytes into the areas of necrosis to remove necrotic cells and prepare for regeneration of the lost tissue. However, an excessive innate immune response may cause additional cell death and exaggerate the original injury. The factors that trigger a proinjury versus a proregenerative innate immune response during drug-induced liver injury remain to be investigated. On the other hand, a prolonged subclinical stress caused by therapeutic doses of certain drugs can trigger activation of T and B lymphocytes and an adaptive immune-mediated liver injury in susceptible individuals. Although specific HLA alleles have been identified as risk factors for drug hepatotoxicity, there is still limited understanding of the mechanisms of adaptive immune cell activation, the development of immune tolerance and the mechanisms of cell death in patients. The chapter summarizes the current knowledge on innate and adaptive immune-mediated liver injury mechanisms in drug hepatotoxicity.

Key words Drug-induced liver injury, Acetaminophen, Innate immunity, Neutrophils, Monocytes, Adaptive immunity, T cells, IgG, Flucloxacillin

1 Introduction

Drug-induced liver injury is a significant clinical problem and a major challenge during drug development. It is generally agreed on that the metabolism of a drug or chemical in hepatocytes, and in rare cases the parent drug itself, causes an intracellular stress [1]. In the case of drugs that directly cause hepatotoxicity in patients, e.g., acetaminophen (APAP), the initial stress coming from the formation of a reactive metabolite that binds to cellular proteins triggers intracellular signaling pathways leading to cell death and severe liver injury [2]. The extensive release of cellular content

Minjun Chen and Yvonne Will (eds.), *Drug-Induced Liver Toxicity*, Methods in Pharmacology and Toxicology,
https://doi.org/10.1007/978-1-4939-7677-5_25, © Springer Science+Business Media, LLC, part of Springer Nature 2018

induces a rapid innate immune response, with the main purpose of removing the cellular debris and promotion of regeneration [3]. However, a misguided and exaggerated innate immune response can also greatly enhance the original injury and lead to acute liver failure [3–5]. On the other hand, in cases of drugs that induce idiosyncratic hepatotoxicity in patients, the initial stress may be much more subtle and more difficult to detect, especially in preclinical models [6]. However, the more subtle chronic stress can eventually trigger an adaptive immune response, which may cause liver injury [6]. This chapter discusses mechanisms and examples of both innate and adaptive immune responses during the development of drug-induced liver injury.

2   Innate Immune Mechanisms and Drug Hepatotoxicity

Innate immune cells that are present in the liver include the largest resident macrophage pool (Kupffer cells) and various lymphocyte populations including natural killer (NK), NK T cells, and dendritic cells [7]. In addition, inflammatory mediators can activate and recruit neutrophils and monocyte into the liver. Each of these cell types has been implicated in drug-induced liver injury either as proinflammatory cell type exaggerating the initial injury or being involved in the resolution of the inflammatory response and promoting liver repair. Although an innate immune response has been implicated in a number of drug- and chemical-induced liver injury models [4, 8], the by far most-studied and mechanistically best-described example is the direct hepatotoxin acetaminophen (APAP) [5, 9]. In addition to the preclinical investigations, APAP overdose is also the clinically most relevant cause of drug hepatotoxicity and acute liver failure in the Western world [10], and thus allows the direct assessment of mechanisms derived from preclinical models in patients [11].

2.1   Initiation of the Innate Immune Response in Drug Hepatotoxicity

Extensive cell necrosis causes the release of cell contents including molecules that are collectively termed damage-associated molecular patterns (DAMPs) (Fig. 1a). Compounds identified as DAMPs include high mobility group box 1 (HMGB1) protein, nuclear DNA fragments, mitochondrial DNA, ATP, and many others [4, 5, 9]. These DAMPs are recognized by pattern recognition receptors such as toll-like receptors (TLRs), which are located on all liver cells including macrophages [12]. Stimulation of TLRs induces the transcriptional activation of cytokines and chemokines [12], which can induce adhesion molecules on hepatic cells [13], directly prime and activate neutrophils and monocytes but also, when generated by hepatocytes, provide a chemotactic gradient for neutrophil and monocyte extravasation [14].

After an APAP overdose resulting in severe liver injury, extensive release of DAMPs including nonacetylated HMGB1 [15], nuclear DNA fragments and mitochondrial DNA [16], heat shock proteins [17], and uric acid [18] have been observed in experimental models but also in humans [17, 19] (Fig. 1b). Furthermore, cytokine and chemokine levels are increased in serum of APAP-treated animals [20–24]. The increase in cytokine formation was attributed in part to TLR9, which is mainly activated by mtDNA or DNA fragments [25, 26] and in part to TLR4, which can be activated by HMGB1 and other DAMPs [23]. However, others have argued that HMGB1 does not act through TLR4 but through the receptor for advanced glycation end products (RAGE) instead [27].

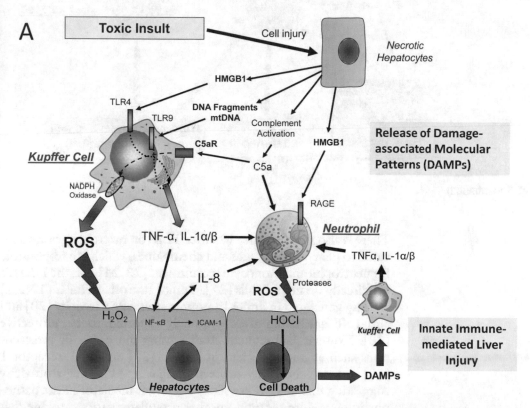

Fig. 1 Mechanisms of a sterile inflammatory response after cell necrosis causing additional inflammatory liver injury or supporting liver regeneration. General scheme of the initiation of a sterile inflammatory response by release of damage associated molecular patterns (DAMPs) by necrotic cells, the promotion of cytokine and chemokine formation by activating pattern recognition receptors such as toll-like receptors (TLRs), and the consequent activation and recruitment of inflammatory cells, which can aggravate the initial injury (see text for details) (**a**). The sterile inflammatory response after acetaminophen-induced liver injury, which does not aggravate the original injury, promotes the removal of necrotic cell debris and supports regeneration (see text for details) (**b**). Abbreviations: *C5aR* complement fragment C5a receptor, *HMGB1* high mobility group box 1 protein, *HOCl* hypochlorous acid, *ICAM-1* intercellular adhesion molecule-1, *IL* interleukin, *MCP-1* monocyte chemoattractant protein-1, *mtDNA* mitochondrial DNA, *RAGE* receptor for advanced glycation end products

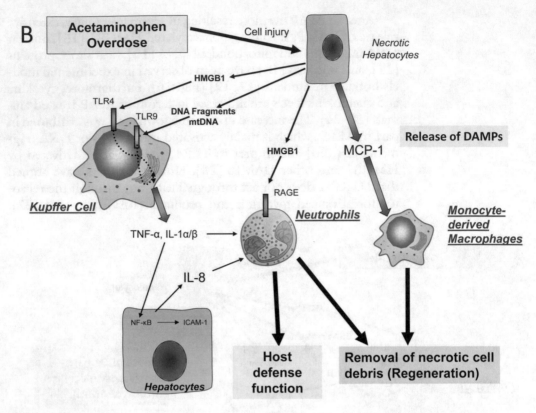

Fig. 1 (continued)

There is also a controversy whether TLRs on macrophages are activated to generate cytokines and chemokines, which are responsible for neutrophil and monocyte recruitment [23, 24] or if the DAMPs act directly on neutrophils [27]. Tumor necrosis factor-α (TNF-α) is being generated in limited amounts after APAP toxicity [20] and anti-TNF antibodies were originally reported to be protective [28]. However, subsequent studies using more specific interventions such as mice deficient in TNF-α [29] and TNF-receptor 1 [30] did not show any protection against APAP hepatotoxicity suggesting that TNF is not likely a relevant mediator in the pathophysiology. More recently, another proinflammatory cytokine that received attention in APAP hepatotoxicity is interleukin-1β (IL-1β). The formation of this cytokine not only requires the transcriptional activation of pro-IL-1β through TLR9 but also the cleavage of pro-IL-1β to the active cytokine by caspase-1 [25]. DAMPs such as ATP act on the purinergic receptor P2X7 and activate the Nalp3 inflammasome, which results in activation of caspase-1 [4, 9]. Although the TLR9-dependent transcriptional formation of pro-IL-1β [25] and the caspase-dependent formation of the actual cytokine IL-1β [22] was shown, the relevance of this cytokine as activator of neutrophils has been questioned due to the very low levels formed during APAP hepatotoxicity in mice [22] and in humans [9]. The limited formation of IL-1β was recently confirmed and it was suggested that IL-1α, a cytokine that does not require the inflammasome activation, is the dominant IL-1 responsible for neutrophil recruitment during APAP hepatotoxicity [23]. Despite these somewhat controversial reports about which cytokine is actually responsible for the activation and the recruitment of neutrophils, the innate immune cells accumulating first in the liver during the development of APAP-induced liver injury, there is much more consensus that MCP1 is the driving force for the later accumulating monocyte-derived macrophages in mice [24, 31] and also in humans [32].

2.2 Neutrophil-Induced Liver Injury and Drug Hepatotoxicity

The mechanisms of neutrophil-induced liver injury has been studied extensively and is well established for the pathophysiology of hepatic ischemia–reperfusion injury [33], endotoxemia [34] and obstructive cholestasis [35]. Despite the different insults, the general characteristics of tissue injury by neutrophils are very similar and include neutrophil activation (CD11b, reactive oxygen) by proinflammatory mediators in circulation [36], the accumulation in sinusoids and subsequent transmigration dependent mainly on β2 integrins (CD11/CD18) and intercellular adhesion molecule-1 (ICAM-1) and the adhesion to hepatocytes with prolonged reactive oxygen formation leading to an oxidant stress-mediated cell death in the target cell [14]. Because neutrophils generate the potent oxidant hypochlorous acid through the enzyme myeloperoxidase, specific products such as chlorotyrosine [35, 37] and hypochlorous acid-modified proteins [38] can be detected in cells subjected to a neutrophil-induced oxidant stress.

Neutrophils accumulate in the liver shortly after the APAP-induced liver injury starts around 4–6 h after an overdose in mice [20, 39] and it has been suggested that they aggravate liver injury over the next 15–20 h [23, 26, 40]. However, fundamental features of the mechanism could not be verified. First, systemic neutrophil priming was not observed during the early injury [41]. Second, many different interventions that directly affected the capacity for the neutrophil to transmigrate and attack a target cells such as antibodies that cause neutropenia or functionally block CD18, or the use of knockout mice of CD18 or ICAM-1 all had no effect on the injury [20, 39, 41]. Furthermore, using inhibitors of NADPH oxidase, the enzyme responsible for reactive oxygen formation by neutrophils and other phagocytes, or mice deficient in NADPH oxidase genes, showed both similar APAP-induced liver injury and oxidant stress as the respective controls and wild type animals [39, 42, 43]. In addition, no direct evidence (hypochlorite-modified proteins) for a neutrophil-induced oxidant stress was observed during APAP hepatotoxicity [39]. The consistent absence of any protective effect with direct interventions against neutrophils, all of which are effective against hepatic ischemia–reperfusion injury, endotoxemia, and obstructive cholestasis [33–35], make it highly unlikely that neutrophils, despite the recruitment and inflammatory mediator production, actively contribute to APAP-induced liver injury [2, 5, 9] (Fig. 1b).

How can we explain some of the other reports that appear to favor a neutrophil-induced injury phase? Most of these studies are based on neutropenia experiments where the Gr-1 or Ly6G antibody was injected 24 h before APAP administration [23, 26, 40]. Due to the Kupffer cell activation that is caused by the inactivated neutrophils in sinusoids and the resulting preconditioning effect with upregulation of protective genes including metallothionein and heat shock proteins [44], the hepatoprotection is not caused by neutrophils but by the off-target effect of the interventions [2, 9]. Moreover, many other interventions that affect upstream cytokines or their receptors [23, 25] may have only indirect effects on neutrophils potentially due to the reduced injury. However, some of these cytokines can modulate the injury through induction of inducible nitric oxide synthase [45], which contribute to the peroxynitrite formation critical for the APAP-induced cell death mechanisms [2, 46]. Another reason for variable results can be the background strains of gene knockout mice. Unless littermates are being used as wild type controls, there is always a chance that even a slight mismatch of the genetic background between wild type and gene knockout mice can lead to results that reflect the different susceptibility of the different background strains rather than the gene deficiency [47, 48]. Thus, a detailed knowledge of the pathophysiology of APAP-induced liver injury and potential off-target effects of therapeutic interventions need to be considered when interpreting data from experiments assessing the innate immunity in drug toxicity.

Independent of the controversial studies in mice, the critical question remains how these immune mechanisms translate to patients. A recent study has shown that neutrophil activation, assessed as CD11b upregulation, ROS priming and increased phagocytosis, is only observed after the peak of injury as indicated by declining plasma ALT levels [43]. This suggests that neutrophils are unlikely to be involved in the injury phase in humans but are more likely recruited to promote recovery (Fig. 1b). This is consistent with the lack of a relevant formation of proinflammatory cytokines such as TNF-α and IL-1β and only limited generation of IL-8 during the injury phase [49].

2.3 Role of Kupffer Cells and Monocytes in Drug Hepatotoxicity

Early studies have suggested that Kupffer cells are activated after APAP-induced liver injury [50] and follow-up studies using general inhibitors of these phagocytes such as gadolinium chloride have reported protective effects [51, 52]. However, these reports could not be confirmed [53–55]; in fact, a more specific elimination of Kupffer cells with clodronate liposomes demonstrated beneficial effects of Kupffer cell activation [55], most likely due to anti-inflammatory cytokine (IL-10) formation [45]. An argument against a Kupffer cell-induced oxidant stress as the main reason for APAP-induced injury as postulated [52] is the fact that the most active Kupffer cells are located in the periportal area, which would make it difficult to selectively cause centrilobular necrosis, and the fact that a NADPH-deficient mouse shows similar oxidant stress and injury as wild type animals [42]. However, more recent studies have also implicated Kupffer cells as the major source of IL-1α and an IL-1α-mediated injury phase [23], which contradicts a previous study implicating IL-1β and the inflammasome activation in Kupffer cells [25]. Although the limited inflammasome activation and IL-1β formation as reported by Zhang and coworkers [23] agrees with other previous studies [22, 56, 57], it still assumes an IL-1 receptor-dependent neutrophil activation and injury, which has been already disputed [22].

In addition to the resident Kupffer cells, it is well established that monocyte-derived macrophages accumulate in the liver, mainly in the area of necrosis, after APAP overdose [24]. The main chemokine responsible for their activation and recruitment is monocyte chemoattractant protein-1 (MCP-1, CCL2), which is generated by both macrophages and damaged hepatocytes during APAP hepatotoxicity [24]. The receptor for MCP-1 is the chemokine receptor CCR2 located on monocytes and macrophages [24]. Mice deficient in CCR2 and MCP-1 showed reduced accumulation of monocyte-derived macrophages in the liver but no protection against APAP-induced liver injury [24, 31]. Interestingly, the resolution of the injury and recovery was significantly delayed in CCR2-deficient mice [24, 31, 58], suggesting that these monocytes are recruited mainly for removal of cell debris in preparation for regeneration [24, 31]. However, since neutrophil accumulation was also reduced in CCR2-deficient mice [31], it is likely that the removal of cell debris involves both monocyte-derived macrophages and neutrophils (Fig. 1b).

In human APAP overdose patients, the minimal formation of classical proinflammatory mediators including TNF-α and IL-1β together with formation of the anti-inflammatory cytokine IL-10 [21, 49] suggests a limited inflammatory response of macrophages (M1 phenotype). In contrast, high levels of MCP-1 promote monocyte-derived macrophage infiltration into the liver that appears to be mainly of the proregenerative phenotype (M2) [32]. Interestingly, MCP-1 levels decline over time in patients who regenerate damaged tissue and recover but remain substantially elevated in patients who do not recover and progress to acute liver failure [49]. This observation suggests that the limited removal of necrotic tissue leads to a prolonged formation of MCP-1 and recruitment of monocyte-derived macrophages [49], which may be the reason for the more pronounced depletion of monocytes in APAP-induced liver failure patients with poor outcome [32].

Overall, both the studies in mice and in humans strongly support a pro-regenerative inflammatory response after APAP-induced liver injury that is critical for the recovery.

2.4 NK, NKT and Dendritic Cells in Drug Hepatotoxicity

A role of NK and NKT cells in APAP hepatotoxicity has been suggested based on the reduced injury observed in mice where both NK and NKT cells were depleted with an anti-NK1.1 monoclonal antibody [59]. However, the relevance of these results has been questioned because the protective effect was only observed when the animals were cotreated with dimethyl sulfoxide, which appears to recruit and activate NK and NKT cells [60]. The story is further complicated by conflicting observations that NKT cell-deficient mice [CD1d(−/−) and Jα18(−/−) mice] showed increased APAP hepatotoxicity due to enhanced ketone body formation during starvation, which induced Cyp2E1 levels [61]. In contrast, fed Jα18(−/−) mice were more resistant to APAP due to enhanced GSH levels and the improved scavenging capacity for the reactive metabolite [62]. A recent study on dendritic cells showed that depletion of these immune cells exacerbated APAP toxicity [63], however, the mechanism by which dendritic cells limit APAP hepatotoxicity remained unclear. The enhanced liver injury was independent of neutrophils or NK cells [63], which also confirmed previous studies showing that neither neutrophils [20, 39, 41] nor NK cells affect APAP hepatotoxicity [60].

2.5 Summary and Conclusions Regarding the Innate Immune Response in Drug Hepatotoxicity

Severe cell necrosis induced by drug hepatotoxicity causes the release of DAMPs, which can trigger cytokine and chemokine formation through stimulation of TLRs and other pattern recognition receptors on macrophages, neutrophils and hepatocytes. These mediators activate a number of resident and circulating leukocytes including neutrophils and monocytes. Although the main purpose of this sterile inflammatory response is to remove necrotic cells and assist in tissue recovery, there is the possibility that such an inflammatory response can also cause additional tissue injury (Fig. 1a). As outlined for the example of APAP hepatotoxicity in mice and humans, selective interventions and their interpretations are not always straightforward and can be affected by off-target effects. Clearly, multiple experimental approaches need to be applied and any conclusion should not only narrowly focus on the results of individual experiments but should consider the entire body of literature on the subject.

3   Adaptive Immune Mechanisms and Drug Hepatotoxicity

The adaptive immune system is made up of specialized cells designed to eliminate infectious pathogens. T and B lymphocytes are the primary cells involved in the adaptive immune response.

When T cells are activated they secrete a plethora of mediators (e.g., cytokines, chemokines) that help to control the nature of the immune response and the recruitment and activation of innate immune cells. Furthermore, T cells have the capacity to cause cytotoxicity directly through the release of cytolytic mediators. In contrast, activation of B cells results in secretion of antibodies that migrate through the blood and bind to foreign material preventing binding to host tissue. The total mass of lymphocytes in the body is similar to that of the liver; a small portion travels through the bloodstream, but much larger numbers reside in tissues [64]. Immunological memory is the key defining characteristic that separates innate and adaptive immune responses. Following exposure to a pathogen there is a process of clonal expansion where large numbers of lymphocytes are generated that recognize a specific pathogen, commonly referred to as the antigen. These cells migrate to the site of an immune response where they become actively involved in elimination of the pathogen. Afterward, the majority of lymphocytes die by apoptosis. However, a small number survive often for the lifespan of the host and are primed to respond rapidly in a highly efficient manner. This concept of immunological memory allows researchers to isolate and study the drug-specific lymphocyte response in patients with liver injury many years after the adverse event.

The clinical observation that certain forms of liver injury have a long delay in onset and sometimes occur rapidly on rechallenge forced early researchers to speculate that the adaptive immune system participates in the reaction. A number of review articles discuss the possible role of the adaptive immune system in drug-induced liver injury (e.g., [65, 66]); however, until recently, direct evidence of drug-specific T and/or B lymphocyte responses in patients has been lacking. Below we discuss how drugs activate lymphocytes, the discovery of specific HLA alleles as risk factors and specific drug examples where it has been possible to delve into patient blood and isolate and characterize antigen-specific lymphocyte responses.

3.1 HLA Alleles in Drug Hepatotoxicity

Hypersensitivity reactions to the antiviral drug abacavir were the first to be strongly associated with expression of a single human leukocyte antigen (HLA) allele, HLA-B*57:01 [67]. Very rapidly immunologically confirmed reactions to abacavir were shown to develop only in patients expressing this HLA allele [68]. The strength of the positive predictive value (100%) and negative predictive value (48%) led to the employment of a cost-effective pharmacogenetic test prior to abacavir use [69], which effectively prevents abacavir hypersensitivity. Over the past 10 years, genome-wide association studies have identified HLA associations with several drugs associated with liver injury (Fig. 2; e.g., ximelagatran [70], flucloxacillin [71], amoxicillin-clavulanate [72], ticlopidine

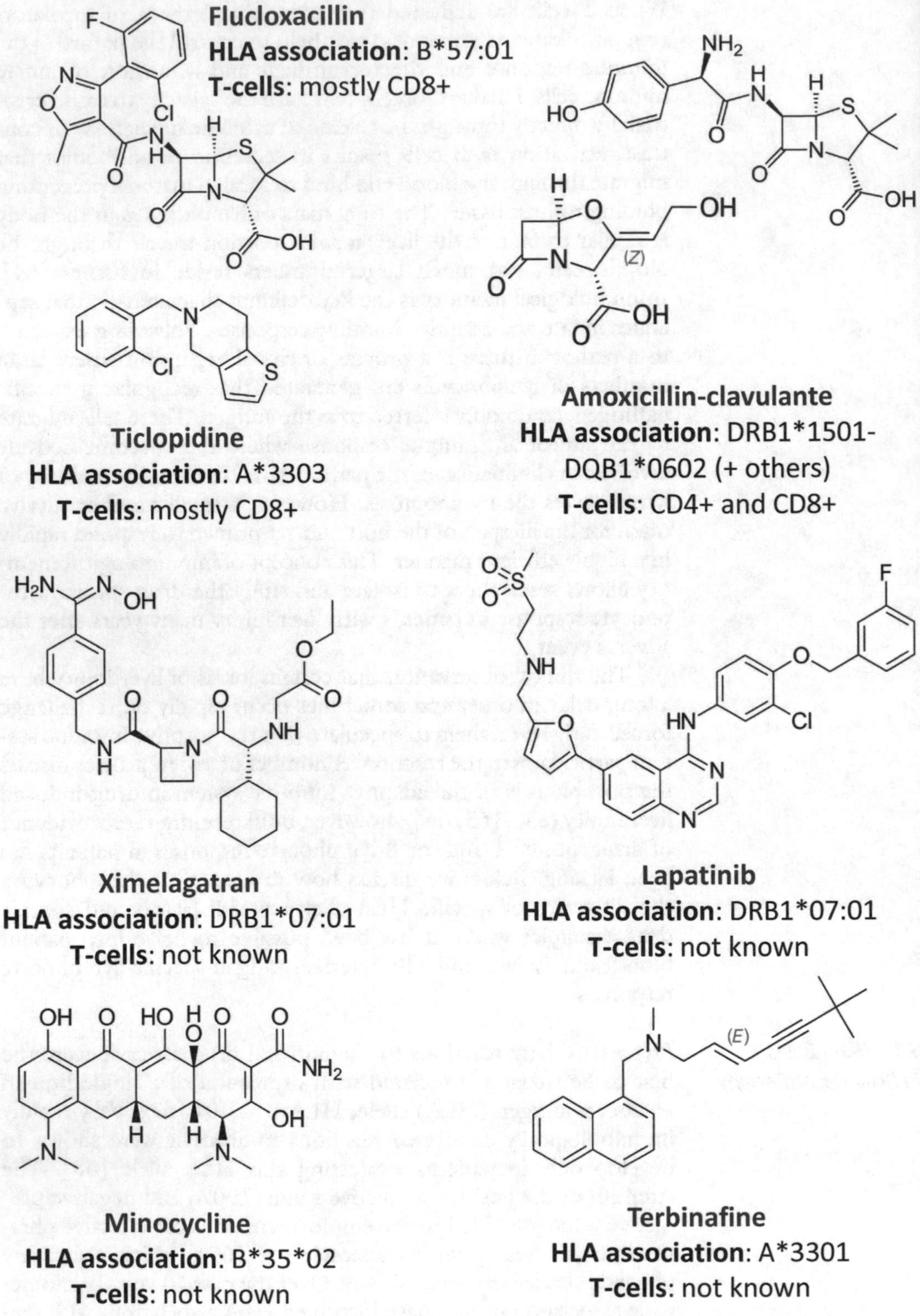

Fig. 2 Examples of several drugs that cause liver injury related to HLA associations

[73], lapatinib [74], minocycline [75], and terbinafine [76]). In most of these studies, carriage of the HLA allele was identified as a strong risk factor (i.e., most individuals with liver injury express the HLA allele); however, only small numbers of individuals expressing the HLA allele go on to develop liver injury when exposed to the culprit drug. For example, with flucloxacillin, only 1 in 500–1000 HLA-B*57:01 positive patients prescribed flucloxacillin will go on to develop liver injury [71]. As such, unlike abacavir, genotyping prior to drug use offers little benefit.

These genetic association studies suggest that drug-derived antigens bind selectively to protein encoded by the HLA allele to activate T cell responses that presumably participate in the adverse event (see detailed discussion below). However, it is important that future research explores why most drug-exposed individuals expressing HLA risk alleles do not develop liver injury. It is possible that environmental factors act synergistically with drug-induced stress signaling to activate the innate immune system and/or modulate costimulatory/coinhibitory signaling, to drive the antigen-specific T cell response in genetically predisposed individuals.

For a drug to activate T cells it must be presented to the T cell receptor in the context of major histocompatibility complex (MHC) molecules encoded by HLA alleles. Endogenous MHC molecules traditionally bind short peptides in a linear confirmation prior to display on the surface of antigen presenting cells and activation of T cells. In in vitro systems, drugs have been shown to interact directly with MHC peptide complexes expressed on the surface of antigen presenting cells to activate T cells [77, 78]. The nature of the drug MHC T-cell receptor binding interaction has not been fully defined and as such it is possible to develop multiple scenarios that explain how the combination of MHC molecule, drug and peptide trigger signal transduction events that result in T cell activation [79–81]. Drugs and drug metabolites also trigger T cell responses by binding irreversibly to non-MHC-associated protein through a hapten mechanism originally proposed by Landsteiner and Jacobs [82–84]. Protein processing within antigen presenting cells is thought to liberate T-cell stimulatory MHC binding drug-modified peptides. However, it is also possible that drug binding alters proteosomal processing of the protein with the subsequent T cell response being directed against novel peptide sequences.

3.2 T Lymphocytes in Drug Hepatotoxicity

Maria and Victorino [85] demonstrated that one could use the lymphocyte transformation test to detect drug-responsive T cells in the peripheral blood of approximately 50% of patients with drug-induced liver injury. Similar responses were not detected with peripheral blood mononuclear cells (PBMCs) from drug-tolerant controls or drug-naïve donors. The lymphocyte transformation test is a simple assay that uses proliferation as readout for T cell activation. PBMCs are cultured with drug and a positive control antigen for 5–6 days prior to addition of [³H]thymidine for the final 16 h of the experiment. A stimulation index (proliferation in test incubations/proliferation in control incubations) of two or more indicates the presence of drug-responsive memory T-cells in the patient. Similarly, Warrington found that the lymphocyte transformation test was positive in 85–95% of isoniazid liver injury cases [86, 87]. Unfortunately, in neither study was the nature of the T cell response studied.

3.2.1 Flucloxacillin Hepatotoxicity

Flucloxacillin is a β-lactam antibiotic associated with a high incidence of delayed-onset liver injury. Approximately 85% of patients with flucloxacillin-induced liver injury express HLA-B*57:01 [71], which suggests that the flucloxacillin antigen interacts selectively with the HLA-B*57:01 protein promoting T-cell responses. Flucloxacillin-specific T cells from blood of patients with liver injury have been isolated, cloned and characterized in terms of cellular phenotype and function. Drug-specific T-cells were for the most part CD8+ and the T cell response was MHC class I restricted and dependent on processing of a drug-derived protein adduct by antigen presenting cells [83, 84]. Flucloxacillin treatment of T cells resulted in the secretion of IFN-γ and cytolytic molecules.

Mass spectrometry has been used to show that flucloxacillin binds irreversibly to selective lysine residues on model proteins such as human serum albumin [88]. Moreover, flucloxacillin binds to multiple hepatic proteins in rodent models [89] and primary human hepatocytes (unpublished data). Thus, the search is on to identify and characterize the protein adducts and derived peptide fragments that stimulate the T cell response.

Flucloxacillin-specific CD8+ T-cell responses are also detectable using PBMC from drug-naïve donors expressing HLA-B*57:01 [77, 83, 90]. HLA-deficient cell lines transfected with HLA-B*57:01 and a panel of antigen presenting cells expressing different HLA B alleles were used to show that flucloxacillin does indeed interact selectively with HLA-B*57:01 to activate T cells. Immunohistochemical staining of a liver biopsy from a patient with flucloxacillin-induced liver injury showed the infiltration of granzyme B-secreting CD8+ T cells into the liver [91]; however, the way in which T cells participate in liver injury that manifests in patients remains to be addressed.

Burban et al. [92] have recently shown that flucloxacillin induces non-immune-mediated cholestatic features in human hepatocytes from HLA-B*57:01 negative and positive donors. Thus, it will be important to develop in vitro models to study how this direct effect of flucloxacillin impacts on its disposition and the provision of antigenic and stress signals to the adaptive and innate immune system, respectively.

3.2.2 Amoxicillin-Clavulanate Hepatotoxicity

The combination of amoxicillin and clavulanic acid is an effective treatment for a wide spectrum of bacterial infections including resistant bacteria that produce β-lactamase. The incidence of amoxicillin-clavulanate-induced liver injury has been estimated to be 1 in 2350 patients [93]. Since more than 70 million people in the USA alone are treated with amoxicillin-clavulanate, the drug combination represents one of the most common causes of drug-induced liver injury. Several HLA class I and II alleles are associated with an altered susceptibility to amoxicillin-clavulanate-mediated liver injury [94–96].

Amoxicillin-specific T cells are known to participate in amoxicillin-induced skin reactions [97]. Thus, it has been proposed clavulanic acid might skew or redirect the amoxicillin-specific T cells toward liver. To investigate this, we recently characterized the phenotype and drug-specificity of T cells cloned from patients with amoxicillin-clavulanate-mediated liver injury [98]. Amoxicillin- and clavulanic acid-responsive T cells were detected, but no cross-reactivity was observed with the two structurally diverse compounds that form distinct multiple haptenic structures in patients [99]. In contrast to flucloxacillin, amoxicillin- and clavulanic acid-derived antigens interact with multiple MHC class I and II molecules to activate T cells, with little apparent preference for those detected in genome-wide association studies.

3.2.3 Tuberculosis Medication Hepatotoxicity

A combination of isoniazid, rifampicin, pyrazinamide and/or ethambutol is commonly used for the treatment of tuberculosis. Drug treatment is associated with a mild elevation of liver enzymes in between 2 and 28% of patients that occasionally develops into liver failure. A strong association between expression of HLA alleles and susceptibility to liver injury has not been described. Since identification of the culprit drug is often difficult due to multiple medications being taken simultaneously we recently investigated whether drug-specific T cells were detectable in patients with liver injury [100, 101]. Isoniazid, but not the other antituberculosis drugs, was found to activate CD4+ T cell clones from patients with mild–moderate liver injury via an MHC class II-restricted pathway through the drug binding directly to MHC molecules. Somewhat surprisingly, T cells from a patient with fatal antituberculosis drug-mediated liver injury were activated with ethambutol and rifampicin, but not isoniazid. These data show that individual antituberculosis drugs each have the capacity to activate T cells and as such personalized treatment strategies for liver injury patients should be designed with care.

3.3 B Lymphocytes in Drug Hepatotoxicity

Halothane-induced hepatotoxicity is an immunological event thought to be initiated by oxidative metabolism of halothane. Blood from patients with hepatotoxicity contains B cell-derived IgG antibodies directed against microsomal proteins modified with a trifluoroacetyl halide metabolite [102–105]. The role of metabolic activation and protein binding in the hepatotoxicity of halothane is best illustrated by consideration of the relationship between the in vivo metabolism of general anesthetics and the observed incidence of the adverse drug reactions in humans (see [106] for a detailed discussion). The extent of metabolism correlates directly with the incidence of toxicity. Halothane-induced liver injury can be modeled in rodent systems [107–109], where CD4+ and CD8+ T are activated against trifluoroacetyl-modified proteins and eosinophils accumulate in liver and mediate the pathogenesis.

Metushi et al. [110, 111] identified a range of antidrug and autoantibodies in patients with isoniazid-induced liver failure. Antibodies were not detected in tolerant patients. The dominant isotype of the anti-isoniazid antibody was IgG, with IgG3 being most highly expressed. These studies suggest that B cells are selectively activated by drug-induced liver injury causing drugs and that IgG antibodies participate in the disease pathogenesis. However, it is unclear whether the antibodies are responsible for the tissue injury. It is equally likely that antibody binding negatively regulates the disease through neutralization (limiting the availability) of the T cell antigen or through other immune mechanisms.

3.4 Animal Models of Drug Hepatotoxicity Involving the Adaptive Immune System

Several mouse models of drug-induced hepatotoxicity have been developed to investigate the importance of immune components in the disease, but most do not mimic the clinical features seen in human patients (e.g., delayed onset). To address this, a CD4-deficient mouse strain has been used to study CD8+ T cell responses against flucloxacillin and whether activated T cells target hepatocytes [112]. CD8+ T cells from flucloxacillin-sensitized mice were stimulated to proliferate and secrete granzyme B in vitro when restimulated with the drug. Furthermore, T cell activation resulted in the killing of primary hepatocytes. Although oral exposure to flucloxacillin resulted in a marked swelling of the gall bladder, only mild elevations in alanine aminotransferase were observed.

An important advance in drug hepatotoxicity model development was recently presented by Uetrecht and coworkers. They have shown that blockade of immune checkpoints PD1 and CTLA4 prior to exposure to drugs (amodiaquine, isoniazid, nevirapine) leads to liver injury with similar characteristics to the human disease such as delayed onset and a mononuclear inflammatory infiltrate with necrosis [113–116]. Liver injury was not observed when drugs were administered without checkpoint inhibition, which provides strong evidence that immune regulatory mechanisms dampen unwanted immune responses to drugs in the animal model, but also potentially in human subjects. Further work should be conducted to characterize drug-specific T cells and how they contribute to the liver injury when activated. Furthermore, it will be interesting to see whether drugs associated with other forms in immunological reactions in humans cause unexpected liver injury in the animal model.

3.5 Conclusion and Future Directions Regarding the Adaptive Immune Response in Drug Hepatotoxicity

To summarize, components of the innate immune system are now believed to be activated in patients with DILI. Furthermore, there is an emerging body of evidence to suggest that severe cases of DILI involve the synergistic actions of the innate and adaptive immune systems to bring about the tissue injury. A comprehensive understanding of innate pathways activated by drugs and how these pathways promote adaptive immune responses is urgently needed. Only a few in vitro studies have attempted to explore the relationship between activation of the immune system and drug-induced hepatocyte death. Oda and colleagues developed a cell-based assay that evaluated immune and inflammatory gene expressions [117]. The human hepatoma HepaRG or HepG2 were exposed to 96 drugs and supernatants were then cultured with human promyelocytic neutrophil-derived cells (HL-60) followed by the evaluation of immune and inflammatory genes. Using an integrated score of S100 calcium-binding protein A9 (S100A9), IL-1β, and IL-8 gene expression, the authors successfully classified test drugs into positive and negative compounds. More recently, freshly isolated primary human hepatocytes have been used to characterize drug-specific signaling between the liver and innate immune cells [118]. Drug-treated primary human hepatocytes released damage associated molecular patterns, particularly HMGB1, in a drug- and dose-dependent manner. Furthermore, hepatocyte-conditioned media stimulated dendritic cells to secrete proinflammatory cytokines. Work is now urgently needed to explore whether it might be possible to develop these models systems to incorporate the adaptive immune system. The study of the cellular mechanisms of immune-mediated DILI in vitro requires a fully autologous system. To overcome this hurdle, an HLA-typed PBMC bank from 1000 healthy volunteers has been established [119], and cell culture methods to assess the immunogenicity of drugs has been developed [90, 120–122]. In the near future, it might be possible to incorporate iPS-derived hepatocyte-like cells from the same HLA-typed donors into immune assays.

Acknowledgments

The authors' laboratory was supported in part by the National Institutes of Health grants R01 DK070195 (to H.J.), and by grants P20 GM103549 and P30 GM118247 (to H.J.) from the National Institute of General Medical Sciences of the National Institutes of Health and the UK Medical Research Council (Centre for Drug Safety Science grant G0700654) (to D.J.N.).

References

1. Park BK, Boobis A, Clarke S, Goldring CE, Jones D, Kenna JG, Lambert C, Laverty HG, Naisbitt DJ, Nelson S, Nicoll-Griffith DA, Obach RS, Routledge P, Smith DA, Tweedie DJ, Vermeulen N, Williams DP, Wilson ID, Baillie TA (2011) Managing the challenge of chemically reactive metabolites in drug development. Nat Rev Drug Discov 10:292–306

2. Jaeschke H, McGill MR, Ramachandran A (2012) Oxidant stress, mitochondria, and cell death mechanisms in drug-induced liver injury: lessons learned from acetaminophen hepatotoxicity. Drug Metab Rev 44:88–106

3. Jaeschke H, Williams CD, Ramachandran A, Bajt ML (2012) Acetaminophen hepatotoxicity and repair: the role of sterile inflammation and innate immunity. Liver Int 32:8–20

4. Kubes P, Mehal WZ (2012) Sterile inflammation in the liver. Gastroenterology 143:1158–1172

5. Woolbright BL, Jaeschke H (2017) The impact of sterile inflammation in acute liver injury. J Clin Transl Res 3(Suppl 1):170–188

6. Uetrecht J, Naisbitt DJ (2013) Idiosyncratic adverse drug reactions: current concepts. Pharmacol Rev 65:779–808

7. Bogdanos DP, Gao B, Gershwin ME (2013) Liver immunology. Compr Physiol 3:567–598

8. Zimmermann HW, Trautwein C, Tacke F (2012) Functional role of monocytes and macrophages for the inflammatory response in acute liver injury. Front Physiol 3:56

9. Woolbright BL, Jaeschke H (2017) Role of the inflammasome in acetaminophen-induced liver injury and acute liver failure. J Hepatol 66:836–848

10. Larson AM, Polson J, Fontana RJ, Davern TJ, Lalani E, Hynan LS, Reisch JS, Schiødt FV, Ostapowicz G, Shakil AO, Lee WM, Acute Liver Failure Study Group (2005) Acetaminophen-induced acute liver failure: results of a United States multicenter, prospective study. Hepatology 42:1364–1372

11. Jaeschke H, Xie Y, McGill MR (2014) Acetaminophen-induced liver injury: from animal models to humans. J Clin Transl Hepatol 2:153–161

12. Petrasek J, Csak T, Szabo G (2013) Toll-like receptors in liver disease. Adv Clin Chem 59:155–201

13. Jaeschke H (1997) Cellular adhesion molecules: regulation and functional significance in the pathogenesis of liver diseases. Am J Physiol 273:G602–G611

14. Jaeschke H (2006) Mechanisms of liver injury. II. Mechanisms of neutrophil-induced liver cell injury during hepatic ischemia-reperfusion and other acute inflammatory conditions. Am J Physiol Gastrointest Liver Physiol 290:G1083–G1088

15. Antoine DJ, Williams DP, Kipar A, Jenkins RE, Regan SL, Sathish JG, Kitteringham NR, Park BK (2009) High-mobility group box-1 protein and keratin-18, circulating serum proteins informative of acetaminophen-induced necrosis and apoptosis in vivo. Toxicol Sci 112:521–531

16. Martin-Murphy BV, Holt MP, Ju C (2010) The role of damage associated molecular pattern molecules in acetaminophen-induced liver injury in mice. Toxicol Lett 192:387–394

17. McGill MR, Sharpe MR, Williams CD, Taha M, Curry SC, Jaeschke H (2012) The mechanism underlying acetaminophen-induced hepatotoxicity in humans and mice involves mitochondrial damage and nuclear DNA fragmentation. J Clin Invest 122:1574–1583

18. Kono H, Chen CJ, Ontiveros F, Rock KL (2010) Uric acid promotes an acute inflammatory response to sterile cell death in mice. J Clin Invest 120:1939–1949

19. Antoine DJ, Jenkins RE, Dear JW, Williams DP, McGill MR, Sharpe MR, Craig DG, Simpson KJ, Jaeschke H, Park BK (2012) Molecular forms of HMGB1 and keratin-18 as mechanistic biomarkers for mode of cell death and prognosis during clinical acetaminophen hepatotoxicity. J Hepatol 56:1070–1079

20. Lawson JA, Farhood A, Hopper RD, Bajt ML, Jaeschke H (2000) The hepatic inflammatory response after acetaminophen overdose: role of neutrophils. Toxicol Sci 54:509–516

21. James LP, Simpson PM, Farrar HC, Kearns GL, Wasserman GS, Blumer JL, Reed MD, Sullivan JE, Hinson JA (2005) Cytokines and toxicity in acetaminophen overdose. J Clin Pharmacol 45:1165–1171

22. Williams CD, Farhood A, Jaeschke H (2010) Role of caspase-1 and interleukin-1beta in acetaminophen-induced hepatic inflammation and liver injury. Toxicol Appl Pharmacol 247:169–178

23. Zhang C, Feng J, Du J, Zhuo Z, Yang S, Zhang W, Wang W, Zhang S, Iwakura Y, Meng G, Fu YX, Hou B, Tang H (2017) Macrophage-derived IL-1α promotes sterile inflammation in a mouse model of acetaminophen hepatotoxicity. Cell Mol Immunol. https://doi.org/10.1038/cmi.2017.22. [Epub ahead of print]

24. Dambach DM, Watson LM, Gray KR, Durham SK, Laskin DL (2002) Role of CCR2 in macrophage migration into the liver

during acetaminophen-induced hepatotoxicity in the mouse. Hepatology 35:1093–1103

25. Imaeda AB, Watanabe A, Sohail MA, Mahmood S, Mohamadnejad M, Sutterwala FS, Flavell RA, Mehal WZ (2009) Acetaminophen-induced hepatotoxicity in mice is dependent on Tlr9 and the Nalp3 inflammasome. J Clin Invest 119:305–314

26. Marques PE, Amaral SS, Pires DA, Nogueira LL, Soriani FM, Lima BH, Lopes GA, Russo RC, Avila TV, Melgaço JG, Oliveira AG, Pinto MA, Lima CX, De Paula AM, Cara DC, Leite MF, Teixeira MM, Menezes GB (2012) Chemokines and mitochondrial products activate neutrophils to amplify organ injury during mouse acute liver failure. Hepatology 56:1971–1982

27. Huebener P, Pradere JP, Hernandez C, Gwak GY, Caviglia JM, Mu X, Loike JD, Jenkins RE, Antoine DJ, Schwabe RF (2015) The HMGB1/RAGE axis triggers neutrophil-mediated injury amplification following necrosis. J Clin Invest 125:539–550

28. Blazka ME, Wilmer JL, Holladay SD, Wilson RE, Luster MI (1995) Role of proinflammatory cytokines in acetaminophen hepatotoxicity. Toxicol Appl Pharmacol 133:43–52

29. Boess F, Bopst M, Althaus R, Polsky S, Cohen SD, Eugster HP, Boelsterli UA (1998) Acetaminophen hepatotoxicity in tumor necrosis factor/lymphotoxin-alpha gene knockout mice. Hepatology 27:1021–1029

30. Gardner CR, Laskin JD, Dambach DM, Chiu H, Durham SK, Zhou P, Bruno M, Gerecke DR, Gordon MK, Laskin DL (2003) Exaggerated hepatotoxicity of acetaminophen in mice lacking tumor necrosis factor receptor-1. Potential role of inflammatory mediators. Toxicol Appl Pharmacol 192:119–130

31. Holt MP, Cheng L, Ju C (2008) Identification and characterization of infiltrating macrophages in acetaminophen-induced liver injury. J Leukoc Biol 84:1410–1421

32. Antoniades CG, Quaglia A, Taams LS, Mitry RR, Hussain M, Abeles R, Possamai LA, Bruce M, McPhail M, Starling C, Wagner B, Barnardo A, Pomplun S, Auzinger G, Bernal W, Heaton N, Vergani D, Thursz MR, Wendon J (2012) Source and characterization of hepatic macrophages in acetaminophen-induced acute liver failure in humans. Hepatology 56:735–746

33. Jaeschke H (2003) Molecular mechanisms of hepatic ischemia-reperfusion injury and preconditioning. Am J Physiol Gastrointest Liver Physiol 284:G15–G26

34. Jaeschke H, Fisher MA, Lawson JA, Simmons CA, Farhood A, Jones DA (1998) Activation of caspase 3 (CPP32)-like proteases is essential

for TNF-alpha-induced hepatic parenchymal cell apoptosis and neutrophil-mediated necrosis in a murine endotoxin shock model. J Immunol 160:3480–3486

35. Gujral JS, Farhood A, Bajt ML, Jaeschke H (2003) Neutrophils aggravate acute liver injury during obstructive cholestasis in bile duct-ligated mice. Hepatology 38:355–363

36. Bajt ML, Farhood A, Jaeschke H (2001) Effects of CXC chemokines on neutrophil activation and sequestration in hepatic vasculature. Am J Physiol Gastrointest Liver Physiol 281:G1188–G1195

37. Gujral JS, Hinson JA, Farhood A, Jaeschke H (2004) NADPH oxidase-derived oxidant stress is critical for neutrophil cytotoxicity during endotoxemia. Am J Physiol Gastrointest Liver Physiol 287:G243–G252

38. Hasegawa T, Malle E, Farhood A, Jaeschke H (2005) Generation of hypochlorite-modified proteins by neutrophils during ischemia-reperfusion injury in rat liver: attenuation by ischemic preconditioning. Am J Physiol Gastrointest Liver Physiol 289:G760–G767

39. Cover C, Liu J, Farhood A, Malle E, Waalkes MP, Bajt ML, Jaeschke H (2006) Pathophysiological role of the acute inflammatory response during acetaminophen hepatotoxicity. Toxicol Appl Pharmacol 216:98–107

40. Liu ZX, Han D, Gunawan B, Kaplowitz N (2006) Neutrophil depletion protects against murine acetaminophen hepatotoxicity. Hepatology 43:1220–1230

41. Williams CD, Bajt ML, Farhood A, Jaeschke H (2010) Acetaminophen-induced hepatic neutrophil accumulation and inflammatory liver injury in CD18-deficient mice. Liver Int 30:1280–1292

42. James LP, McCullough SS, Knight TR, Jaeschke H, Hinson JA (2003) Acetaminophen toxicity in mice lacking NADPH oxidase activity: role of peroxynitrite formation and mitochondrial oxidant stress. Free Radic Res 37:1289–1297

43. Williams CD, Bajt ML, Sharpe MR, McGill MR, Farhood A, Jaeschke H (2014) Neutrophil activation during acetaminophen hepatotoxicity and repair in mice and humans. Toxicol Appl Pharmacol 275:122–133

44. Jaeschke H, Liu J (2007) Neutrophil depletion protects against murine acetaminophen hepatotoxicity: another perspective. Hepatology 45:1588–1589

45. Bourdi M, Masubuchi Y, Reilly TP, Amouzadeh HR, Martin JL, George JW, Shah AG, Pohl LR (2002) Protection against acetaminophen-induced liver injury and

lethality by interleukin 10: role of inducible nitric oxide synthase. Hepatology 35:289–298

46. Du K, Ramachandran A, Jaeschke H (2016) Oxidative stress during acetaminophen hepatotoxicity: sources, pathophysiological role and therapeutic potential. Redox Biol 10:148–156

47. Duan L, Davis JS, Woolbright BL, Du K, Cahkraborty M, Weemhoff J, Jaeschke H, Bourdi M (2016) Differential susceptibility to acetaminophen-induced liver injury in substrains of C57BL/6 mice: 6N versus 6J. Food Chem Toxicol 98:107–118

48. Bourdi M, Davies JS, Pohl LR (2011) Mispairing C57BL/6 substrains of genetically engineered mice and wild-type controls can lead to confounding results as it did in studies of JNK2 in acetaminophen and concanavalin a liver injury. Chem Res Toxicol 24(6):794–796

49. Woolbright BL, McGill MR, Sharpe MR, Jaeschke H (2015) Persistent generation of inflammatory mediators after acetaminophen overdose in surviving and non-surviving patients (abstract). Hepatology 62:500A

50. Laskin DL, Pilaro AM (1986) Potential role of activated macrophages in acetaminophen hepatotoxicity. I. Isolation and characterization of activated macrophages from rat liver. Toxicol Appl Pharmacol 86:204–215

51. Laskin DL, Gardner CR, Price VF, Jollow DJ (1995) Modulation of macrophage functioning abrogates the acute hepatotoxicity of acetaminophen. Hepatology 21:1045–1050

52. Michael SL, Pumford NR, Mayeux PR, Niesman MR, Hinson JA (1999) Pretreatment of mice with macrophage inactivators decreases acetaminophen hepatotoxicity and the formation of reactive oxygen and nitrogen species. Hepatology 30:186–195

53. Knight TR, Jaeschke H (2004) Peroxynitrite formation and sinusoidal endothelial cell injury during acetaminophen-induced hepatotoxicity in mice. Comp Hepatol 3(Suppl 1):S46

54. Ito Y, Bethea NW, Abril ER, McCuskey RS (2003) Early hepatic microvascular injury in response to acetaminophen toxicity. Microcirculation 10:391–400

55. Ju C, Reilly TP, Bourdi M, Radonovich MF, Brady JN, George JW, Pohl LR (2002) Protective role of Kupffer cells in acetaminophen-induced hepatic injury in mice. Chem Res Toxicol 15:1504–1513

56. Williams CD, Antoine DJ, Shaw PJ, Benson C, Farhood A, Williams DP, Kanneganti TD, Park BK, Jaeschke H (2011) Role of the Nalp3 inflammasome in acetaminophen-induced sterile inflammation and liver injury. Toxicol Appl Pharmacol 252:289–297

57. Jaeschke H, Cover C, Bajt ML (2006) Role of caspases in acetaminophen-induced liver injury. Life Sci 78:1670–1676

58. You Q, Holt M, Yin H, Li G, Hu CJ, Ju C (2013) Role of hepatic resident and infiltrating macrophages in liver repair after acute injury. Biochem Pharmacol 86:836–843

59. Liu ZX, Govindarajan S, Kaplowitz N (2004) Innate immune system plays a critical role in determining the progression and severity of acetaminophen hepatotoxicity. Gastroenterology 127:1760–1774

60. Masson MJ, Carpenter LD, Graf ML, Pohl LR (2008) Pathogenic role of natural killer T and natural killer cells in acetaminophen-induced liver injury in mice is dependent on the presence of dimethyl sulfoxide. Hepatology 48:889–897

61. Martin-Murphy BV, Kominsky DJ, Orlicky DJ, Donohue TM Jr, Ju C (2013) Increased susceptibility of natural killer T-cell-deficient mice to acetaminophen-induced liver injury. Hepatology 57:1575–1584

62. Downs I, Aw TY, Liu J, Adegboyega P, Ajuebor MN (2012) Vα14iNKT cell deficiency prevents acetaminophen-induced acute liver failure by enhancing hepatic glutathione and altering APAP metabolism. Biochem Biophys Res Commun 428:245–251

63. Connolly MK, Ayo D, Malhotra A, Hackman M, Bedrosian AS, Ibrahim J, Cieza-Rubio NE, Nguyen AH, Henning JR, Dorvil-Castro M, Pachter HL, Miller G (2011) Dendritic cell depletion exacerbates acetaminophen hepatotoxicity. Hepatology 54:959–968

64. Alberts B, Wilson JH, Hunt T (2008) Molecular biology of the cell. Garland Science, New York

65. Adams DH, Ju C, Ramaiah SK, Uetrecht J, Jaeschke H (2010) Mechanisms of immune-mediated liver injury. Toxicol Sci 115:307–321

66. Uetrecht J (2009) Immunoallergic drug-induced liver injury in humans. Semin Liver Dis 29:383–392

67. Mallal S, Nolan D, Witt C, Masel G, Martin AM, Moore C, Sayer D, Castley A, Mamotte C, Maxwell D, James I, Christiansen FT (2002) Association between presence of HLA-B*5701, HLA-DR7, and HLA-DQ3 and hypersensitivity to HIV-1 reverse-transcriptase inhibitor abacavir. Lancet 359:727–732

68. Mallal S, Phillips E, Carosi G, Molina JM, Workman C, Tomazic J, Jagel-Guedes E, Rugina S, Kozyrev O, Cid JF, Hay P, Nolan D, Hughes S, Hughes A, Ryan S, Fitch N,

Thorborn D, Benbow A (2008) HLA-B*5701 screening for hypersensitivity to aba-cavir. N Engl J Med 358:568–579

69. Hughes DA, Vilar FJ, Ward CC, Alfirevic A, Park BK, Pirmohamed M (2004) Cost-effectiveness analysis of HLA B*5701 geno-typing in preventing abacavir hypersensitivity. Pharmacogenetics 14:335–342

70. Kindmark A, Jawaid A, Harbron CG, Barratt BJ, Bengtsson OF, Andersson TB, Carlsson S, Cederbrant KE, Gibson NJ, Armstrong M, Lagerstrom-Fermer ME, Dellsen A, Brown EM, Thornton M, Dukes C, Jenkins SC, Firth MA, Harrod GO, Pinel TH, Billing-Clason SM, Cardon LR, March RE (2008) Genome-wide pharmacogenetic investigation of a hepatic adverse event without clinical signs of immunopathology suggests an underlying immune pathogenesis. Pharmacogenomics J 8:186–195

71. Daly AK, Donaldson PT, Bhatnagar P, Shen Y, Pe'er I, Floratos A, Daly MJ, Goldstein DB, John S, Nelson MR, Graham J, Park BK, Dillon JF, Bernal W, Cordell HJ, Pirmohamed M, Aithal GP, Day CP (2009) HLA-B*5701 genotype is a major determinant of drug-induced liver injury due to flucloxacillin. Nat Genet 41:816–819

72. Lucena MI, Molokhia M, Shen Y, Urban TJ, Aithal GP, Andrade RJ, Day CP, Ruiz-Cabello F, Donaldson PT, Stephens C, Pirmohamed M, Romero-Gomez M, Navarro JM, Fontana RJ, Miller M, Groome M, Bondon-Guitton E, Conforti A, Stricker BH, Carvajal A, Ibanez L, Yue QY, Eichelbaum M, Floratos A, Pe'er I, Daly MJ, Goldstein DB, Dillon JF, Nelson MR, Watkins PB, Daly AK, Spanish, Eudragene, Dilin, Diligen, and S. International (2011) Susceptibility to amoxicillin-clavulanate-induced liver injury is influenced by multiple HLA class I and II alleles. Gastroenterology 141:338–347

73. Hirata K, Takagi H, Yamamoto M, Matsumoto T, Nishiya T, Mori K, Shimizu S, Masumoto H, Okutani Y (2008) Ticlopidine-induced hepatotoxicity is associated with specific human leukocyte antigen genomic subtypes in Japanese patients: a prelimi-nary case-control study. Pharmacogenomics J 8:29–33

74. Spraggs CF, Budde LR, Briley LP, Bing N, Cox CJ, King KS, Whittaker JC, Mooser VE, Preston AJ, Stein SH, Cardon LR (2011) HLA-DQA1*02:01 is a major risk factor for lapatinib-induced hepatotoxicity in women with advanced breast cancer. J Clin Oncol 29:667–673

75. Urban TJ, Nicoletti P, Chalasani N, Serrano J, Stolz A, Daly AK, Aithal GP, Dillon J, Navarro V, Odin J, Barnhart H, Ostrov D, Long N, Cirulli ET, Watkins PB, Fontana N, Drug-Induced Liver Injury, g. Pharmacogenetics of Drug-Induced Liver Injury. International Serious Adverse Events (2017) Minocycline hepatotoxicity: clinical characterization and identification of HLA-B *35:02 as a risk fac-tor. J Hepatol 67:137–144

76. Nicoletti P, Aithal GP, Bjornsson ES, Andrade RJ, Sawle A, Arrese M, Barnhart HX, Bondon-Guitton E, Hayashi PH, Bessone F, Carvajal A, Cascorbi I, Cirulli ET, Chalasani N, Conforti A, Coulthard SA, Daly MJ, Day CP, Dillon JF, Fontana RJ, Grove JI, Hallberg P, Hernandez N, Ibanez L, Kullak-Ublick GA, Laitinen T, Larrey D, Lucena MI, Maitland-van der Zee AH, Martin JH, Molokhia M, Pirmohamed M, Powell ME, Qin S, Serrano J, Stephens C, Stolz A, Wadelius M, Watkins PB, Floratos A, Shen Y, Nelson MR, Urban TJ, Daly AK, I. L. I. N. I. International Drug-Induced Liver Injury Consortium. International Serious Adverse Events (2017) Association of liver injury from specific drugs, or groups of drugs, with polymorphisms in HLA and other genes in a genome-wide association study. Gastroenterology 152:1078–1089

77. Wuillemin N, Adam J, Fontana S, Krahenbuhl S, Pichler WJ, Yerly D (2013) HLA haplotype determines hapten or p-i T cell reactivity to flucloxacillin. J Immunol 190:4956–4964

78. Yun J, Marcaida MJ, Eriksson KK, Jamin H, Fontana S, Pichler WJ, Yerly D (2014) Oxypurinol directly and immediately acti-vates the drug-specific T cells via the pref-erential use of HLA-B*58:01. J Immunol 192:2984–2993

79. Pichler WJ, Hausmann O (2016) Classification of drug hypersensitivity into allergic, p-i, and pseudo-allergic forms. Int Arch Allergy Immunol 171:166–179

80. Pichler WJ, Adam J, Watkins S, Wuillemin N, Yun J, Yerly D (2015) Drug hypersensitivity: how drugs stimulate T cells via pharmacologi-cal interaction with immune receptors. Int Arch Allergy Immunol 168:13–24

81. Pavlos R, Mallal S, Ostrov D, Buus S, Metushi I, Peters B, Phillips E (2015) T cell-mediated hypersensitivity reactions to drugs. Annu Rev Med 66:439–454

82. Landsteiner K, Jacobs J (1935) Studies on the sensitization of animals with simple chemical compounds. J Exp Med 61:643–656

83. Monshi MM, Faulkner L, Gibson A, Jenkins RE, Farrell J, Earnshaw CJ, Alfirevic A, Cederbrant K, Daly AK, French N, Pirmohamed M, Park BK, Naisbitt DJ (2013) Human leukocyte antigen (HLA)-B*57:01-restricted activation of drug-specific

T cells provides the immunological basis for flucloxacillin-induced liver injury. Hepatology 57:727–739

84. Yaseen FS, Saide K, Kim SH, Monshi M, Tailor A, Wood S, Meng X, Jenkins R, Faulkner L, Daly AK, Pirmohamed M, Park BK, Naisbitt DJ (2015) Promiscuous T-cell responses to drugs and drug-haptens. J Allergy Clin Immunol 136:474–476

85. Maria VA, Victorino RM (1997) Diagnostic value of specific T cell reactivity to drugs in 95 cases of drug induced liver injury. Gut 41:534–540

86. Warrington RJ, McPhilips-Feener S, Rutherford WJ (1982) The predictive value of the lymphocyte transformation test in isoniazid-associated hepatitis. Clin Allergy 12:217–222

87. Warrington RJ, Tse KS, Gorski BA, Schwenk R, Sehon AH (1978) Evaluation of isoniazid-associated hepatitis by immunological tests. Clin Exp Immunol 32:97–104

88. Jenkins RE, Meng X, Elliott VL, Kitteringham NR, Pirmohamed M, Park BK (2009) Characterisation of flucloxacillin and 5-hydroxymethyl flucloxacillin haptenated HSA in vitro and in vivo. Proteomics Clin Appl 3:720–729

89. Carey MA, van Pelt FN (2005) Immunochemical detection of flucloxacillin adduct formation in livers of treated rats. Toxicology 216:41–48

90. Faulkner L, Gibson A, Sullivan A, Tailor A, Usui T, Alfirevic A, Pirmohamed M, Naisbitt DJ, Park BK (2016) Detection of primary T cell responses to drugs and chemicals in HLA-typed volunteers: implications for the prediction of drug immunogenicity. Toxicol Sci 154:416–429

91. Wuillemin N, Terracciano L, Beltraminelli H, Schlapbach C, Fontana S, Krahenbuhl S, Pichler WJ, Yerly D (2014) T cells infiltrate the liver and kill hepatocytes in HLA-B(*)57:01-associated floxacillin-induced liver injury. Am J Pathol 184:1677–1682

92. Burban A, Sharanek A, Hue R, Gay M, Routier S, Guillouzo A, Guguen-Guillouzo C (2017) Penicillinase-resistant antibiotics induce non-immune-mediated cholestasis through HSP27 activation associated with PKC/P38 and PI3K/AKT signaling pathways. Sci Rep 7:1815

93. Bjornsson ES, Bergmann OM, Bjornsson HK, Kvaran RB, Olafsson S (2013) Incidence, presentation, and outcomes in patients with drug-induced liver injury in the general population of Iceland. Gastroenterology 144:1419–1425

94. Stephens C, Lopez-Nevot MA, Ruiz-Cabello F, Ulzurrun E, Soriano G, Romero-Gomez M, Moreno-Casares A, Lucena MI, Andrade RJ (2013) HLA alleles influence the clinical signature of amoxicillin-clavulanate hepatotoxicity. PLoS One 8:e68111

95. Lucena MI, Molokhia M, Shen Y, Urban TJ, Aithal GP, Andrade RJ, Day CP, Ruiz-Cabello F, Donaldson PT, Stephens C, Pirmohamed M, Romero-Gomez M, Navarro JM, Fontana RJ, Miller M, Groome M, Bondon-Guitton E, Conforti A, Stricker BH, Carvajal A, Ibanez L, Yue QY, Eichelbaum M, Floratos A, Pe'er I, Daly MJ, Goldstein DB, Dillon JF, Nelson MR, Watkins PN, Daly AK (2011) Susceptibility to amoxicillin-clavulanate-induced liver injury is influenced by multiple HLA class I and II alleles. Gastroenterology 141:338–347

96. Donaldson PT, Daly AK, Henderson J, Graham J, Pirmohamed M, Bernal W, Day CP, Aithal GP (2010) Human leucocyte antigen class II genotype in susceptibility and resistance to co-amoxiclav-induced liver injury. J Hepatol 53:1049–1053

97. Rozieres A, Hennino A, Rodet K, Gutowski MC, Gunera-Saad N, Berard F, Cozon G, Bienvenu J, Nicolas JF (2009) Detection and quantification of drug-specific T cells in penicillin allergy. Allergy 64:534–542

98. Kim SH, Saide K, Farrell J, Faulkner L, Tailor A, Ogese M, Daly AK, Pirmohamed M, Park BK, Naisbitt DJ (2015) Characterization of amoxicillin- and clavulanic acid-specific T cells in patients with amoxicillin-clavulanate-induced liver injury. Hepatology 62:887–899

99. Meng X, Earnshaw CJ, Tailor A, Jenkins RE, Waddington JC, Whitaker P, French NS, Naisbitt DJ, Park BK (2016) Amoxicillin and clavulanate form chemically and immunologically distinct multiple haptenic structures in patients. Chem Res Toxicol 29:1762–1772

100. Usui T, Meng X, Saide K, Farrell J, Thomson P, Whitaker P, Watson J, French NS, Park BK, Naisbitt DJ (2017) Characterization of isoniazid-specific T-cell clones in patients with anti-tuberculosis drug-related liver and skin injury. Toxicol Sci 155:420–431

101. Usui T, Whitaker P, Meng X, Watson J, Antoine DJ, French NS, Park BK, Naisbitt DJ (2016) Detection of drug-responsive T-lymphocytes in a case of fatal antituberculosis drug-related liver injury. Chem Res Toxicol 29:1793–1795

102. Kenna JG, Knight TL, van Pelt FN (1993) Immunity to halothane metabolite-modified proteins in halothane hepatitis. Ann N Y Acad Sci 685:646–661

103. Pohl LR, Thomassen D, Pumford NR, Butler LE, Satoh H, Ferrans VJ, Perrone A, Martin BM, Martin JL (1990) Hapten carrier con-

jugates associated with halothane hepatitis. In: Witmer RRSCM, Jollow DJ, Kalf GF, Kocsis JJ, Sipes IG (eds) Biological reactive intermediates IV. Plenum Press, New York, pp 111–120

104. Satoh H, Martin BM, Schulick AH, Christ DD, Kenna JG, Pohl LR (1989) Human anti-endoplasmic reticulum antibodies in sera of patients with halothane-induced hepatitis are directed against a trifluoroacetylated carboxylesterase. Proc Natl Acad Sci U S A 86:322–326

105. Kenna JG, Neuberger J, Williams R (1988) Evidence for expression in human liver of halothane-induced neoantigens recognized by antibodies in sera from patients with halothane hepatitis. Hepatology 8:1635–1641

106. Park BK, Pirmohamed M, Kitteringham NR (1998) Role of drug disposition in drug hypersensitivity: a chemical, molecular and clinical perspective. Chem Res Toxicol 9:969–988

107. Proctor WR, Chakraborty M, Chea LS, Morrison JC, Berkson JD, Semple K, Bourdi M, Pohl LR (2013) Eosinophils mediate the pathogenesis of halothane-induced liver injury in mice. Hepatology 57:2026–2036

108. Uetrecht J, Kaplowitz N (2015) Inhibition of immune tolerance unmasks drug-induced allergic hepatitis. Hepatology 62:346–348

109. You Q, Cheng L, Ju C (2010) Generation of T cell responses targeting the reactive metabolite of halothane in mice. Toxicol Lett 194:79–85

110. Metushi IG, Lee WM, Uetrecht J (2014) IgG3 is the dominant subtype of anti-isoniazid antibodies in patients with isoniazid-induced liver failure. Chem Res Toxicol 27:738–740

111. Metushi IG, Sanders C, Lee WM, Uetrecht J (2014) Detection of anti-isoniazid and anti-cytochrome P450 antibodies in patients with isoniazid-induced liver failure. Hepatology 59:1084–1093

112. Nattrass R, Faulkner L, Vocanson M, Antoine DJ, Kipar A, Kenna G, Nicolas JF, Park BK, Naisbitt DJ (2015) Activation of flucloxacillin-specific CD8+ T-cells with the potential to promote hepatocyte cytotoxicity in a mouse model. Toxicol Sci 146:146–156

113. Liu F, Cai P, Metushi I, Li J, Nakayawa T, Vega L, Uetrecht J (2016) Exploring an animal model of amodiaquine-induced liver injury in rats and mice. J Immunotoxicol 13:694–712

114. Mak A, Uetrecht J (2015) The combination of anti-CTLA-4 and PD1−/− mice unmasks the potential of isoniazid and nevirapine to cause liver injury. Chem Res Toxicol 28:2287–2291

115. Mak A, Uetrecht J (2015) The role of CD8 T cells in amodiaquine-induced liver injury in PD1−/− mice cotreated with anti-CTLA-4. Chem Res Toxicol 28:1567–1573

116. Metushi IG, Hayes MA, Uetrecht J (2015) Treatment of PD-1(−/−) mice with amodiaquine and anti-CTLA4 leads to liver injury similar to idiosyncratic liver injury in patients. Hepatology 61:1332–1342

117. Oda S, Matsuo K, Nakajima A, Yokoi T (2016) A novel cell-based assay for the evaluation of immune- and inflammatory-related gene expression as biomarkers for the risk assessment of drug-induced liver injury. Toxicol Lett 241:60–70

118. Ogese MO, Faulkner L, Jenkins RE, French NS, Copple IM, Antoine DJ, Elmasry M, Malik H, Goldring CE, Park BK, Betts C, Naisbitt DJ (2017) Characterisation of drug-specific signalling between primary human hepatocytes and immune cells. Toxicol Sci 158(1):76–89

119. Alfirevic A, Gonzalez-Galarza F, Bell C, Martinsson K, Platt V, Bretland G, Evely J, Lichtenfels M, Cederbrant K, French N, Naisbitt D, Park BK, Jones AR, Pirmohamed M (2012) In silico analysis of HLA associations with drug-induced liver injury: use of a HLA-genotyped DNA archive from healthy volunteers. Genome Med 4:51

120. Faulkner L, Martinsson K, Santoyo-Castelazo A, Cederbrant K, Schuppe-Koistinen I, Powell H, Tugwood J, Naisbitt DJ, Park BK (2012) The development of in vitro culture methods to characterize primary T-cell responses to drugs. Toxicol Sci 127:150–158

121. Gibson A, Ogese M, Sullivan A, Wang E, Saide K, Whitaker P, Peckham D, Faulkner L, Park BK, Naisbitt DJ (2014) Negative regulation by PD-L1 during drug-specific priming of IL-22-secreting T cells and the influence of PD-1 on effector T cell function. J Immunol 192:2611–2621

122. Gibson A, Faulkner L, Lichtenfels M, Ogese M, Al-Attar Z, Alfirevic A, Esser PR, Martin SF, Pirmohamed M, Park BK, Naisbitt DJ (2017) The effect of inhibitory signals on the priming of drug hapten-specific T cells that express distinct vbeta receptors. J Immunol 199:1223–1237

Chapter 26

Translational and Mechanistic Biomarkers of Drug-Induced Liver Injury – Candidates and Qualification Strategies

Daniel J. Antoine

Abstract

Drug-induced liver injury (DILI) represents a major medical concern associated with significant patient morbidity and mortality. However, currently used biomarkers are insufficient, not fit for purpose and lack sensitivity and specificity. Recently studies from preclinical and clinical DILI have revealed candidates that hold transformative potential for the sensitive identification of DILI and its prognostic assessment. Promising biomarkers provide increased hepatic specificity (miR-122), mechanistic insight (Keratin-18), and prognostic information (HMGB1, KIM-1, CSF-1). Moreover, given their inherent mechanistic basis, these candidate biomarkers have led to promising mechanism-based therapeutic interventions. Such candidate molecules have recently received regulatory endorsement and their further qualification is to be assessed in formal clinical trial settings. Here the integrated use of such candidates is discussed with respect to roadblocks to clinical adoption and their use for understanding fundamental hepatic drug safety science to improve patient safety.

Key words Acetaminophen, DILI, Hepatotoxicity, Qualification, Sensitivity, Specificity, Validation

1 Introduction

Drug-induced liver injury (DILI) represents a major medical concern associated with significant patient morbidity and mortality. Within drug development, attrition due to DILI occurs in all phases of the pipeline, from preclinical testing to clinical trials, to the marketplace. In cases where the frequency is high in either animal species or in humans, DILI is considered "intrinsic" in that it is assumed to result from direct hepatocellular damage [1]. Acetaminophen (paracetamol) induced liver injury is a well cited example here. However, another concerning manifestation of DILI, termed "idiosyncratic," occurs very rarely in susceptible individuals exposed to therapeutic doses [2]. Idiosyncratic DILI is difficult to predict due to the complex nature of the mechanisms of the disease and is one of most feared adverse drug reactions.

Minjun Chen and Yvonne Will (eds.), *Drug-Induced Liver Toxicity*, Methods in Pharmacology and Toxicology,
https://doi.org/10.1007/978-1-4939-7677-5_26, © Springer Science+Business Media, LLC, part of Springer Nature 2018

The prediction of DILI in humans from preclinical models remains difficult, particularly in cases characterized by marked interindividual variation. To date, only a relatively small number of blood-based tests are used to assess DILI while the assessment of DILI in preclinical drug development is heavily dependent upon hepatic histological interpretation [3]. For causality assessment, different tools such as the Roussel Uclaf Causality Assessment Method (RUCAM) or Maria and Victorino score are available that provide a robust initial assessment. However, consensus within the community is that "Expert Opinion" is the current gold standard [4]. A lack of sensitivity, specificity and an indirect mechanistic basis of currently used biomarkers of hepatic injury remains a factor for the delayed identification of DILI. The potential of novel mechanistic biomarkers to improve the prediction of DILI is widely acknowledged and significant investment and progress has been made in this area [5–7].

2 Methods

2.1 Current Biomarkers and Methods to Assess DILI

The US National Institute of Health (NIH) defined a biomarker (for example an oligonucleotide, protein or metabolite) in 2001 as a characteristic that is objectively measured and evaluated as an indicator of normal biological process, a pathogenic process or a pharmacological response to a therapeutic intervention [8]. Biomarkers can be subdivided according to their intended use and function (Table 1). Biomarkers have also been classified by the US Food and Drug Administration (FDA) as exploratory, probable valid and known valid to aid the qualification process (see later) [9].

- Known valid biomarker—a biomarker that is measured in an analytical test system with well-established performance characteristics. A biomarker for which there is widespread agreement in the medical or scientific community about the physiological, toxicological, pharmacological, or clinical significance of the results

- Probable valid biomarker—as above but a probable valid biomarker may not have reached the status of a known valid biomarker because, for example, any one of the following reasons:

  - Data elucidating significance may have been generated within a single company and may not be publically available for scientific scrutiny

  - The data, although highly suggestive, may not be conclusive

  - Independent verification of the results may not have occurred

Table 1
Biomarker classification and relevance to DILI

Biomarker type	Definition and relevance to DILI
Screening	Early detection of phenotype in general or at risk population
Diagnostic	Definition of phenotype subtype, stage, grade
Prognostic	Definition of likely phenotype course and hence appropriate therapeutic approach
Predictive	In vitro, in vivo, or patient enrichment to maximize benefit from specific therapy
Pharmacological/ toxicological	Demonstrate active therapy concentration at site, therapy-target interaction (PD/ TD—Proof of mechanism), phenotypic effect (PD/TD—Proof of concept)
Surrogate response	Early prediction of ultimate efficacy and safety

- Exploratory biomarker—a biomarker that does not match either of the above categories

Since the publishing of these criteria, recommendations have been set to avoid confusion that the term "validation" should refer to the technical characterization and documentation of methodological performances, and the term "qualification" refer to the evidentiary process of linking a biomarker to a clinical end point or biological process [10].

DILI is categorized into hepatocellular (injury predominantly to hepatocytes), cholestatic (injury to bile ducts or affecting bile flow) or mixed (hepatocellular and cholestatic injury). The R-value is the main metric for phenotypic assessment of DILI and is based on the measurement of the enzymes alkaline phosphatase (ALP) and alanine aminotransferase (ALT) in blood and their ratio to the upper limits of normal (ULN). Hepatocellular is classified with an R-value ≥ 5 [ALT/ULN $\div$ ALP/ULN], cholestatic with an R-value ≤ 2 and mixed-type injury with an R-value of 2–5.

Currently, blood-based markers such as ALT are often combined with the liver-specific functional assessment of the clearance of total bilirubin (TBL) as part of Hy's law. Hy Zimmerman first noted that a patient who presents with jaundice as a result of hepatocellular DILI has at least a 10% chance of developing ALF, regardless of which drug has caused the hepatocellular injury [11]. Hy's law is currently the only accepted regulatory model to assess significant, acute DILI [12–14]. Staffs at the FDA have developed a liver safety data management tool call eDISH (evaluation of Drug-Induced Serious Liver Injury) which involves data visualization by plotting the peak serum ALT versus the peak serum TBL for each subject in a clinical trial [14]. Although eDISH has revolutionized the standardization and transparent means of displaying and organizing relevant liver safety data from a clinical trial, it remains limited by its reliance on Hy's law although various modified eDISH plots have been proposed to take into account the temporal relationship of peak values and R value amongst other variables [15–17]. In the context of hepatocellular DILI, TBL most likely only rises once there has been a substantial loss of functioning hepatocytes, placing the patient in danger of liver failure. Therefore, at the individual patient level, serum TBL is not a biomarker that predicts severe toxicity potential, but instead a confirmation that severe hepatotoxicity has occurred.

Although ALT activity is widely used, it is not without its limitations for the assessment of human DILI. Changes in ALT activity are not specific for DILI and can occur in a number of disease processes, including viral hepatitis, fatty liver disease, and liver cancer [18]. Nor are elevations in the aminotransferases unique to liver injury since increases in ALT in circulation can also result from myocardial damage, muscle damage or extreme exercise. The methods used to quantify ALT activity have not been standardized and a robust definition of normal reference ranges have not been agreed upon; these ranges inevitably depend upon the population group defined as normal and assay measurements will vary between laboratories. Although ALT activity is regarded as generally sensitive for detecting liver injury when it occurs, it is not sensitive with respect to time/kinetics. Furthermore, ALT activity has often been described as having little prognostic value due to the fact that an ALT elevation represents probable injury to the liver after it has occurred. From the regulatory point of view, elevations in ALT activity are also worrisome with respect to establishing liver safety during drug treatment. Frequent and relatively large elevations in ALT activity are associated with treatments that do not pose a clinical liver safety issue, such as heparins and tacrine [19, 20]. The challenge here is to distinguish between benign elevations in ALT activity and the potential for a serious DILI outcome. However, despite their shortcomings, the combined approach of ALT and TBL represent the current standard any novel biomarker must surpass or provide added value.

2.2 Statistical Considerations

It has been widely acknowledged that one of the most powerful tools to assess the performance of a biomarker is through the Receiver Operator Characteristic (ROC) analysis. The concept originated based on the analyses of radar signals for detecting enemy airplanes during World War II when it was vital to determine how far a plane was and if in fact the signal detected was a plane. Later these concepts have been applied to many medical fields for the performance evaluation of a biomarker. The test relies on determining the trade-off between sensitivity (the ability of a biomarker to correctly identify toxicity when it occurs) and specificity (the ability of a biomarker to correctly identify individuals who do not have toxicity). An area under the curve (AUC) can be generated by plotting sensitivity against 1-specificity for a range of changing thresholds which can be used to directly compare biomarkers. Although widely used, there are some important considerations which need to be thought through when applied these analyses to toxicological research. Care should be taken to consider incidence (new finding) or prevalence (present finding) of the effect being sought by the test or biomarker. A test that looks powerful for high incidence/prevalence is not always strong when used to look for rare events such as idiosyncratic DILI.

Given concerns surrounding the prevalence of the event to impact on the performance power of a biomarker, additional metrics such as the negative (proportion of subjects with negative test that are correctly diagnosed) and positive (precision rate or proportion of positive test results that are true positives) predictive value are useful tools to aid interpretation. Therefore, if a biomarker is going to be useful in general, you would expect that the proportion of times it predicts a subject to reach a predefined primary end point or gold standard would be similar to the proportion of subjects who actually reach this end point; Moreover the proportion of times the biomarker predicts a subject not to have the primary end point would be similar to the proportion who actually do not have the primary end point.

Over the past decade, investigators have become familiar the ROC AUC as it is easy to interpret. An AUC of 1 characterizes perfect discrimination between the patients with toxicity and those without and therefore all patients are correctly classified by that particular biomarker. An AUC of 0.5 demonstrates that the biomarker provides no discrimination between toxicity and not and therefore patients are correctly classified no more frequently than random chance. One disadvantage with the AUC is that it is an insensitive measure of the ability of a new marker to add value to a preexisting risk prediction model; it does not provide good information on whether adding this biomarker to the other relevant diagnostic information will more accurately identify individual risk. This is particularly important given that serum ALT and total bilirubin are widely used. Two new metrics, the integrated discrimination improvement (IDI) and net reclassification improvement (NRI), have recently been introduced to assess the added value of a candidate biomarker to preexisting risk prediction models. In the context of acute kidney injury [21], these methodologies have provided significant added value to determine the clinical utility of novel biomarkers that have undergone preclinical qualification [22, 23]. However, the application and utility has still not been investigated within the context of DILI.

2.3 Qualification Considerations

As previously mentioned, the term "qualification" refers to the evidentiary process of linking a biomarker to a clinical end point or biological process. However, until recently there has been no systematic scientific qualification strategy or guidance in place allowing for the accumulation of sufficient clinical and biological evidence for the acceptance of a biomarker independent of a specific drug. Regulatory agencies have now established submission procedures for the regulatory review and endorsement of biomarker qualification, but have not yet defined the scientific standards and approaches needed. The first submission of kidney safety biomarkers by the Predictive Safety Testing Consortium (PSTC) [3] also opened the door to a new framework of fit-for-purpose qualification of biomarkers instead of having an absolute "all or nothing" qualification. With more data and evidence the limited context can be extended. This principle has been referred to as "incremental," "progressive," or "rolling" qualification. Critical to this is the concept of the qualification of a biomarker within a defined context of use (COU). The COU is a statement that describes the manner and purpose of use for the biomarker in a defined situation or within a drug development process. Any supporting data and analysis undertaken during a biomarker qualification process and submission to regulators determines the appropriateness of the proposed qualified COU.

There have been recently published frameworks by consortia and regulators regarding the development of translational safety biomarkers and other drug developmental tools [10]. These frameworks described the critical interaction and interaction between sponsors and regulators to enable the qualification of a proposed biomarker within a prospectively defined COU. Broadly, the qualification process consists of three stages: (1) initiation, (2) consultation and advice stage, and (3) a review stage for the qualification determination. The ultimate goal of the process is to reach a consensus about the suitability of the submitted data to support qualification within a COU. Importantly, there is room to evolve the intended use of the biomarker as scientific advances are made or as clinical/drug developmental need changes. If a biomarker is qualified for a specific use, the COU may be modified or expanded over time.

Given the effort and time required to reach qualification, an important advance in the field and critical to the aforementioned concept of rolling qualification is the regulatory letter of support initiative. A letter of support is issued to a sponsor that briefly describes the regulators opinions on the potential value of a biomarker and encourages its further evaluation and development. The letter does not endorse a specific biomarker but is meant to enhance its visibility, encourage data sharing, and stimulate additional studies to enable the qualification process in a precompetitive collaborative way.

3   Results

3.1   Novel DILI Biomarkers: Current Needs and Knowledge Gaps

There is a current need for new biomarkers to assess the safety of new or existing medicines, especially for DILI. However, the development and clinical integration of potential hepatic biomarkers over the past 60 years has revealed only a limited number of candidates [24]. This concept is perhaps not so surprising given the fact that less focus has been placed on the science of drug safety and the rigorous guidelines we impose on the validation and biological qualification of a potential DILI biomarker [3, 10] compared to drug efficacy [12]. Furthermore, the delayed qualification and ultimate scientific acceptance of a potential DILI biomarker has been hindered by what has been previously thought of as the competing interests between the various stakeholders. Safety assessment within drug development has traditionally focused on reliable clinical–preclinical concordance. Low baseline variability, specificity, and rapid analysis are sought after by clinicians and the ability to provide enhanced mechanistic understanding about toxicological processes is required by the academic community. Public–private consortia were developed to meet this goal consisting of leading academic groups, large pharmaceutical companies, small-medium enterprises, and clinical units of excellence. These consortia include the Predictive Safety Testing Consortium (PSTC) (www.c-path.org/pstc.cfm) and the Safer and Faster Evidence-based Translation (SAFE-T) consortium (www.imi-safe-t.eu). These consortia efforts, coupled with feedback and representation from regulatory authorities as external members and advisors, provide an opportunity for collaborative efforts to aid the identification, validation and qualification of novel translation safety biomarkers (TSBM) for DILI [10]. Due to the multifactorial nature of DILI, it has become clear that through these consortia efforts, no "one size fits all" biomarker will suffice. Recent evidence from clinical and preclinical studies have described the development of such a panel based approach that includes both circulating biomarkers and cell based screening methods to rule in or out liver injury, provide early detection of liver injury, enhanced mechanistic understanding, prognostic information and defining the causative agent. These efforts have recently led to regulatory support from both EMA and FDA for the more systematic use and further qualification [25, 26]. The further development of these markers in well-controlled phase I studies and trials designed to test the ability of the biomarker to guide patient care should remain the focus of new efforts [16]. In addition to these consortia efforts, significant advances have been in terms of developing comprehensive resources for researchers, clinicians and patients that can provide synergy to understanding the overall problem of DILI. One such valuable resource is "LIVERTOX" (www.livertox.nih.gov).

LIVERTOX provides up-to-date and accurate information on the diagnosis, cause, frequency, patterns, and management of liver injury attributable to prescription and nonprescription drugs, herbal and dietary supplements. This resource also includes case registries that can enable scientific analysis and better characterization of the clinical patterns of liver injury that can be used to better understand the utility of novel biomarkers.

The key questions surrounding the development of new biomarkers for the assessment of DILI in humans include:

- Can new biomarkers sensitively identify DILI when it occurs with enhanced specificity?

- Can new biomarkers distinguish between DILI and background occurring liver disease (HCV infection, nonalcoholic fatty liver disease, etc.)?

- Are new biomarkers translational between preclinical models and humans?

- Can we use new biomarkers to report clinical mechanisms of DILI?

- Can new biomarkers be used to predict patient prognosis or stratify treatment?

- Do new investigational biomarkers distinguish benign transaminase elevations from serious DILI to build on "Hy's law"?

- What are the hurdles that could prevent clinical adoption?

With the exception of APAP (APAP-adducts, APAP metabolite ratios [27, 28]), there is no specific, objective, noninvasive test to diagnoses DILI or aid its treatment [29–31]. Therefore, there has been a considerable effort to identify and develop new biomarkers that can inform the mechanistic basis of DILI and provide potential measures for patient management. Below are insights and opinions as to the utility of currently proposed translational safety biomarkers (TSBMs). Table 2 contains a summary of current novel DILI biomarkers and their utility based on existing preclinical and clinical evidence.

3.2 DILI Biomarkers with Improved Hepatic Specificity and Early Detection of Liver Injury

Unfortunately the expression of ALT is not exclusive to the liver. Therefore, elevations in ALT activity in circulation can also result from myocardial damage, muscle damage, or extreme exercise. Therefore, DILI biomarkers with improved hepatic specificity are required to complement and support current tests. MicroRNAs (miRNAs) are small noncoding RNAs approximately 22–25 nucleotides in length which predominantly serve to negatively regulate posttranscriptional gene expression. Circulating microRNAs are stable and provide disease state biomarkers spanning diverse therapeutic areas and have been associated with a wide range of tissue-specific toxicities [32]. Some microRNA species show a high

Table 2
Summary of novel translational DILI biomarkers and their utility

Biomarker	Mechanism	Assay platform	Utility Liver specific	Diagnostic	Organ specific	Early injury detection	Mechanistic	Prognostic
APAP-cys adducts	Reactive metabolite formation	HLPC-Mass spectrometry and Point of Care		X				
miR-122	Cell leakage	PCR	X		X	X		
Total HMGB1	Necrosis	ELISA				X	X	
Keratin-18 (full length and caspase cleaved)	Cell death mode	ELISA				X	X	
Acylcarnitines	Mitochondrial function	LC-MS/MS					X	X
GLDH	Mitochondrial injury	Fluorometric	X				X	
Acetylated HMGB1	Inflammation	LC-MS/MS					X	X
CSF-1	Regeneration	ELISA					X	X

degree of organ specificity and cross-species conservation which makes them attractive candidates as translational safety biomarkers [33]. MicroRNA-122 (miR-122) represents 75% of the total hepatic miRNA content and exhibits exclusive hepatic expression. miR-122 has been shown to be a serum biomarker of APAP-induced ALI in mice, which was more sensitive with respect to dose and time than ALT [34]. The improved tissue specificity of miR-122 versus ALT is supported by the observation that clinical ALT elevations associated with muscle injury are not accompanied by concomitant elevations in miR-122 [35]. MiR-122 has also been previously shown to serve as a clinical indicator of heparin-induced hepatocellular necrosis [20]. Moreover, as observed in mice, miR-122 is elevated in blood following APAP overdose in man and correlates strongly with ALT activity in patients with established acute liver injury. Furthermore miR-122 has been shown to represent a more sensitive biomarker of APAP hepato-toxicity in humans compared to currently used clinical chemistry parameters [36, 37]. In these investigations, elevated miR-122 was observed in patients that present to hospital with normal liver function test values within the normal range but then later develop acute liver injury compared to those that did not develop acute liver injury following APAP overdose [38]. Furthermore, healthy volunteer studies have also demonstrated that miR-122 elevation is associated with individuals that develop liver injury despite only taking the therapeutic APAP dose and that miR-122 rises 24 h before ALT activity [39, 40]. Interestingly, these data are also supported by a recently published case report highlighting that life threating hepatotoxicity following APAP overdose could have potentially been avoided if these biomarkers had been measured [37]. These data demonstrate, for the first time in humans, that miR-122 is a more sensitive biomarker of DILI in a temporal sense compared to currently used indicators and can be used to aid treatment stratification and identify risk.

The release of miRNAs into the extracellular space and circulation has been extensively investigated and thought to serve physiological processes (such as cell-to-cell communication) or indicate liver injury/inflammation [41]. miRNAs circulate in blood either in a protein-bound form (associated with Ago2 or lipoproteins) or encapsulated in extracellular vesicles (EVs) [41]. Three types of EVs have been found in peripheral circulation: exosomes (50–100 nm in diameter), microparticles (100–1000 nm), and larger apoptotic bodies; all of which are thought to carry miRNA species and it may be that these varying compartments are representative of different mechanisms or time points of injury [41]. The translational value of miR-122 as a sensitive circulating biomarker has also been demonstrated in an APAP overdose model in zebrafish [42]. This represents an important observation for translational research and data interpretation given the increasing utility of this organism for earlier drug development studies. Despite, the advantages of miR-122, future efforts should be coordinated to develop cross laboratory validated methods for miRNA isolation and quantification as well as developing a consensus on normalization standards [43].

3.3 DILI Biomarkers with Improved Prognostic Utility

Currently used clinical chemistry parameters offer little sensitivity and specificity with respect to patient prognosis. High Mobility Group Box-1 (HMGB1) is a chromatin binding protein which is passively released by cells undergoing necrosis were it acts as a damage associated molecular pattern (DAMP) molecule by linking cell death to the activation of an immune response by targeting Toll-like receptors and the receptor for advanced glycation end products (RAGE) [44–46]. HMGB1 has activity at the intersection between infectious and sterile inflammation. It is also actively secreted as a cytokine by innate immune cells in a hyper-acetylated form [47, 48] and its biological function is highly dependent upon, and regulated by, post-translational redox modifications of three key cysteine residues [49, 50]. Furthermore, a recently defined nomenclature has been developed to identify these functionally relevant isoforms [51]. Acetylation of lysine residues is also important for the active release of HMGB1 from immune cells and for release in cell death mechanisms such as pyroptosis [47, 48, 52, 53]. HMGB1 is an informative and early serum indicator of cell death processes in preclinical models of APAP poisoning [54, 55] and in the clinic [36, 37]. Circulating levels of total and acetylated HMGB1 displayed different temporal profiles, which in mouse models of APAP toxicity correlate with the onset of necrosis and inflammation, respectively [54]. Serum levels of total HMGB1 correlate strongly with ALT activity and prothrombin time in patients with established acute liver injury following APAP overdose [56]. The prognostic utility of acetylated HMGB1 has also been demonstrated in clinical DILI. In patients with established acute liver injury following APAP overdose, elevations in acetylated HMGB1 associate with a poor prognosis and outcome [56]. As well as being an important biomarker of APAP toxicity, conditional knock out animals for HMGB1 and novel therapeutic targeting of this signaling pathways have demonstrated its importance in the pathogenesis of the disease [57, 58]. Furthermore, HMGB1 has been demonstrated to be a mechanistic player and biomarker in alcoholic liver disease [59], hepatic fibrosis [60] and preclinical and clinical cholestasis [61]. The specific targeting of key DAMP mediators to prevent exacerbation of experimental DILI (such as HMGB1), with antibodies and inhibitory peptides, has proven efficacious in vivo and may lead to potential therapeutic candidates for DILI for further development [55, 58, 62].

Recently, the quantification of acetylated HMGB1 during APAP overdose in parallel with colony stimulating factor-1 (CSF-1) has been shown to offer increased prediction of patient prognosis [63]. Hepatic macrophages are necessary for effective hepatocyte proliferation and for the clearing of gut-derived pathogenic material from the portal system. Maintenance of hepatic macrophages is controlled by macrophage CSF-1 and hepatic regeneration following partial hepatectomy and drug toxicity is stunted in CSF-1 deficient mice and similarly direct depletion of macrophages also impairs regeneration. Increased circulating CSF-1 has been proposed as a biomarker of hepatic regeneration and improved outcome in patients following APAP overdose and partial hepatectomy [63].

The assessment of secondary renal injury is a major determinant of poor prognosis in patients with acute liver failure. Kidney Injury Molecule-1 (KIM-1) is a transmembrane glycoprotein that confers phagocytic activity on the proximal tubule cells of the kidney. During acute kidney injury (AKI), KIM-1 is rapidly upregulated and its ectodomain is shed into urine and blood and has been shown to be a sensitive and specific biomarker of acute kidney injury. Furthermore, KIM-1 has been formally qualified by regulatory authorities for its use to monitor acute renal injury in the preclinical setting [23]. In patients with APAP overdose, secondary injury to the kidney and specifically the proximal tubule epithelia is a major determinate for mortality. Indeed, biomarkers such as serum creatinine are often incorporated into prognostic algorithms such as the King's College Criteria (KCC) [64]. However, serum creatinine is delayed in its onset of increase and data from animal models and humans has repeatedly demonstrated the ability of KIM-1 to elevate earlier after acute kidney injury [65, 66]. In patients with established APAP-induced ALI circulating KIM-1 has been recently demonstrated to be elevated in patients that subsequently died or required a liver transplant compared to spontaneous survivors [67]. The fold change in KIM-1 in this worse prognostic group was higher than creatinine and it also outperformed creatinine in a ROC analysis. Furthermore, circulating KIM-1 was an independent predictor of outcome in a logistic regression model that took into account established markers [67].

Fatty acid-binding proteins (FABPs) are small cytoplasmic proteins with the primary function of transporting intracellular long-chain fatty acids. They are highly expressed in tissue with active fatty acid metabolism such as the liver. Their expression can be induced in conditions such as ischemia/inflammation. Circulating levels of liver FABP (FABP1) have been found to be elevated following hepatocyte injury induced by a range of insults [68]. However, recent reports have described the utility of serum FABP1 as a prognostic biomarker during acute liver failure induced by acetaminophen. This recent nested case-control study elegantly demonstrated that elevated serum FABP1 was associated with significantly higher risk of death when measured at early time points. Moreover, the authors demonstrated that when adjusting for other significant covariates, serum FABP1 is associated with 21-day mortality and improves current prognostic models such as KCC [69].

3.4 Potential DILI Biomarkers That Enhance Mechanistic Understanding

Given the multistep and multicellular process of DILI, panels of biomarkers that have potential to provide insights into the underlying mechanistic basis of DILI are increasingly being recognized as fundamental to efforts in translational research and patient treatment stratification. The understanding of cell death mode dynamics is important from a pathogenic point of view given that the activation of the innate immune response can vary greatly depending on which mode of cell death is triggered and when. The majority of experimental data to date on human DILI mechanistic biomarkers has been obtained from studies of APAP overdose rather than idiosyncratic DILI so these observations have to be considered in this light.

Keratin-18 (K18) is a type I intermediate filament protein expressed in epithelial cells and is responsible for cell structure and integrity [70]. Caspase-mediated cleavage of K18 is an early event in cellular structural rearrangement during apoptosis [71]. Caspases 3, 7, and 9 have been implicated in the cleavage of K18 at the C-terminal DALD/S motif. Full-length K18 is released passively during necrotic cell death whereas fragmented K18 is released with apoptosis [72]. The use of immunoassays directed toward the recognition of caspase-cleaved K18 (apoptosis) and full length K18 (necrosis) have been reported clinically as biomarkers for the therapeutic drug monitoring of chemotherapeutic agents and for the quantification of apoptosis during liver disorders such as nonalcoholic steatohepatitis (NASH) and hepatitis C infection [73, 74] and mutations in K18 predispose toward acute liver failure and hepatotoxicity [75, 76]. Circulating necrosis K18 and apoptosis K18 have been shown to represent indicators of hepatic necrotic and apoptotic events in a mouse model of APAP induced liver injury [54], hypoxic hepatitis [77] and during heparin-induced hepatocellular injury in man [20]. The prognostic utility of K18 has also been demonstrated in clinical DILI and acute liver injury [56, 78]. In patients with established acute liver injury following APAP overdose, elevations in absolute levels of necrosis K18 associate with a poor prognosis (KCC) and outcome and a total percentage of K18 attributed to apoptosis as associates with improved survival [56]. Interestingly, in the first blood sample taken at the point of admission following APAP overdose, when currently used markers of liver injury remained within the normal range and prior to antidote treatment, K18 (and also miR-122 and HMGB1) were significantly elevated in the group of patients that subsequently went on to develop liver injury, even in patients that presented less than 8 h post overdose [36]. Recent evidence also suggests that the modeling of the ratio between full length and caspase cleaved K18 may provide an important tool to aid risk prediction of liver safety signals during clinical trials [79].

The pathogenesis of DILI has been closely associated with mitochondrial dysfunction. Therefore a translational biomarker(s) of mitochondrial dysfunction to add to the currently battery of tests appears logical. Glutamate dehydrogenase (GLDH) is an enzyme present in matrix-rich mitochondria (liver) and not in cristae-rich mitochondria (cardiac and skeletal muscle). It is important to note that while GLDH is also expressed in the brain and in kidney, its release from these tissues enters the cerebrospinal fluid and tubular lumen, respectively, rather than the blood [80, 81]. GLDH is a key enzyme in amino acid oxidation and urea production that is highly conserved across species, making it an attractive biomarker candidate [82]. It is considered relatively liver-specific and provides an indicator of leakage of mitochondrial contents into the circulation [24]. GLDH localization within the liver is regional, with higher concentrations present in the centrilobular area, the region of metabolic activation and site of tissue damage during APAP toxicity. GLDH use as a DILI biomarker is well documented and appears more sensitive and indicative of DILI than other cytosolic enzymes [83]. A recent study in rats subjected to multiple liver injury modalities indicated that GLDH increases were up to tenfold greater and threefold more persistent than ALT elevations [84]. As GLDH is localized to the mitochondrial matrix and due to its relative large size (330 kDa), release of GLDH into the circulation is delayed during hepatocellular necrosis when compared to cytosolic enzymes like the aminotransferases. This property may contribute to increased specificity of GLDH to indicate hepatocellular necrosis. In acute liver injury GLDH is elevated in blood in both preclinical models and clinical cases of DILI and liver impairment [36, 83, 85, 86], highlighting its potential as a translational biomarker. Circulating GLDH has been shown to rise in healthy volunteers treated with heparins and cholestyramine, treatments that are not associated with clinically important liver injury [20, 87] and specific recommendations have been made when drawing conclusions on data regarding sample type and specimen preparation [88]. Measurement of GLDH alone may or may not be useful in distinguishing benign elevations in ALT from those that portent severe DILI potential.

Due to the fact that most of enzymes used to investigate mitochondrial dysfunction track changes in ALT activity [85], a promising approach to the identification of biomarkers of injury that are useful at earlier time points may involve metabolomics. In general, metabolic intermediates are much smaller than proteins and more likely to cross cell membranes and enter blood before the development of injury. In 2009, Chen et al. [89] measured increased levels of acylcarnitines in serum from APAP-treated mice. Acylcarnitines are derivatives of long-chain fatty acids which are required for transport of these fatty acids into mitochondria for β-oxidation. First, a coenzyme A (CoA) group is attached in a reaction catalyzed by acyl-CoA synthetase. The CoA group is then displaced by carnitine through the action of carnitine palmitoyl transferase I (CPT I), forming an acylcarnitine that can enter the mitochondrial matrix through facilitated diffusion with the help of a carnitine-acylcarnitine translocase (CACT). Because acylcarnitines are broken down within mitochondria by carnitine palmitoyl transferase II (CPT II) and beta-oxidation, mitochondrial dysfunction may result in their accumulation. It was been shown that these fatty acid–carnitine conjugates rise in the serum of mice treated with APAP (mitochondrial dependent hepatocyte death) but not with mice treated with furosemide (which has been shown to cause liver injury without primarily affecting mitochondrial function) [90]. Therefore, circulating acylcarnitines have potential as specific biomarkers of mitochondrial dysfunction. It is important to note that acylcarnitines have been shown to not be elevated in patients with APAP overdose [90]. This is most likely due in part to the standard-of-care treatment N-acetylcysteine (NAC). However, it might be useful to measure acylcarnitines in other forms of liver injury or APAP patients that present to the "hospital front door" prior to the treatment with NAC [36, 37, 91].

4   Conclusions and Future Developments

The lack of qualified mechanistic biomarkers has resulted in a significant challenge with regard to defining the true extent and diagnosis of DILI in humans [92]. The development and qualification of sensitive and specific hepatic biomarkers that hold translation between preclinical and clinical studies is urgently required to accelerate the pace of drug development. Improved DILI biomarkers may additionally enable patient and/or DILI specific treatment stratification for marketed therapeutics. Moreover, the potential for novel biomarkers to provide enhanced understanding of the fundamental mechanisms that result in clinical DILI is becoming increasingly recognized. Critical to the development of any novel biomarker is to frame its qualification and understand its utility within a defined context of use. Moreover, to maximize the utility of any DILI biomarker and to interpret data correctly, it is imperative for the end users to have a comprehensive understanding of whether a biomarker is fit for purpose before undertaking translational or clinical studies.

Significant recent progress has been made and clinical utility has been shown regarding "mechanism-based" biomarkers such as acylcarnitines, HMGB1, K18, GLDH and highly liver specific markers such as miR-122 that can be used alongside currently used clinical tests rather than be used to replace them with their added valued determined by new statistical analyses such as IRI and NRI [93]. These biomarkers have been shown to be translational, can report DILI sensitively when it occurs, shed light on mechanistic aspects of clinical DILI and can predict patient prognosis (such as acetylated HMGB1, CSF-1, FABP1 and KIM-1). However, the vast majority of clinical data to date has been obtained from studies of APAP-induced liver injury and has not been assessed in rare cases of idiosyncratic DILI. Moreover, a clear knowledge gap still exists regarding the identification and development of biomarkers that differentiate between serious DILI, transient increases in ALT activity and that reflect hepatic regenerative processes, although promising results have been obtained for CSF-1.

Since it is thought that full understanding and appreciation of the potential value of these biomarkers will only be seen following the measurement of thousands of samples; clinical trials are one important way of carrying out this collection [94] and recent proactive studies are start to gain traction [79]. Moreover, important lessons can be learnt from the recently successful qualification of biomarkers for renal injury.

The qualification of new DILI biomarkers will require adoption of standardized liver safety databases, standardized protocols for biospecimen collection and storage and the initiation of large prospective clinical trials, involving diverse disease populations and treatment with many different drugs. This should now become a high priority within the pharmaceutical industry. It is important that pharmaceutical companies start now to archive samples and link these specimens to the relevant liver safety data. Ideally, liver safety data management tools should be standardized across the industry to facilitate the precompetitive collaborations on biomarker validation and qualification, such as eDISH [14]. Of additional importance is the agreement for sponsors to apply novel DILI biomarkers voluntary in clinical trials without penalty. Clinical trials have the unique advantage of allowing prospective data selection by enrolling a diverse population of healthy volunteers and patients expected to have DILI in the future and through the inclusion of drugs that are both safe and not safe toward the liver. This resource will prove extremely valuable as researchers are thus able to get a sense of the whole picture—before, during and after injury occurs [17].

The utility of clinical trials to assess biomarker performance is not without problems and one that the traditional drug development paradigm is not suited to [95]. Therefore, a recently proposed workflow has been discussed in the context of cancer biomarkers, constituting of phase I (assay assessment in healthy and nonhealthy scenarios as well as determining healthy reference intervals), phase II (retrospective analysis of biomarkers within clinical samples to direct clinical utility), and phase III confirmatory phase (qualifying the biomarker through large, prospective, multicenter RCT trials). This workflow can be easily applicable to the development of DILI biomarkers. However, these current trials do not get to the heart of the question and test the hypothesis that the new biomarker provides real added value and helps with clinical decision-making. Recently reviews have provided suggestions to encourage the development of novel trial designs to aid biomarker-guided decision making for drug safety sciences.

The recently published literature suggests that existing biomarkers for DILI appear ready for safety trials to test the rigor of novel biomarkers. Even marginally effective biomarkers can have dramatically positive impacts on therapeutic trials based on enrichment for events and narrowing in on cases where an intervention will work based on a comprehensive understanding of risk–benefit ratio for drugs. New DILI biomarkers also provide insights into mechanisms of pathophysiology that should not be ignored given that we have no specific therapies for DILI and that we currently rely on imperfect "gold standards" to qualify the biomarker. The further development of these markers in well-controlled phase I studies and trials designed to test the ability of the biomarker to guide patient care should remain the focus of new efforts [5, 6]. A crucial roadblock is the development of clinical grade assays capable of delivering a result within an appropriate time frame. In the example of suspected APAP toxicity, the time from taking blood to result should be no longer than around 1 h. In early phase clinical trials the maximum time to result could be longer, but current ELISA and PCR based analysis is still unsuitable. Total HMGB1, FABP1, CSF1 and K18 are circulating proteins that should be amenable to point-of-care assay development with existing platforms. By contrast, miR-122 rapid and accurate point-of-care detection will require advances on the current technology level. Such technologies are in development, with some showing promise in this field and having potential for use beyond the measurement of only one microRNA species. Measurement of DILI biomarkers out with the hospital or clinical research facility may be desirable in certain scenarios, such as home monitoring for patients taking drugs with a high DILI liability or in the developing world where antimicrobials cause significant morbidity due to DILI. Assay developers could draw on the success with regard to low cost, finger prick, point-of-care ALT measurement [96].

It is clear that significant progress has been made regarding the identification and development of DILI biomarkers. However, there is still significant research to be carried out. DILI is a complex multicellular and multimechanism disease; therefore it is logical that a battery of complimentary biomarkers (both genetic and circulating) that reflect specific cellular processes and predisposition to DILI are required. If the further development of these candidate markers leads to full qualification, the focus of updated regulatory guidance should therefore account for the measurement of such tests. Advances in software, databases and data visualization approaches such as DILIsym®, LiverTox (www.livertox.nih.gov) and eDISH (evaluation of drug-induced serious hepatotoxicity) have added significantly in recent years to the understanding of serious drug-induced liver injury. The application of data sets applying these novel biomarkers will no doubt further realize the promise of these novel and potentially transformative biomarkers.

Acknowledgments

The author declares no conflict of interest and would like to acknowledge the financial support for academic research from the Medical Research Council (MRC).

References

1. Corsini A et al (2012) Current challenges and controversies in drug-induced liver injury. Drug Saf 35(12):1099–1117

2. Sgro C et al (2002) Incidence of drug-induced hepatic injuries: a French population-based study. Hepatology 36(2):451–455

3. Moggs J et al (2012) Investigative safety science as a competitive advantage for Pharma. Expert Opin Drug Metab Toxicol 8(9):1071–1082

4. Rockey DC et al (2010) Causality assessment in drug-induced liver injury using a structured expert opinion process: comparison to the Roussel-Uclaf causality assessment method. Hepatology 51(6):2117–2126

5. Clarke JI, Dear JW, Antoine DJ (2016) Recent advances in biomarkers and therapeutic interventions for hepatic drug safety–false dawn or new horizon? Expert Opin Drug Saf 15(5):625–634

6. Antoine DJ, Dear JW (2017) Transformative biomarkers for drug-induced liver injury: are we there yet? Biomark Med 11(2):103–106

7. Kullak-Ublick GA et al (2017) Drug-induced liver injury: recent advances in diagnosis and risk assessment. Gut 66(6):1154–1164

8. Biomarkers Definitions Working Group (2001) Biomarkers and surrogate endpoints: preferred definitions and conceptual framework. Clin Pharmacol Ther 69(3):89–95

9. Ratner M (2005) FDA pharmacogenomics guidance sends clear message to industry. Nat Rev Drug Discov 4(5):359

10. Matheis K et al (2011) A generic operational strategy to qualify translational safety biomarkers. Drug Discov Today 16(13–14):600–608

11. Zimmerman HJ (1968) The spectrum of hepatotoxicity. Perspect Biol Med 12(1):135–161

12. Watkins PB (2011) Drug safety sciences and the bottleneck in drug development. Clin Pharmacol Ther 89(6):788–790

13. Senior JR (2012) Alanine aminotransferase: a clinical and regulatory tool for detecting liver injury-past, present, and future. Clin Pharmacol Ther 92(3):332–339

14. Watkins PB et al (2011) Evaluation of drug-induced serious hepatotoxicity (eDISH): application of this data organization approach to phase III clinical trials of rivaroxaban after total hip or knee replacement surgery. Drug Saf 34(3):243–252

15. Merz M et al (2014) Methodology to assess clinical liver safety data. Drug Saf 37(Suppl 1):S33–S45

16. Avigan MI et al (2014) Liver safety assessment: required data elements and best practices for data collection and standardization in clinical trials. Drug Saf 37(Suppl 1):S19–S31

17. Watkins PB et al (2014) The clinical liver safety assessment best practices workshop: rationale, goals, accomplishments and the future. Drug Saf 37(Suppl 1):S1–S7

18. Ozer J et al (2008) The current state of serum biomarkers of hepatotoxicity. Toxicology 245(3):194–205

19. Watkins PB et al (1994) Hepatotoxic effects of tacrine administration in patients with Alzheimer's disease. JAMA 271(13):992–998

20. Harrill AH et al (2012) The effects of heparins on the liver: application of mechanistic serum biomarkers in a randomized study in healthy volunteers. Clin Pharmacol Ther 92(2):214–220

21. Pickering JW, Endre ZH (2012) New metrics for assessing diagnostic potential of candidate biomarkers. Clin J Am Soc Nephrol 7(8):1355–1364

22. Bonventre JV et al (2010) Next-generation biomarkers for detecting kidney toxicity. Nat Biotechnol 28(5):436–440

23. Vaidya VS et al (2010) Kidney injury molecule-1 outperforms traditional biomarkers of kidney injury in preclinical biomarker qualification studies. Nat Biotechnol 28(5):478–485

24. Antoine DJ et al (2009) Mechanism-based bio-analysis and biomarkers for hepatic chemical stress. Xenobiotica 39(8):565–577

25. EMA (2016) http://www.ema.europa.eu/docs/en_GB/document_library/Other/2016/09/WC500213479.pdf

26. FDA (2016) http://www.fda.gov/Drugs/DevelopmentApprovalProcess/ucm434382.htm

27. Davern TJ 2nd et al (2006) Measurement of serum acetaminophen-protein adducts in patients with acute liver failure. Gastroenterology 130(3):687–694

28. Vliegenthart A et al (2017) Circulating acetaminophen metabolites are toxicokinetic biomarkers of acute liver injury. Clin Pharmacol Ther 101(4):531–540

29. Antoine DJ, Dear JW (2016) How to treat paracetamol overdose and when to do it. Expert Rev Clin Pharmacol 9(5):633–635

30. Park BK, Dear JW, Antoine DJ (2015) Paracetamol (acetaminophen) poisoning. BMJ Clin Evid 2015:pii: 2101

31. Dear JW, Antoine DJ, Park BK (2015) Where are we now with paracetamol? BMJ 351:h3705

32. Starkey Lewis PJ et al (2012) Serum microRNA biomarkers for drug-induced liver injury. Clin Pharmacol Ther 92(3):291–293

33. Zen K, Zhang CY (2012) Circulating microR-NAs: a novel class of biomarkers to diagnose and monitor human cancers. Med Res Rev 32(2):326–348

34. Wang K et al (2009) Circulating microRNAs, potential biomarkers for drug-induced liver injury. Proc Natl Acad Sci U S A 106(11):4402–4407

35. Zhang Y et al (2010) Plasma microRNA-122 as a biomarker for viral-, alcohol-, and chemical-related hepatic diseases. Clin Chem 56(12):1830–1838

36. Antoine DJ et al (2013) Mechanistic biomarkers provide early and sensitive detection of acetaminophen-induced acute liver injury at first presentation to hospital. Hepatology 58(2):777–787

37. Dear JW et al (2013) Letter to the Editor: Early detection of paracetamol toxicity using circulating liver microRNA and markers of cell necrosis. Br J Clin Pharmacol 77(5):904–905. https://doi.org/10.1111/bcp.12214

38. Dear JW et al (2017) Risk stratification after paracetamol overdose using mechanistic biomarkers: results from two prospective cohort studies. Lancet Gastroenterol Hepatol. pii: S2468-1253(17)30266-2. https://doi.org/10.1016/S2468-1253(17)30266-2. [Epub ahead of print]. PMID: 29146439

39. Thulin P et al (2013) Keratin-18 and microRNA-122 complement alanine aminotransferase as novel safety biomarkers for drug-induced liver injury in two human cohorts. Liver Int 34(3):367–378

40. Vliegenthart AD et al (2015) Comprehensive microRNA profiling in acetaminophen toxicity identifies novel circulating biomarkers for human liver and kidney injury. Sci Rep 5:15501

41. Arrese M, Eguchi A, Feldstein AE (2015) Circulating microRNAs: emerging biomarkers of liver disease. Semin Liver Dis 35(1):43–54

42. Vliegenthart AD et al (2014) Retro-orbital blood acquisition facilitates circulating microRNA measurement in Zebrafish with Paracetamol hepatotoxicity. Zebrafish 11(3):219–226

43. Sharkey JW, Antoine DJ, Park BK (2012) Validation of the isolation and quantification of kidney enriched miRNAs for use as biomarkers. Biomarkers 17(3):231–239

44. Scaffidi P, Misteli T, Bianchi ME (2002) Release of chromatin protein HMGB1 by necrotic cells triggers inflammation. Nature 418(6894):191–195

45. Wang H et al (1999) HMG-1 as a late mediator of endotoxin lethality in mice. Science 285(5425):248–251

46. Yang H et al (2013) The many faces of HMGB1: molecular structure-functional activity in inflammation, apoptosis, and chemotaxis. J Leukoc Biol 93(6):865–873

47. Nystrom S et al (2013) TLR activation regulates damage-associated molecular pattern isoforms released during pyroptosis. EMBO J 32(1):86–99

48. Lu B et al (2012) Novel role of PKR in inflammasome activation and HMGB1 release. Nature 488(7413):670–674

49. Yang H et al (2012) Redox modification of cysteine residues regulates the cytokine activity of high mobility group box-1 (HMGB1). Mol Med 18(1):250–259

50. Venereau E et al (2012) Mutually exclusive redox forms of HMGB1 promote cell recruitment or proinflammatory cytokine release. J Exp Med 209(9):1519–1528

51. Antoine DJ et al (2014) A systematic nomenclature for the redox states of high mobility group box (HMGB) proteins. Mol Med 20(1):135–137

52. Bonaldi T et al (2003) Monocytic cells hyperacetylate chromatin protein HMGB1 to redirect it towards secretion. EMBO J 22(20):5551–5560

53. Lu B et al (2014) JAK/STAT1 signaling promotes HMGB1 hyperacetylation and nuclear translocation. Proc Natl Acad Sci U S A 111(8):3068–3073

54. Antoine DJ et al (2009) High-mobility group box-1 protein and keratin-18, circulating serum proteins informative of acetaminophen-induced necrosis and apoptosis in vivo. Toxicol Sci 112(2):521–531

55. Antoine DJ et al (2010) Diet restriction inhibits apoptosis and HMGB1 oxidation and promotes inflammatory cell recruitment during acetaminophen hepatotoxicity. Mol Med 16(11–12):479–490

56. Antoine DJ et al (2012) Molecular forms of HMGB1 and keratin-18 as mechanistic biomarkers for mode of cell death and prognosis during clinical acetaminophen hepatotoxicity. J Hepatol 56(5):1070–1079

57. Huebener P et al (2015) The HMGB1/RAGE axis triggers neutrophil-mediated injury amplification following necrosis. J Clin Invest 125(2):539–550

58. Yang H et al (2015) MD-2 is required for disulfide HMGB1-dependent TLR4 signaling. J Exp Med 212(1):5–14

59. Ge X et al (2014) High mobility group box-1 (HMGB1) participates in the pathogenesis of alcoholic liver disease (ALD). J Biol Chem 289(33):22672–22691

60. Arriazu E et al (2016) Signalling via the osteopontin and high mobility group box-1 axis drives the fibrogenic response to liver injury. Gut 66(6):1123–1137

61. Woolbright BL et al (2013) Plasma biomarkers of liver injury and inflammation demonstrate a lack of apoptosis during obstructive cholestasis in mice. Toxicol Appl Pharmacol 273(3):524–531

62. Lundback P et al (2016) A novel high mobility group box 1 neutralizing chimeric antibody attenuates drug-induced liver injury and postinjury inflammation in mice. Hepatology 64(5):1699–1710

63. Stutchfield BM et al (2015) CSF1 restores innate immunity after liver injury in mice and serum levels indicate outcomes of patients with acute liver failure. Gastroenterology 149(7):1896–1909.e14

64. Chalasani N et al (2002) Model for end-stage liver disease (MELD) for predicting mortality in patients with acute variceal bleeding. Hepatology 35(5):1282–1284

65. McWilliam SJ et al (2012) Mechanism-based urinary biomarkers to identify the potential for aminoglycoside-induced nephrotoxicity in premature neonates: a proof-of-concept study. PLoS One [Electronic Resource] 7(8):e43809

66. Sabbisetti VS et al (2014) Blood kidney injury molecule-1 is a biomarker of acute and chronic kidney injury and predicts progression to ESRD in type I diabetes. J Am Soc Nephrol 25(10):2177–2186

67. Antoine DJ et al (2015) Circulating kidney injury molecule 1 predicts prognosis and poor outcome in patients with acetaminophen-induced liver injury. Hepatology 62(2):591–599

68. Pelsers MM, Hermens WT, Glatz JF (2005) Fatty acid-binding proteins as plasma markers of tissue injury. Clin Chim Acta 352(1-2):15–35

69. Karvellas CJ et al (2017) Elevated FABP1 serum levels are associated with poorer survival in acetaminophen-induced acute liver failure. Hepatology 65(3):938–949

70. Ku NO et al (2007) Keratins let liver live: mutations predispose to liver disease and cross-linking generates Mallory-Denk bodies. Hepatology 46(5):1639–1649

71. Caulin C, Salvesen GS, Oshima RG (1997) Caspase cleavage of keratin 18 and reorganization of intermediate filaments during epithelial cell apoptosis. J Cell Biol 138(6):1379–1394

72. Schutte B et al (2004) Keratin 8/18 breakdown and reorganization during apoptosis. Exp Cell Res 297(1):11–26

73. Wieckowska A et al (2006) In vivo assessment of liver cell apoptosis as a novel biomarker of disease severity in nonalcoholic fatty liver disease. Hepatology 44(1):27–33

74. Cummings J et al (2008) Preclinical evaluation of M30 and M65 ELISAs as biomarkers of drug induced tumor cell death and antitumor activity. Mol Cancer Ther 7(3):455–463

75. Ku NO et al (1996) Susceptibility to hepatotoxicity in transgenic mice that express a dominant-negative human keratin 18 mutant. J Clin Invest 98(4):1034–1046

76. Strnad P et al (2010) Keratin variants predispose to acute liver failure and adverse outcome: race and ethnic associations. Gastroenterology 139(3):828–835. 835.e1–3

77. Weemhoff JL et al (2017) Plasma biomarkers to study mechanisms of liver injury in patients with hypoxic hepatitis. Liver Int 37(3):377–384

78. Bechmann LP et al (2010) Cytokeratin 18-based modification of the MELD score improves prediction of spontaneous survival after acute liver injury. J Hepatol 53(4):639–647

79. Longo DM et al (2017) Refining liver safety risk assessment: application of mechanistic modeling and serum biomarkers to Cimaglermin alfa (GGF2) clinical trials. Clin Pharmacol Ther 102(6):961–969

80. Feldman BF (1989) Cerebrospinal fluid. In: Kaneko J (ed) Clinical biochemistry of domestic animals. Academic, San Diego, pp 835–865

81. Stonard MD (1996) Assessment of nephrotoxicity. In: Evans GO (ed) Animal clinical chemistry. Taylor & Francis, London, pp 87–89

82. Schmidt ES, Schmidt FW (1988) Glutamate dehydrogenase: biochemical and clinical aspects of an interesting enzyme. Clin Chim Acta 173(1):43–55

83. Schomaker S et al (2013) Assessment of emerging biomarkers of liver injury in human subjects. Toxicol Sci 132(2):276–283

84. O'Brien PJ et al (2002) Advantages of glutamate dehydrogenase as a blood biomarker of acute hepatic injury in rats. Lab Anim 36(3):313–321

85. McGill MR et al (2012) The mechanism underlying acetaminophen-induced hepatotoxicity in humans and mice involves mitochondrial damage and nuclear DNA fragmentation. J Clin Invest 122(4):1574–1583

86. Thulin P et al (2017) A longitudinal assessment of miR-122 and GLDH as biomarkers of drug-induced liver injury in the rat. Biomarkers 22(5):461–469

87. Singhal R, Harrill AH, Menguy-Vacheron F, Jayyosi Z, Benzerdjeb H, Watkins PB. (2014) Benign elevations in serum aminotransferases and biomarkers of hepatotoxicity in healthy volunteers treated with cholestyramine. BMC Pharmacol Toxicol 15:42. https://doi. org/10.1186/2050-6511-15-42. PMID: 25086653

88. Jaeschke H, McGill MR (2013) Serum glutamate dehydrogenase—biomarker for liver cell death or mitochondrial dysfunction? Toxicol Sci 134(1):221–222

89. Chen C et al (2009) Serum metabolomics reveals irreversible inhibition of fatty acid beta-oxidation through the suppression of PPARalpha activation as a contributing mechanism of acetaminophen-induced hepatotoxicity. Chem Res Toxicol 22(4):699–707

90. McGill MR et al (2014) Circulating acylcarnitines as biomarkers of mitochondrial dysfunction after acetaminophen overdose in mice and humans. Arch Toxicol 88(2):391–401

91. Dear JW, Antoine DJ (2014) Stratification of paracetamol overdose patients using new toxicity biomarkers: current candidates and future challenges. Expert Rev Clin Pharmacol 7(2):181–189

92. Aithal GP, Rawlins MD, Day CP (1999) Accuracy of hepatic adverse drug reaction reporting in one English health region. BMJ 319(7224):1541

93. Antoine DJ et al (2013) Are we closer to finding biomarkers for identifying acute drug-induced liver injury? Biomark Med 7(3):383–386

94. Watkins PB et al (2008) Using controlled clinical trials to learn more about acute drug-induced liver injury. Hepatology 48(5):1680–1689

95. Mandrekar SJ, Dahlberg SE, Simon R (2015) Improving clinical trial efficiency: thinking outside the box. Am Soc Clin Oncol Educ Book 35:e141–e147

96. Pollock NR et al (2012) A paper-based multiplexed transaminase test for low-cost, point-of-care liver function testing. Sci Transl Med 4(152):152ra129

Chapter 27

Causality Assessment Methods in Drug-Induced Liver Injury

Rolf Teschke and Gaby Danan

Abstract

A robust causality assessment method (CAM) is not only indispensable for the diagnosis of suspected drug-induced liver injury (DILI) and herb-induced liver injury (HILI) but is also critical for the investigation of the clinical features, risk factors, and incidence in pharmacological or epidemiological studies. RUCAM (Roussel Uclaf Causality Assessment Method) is the most widely used CAM in suspected DILI and HILI cases worldwide, as evidenced by its application in a large number of case reports and case series since RUCAM was first published in 1993. It offers a structured, standardized diagnostic approach specific to liver injury by attributing scores to individual key items that provide final quantitative gradings of causality. In many countries and for more than two decades, physicians, regulatory agencies, case report authors, and pharmaceutical companies have successfully applied this well-validated CAM. The RUCAM update in 2016 clarified a few complicated items such as alcohol use and exclusion of nondrug causes. The intention of this approach was to provide accurately defined and objective core elements to simplify item handling, and therefore reduce interobserver and intraobserver variability. In conclusion, RUCAM should be recommended as the preferred CAM for suspected DILI and HILI cases.

Key words Drug-induced liver injury, DILI, Roussel Uclaf Causality Assessment, RUCAM, Causality assessment methods

1 Introduction

Idiosyncratic drug-induced liver injury (DILI) is a multifaceted disease that continuously attracts the interest of clinicians, scientists, regulatory agencies, and pharmaceutical companies, as evidenced by the wealth of publications summarized recently [1]. Indeed, research in the diagnosis and mechanisms of liver injury by drugs [1–10], herbs [11–14], and dietary supplements [15–17] is encouraged. All suspected adverse reactions require a robust causality assessment method (CAM) in order to help establish the diagnosis and describe key clinical features, risk factors, and incidence.

Idiosyncratic DILI is considered as a rare event with an estimated incidence rate in the general population of 13.9 cases per 100,000 inhabitants-years in France [18] and 19.1 cases per 100,000

Minjun Chen and Yvonne Will (eds.), *Drug-Induced Liver Toxicity*, Methods in Pharmacology and Toxicology,
https://doi.org/10.1007/978-1-4939-7677-5_27, © Springer Science+Business Media, LLC, part of Springer Nature 2018

inhabitants-years in Iceland [19]. These rates differ considerably from the reported incidence rate of 2.4 cases per 100,000 individuals registered in the UK-based Medical Research Practice Database; however, the UK data was not calculated in per inhabitants-years [20]. Incidence variability may be due to different criteria for defining a case and product use, as some studies include cases of intrinsic DILI from acetaminophen overdose and others also considered cases of herb-induced liver injury (HILI) caused by herbal preparations or dietary supplements. A robust liver specific CAM such as RUCAM (Roussel Uclaf Causality Assessment Method), with a transparent scoring system [21] for individual key elements to establish causality was used in one study [19] but not in two other published studies [18, 20]. The reported data should be considered tentative, since underestimation or overreporting may have occurred and confounded the results due to the absence of causality assessment or failure to carefully consider all alternative causes. Similar flaws have been observed in a series of DILI cases [8, 22, 23].

Describing and defining characteristic features of idiosyncratic DILI is a particular challenge due to the small incidence rate or insufficient causality assessment of individual cases. Because individual liver centers have access to only a small number of clinical DILI cases, several DILI registries were established across several countries including USA [7], Spain [24], Serbia [25, 26], Sweden, Iceland [19, 27], and Latin America [10]. With the USA as the single exception [7], all other DILI registries [10, 19, 25–27] aim at studying specific clinical features of DILI cases by using robust CAMs such as RUCAM [6, 21, 28]. Presently, even published cases of DILI characteristics may have to be questioned in the absence of a structured, quantitative, and transparent causality analysis.

The present review analyzes various CAMs regarding their suitability to establish a valid causality in idiosyncratic DILI. RUCAM will be discussed in detail and compared with other CAM approaches in order to highlight their clinical and regulatory advantages and shortcomings.

2   Data Searches and Sources

To identify relevant publications, we searched the PubMed database using the following terms: DILI combined with causality assessment method, which provided around 31,000 hits; DILI combined with expert opinion causality assessment method, 16,000 hits; RUCAM, 48,000 hits; and DILI combined with RUCAM, 13,300 hits. From each searched segment, we analyzed the publications of the first 100 hits.

Additional publications were retrieved on 24 December, 2016 from a large, private scientific archive that contains original full-length publications on DILI including causality assessment method. Prior to the final analysis, the publications were assessed regarding their clinical quality and data completeness. The final compilation consisted of original papers, case series, case reports, consensus reports, and review articles. The most relevant reports were included in the reference list of this review.

3   DILI Case Definition

3.1   Idiosyncratic Versus Intrinsic DILI

DILI commonly refers to idiosyncratic DILI, which is different from intrinsic DILI based on several characteristics (Fig. 1). Specifically, idiosyncratic DILI is typically caused by drugs at therapeutic dosages in a few exposed patients through idiosyncratic, unpredictable drug reactions. In contrast, intrinsic DILI is a predictable reaction related to overdosed drugs, such as acetaminophen [29]. Idiosyncratic and intrinsic DILI share the risk of acute liver failure (ALF) with high mortality rate or need for liver transplantation. According to an Acute Liver Failure (ALF) registry in the USA (http://www.fda. gov/Drugs/ScienceResearch/ResearchAreas/ucm071471.htm, accessed 14 December 2016), almost half of ALF cases caused by

Idiosyncratic DILI	Intrinsic DILI
Unpredictability	Predictability
Dose independency	Clear dose dependency
Long and variable latency period	Short and consistent latency period
Variable liver pathology	Distinctive liver pathology
Low incidence in humans	High incidence in humans
Lack of experimental reproducibility	Experimental reproducibility

↓

Types of idiosyncratic DILI	
- Metabolic type	Duration of exposure: 1 week to 12 months Rarely also some weak dose dependency Lack of hypersensitivity features Delayed response to reexposure (weeks)
- Immunologic type	Duration of exposure: 1-5 weeks Hypersensitivity features Prompt response to reexposure with 1 or 2 doses

Fig. 1 Idiosyncratic DILI versus intrinsic DILI. Adapted from previous reports [6, 21]. *DILI* drug-induced liver injury

Table 1
Scores for individual RUCAM items for hepatocellular injury and cholestatic or mixed liver injury

Data elements assessed in RUCAM	Scores of RUCAM for hepatocellular injury	Scores of RUCAM for cholestatic or mixed liver injury
• Time frame of latency period	From +1 to +2	From +1 to +2
• Time frame of dechallenge	From −2 to +3	From 0 to +2
• Recurrent ALT increase	−2	–
• Recurrent ALP increase	–	0
• Risk factors	0 or +1	0 or +1
• Individual comedication	From −3 to 0	From −3 to 0
• Search for individual alternative causes	From −3 to +2	From −3 to +2
• Verified exclusion of alternative causes	Requires individual scoring	
• Markers of HAV, HBV, HCV, HEV		
• Markers of CMV, EBV, HSV, VZV		
• Evaluation of cardiac hepatopathy		
• Liver and biliary tract imaging		
• Doppler sonography of liver vessels		
• Prior known hepatotoxicity	From 0 to +2	From 0 to +2
• Unintentional reexposure	From −2 to +3	From −2 to +3

Data above are condensed for a quick overview and adapted from a previous report [6]. Details of each criterion and score are given in the RUCAM worksheet, which in its original, not condensed form is to be used for causality assessment [6]
ALT alanine aminotransferase, *ALP* alkaline phosphatase, *CMV* cytomegalovirus, *EBV* Epstein Barr virus, *HAV* Hepatitis A virus, *HBV* Hepatitis B virus, *HCV* Hepatitis C virus, *HEV* Hepatitis E virus, *HSV* Herpes simplex virus, *RUCAM* Roussel Uclaf Causality Assessment Method, *VZV* Varicella zoster virus

drugs are intrinsic DILI by intentional and unintentional overdose of acetaminophen as compared to idiosyncratic DILI caused by a variety of drugs. However, the causality attribution to idiosyncratic DILI(s) is often identified without a transparent approach and quantitative scoring system [30, 31] such as RUCAM (Table 1) [21].

3.2 Liver Injury with Liver Test Thresholds and Liver Injury Pattern

RUCAM was the first CAM that clearly defined criteria of liver injury by using liver test (LT) thresholds [6] based on multiples of LT ULN (upper limit of normal) as a diagnostic criterion (Fig. 2) [6, 21], thereby eliminating cases with trivial increases in liver enzymes lacking clinical relevance. In addition, RUCAM was the first CAM to recognize the importance of various types of suspected DILI [6, 21]. Based on the analysis of clinical feature

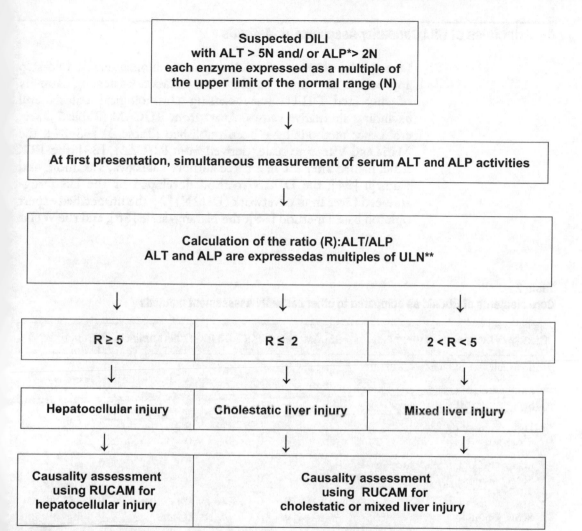

Fig. 2 Classification of liver injury required for causality assessment. *If ALT is within normal range, ensure that ALP is of hepatic origin: increase in GGT or 5′ nucleosidase. **By convention if ALT or ALP <ULN (Upper limit of normal), then the number to retain is 1. RUCAM allows for causality of the types of liver injury that differ on few items and scores (Table 2). *ALP* alkaline phosphatase, *ALT* alanine aminotransferase, *DILI* drug-induced liver injury, *RUCAM* Roussel Uclaf Causality Assessment Method

variability in DILI cases, three types of liver injury pattern are recognized: hepatocellular, cholestatic, and mixed liver injury (Fig. 2, Table 1) [6, 21]. For RUCAM causality assessment, only two of the three injury types are considered, i.e., hepatocellular injury and cholestatic/mixed liver injury (Fig. 2, Table 1) [6, 21]. Specific and individual scores had to be defined for each liver injury type as each shows different clinical features and courses, especially in regard to challenge, dechallenge, and rechallenge characteristics and patient demographics (e.g., age) [32].

4 Principles of DILI Causality Assessment Methods

Due to the absence of valid diagnostic biomarkers, a two-step approach is commonly employed in CAMs for assessing causality of suspected DILI cases: assessing chronological criteria and excluding alternative causes. Apart from RUCAM (Table 2), several other methods have been published (Table 2) [33–37]: the Maria and Victorino scale (derived from RUCAM) [33]; the TTK scale, named after the first three authors Takikawa, Takamori, and Kumagi [34]; the DILIN method developed by the US Drug-Induced Liver Injury Network (DILIN) [7]; the unspecified expert opinion based method [35]; the Naranjo scale [36]; and the WHO

Table 2
Core elements of RUCAM as compared to other causality assessment methods

Clearly defined core elements	RUCAM	MV	TKK	DILIN	Expert opinion	Naranjo	WHO
Individually scored items							
• Time frame of latency period	+	+	?	?	0	0	0
Scored item	+	+	0	0	0	0	0
• Time frame of dechallenge	+	+	?	?	0	0	0
Scored item	+	+	0	0	0	0	0
• Recurrent ALT or ALP increase	+	0	0	?	0	0	0
Scored item	+	0	0	0	0	0	0
• Risk factors	+	0	0	?	0	0	0
Scored items	+	0	0	0	0	0	0
• All comedications	+	0	0	?	0	+	0
Scored items	+	0	0	0	0	+	0
• Individual comedication	+	0	0	?	0	0	0
Scored item	+	0	0	0	0	0	0
• Exclusion of alternative causes	+	+	0	?	0	0	0
Scored items	+	+	0	0	0	0	0
• Markers of HAV, HBV, HCV, HEV	+	0	0	?	0	0	0
Scored items	+	0	0	0	0	0	0
• Markers of CMV, EBV, HSV, VZV	+	0	0	?	0	0	0
Scored items	+	0	0	0	0	0	0
• Cardiac hepatopathy	+	+	0	?	0	0	0
Scored item	+	?	0	0	0	0	0
• Liver and biliary tract imaging	+	+	0	?	0	0	0
Scored item	+	?	0	0	0	0	0

(continued)

Table 2
(continued)

Clearly defined core elements	RUCAM	MV	TKK	DILIN	Expert opinion	Naranjo	WHO
• Doppler sonography of liver vessels	+	0	0	?	0	0	0
Scored item	+	0	0	0	0	0	0
• Prior known hepatotoxicity of drug	+	+	0	?	0	+	0
Scored item	+	+	0	0	0	+	0
• Unintentional reexposure	+	+	0	?	0	+	0
Scored item	+	+	0	0	0	+	0
• Laboratory hepatotoxicity criteria	+	+	0	+	0	0	0
• Laboratory hepatotoxicity pattern	+	+	+	?	0	0	0
• Hepatotoxicity specific method	+	+	+	+	0	0	0
• Structured, liver related method	+	+	+	0	0	0	0
• Quantitative, liver related method	+	+	+	0	0	0	0
• Validated method (gold standard)	+	0	0	0	0	0	0

Listing compilation of core elements of RUCAM and other CAMs, which are adapted from a previous report containing additional details [6]. The table includes RUCAM [6], the MV scale from the report of Maria and Victorino [33], the TKK scale named after the first three authors Takikawa, Takamori, Kumagi et al. [34], the DILIN method of the Drug-Induced Liver Injury Network [7], the unspecified expert opinion based method or ad-hoc approach as outlined by Kaplowitz [35], the Naranjo scale based on the report of Naranjo et al. [36], and the WHO method from the WHO database [37]. The symbol "+" shows that this specific item is published, and the symbol "0" indicates that the item lacks publication, and the symbol "?" refers to uncertain documentation

ALT alanine aminotransferase, *ALP* alkaline phosphatase, *CMV* cytomegalovirus, *EBV* Epstein Barr virus, *HAV* Hepatitis A virus, *HBV* Hepatitis B virus, *HCV* Hepatitis C virus, *HEV* Hepatitis E virus, *HSV* Herpes simplex virus, *VZV* Varicella zoster virus

method [37]. For most methods [33–37], shortcomings have been found [6, 25, 29, 38].

As a general rule, DILI causality assessment should consider defined core elements of important in the diagnosis of DILI, and provide an individual score for each item; however, only a few methods followed this diagnostic and quantitative approach (Table 2) [6]. Structured core items with individual and final scores, which provide transparent data for reevaluation by other professionals, should be the ultimate goal of any publication of DILI cases. Clinicians and regulators attempting to establish DILI as a firm diagnosis must confirm or exclude alternative causes, such as those listed in Fig. 3 [6]. Such listing presents alternative causes and diagnoses that should be suspected, depending on the patient characteristics and clinical context [6]; indeed, many liver injury cases are not DILI or HILI [8, 22, 23].

**Clinical evaluation of a case with suspected DILI
Causality assessment using RUCAM**

↓

**Exclusion of alternative causes
A reminder for physicians
to ensure data completeness**

↓   ↓

Differential diagnosis	Diagnostic parameters
• Hepatitis A virus (HAV)	Anti-HAV-IgM
• Hepatitis B virus (HBV)	HBV-DNA, anti-HBc-IgM
• Hepatitis C virus (HCV)	HCV-RNA, anti-HCV
• Hepatitis E virus (HEV)	HEV-RNA , titer change for anti-HEV-IgM/anti-HEV-IgG
• Cytomegalovirus (CMV)	CMV-PCR, titer change for anti-CMV-IgM/anti-CMV-IgG
• Epstein Barr virus (EBV)	EBV-PCR, titer change for anti-EBV-IgM/anti-EBV-IgG
• Herpes simplex virus (HSV)	HSV-PCR, titer change for anti-HSV-IgM/anti-HSV-IgG
• Varicella zoster virus (VZV)	VZV-PCR, titer change for anti-VZV-IgM/anti-VZV-IgG
• Other viral infections according to the clinical context	Specific serology of Adenovirus, Coxsackie-B-Virus, Echovirus, Measles virus, Rubella virus, Flavivirus, Arenavirus, Filovirus, Parvovirus, HIV, and others
• Other infectious diseases	Specific assessment of bacteria, fungi, parasites, and others
• Autoimmune hepatitis (AIH) type I	Gamma globulins, ANA, SMA, AAA, SLA/LP, Anti-LSP, Anti-ASGPR
• Autoimmune hepatitis (AIH) type II	Gamma globulins, Anti-LKM-1 (CYP 2D6), Anti-LKM-2 (CYP 2C9), Anti-LKM-3
• Primary biliary cholangitis (PBC)	AMA, Anti PDH-E2
• Primary sclerosing cholangitis (PSC)	p-ANCA, MRC
• Autoimmune cholangitis (AIC)	ANA, SMA
• Overlap syndromes	See AIH, PBC, PSC, and AIC
• Non alcoholic steatohepatitis (NASH)	BMI, insulin resistance, hepatomegaly, echogenicity of the liver
• Alcoholic liver disease (ALD)	Patient's history, clinical and laboratory assessment, other alcoholic disease(s)
• Cocaine, ecstasy and other amphetamines	Toxin screening

Fig. 3 Checklist of differential diagnoses in cases of suspected DILI. This tabular listing is adapted and derived from a previous publication [6]. Although not comprehensive, it is to be used as a guide and in connection with RUCAM [6]. *AAA* anti-actin antibodies, *AMA* antimitochondrial antibodies, *ANA* antinuclear antibodies, *ASGPR* Asialo-glycoprotein-receptor, *BMI* body mass index, *CT* computed tomography, *CYP* cytochrome P450, *DILI* drug-induced liver injury, *DPH* pyruvate dehydrogenase, *HAV* Hepatitis A virus, *HBc* Hepatitis B core, *HBV* Hepatitis B virus, *HCV* Hepatitis C virus, *HEV* Hepatitis E virus, *HIV* human immunodeficiency virus, *LKM* liver kidney microsomes, *LP* Liver-pancreas antigen, *LSP* liver specific protein, *MRC* magnetic resonance cholangiography, *MRT*

• Rare intoxications	Toxin screening for household and occupational toxins
• Hereditary hemochromatosis	Serum ferritin, total iron-binding capacity, genotyping for C2824 and H63D mutation, hepatic iron content
• Wilson disease	Copper excretion (24 h urine), ceruloplasmin in serum, free copper in serum, Coombs-negative hemolytic anemia, hepatic copper content, Kayser-Fleischer-ring, neurologic-psychiatric work-up, genotyping
• Porphyria	Porphobilinogen in urine, total porphyrines in urine
• α_1-Antitrypsin deficiency	α_1 – Antitrypsin in serum
• Biliary diseases	Clinical and laboratory assessment, hepatobiliary sonography, and other imaging (CT, MRC)
• Pancreatic diseases	Clinical and laboratory assessment, sonography, CT, MRT
• Celiac disease	TTG antibodies, endomysium antibodies, duodenal biopsy
• Anorexia nervosa	Clinical context
• Parenteral nutrition	Clinical context
• Cardiopulmonary diseases	Cardiopulmonary assessment of congestive heart disease, myocardial infarction, cardiomyopathy, cardiac valvular dysfunction, pulmonary embolism, pericardial diseases, arrhythmia, hemorrhagic shock, and various other conditions
• Addison disease	Plasma cortisol
• Thyroid diseases	TSH basal, T4, T3
• Grand mal seizures	Clinical context of epileptic seizure (duration >30 min)
• Heat stroke	Shock, hyperthermia
• Polytrauma	Shock, liver injury
• Systemic diseases	Specific assessment of sarcoidosis, amyloidosis, metastatic tumor, sepsis, and others
• Other diseases	Clinical context

Fig. 3 (continued) magnetic resonance tomography, *p-ANCA* perinuclear antineutrophil cytoplasmatic antibodies, *PCR* polymerase chain reaction, *RUCAM* Roussel Uclaf Causality Assessment Method, *SLA* soluble liver antigen, *SMA* smooth muscle antibodies, *TSH* thyroid stimulating hormone, *TTG* tissue transglutaminase

5   Roussel Uclaf Causality Assessment Method (RUCAM)

RUCAM was developed in the late 80s as a result of international consensus meetings of experts [6, 21]. The core items and specific details included in RUCAM were designed to resolve the problems that experts and clinicians encountered in poorly defined existing CAMs, which lacked defined and scored items and often resulted in endless discussion on causality assignments. First, definitions of terms related to liver injury and chronological criteria were developed in a consensus meeting of experts in hepatology, who provided their expertise on liver injury pattern; some chronological quantitative criteria such as time to onset and other criteria for additional items including drug rechallenge [39]. Second, some specific and quantitative items like alcohol consumption details were added, and all the items were scored in order to standardize causality assessment of liver injury [21]. Finally, RUCAM-based approach has high sensitivity (86%) and specificity (89%), with high positive (93%) and negative (78%) predictive values, based on 77 case reports [28].

The global use of and experience with the original RUCAM since its publication in 1993 [21, 28] led to an updated version of RUCAM published in 2016 [6]. A few core items such as alcohol usage were specified, and recent diagnostic developments related to HEV exclusion were considered. The updated RUCAM can be used for DILI as well as HILI. Recently, this version of RUCAM was applied in a cohort study of ten patients with suspected but disproved liver injury caused by an herbal drug, manufactured as extract from *Petasites hybridus* for migraine prophylaxis (Table 3) [40].

5.1 Specific Key Items of RUCAM

DILI cases considered for causality must fulfil the criteria of liver injury (Fig. 2) and laboratory-based liver injury pattern (also called phenotype) (Fig. 2) [6]. A stepwise approach is indispensable: first, a careful clinical evaluation needs to be conducted and second, the RUCAM assessment with its key items need to be scored according to clinical and laboratory data (Tables 1 and 3) [6]. The RUCAM items are defined clearly enough to allow for fast collection of diagnostic data, while the patient is still under medical care. Conceptualized for ongoing use, RUCAM provides best results if applied in real-time rather than retrospectively, ensuring completeness of case data sets and unbiased case evaluation (Table 4). Otherwise, late assessment may cause major problems in collecting relevant data used to assess the cases, resulting in interobserver and intraobserver variability [6].

5.2 Time to Onset from the Beginning of the Drug Administration

It is a challenge to define and score with a time interval between beginning of the drug usage, with day 0 as the first day of intake, and the onset of increased liver enzymes or symptoms if they are likely related to the liver injury [6]. This period is sometimes also called the latency period. Termination of drug use prior to the onset of the liver injury requires alternative scoring, and slowly metabolized chemicals with prolonged half-lives are specifically to be considered (Table 3) [6].

5.3 Course of ALT or ALP After Cessation of the Drug

An important part of the RUCAM assessment are the precise dechallenge criteria with individual scores that reflect the course of serum ALT and/or ALP observed after cessation of the suspected product, which are cornerstones of RUCAM to facilitate causality assessment [6]. During the dechallenge phase in patients experiencing DILI, assessing the natural course of LTs (i.e., not confounded by any external factors) is essential. For instance, treatment

Table 3

Example of a RUCAM-based causality assessment in a study cohort of 10 patients who used a herbal drug, made from an extract of *Petasites hybridus* (PH)

Items	Score	Case 1		Case 2		Case 3		Case 4		Case 5	Case 6		Case 7	Case 8	Case 9	Case 10
		PH	Other drugs	PH	Other drug	PH	Other drug	PH	Other drug	PH	PH	Other drugs	PH	PH	PH	PH
1. Time to onset from the beginning of the drug/herb																
• 5–90 d, rechallenge: 1–15 d	+2	+2	?	+2				+2				+2				
• <5 or >90 d, rechallenge: >15 d	+1	+1			+1	+1	+1		+1	+1	+1		+1	+1	+1	+1
Alternative: time to onset from cessation of the drug/herb																
• ≤15 d (except for slowly metabolized chemicals: >15 d)	+1														?	
2. Course of ALT after cessation of the drug/herb																
Percentage difference between ALT peak and ULN																
• Decrease ≥50% within 8 d	+3			+3	+3					+3						
• Decrease ≥50% within 30 d	+2							+2	+2					+2		
• No information or continued drug use	0										0	0	0		0	
• Decrease ≥50% after 30 d	0															
• Decrease <50% after the 30th day or recurrent increase	–2	–2	–2			–2	–2				–2	–2		–2	–2	

(continued)

Table 3
(continued)

Items	Score	Case 1		Case 2		Case 3		Case 4		Case 5	Case 6		Case 7	Case 8	Case 9	Case 10
		PH	Other drugs	PH	Other drug	PH	Other drug	PH	Other drug	PH	PH	Other drugs	PH	PH	PH	PH
3. Risk factors																
• Alcohol use (current drinks/d: >2 for women, >3 for men)	+1															
• Alcohol use (current drinks/d: ≤2 for women, ≤3 for men)	0	0	0	0	0	0	0	0	0	0	0	0	0	0	0	0
• Age ≥55 years	+1															
• Age <55 years	0	0	0	0	0	0	0	0	0	0	0	0	+1	0	0	0
4. Concomitant drug–herb																
• None or no information	0									0				0		
• Concomitant drug–herb with incompatible time to onset	0	?	?			0	0				0	0	0?			0
• Concomitant drug–herb with compatible or suggestive time to onset	−1			−1	−1			−1	−1		−1					
• Concomitant drug–herb known as hepatotoxin and with compatible or suggestive time to onset	−2															
• Concomitant drug–herb with evidence for its role in this case (positive rechallenge or validated test)	−3															

5. Search for alternative causes											
Group I (seven causes)											
• HAV: Anti-HAV-IgM	–	–	–?	–	–	–	–	–	–	n.a.	–	n.a.
• HBV: HBsAg, anti-HBc-IgM, HBV-DNA	+?	+?	–?	–	–	–	–	–	–	n.a.	–	n.a.
• HCV: Anti-HCV, HCV-RNA	–	–	–?	–	–	–	–	–	–	n.a.	–	n.a.
• HEV: Anti-HEV-IgM, anti-HEV-IgG, HEV-RNA	n.a. n.a.	n.a.	n.a. r.a.	n.a. n.a.	n.a. n.a.	n.a. n.a.	n.a. n.a.	n.a. n.a.	n.a. n.a.	n.a.	n.a.?	n.a.
• Hepatobiliary sonography/color Doppler sonography of liver vessels/endosonography/CT/MRC	–	–	–	+	+	+	+	–	–	+	–	+
• Alcoholism (AST/ALT ≥2)	–	–	–	–	–	–	–	–	–	–	–	–
• Acute recent hypotension history (particularly if underlying heart disease)	–	–	–	–	–	–	–	–	–	–	–	–
Group II (six causes)											
• Complications of underlying disease(s) such as sepsis, metastatic malignancy, autoimmune hepatitis, chronic hepatitis B or C, primary biliary cholangitis or sclerosing cholangitis, genetic liver diseases	–	–	–	–	–	–	–	–	–	–	–	–

(continued)

Table 3
(continued)

Items	Score	Case 1		Case 2		Case 3		Case 4		Case 5		Case 6		Case 7	Case 8	Case 9	Case 10
		PH	Other drugs	PH	Other drug	PH	Other drug	PH	Other drug	PH	Other	PH	Other drugs	PH	PH	PH	PH
Infection suggested by titer changes and PCR:																	
• CMV (anti-CMV-IgM, anti-CMV-IgG, CMV PCR)		−	−	?	?	n.a.	n.a.	−	−	n.a.	n.a.	n.a.	n.a.	n.a.	+?	n.a.?	n.a.
• EBV (anti-EBV-IgM, anti-EBV-IgG, EBV PCR)		−	−	+	+	(+)?	(+)?	n.a.	n.a.	−		−	−	n.a.	−	?	n.a.
• HSV (anti-HSV-IgM, anti-HSV-IgG, HSV PCR)		n.a.	n.a.	n.a.	n.a.	n.a.	n.a.	+?	+?	n.a.	n.a.	n.a.		n.a.?	n.a.?	n.a.?	n.a.
• VZV (anti-VZV-IgM, anti-VZV-IgG, VZV PCR)		n.a.	n.a.	n.a.	n.a.	n.a.	n.a.	n.a.	n.a.	n.a.	n.a.	n.a.		n.a.	n.a.	n.a.?	n.a.
Evaluation of groups I and II																	
• All causes—groups I and II—reasonably ruled out	+2																
• The seven causes of group I ruled out	+1																
• Six or five causes of group I ruled out	0	0	0			0	0			0		0	0			0	
• Less than five causes of group I ruled out	−2													−2			
• Alternative cause highly probable	−3			−3	−3			−3	−3		−3				−3		−3

	Score													
6. Previous hepatotoxicity of the drug/herb														
• Reaction labeled in the product characteristics	+2	+2	+2	+2	+2	+2	+2	?	+2	+2	+2	+2	+2	+2
• Reaction published but unlabelled	+1													
• Reaction unknown	0													
7. Response to unintentional reexposure														
• Doubling of ALT with the drug/herb alone, provided ALT below 5 ULN before reexposure	+3													
• Doubling of ALT with the drug(s)/herb(s) already given at the time of first reaction	+1													
• Increase of ALT but less than ULN in the same conditions as for the first administration	−2													
• Other situations	0	0	0	0	0	0	0	0	0	0	0	0	0	0
Total score for patient		+2	0?	+3	+2	+1	+1	+2	+1	+3	0	+2	0	+1

Additional case details are provided in another publication [40]. Details of RUCAM are presented in a recent report [6], whereby for this cohort the RUCAM subscale was used that is specifically reserved for the hepatocellular injury. The symbol "+" indicates that an abnormal result was obtained, whereas "−" indicates a normal result

ALT alanine aminotransferase, *AST* aspartate aminotransferase, *CMV* cytomegalovirus, *CT* computer tomography, *DILI* drug-induced liver injury, *EBV* Epstein Barr virus, *HAV* Hepatitis A virus, *HBc* Hepatitis B core, *HBsAg* Hepatitis B antigen, *HBV* Hepatitis B virus, *HCV* Hepatitis C virus, *HEV* Hepatitis E virus, *HILI* herb induced liver injury, *HSV* Herpes simplex virus, *MRC* magnetic resonance cholangiography, *n.a.* not assessed or not available, *PH* Petasites hybridus, from which the herbal drug Petadolex® was manufactured, *RUCAM* Roussel Uclaf Causality Assessment Method, *ULN* upper limit of the normal range, *VZV* Varicella zoster virus

Total score and resulting causality grading: ≤0, excluded; 1–2, unlikely; 3–5, possible; 6–8, probable; ≥9, highly probable

Table 4
Advantages and limitations of RUCAM

Advantages of RUCAM

- Prospective use and timely decision
- Stepwise first clinical approach, followed by RUCAM
- User-friendly and cost-saving method
- Effective use without the need of an expert panel
- Timely use at the bedside of the patient
- Clearly defined key items of clinical features and course
- Full consideration of comedication and alternative causes
- Consideration of prior known hepatotoxicity
- Incorporation of unintentional reexposure results
- Hepatotoxicity specific method
- Structured, liver related method
- Individual scoring system of all key items
- Quantitative, liver related method
- Validated method (gold standard)
- Worldwide use
- Use by international registries
- Use by regulatory agencies
- Use by DILI case reports and case series
- Transparent documentation
- Possible reevaluation by peers

Limitations of RUCAM

- RUCAM was not designed for suspected chronic DILI, which is mostly an unrecognized preexisting liver disease
- RUCAM was also not designed when a suspected injury occurs on preexisting liver diseases, a complex condition where expert hepatologists are required

DILI drug-induced liver injury, *RUCAM* Roussel Uclaf Causality Assessment Method

with drugs like corticosteroids or ursodesoxycholic acid may accelerate and thereby mask the natural course of liver enzyme decline, providing no correct information of the natural LT course and leading to a score of 0 (Table 3). In cases of hepatocellular injury, prospective ordering of serial ALT determinations on day 8 and 30 after cessation of the suspect product ensures completeness of data collection. For cholestatic and mixed liver injury, dechallenge results of serial ALP within 180 days after cessation are required for causality assessment [6]. All possible situations are scored, and the resulting scores are placed in the appropriate column of RUCAM according to the type of liver injury (Tables 1 and 3) [6].

5.4   Alcohol Use

According to data obtained, analyzed, and validated during the creation of the original RUCAM, amounts of alcohol usage were further specified and defined separately for women (two drinks per day) and men (three drinks per day), using an average 10 g ethanol for each drink (Table 3) [6]. Other studies also confirmed alcohol use as risk factor of DILI [20, 29]. For instance, according to a British population-based case–control study of DILI, alcohol usage was a potential confounder of DILI among 128 assessable cases, with an odds ratio (OR) ≤2.0, achieved if >10 units were consumed within a week, where 1 unit corresponded to one glass of wine [20]. In line with this study, other reports considered alcohol use as a risk factor of DILI [41–45], especially when alcohol use coincided with acetaminophen use [42]. The increased risk of DILI in alcoholic patients was observed when receiving drugs such as halothane [41, 43], isoflurane [41, 43], and isoniazid [41], various antituberculosis drugs [44, 45], including rifampicin and isoniazid in combination [44], and drug treatment for multidrug-resistant tuberculosis [45], methotrexate, and other drugs [41]. In a study of patients with pulmonary tuberculosis treated with antituberculosis drugs, a multivariate analysis revealed prior alcohol consumption as a significant risk factor of recurrent DILI with an odds ratio (OR) of 2.2 [44]. These observations justify the inclusion of alcohol usage as a risk factor of DILI, and as such alcohol use is awarded one point in the original RUCAM [21] as well as in the RUCAM update of 2016 (Table 3) [6].

5.5   Age and Pregnancy

Age ≥55 years is included as a risk factor for DILI with its respective score (Table 3) [6]. Pregnancy lowers the threshold for cholestasis due to high estrogen concentrations and represents a risk factor for cholestatic/mixed liver injury but not for hepatocellular injury [6].

5.6   Concomitant Drug(s) and Herb(s)

Concomitant usage of drugs and herbs is a crucial item that is best inquired and documented at first presentation whenever DILI is suspected. Details of a temporal association and potential hepatotoxic features of the concomitant product should be assessed and documented [6]. For reasons of comparison and transparency, each concomitant drug or herb requires a separate analysis using RUCAM. For patients given multiple drugs or herbs, the final causality should be attributed primarily to the product with the highest score achieved using RUCAM [6].

5.7   Search for Alternative Causes

DILI assessment is impeded by overlooked potential causes [8, 22, 23] and incomplete case data, a matter stressed by the DILIN group [46], but these flaws can be prevented by the prospective use of RUCAM [6]. RUCAM considers the clinically most relevant alternative causes and the involvement of underlying disease(s) (Fig. 3 and Table 3) [6]. Infections by hepatitis E virus (HEV) are now recognized to sometimes masquerade as DILI, even if the US anti-HEV antibody tests are not currently FDA-approved [5, 6, 16, 29, 40, 47–51]. In many suspected liver injury cases, analysis of HEV RNA was missed [5, 6, 16, 29, 40, 46, 48–51]. Most importantly, in suspected viral infections, titer changes of antibodies should be evaluated in the clinical course to confirm, or refute an ongoing virus infection, but this is rarely practiced in the DILI and HILI series.

Alternative causes are also included in the checklist (Fig. 3) [6]. They should be excluded or verified depending on the clinical context and the benefit for the patient. Discovery of alternative causes for the liver injury may indicate specific treatments. Moreover, suspected autoimmune hepatitis (AIH) in a DILI setting should resolve with drug discontinuation [6, 40], whereas genuine AIH will worsen, remain stable, or relapse [52].

5.8 Previous Hepatotoxicity

The risk of hepatotoxicity listed in the product information sheet (e.g., Summary of product characteristics in the EU or product information in the USA) must be checked, although the terms used to indicate liver injury may vary and usually do not refer to specific definitions. If it is mentioned, then the hepatotoxicity is considered known for that compound. If this hepatotoxicity is not declared, a quick literature search is recommended in PubMed and the NIH LiverTox website [53], although this site lacks an actualized CAM section especially regarding RUCAM and its updated version [6].

5.9 Response to Unintentional Rechallenge

A positive rechallenge test result is viewed as the gold standard to determine the culprit drug in DILI cases [6]. To classify a rechallenge test as positive, certain criteria are required, as specified (Fig. 4) [6]. For hepatocellular injury, the defining criteria are based on ALT levels immediately before rechallenge (designated as baseline ALT or ALTb), and peak ALT levels after rechallenge (designated as ALTr). The rechallenge test is positive if ALTb is <5× ULN and ALTr is ≥2 ALTb, negative if one or both criteria are not fulfilled, and uninterpretable if data are lacking for one or both criteria. For cholestatic/ mixed liver injury, the assessment criteria and interpretation of results are similar, with ALT replaced by ALP (Fig. 4).

5.10 Individual and Final Scores

Each RUCAM item receives an individual score ranging maximum from +3 to −3, and the sum of the individual scores provides the final score for the patient (Tables 1 and 3) [6]. The range of the final scores from +14 to −9 allows for grading causality: ≤0, relationship excluded; 1–2, unlikely; 3–5, possible; 6–8, probable; ≥9, highly probable [6].

5.11 Advantages and Limitations of RUCAM

Advantages and limitations of RUCAM have been discussed previously [6] and are outlined here, as well as summarized in Table 4. RUCAM yields certain advantages as compared to other methods (Table 2) [6].

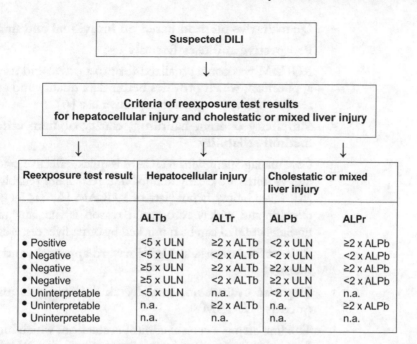

Fig. 4 Conditions and criteria for an unintentional rechallenge test, actualized and adapted from a previous report [6]. Accordingly, required data for the hepatocellular type of liver injury are the ALT levels just before reexposure, designed as baseline ALT or ALTb, and the ALT levels during reexposure, designed as ALTr. Response to reexposure is positive, if both criteria are met: first, ALTb is below 5 × ULN with ULN as the upper limit of the normal value, and second ALTr $\geq$2 × ALTb. Other variations lead to negative or uninterpretable results. For the cholestatic ($\pm$hepatocellular) type of liver injury, corresponding values of ALP are to be used rather than of ALT. *ALP* alkaline phosphatase, *ALT* alanine aminotransferase, *n.a.* not available

5.11.1 *Advantages*   • **Mandatory definition and classification of the liver injury**

RUCAM requires the fulfillment of specific liver injury criteria including thresholds for liver tests (Figs. 1 and 2) [6]. This ensures the a priori elimination of non-liver injury cases and differentiates RUCAM assessment according to the type of liver injury.

• **Algorithm**

RUCAM is based on a sophisticated diagnostic algorithm due to the evaluation of DILI a complex process (Figs. 2, 3, 4 and Tables 1, 2, 3, 4) [6]; another specific algorithm was also used previously for AIH [52]. The usage of such diagnostic algorithms facilitates a uniform approach to a valid diagnosis of these difficult diagnoses.

• **Structured presentation and validation**

RUCAM presents seven categories of criteria that should be systematically scored according to the clinical and lab data (Table 3) [6]. Its validation, including positive rechallenge cases as gold standard (Tables 2 and 4) [6, 28], has been detailed elsewhere [28].

- **Quantitative method based on individual and final scores**
- **Prospective and user-friendly use**

  RUCAM was conceptualized for prospective and user-friendly application, which provides better data quality and assessment results than any vague retrospective use [6].

- **Simplicity of item handling, clarity of item criteria, and method reliability**

  Case management with RUCAM is quick, effective, and cost saving, as items are clearly defined and results are reliably obtained [6]. Liver biopsy is not part of RUCAM [6, 21, 54]; the most relevant and widely recognized reason is that any histological findings in DILI can be mimicked by other liver diseases [21, 54].

- **Robust framework, straightforward approach, and real-time method**
- **Stepwise evaluation, initially clinical analysis and subsequently RUCAM**

  The first step is a careful clinical evaluation, which includes the data collection guided by the items required in RUCAM. This can be drawn from the case narrative that also provides information of the clinical course [55]. Subsequently, RUCAM should be applied (Tables 1 and 3) with a focus on the checklist of differential diagnoses (Fig. 3). If uncertainty remains, an expert opinion may follow using the RUCAM items [6]. RUCAM is applicable even in cases with preexisting liver disease if a new DILI event is suspected [29, 56].

- **Mandatory systematic documentation and data transparency**

  For DILI case assessment, a systematic documentation is mandatory for case reports, regulatory purposes, and reassessment by independent experts [6, 55]. Documentation should start with the narrative, the listing table with all RUCAM data (Table 3), and a table of excluded alternative causes (Fig. 3) [55].

- **Epidemiological, clinical, and genotyping studies**

  RUCAM has been used to identify DILI and HILI in studies of prescription drugs, herbal medications, regulatory evaluations including phase I/II/III clinical studies, long-term post marketing clinical trials, and epidemiological studies, and genotyping studies, just to name a few examples as referenced in detail [6].

- **International appreciation and worldwide usage**

  Experience to date with RUCAM shows that it is the most commonly used CAM by international registries, regulatory agencies, and in case reports to identify suspected DILI and HILI cases worldwide, as evidenced by an increase in publications within the past years (Tables 5 and 6) [19, 57–166].

Table 5
Listing of selected international registries and regulatory agencies, and associated groups that applied RUCAM in suspected DILI and HILI cases

Cases	Suspected products	Country/region	Group/agency	Year	First author
DILI	Multiple synthetic drugs	Spain Europe	Spanish Group for the Study of the Drug-Induced Liver Disease, Malaga	2005	Andrade [57]
DILI	Multiple synthetic drugs	Spain Europe	Spain Hepatotoxicity Registry, Grupo de Estudio Para las Hepatopatías Asociadas a Medicamentos, Malaga	2006	Andrade [24]
HILI DILI	Various herbal TCM, synthetic drugs	Singapore Asia	National University of Singapore	2006	Wai [58]
HILI	Lu Cha (Green tea extract)	Sweden Europe	Swedish Adverse Drug Reactions Advisory Committee	2007	Björnsson [59]
HILI	Black cohosh	Various countries Europe	European Medicines Agency	2007	EMA [60]
HILI	Herbs	Spain Europe	Spanish Liver Toxicity Registry	2008	Garcia-Cortés [61]
DILI, HILI	Multiple synthetic drugs, few herbs	Spain Europe	Spanish Group for the Study of Drug-induced Liver Disease	2008	García-Cortés [62]
DILI	Flucloxacillin	UK, other countries	DILIGEN Study and International SAE Consortium	2009	Daly [63]
DILI	Synthetic drugs	Serbia Europe	Medicines and Medical Devices Agency of Serbia, Belgrade	2011	Miljkovic [25]
HILI	*Polygonum multiflorum*	Korea Asia	Gyeongsang National University School of Medicine, Jinju/ Sungkyunkwan University School of Medicine, Changwon	2011	Jung [64]
HILI	Various herbal TCM	Hong Kong	Hong Kong Herb-Induced Liver Injury Network (HK-HILIN), Hong Kong	2011	Chau [65]
DILI	Multiple synthetic drugs	Spain, other countries	Spanish DILI Registry, EUDRAGENE, DILIN, DILIGEN, and International SAEC	2011	Lucena [66]

(continued)

Table 5
(continued)

Cases	Suspected products	Country/ region	Group/agency	Year	First author
DILI	Synthetic drugs	Serbia Europe	Medicines and Medical Devices Agency of Serbia, Belgrade	2012	Miljkovic [26]
DILI	Statins	Iceland/ Sweden Europe	National University Hospital Reykjvik/University of Gothenburg/Swedish Adverse Drug Reactions Advisory Committee (SADRAC)	2012	Björnsson [27]
DILI	Various synthetic drugs (expected)	Spain Latin America	Spanish-Latin American Network on drug-induced liver Injury, in progress	2012	Bessone [10]
DILI	Flupirtine	Germany Europe	Drug Commission of the German Medical Association	2012	Stammschulte [67]
DILI	Flupirtine	Germany Europe	Berlin Case-control Surveillance Study, German drug reaction reporting database	2014	Douros [68]
DILI	Anabolic and androgenic steroids	Spain Latin America	Spanish DILI Registry and Spanish-Latin-American DILI Network	2015	Robles-Diaz [69]
DILI	Multiple synthetic drugs	Germany Europe	Berlin Case-control Surveillance Study	2015	Douros [70]

DILI drug-induced liver injury, *HILI* herb-induced liver injury, *RUCAM* Roussel Uclaf Causality Assessment Method, *TCM* traditional Chinese medicine

5.11.2 Limitations of RUCAM

- **Poor quality of case data**

  To obtain qualified RUCAM-based results, physicians and assessors are encouraged to adhere to this method carefully [6] and consider basic liver tests for the liver injury classification (Figs. 1 and 2). They should follow the specific operational information, details of core elements and their scoring (Table 3), differential diagnoses (Fig. 3), and the rechallenge criteria (Fig. 4). However, RUCAM cannot compensate for flaws from improper clinical or regulatory case analyses, incomplete case data, or poor quality data transfer from medical records to the RUCAM scale [16, 49–51]. The problem of missing essential elements will remain [46] unless rigorous efforts are undertaken to improve case documentation approaches [50, 51].

- **Chronic DILI**

  RUCAM has been conceptualized for acute DILI but not for complex conditions, such as chronic DILI or suspected DILI in

Table 6
Listing of selected individual reports using RUCAM in suspected DILI and HILI cases

Cases	Products	Country/region	Year	First author
DILI	Various synthetic drugs	France Europe	1993	Danan [21]
DILI	Various synthetic drugs	France Europe	1993	Bénichou [28]
DILI	Ketoprofen	France Europe	1998	Flamenbaum [71]
DILI	NSAIDs	Europe Europe	2003	Lucena [72]
HILI	Kava	Germany Europe	2003	Stickel [73]
DILI	Various synthetic drugs	Japan Asia	2003	Masumotuo [74]
DILI	Multiple synthetic drugs	Spain Europe	2004	Andrade [75]
DILI	Pioglitazone	France Europe	2004	Arotcarena [76]
DILI	Ximelagatran	USA, France, Sweden	2005	Lee [77]
HILI	Ji Xue Cao	Argentina South America	2005	Jorge [78]
HILI	Lu Cha (Green tea, *Camellia sinensis*)	France Europe	2005	Gloro [79]
DILI	Amoxicillin, Amoxicillin/Clavulanate	USA	2005	Fontana [80]
DILI	Various synthetic drugs	Sweden Europe	2006	De Valle [81]
HILI	Bo He, Chuan Lian Zi, and various other herbal TCM	Korea Asia	2006	Yuen [82]
HILI	Lu Cha	Spain Europe	2006	Jimenez-Saenz [83]
HILI	*Polygonum multiflorum*	Columbia South America	2006	Cárdenas [84]
DILI	Rofecoxib	Canada North America	2006	Yan [85]
DILI	Antibiotics	UK Europe	2007	Hussaini [86]
DILI	Atomoxetine	USA	2007	Stojanovski [87]
DILI	Varioussyntheticdrugs	Sweden Europe	2007	Björnsson [88]

(continued)

Table 6
(continued)

Cases	Products	Country/region	Year	First author
DILI	Flavoxate	Italy Europe	2007	Rigato [89]
HILI	Kava	Germany Europe	2008	Teschke [90]
HILI	Bai Xian Pi, Kudzu, Lu Cha, Yin Chen Hao	Korea Asia	2008	Kang [91]
HILI	Bai Xian Pi, Ci Wu Jia, Shou Wu Pian, Yin Chen Hao	Korea Asia	2008	Sohn [92]
DILI	Albedazole	Korea Asia	2008	Choi [93]
HILI	Indian Ayurvedic herbs	Germany Europe	2009	Teschke [94]
HILI	Green tea (*Camellia sinensis*)	Italy Europe	2009	Mazzanti [95]
HILI	Herbalife	Switzerland Europe	2009	Stickel [96]
HILI	*Corydalis speciosa*	Korea Asia	2009	Kang [97]
DILI	Black cohosh	Germany Europe	2009	Teschke [98]
HILI	Black cohosh	Germany Europe	2009	Teschke [99]
HILI	Ge Gen	Korea Asia	2009	Kim [100]
DILI	Montelukast	India Asia	2009	Harugeri [101]
DILI	Nimesulide	Italy Europe	2010	Licata [102]
DILI	Tadalafil	Morocco Africa	2010	Essaid [103]
HILI	Herbalife	Iceland Europe	2010	Jóhannsson [104]
HILI	HeShou Wu	Korea Asia	2010	Bae [105]
DILI	Antimicrobial agents	Thailand Asia	2010	Treeprasertsuk [106]

(continued)

Table 6
(continued)

Cases	Products	Country/region	Year	First author
HILI	Aloe	Korea Asia	2010	Yang [107]
DILI	Cephalexin	USA	2010	Singla [108]
HILI	Kava	Germany Europe	2010	Teschke [109]
HILI	*Gynura segetum*	Hong Kong Asia	2011	Lin [110]
DILI	Amiodarone	Israel Europe	2011	Gluck [111]
DILI	Paracetamol	Spain Europe	2011	Sabaté [112]
HILI	Greater Celandine	Germany Europe	2011	Teschke [113]
HILI	Black cohosh	Germany Europe	2011	Teschke [114]
HILI	*Pelargonium sidoides*	Germany Europe	2012	Teschke [115]
DILI	Various dietary supplements	Iran Asia	2012	Timcheh-Hariri [116]
HILI	Greater Celandine	Germany Europe	2012	Teschke [117]
DILI	Etifoxine	France Europe	2012	Moch [118]
HILI	Juguju	Korea Asia	2012	Kim [119]
HILI	*Gynura segetum*	Hong Kong Asia	2012	Gao [120]
DILI	Varenicline	USA	2012	Sprague [121]
DILI HILI	Multiple synthetic drugs and herbs	Korea	2012	Suk [122]
DILI	Multiple synthetic drugs	China Asia	2012	Hou [123]
DILI	Etravirine	USA	2012	Nabha [124]
HILI	*Pelargonium sidoides*	Germany Europe	2012	Teschke [125]
DILI	Crizotinib	France Europe	2013	Ripault [126]

(continued)

Table 6
(continued)

Cases	Products	Country/region	Year	First author
DILI	Methylprednisolone	France Europe	2013	Carrier [127]
DILI	Albendazole	Colombia South America	2013	Ríos [128]
HILI	Herbalife	Germany Europe	2013	Teschke [129]
DILI	Ibandronate	Belgium Europe	2013	Goossens [130]
DILI	Bosentan	USA	2013	Markova [131]
DILI	Cyproterone acetate	Italy Europe	2013	Abenavoli [132]
DILI	Various synthetic drugs	Iceland Europe	2013	Björnsson [19]
DILI	NSAID (investigational)	USA	2013	Marumoto [133]
HILI	Black cohosh	USA	2014	Adnan [134]
DILI	Volatile anesthetics	Australia	2014	Lin [135]
DILI	Multiple synthetic drugs	USA	2014	Cheetham [136]
DILI	Rivaroxaban	Switzerland Europe	2014	Russmann [137]
DILI	Daptomycin	USA	2014	Bohm [138]
DILI	Anastrazole	UK Europe	2014	Saiful-Islam [139]
HILI	Greater Celandine	Korea Asia	2014	Im [140]
DILI	Various synthetic drugs	USA	2014	Lim [141]
DILI HILI	Multiple synthetic drugs and herbal TCM	China Asia	2014	Hao [142]
DILI	Pomalidomide	USA	2014	Veluswamy [143]
HILI	Green tea (*Camellia sinensis*)	Germany Europe	2014	Teschke [144]
HILI	Green tea (*Camellia sinensis*)	Germany Europe	2014	Pillukat [145]
HILI	Herbal TCM	Korea Asia	2015	Lee [146]
DILI HILI	Multiple synthetic drugs and dietary supplements	Germany Europe	2015	Teschke [49, 50]

(continued)

Table 6
(continued)

Cases	Products	Country/region	Year	First author
HILI	Lesser Celandine	Turkey Europe	2015	Yilmaz [147]
HILI	Green tea (*Camellia sinensis*)	Italy Europe	2015	Mazzanti [148]
DILI	Ipimimumab	Australia	2015	Tauquer [149]
DILI	Meloxicam	Korea Asia	2015	Son [150]
DILI	Rivaroxaban	USA	2015	Baig [151]
DILI	Bupropion, doxycycline	USA	2015	Tang [152]
HILI	Herbalife	Brazil South America	2015	Zambrone [153]
DILI HILI	Multiple synthetic drugs and herbs	Korea Asia	2015	Woo [154]
HILI	*Polygonum multiflorum*	China Asia	2015	Wang [155]
DILI HILI	Various drugs and TCM herbs	China Asia	2015	Zhu [156]
HILI	*Polygonum multiflorum*	China Asia	2015	Zhu [157]
DILI HILI	Various drugs and TCM herbs	China Asia	2016	Zhu [158]
HILI	TCM herbs	China Asia	2016	Zhu [159]
DILI HILI	Multiple synthetic drugs and dietary supplements	Germany Europe	2016	Teschke [16]
DILI	Multiple synthetic drugs	Icelandic Europe	2016	Björnsson [8]
HILI	Various herbs	Germany Europe	2016	Douros [13]
HILI	Chinese Skullcap Black Catechu	USA	2016	Papafragkakis [160]
HILI	Multiple herbal TCM	China Asia	2016	Zhang [161]
HILI	Petadolex	Germany Europe	2016	Teschke [40]
HILI	Rheishi fungus	Turkey Europe	2016	Ocak [162]

(continued)

Table 6
(continued)

Cases	Products	Country/region	Year	First author
HILI	Herbal TCM	Germany Europe	2016	Melchart [163]
DILI	Sofosbuvir	UK Europe	2016	Dyson [164]
DILI	Etodolac	India Asia	2017	Taneja [165]
DILI	Antibiotics	Italy, Netherlands Europe	2017	Ferrajolo [166]

DILI drug-induced liver injury, *HILI* herb induced liver injury, *NSAIDs* nonsteroidal anti-inflammatory drugs, *RUCAM* Roussel Uclaf Causality Assessment Method, *TCM*, traditional Chinese medicine

patients with preexisting liver disease [6], where expert hepatologists would provide a more accurate approach [29]. Indeed, RUCAM can be used by experts considering the abnormal baseline of liver tests due to and depending on the preexisting liver disease, the time course of events and the exclusion of alternative causes. Chronic DILI should always be considered as a potential cause of preexisting chronic liver disease [29, 56].

- **Alternative diagnoses**

  It is still difficult to develop high quality algorithms to cover all the possible alternative diagnoses in hepatology and complex diseases. Although attempts are made for DILI (Fig. 3 and Table 3), physicians are encouraged to resolve a few remaining diagnostic problems and consider additional etiologies on a case-by-case basis.

- **Additional data elements**

  Extrahepatic signs like fever, rash, eosinophilia usually accompanying an immune-allergic DILI were not included as such into RUCAM [6]. These data elements are not discriminating enough to generally distinguish DILI from non-DILI causes in favor or against the role of a suspect drug and therefore were not included in RUCAM.

6   Other Causality Assessment Methods

Six methods merit attention (Table 2). Based on some principles of the original RUCAM [21, 28], three liver specific methods were developed: the MV scale [33], the TTK scale [34], and the DILIN method [7]. Three other CAMs do not detail specific and individual DILI items: the unspecified expert opinion based approach [35], the Naranjo scale [36], and the WHO method [37].

6.1 MV Scale

In an attempt to improve the original RUCAM [21], the MV scale removed laboratory items, added clinical elements, and simplified the weight of data elements [6, 33, 38, 53, 167]. As a shortened version of the original RUCAM [21], the MV scale has fewer criteria; evaluates dechallenge as the time necessary for ALT or ALP to fall below 2× ULN; and considers a shorter latency period [33]. It also accepts less accurate exclusion criteria of alternative causes; ignores concomitant drug or herb use; emphasizes drugs with more than 5 years marketing without published hepatotoxicity and overestimates extrahepatic manifestations [33]. Despite these major modifications, performance indicators (specificity, sensitivity) including predictive values, and validation using a gold standard are not available for this scale [33]. The major differences between RUCAM and the MV scale are shown in Table 2. The MV scale is not recommended for assessing causality in suspected DILI cases and is certainly not a substitute for RUCAM [6].

6.2 TTK Scale

The TTK scale was established for DILI cases in Japan [34] and is another attempt to modify the original RUCAM [21], with different evaluations of the chronology, exclusion of comedications, and inclusion of the drug lymphocyte stimulation test (DLST) and eosinophilia in their assessment [34, 168]. Limited access to DLST, difficulties with false positive and false negative predictions [168, 169], and lack of standardization have prevented its clinical use, and consequently the TTK scale has received limited applications outside Japan [6, 167, 169].

6.3 DILIN Method

DILIN members established their own CAM [7, 170]. It is liver specific and considers a few items from the original RUCAM [21], but relies on "expert opinion," does not follow a particular algorithm, arrives at subjective causality gradings expressed as percentage ranges, ignores important items as detailed listed in Table 2, and leaves all elements unscored as also outlined in Table 2 [6]. Some shortcomings of this method have been discussed in detail [6, 38, 51]. A recent analysis also revealed that the DILIN method does substantially upgrade causality levels as compared to RUCAM, which suggests unjustified overdiagnoses and case overreporting in cases of suspected liver injury, a major diagnostic dilemma of DILIN [51]. Such upgrading might be due to the failure of the DILIN method to consider each of the elements in the RUCAM in a systematic fashion to prevent inadvertently overlooking confounding variables. These variables include comedications by numerous drugs and dietary supplements, incomplete exclusion of nondrug causes such as preexisting liver disease and withholding of antivirals in hepatitis B flares causing ALF, intermittent use of the suspected product; incomplete case data, and lack of HEV exclusion by HEV-DNA analyses. The lack of a systematic algorithm for case assessment might raise concern on the overall validity of the DILIN method [51].

Compared to the worldwide applied RUCAM (Tables 5 and 6), the use of the DILIN method is restricted to the US network (Table 2) [6, 51]. In addition, DILIN decisions are based on subjective experts' opinion, which provides percentage ranges of causality likelihood without a structured approach and individual item scoring [6, 7, 51]. By definition, such experts' approach lacks both validation by a gold standard [7] as opposed to RUCAM [6, 21], as well as transparency of how final causality assessment was reached [6, 51]. This impedes reassessment of the US-based DILIN method by outside peers [51]. Indeed, a DILIN member critically analyzed the weaknesses of the DILIN method [7], briefly summarized as follows: [1] process is described as cumbersome, time-consuming, and costly; [2] is an expert-opinion process of imperfect standard without translation into daily clinical practice; [3] takes at least 6 months after case enrolment until final assessments are available; [4] inaccessibility of data to the clinician needing a causality assessment in time; [5] monthly meetings are needed in a teleconference fashion; [6] requires consensus among three hepatologists, avoiding minority votes; [7] even when by consensus, expert opinion is still a subjective opinion; and [8] lengthy and lively conversations often occur, related to overlooked data, weakness of reasoning, or data from new publications [7]. It is therefore not applicable in DILI causality assessment outside of research studies.

6.4 Unspecified Expert Opinion Based Approach

In around two thirds of published DILI cases, no specific CAM is referenced [171]. The reporting authors presumably assessed the timing of events and estimated the likelihood of a hepatotoxic reaction but not clearly in a systematic fashion [35]. Results of such first evaluations are fragile, disputed, not transparent, and not reassessable, as shown for the assessments by the Germany regulatory agency BfArM (Bundesinstitut für Arzneimittel und Medizinprodukte, Federal Institute for Drugs and Medicinal Products) [113, 172, 173] and the FDA in the USA using MedWatch cases, as discussed recently [16]. Their poor data quality including case overreporting is well known; indeed, mostly nonprofessionals are not familiar with liver injury and not aware of the liver specific issues when they reported such cases. This unspecified CAM should be neither applied nor recommended for causality assessment in suspected liver injury.

6.5 Naranjo Scale

The Naranjo scale was developed for any adverse drug reaction [36] but its use in suspected DILI and HILI cases is problematic [38, 62, 114, 167, 174–179]. Indeed, criteria of liver injury, specific time to onset, criteria for recovery time, diagnoses to exclude, and reexposure conditions are not even considered (Table 2) [36]. The items include drug concentrations and monitoring, dose relationship including decreasing dose, placebo response, and cross-reactivity, using unidentified subjective evidence. Since idiosyncratic reactions are prevalent in liver injury, these items are irrelevant for DILI and HILI [36, 38]. Even in the absence of essential data, this scale can result in possible causality simply based on whether the patient took the suspect agent [38, 174]. Problems related to the Naranjo scale were also not resolved [38] when the US Pharmacopeia (USP) used its own modified, shortened, and not validated Naranjo version with only five instead of the original ten items [178]. As this method lacks validation and reproducibility testing [62], the USP has raised concerns about its validity [174, 175]. In essence, the use of the Naranjo scale for suspected DILI and HILI is not recommended.

6.6 WHO Method

The WHO method was also developed for general adverse reactions [37] and does not consider specific characteristics of liver injury (Table 2). These shortcomings led to the conclusion that this scale is neither appropriate for causality assessment in suspected hepatotoxicity cases nor has the advantages over other causality algorithms [38]. The WHO method has been heavily disputed [38, 59, 115, 125, 167, 172, 180, 181] and has not been mentioned on the NIH LiverTox website [53]. For causality assessment of suspected DILI and HILI cases, the WHO should use RUCAM rather than the obsolete WHO method.

7 Perspectives

It is important to maintain an internationally harmonized causality assessment approach that uses the case narrative with clinical characteristics as a basic tool [50], the quantified RUCAM items (Tables 1 and 3), and the checklist for differential diagnoses (Fig. 3). Optionally, an expert panel may reassess the case narrative, RUCAM items, and checklist as obtained and presented by the treating physician. This stepwise approach will ensure completeness, transparency, and comparability of case data. It is also critical for an internationally harmonized approach to causality assessment and improves the acceptance of published case reports or case series on DILI and HILI. Published data across countries and their registries can be harmonized and easily interpreted across populations [5, 182]. Moreover, the use of RUCAM may identify DILI and HILI cases early in the clinical development process, enabling companies and regulatory agencies to reassess the cases and take steps to minimize the risk of severe hepatic reactions.

8 Notes

As a complex disease, DILI has numerous facets, which are difficult to diagnose and are poorly handled validly by most of the published CAMs which lack defined and validated criteria. Opposed to the flaws inherited in most methods, RUCAM does not share these shortcomings and is therefore the focus of the present chapter as the preferred method for assessing causality of DILI. Nevertheless, other CAMs are discussed to provide a balanced overview on the problems of assessing causality.

9   Conclusion

Causality assessment in DILI is challenging since most methods are unable to provide reliable results due to lack of liver specificity, absence of validation, and/or item scoring. Instead, and although not perfect, RUCAM meets the quality requirements including validation against a gold standard using positive DILI responses from experienced drug rechallenge. This justifies that RUCAM is the worldwide most used CAM for DILI as a standard method by attending physicians, regulatory agencies, epidemiologists, regulatory agencies, expert panels, and the scientific community. It provides a straightforward application and allows for data comparability and transparency, reassessment by peers, discussions among experts, and support for case reports to be published.

References

1. Sarges P, Steinberg JM, Lewis JH (2016) Drug-induced liver injury: highlights from a review of the 2015 literature. Drug Saf 39:561–575. https://doi.org/10.1007/s4026401604278

2. Chen M, Borlak J, Tong W (2013) High lipophilicity and high daily dose of oral medications are associated with significant risk for drug-induced liver injury. Hepatology 58:388–396

3. Chen M, Borlak J, Tong W (2014) Predicting idiosyncratic drug-induced liver injury—some recent advances. Expert Rev Gastroenterol Hepatol 8:721–723. https://doi.org/10.1586/17474124.922871

4. Teschke R, Andrade RJ (2016) Special issue "Drug, Herb, and Dietary Supplement Hepatotoxicity". Int J Mol Sci. http://www.mdpi.com/journal/ijms/special_issues/Hepatotoxicity. Last Accessed 15 Dec 1016

5. Teschke R, Andrade RJ (2016) Editorial: drug, herb, and dietary supplement hepatotoxicity. Int J Mol Sci 17:1488. https://doi.org/10.3390/ijms17091488

6. Danan G, Teschke R (2016) RUCAM in drug and herb induced liver injury: the update. Int J Mol Sci 17:14. https://doi.org/10.3390/ijms17010014

7. Hayashi PH (2016) Drug-induced Liver Injury Network causality assessment: criteria and experience in the United States. Int J Mol Sci 17:201. https://doi.org/10.3390/ijms17020201

8. Björnsson ES (2016) Hepatotoxicity by drugs: the most common implicated agents. Int J Mol Sci 17:224. https://doi.org/10.3390/ijms17020224

9. Ortega-Alonso A, Stephens C, Lucena MI, Andrade RJ (2016) Case characterization, clinical features and risk factors in drug-induced liver injury. Int J Mol Sci 17:714. https://doi.org/10.3390/ijms17050714

10. Bessone F, Hernandez N, Lucena MI, Andrade RJ, on behalf of the Latin DILI Network (LATINDILIN) and Spanish DILI Registry (2016) The Latin American DILI registry experience: a successful ongoing collaborative strategic initiative. Int J Mol Sci 17:313. https://doi.org/10.3390/ijms17030313

11. Frenzel C, Teschke R (2016) Herbal hepatotoxicity: clinical characteristics and listing compilation. Int J Mol Sci 17:588. https://doi.org/10.3390/ijms17050588

12. Valdivia-Correa B, Gómez-Gutiérrez C, Uribe M, Méndez-Sánchez N (2016) Herbal medicine in Mexico: a cause of hepatotoxicity. A critical review. Int J Mol Sci 17:235. https://doi.org/10.3390/ijms17020235

13. Douros A, Bronder E, Andersohn F, Klimpel A, Kreutz R, Garbe E, Bolbrinker J (2016) Herb-induced liver injury in the Berlin Case-Control Surveillance Study. Int J Mol Sci 17:114. https://doi.org/10.3390/ijms17010114

14. Pantano F, Tittarelli R, Mannocchi G, Zaami S, Ricci S, Giorgetti R, Terranova D, Busardò

FP, Marinelli E (2016) Hepatotoxicity induced by "the 3Ks": Kava, Kratom and Khat. Int J Mol Sci 17:580. https://doi.org/10.3390/ijms17040580

15. García-Cortés M, Robles-Díaz M, Ortega-Alonso A, Medina-Caliz I, Andrade RJ (2016) Hepatotoxicity by dietary supplements: a tabular listing and clinical characteristics. Int J Mol Sci 17:537. https://doi.org/10.3390/ijms17040537

16. Teschke R, Eickhoff A (2016) The Honolulu liver disease cluster at the medical center: its mysteries and challenges. Int J Mol Sci 17:476. https://doi.org/10.3390/ijms17040476

17. Avigan MI, Mozersky RP, Seeff LB (2016) Scientific and regulatory perspectives in herbal and dietary supplement associated hepatotoxicity in the United States. Int J Mol Sci 17:331. https://doi.org/10.3390/ijms17030331

18. Sgro C, Clinard F, Ouazir K, Chanay H, Allard C, Guilleminet C, Lenoir C, Lemoine A, Hillon P (2002) Incidence of drug-induced hepatic injuries: a French population-based study. Hepatology 36:451–455

19. Björnsson ES, Bergmann OM, Björnsson HK, Kvaran RB, Olafsson S (2013) Incidence, presentation and outcomes in patients with drug-induced liver injury in the general population of Iceland. Gastroenterology 144:1419–1425

20. de Abajo FJ, Montero D, Madurga M, García Rodríguez LA (2004) Acute and clinically relevant drug-induced liver injury: population based case–control study. Br J Clin Pharmacol 58:71–80

21. Danan G, Bénichou C (1993) Causality assessment of adverse reactions to drugs—I. A novel method based on the conclusions of international consensus meetings: application to drug-induced liver injuries. J Clin Epidemiol 46:1323–1330

22. Aithal GP, Rawlins MD, Day CP (1999) Accuracy of hepatic adverse drug reactions reported in one English health region. Br Med J 319:1541

23. Teschke R, Frenzel C, Wolff A, Eickhoff A, Schulze J (2014) Drug induced liver injury: accuracy of diagnosis in published reports. Ann Hepatol 13:248–255

24. Andrade RJ, Lucena MI, Kaplowitz N, García-Muñoz B, Borraz Y, Pachkoria K, García-Cortés M, Fernández MC, Pelaez G, Rodrigo L, Durán JA, Costa J, Planas R, Barriocanal A, Guaner C, Romero-Gomez M, Muñoz-Yagüe T, Salmerón J, Hidalgo R (2006) Outcome of acute idiosyncratic drug-induced liver injury: long term follow-up in a hepatotoxicity registry. Hepatology 44:1581–1588

25. Miljkovic MM, Dobric S, Dragojevic-Simic V (2011) Consistency between causality assessments obtained with two scales and their agreement with clinical judgments in hepatotoxicity. Pharmacoepidemiol Drug Saf 20:272–285

26. Miljkovic MM, Dobric S, Dragojevic-Simic V (2012) Accuracy and reproducibility of two scales in causality assessment of unexpected hepatotoxicity. J Clin Pharm Ther 37:196–203

27. Björnsson E, Jacobsen EI, Kalaitzakis E (2012) Hepatotoxicity associated with statins: reports of idiosyncratic liver injury post-marketing. J Hepatol 56:374–380. https://doi.org/10.1016/j.jhep.2011.07.023

28. Bénichou C, Danan G, Flahault A (1993) Causality assessment of adverse reactions to drugs—II. An original model for validation of drug causality assessment methods: case reports with positive rechallenge. J Clin Epidemiol 46:1331–1336

29. Teschke R, Danan G (2017) Drug-induced liver injury: is chronic liver disease a risk factor and a clinical issue? Expert Opin Drug Metab Toxicol 13:425–438. https://doi.org/10.1080/17425255.2017.1252749

30. Reuben A, Koch DG, Lee WM, the Acute Liver Failure Study Group (2010) Drug-induced acute liver failure: results of a U.S. multicenter, prospective study. Hepatology 52:2065–2076

31. Larson AM, Polson J, Fontana RJ, Davern TJ, Lalani E, Hynan LS, Reisch JS, Schiodt FV, Ostapowicz G, Shakil AO, Lee WM, the Acute Liver Failure Study Group (2005) Acetaminophen-induced acute liver failure: results of a United States multicentre, prospective study. Hepatology 42:1364–1372

32. Chalasani N, Bonkovsky HL, Fontana R, Lee W, Stolz A, Talwalkar J, Reddy KR, Watkins PB, Navarro V, Barnhart H, Gu J, Serrano J (2015) Features and outcomes of 889 patients with drug-induced liver injury: the DILIN prospective study. Gastroenterology 148:1340–1352. https://doi.org/10.1053/j.gastro.2015.03.006

33. Maria VAJ, Victorino RMM (1997) Development and validation of a clinical scale for the diagnosis of drug-induced hepatitis. Hepatology 26:664–669

34. Takikawa H, Takamori Y, Kumagi T, Onji M, Watanabe M, Shibuya A, Hisamochi A, Kumashiro R, Ito T, Mitsumoto Y, Nakamura A, Sakaguchi T (2003) Assessment of 287 Japanese cases of drug induced liver injury by the diagnostic scale of the International Consensus Meeting. Hepatol Res 27:192–195

35. Kaplowitz N (2001) Causality assessment versus guilt-by-association in drug hepatotoxicity. Hepatology 33:308–310

36. Naranjo CA, Busto U, Sellers EM, Sandor P, Ruiz I, Roberts EA, Janecek E, Domecq C, Greenblatt DJ (1981) A method for estimating the probability of adverse drug reactions. Clin Pharmacol Ther 30:239–245

37. WHO, World Health Organization (2000) The use of the WHO-UMC system for standardised case causality assessment. WHO Collaborating Centre for International Drug Monitoring (Uppsala Monitoring Centre, UMC), Database 2000. http://who-umc.org/Graphics/24734.pdf Last accessed 15 Dec 2016

38. Teschke R, Frenzel C, Schulze J, Eickhoff A (2013) Herbal hepatotoxicity: challenges and pitfalls of causality assessment methods. World J Gastroenterol 19:2864–2882

39. Bénichou C (1990) Criteria of drug-induced liver disorders. Report of an international Consensus meeting. J Hepatol 11:272–276

40. Teschke R, Eickhoff A, Schulze J, Wolff A, Frenzel C, Melchart D (2016) Petadolex®, a herbal extract for migraine prophylaxis with spontaneous case reports of disputed liver injury: robust causality evaluation by RUCAM, the Roussel Uclaf Causality Assessment Method. Eur J Pharmaceut Med Res 3(12):154–177

41. Zimmerman HJ (1999) Hepatotoxicity, 2nd edn. Lippincott Williams & Wilkins, Philadelphia

42. Yoon E, Babar A, Choudhary M, Kutner M, Pyrsopoulos N (2016) Acetaminophen-induced hepatotoxicity: a comprehensive update. J Clin Translat Hepatol 4:131–142

43. Safari S, Motavaf M, Siamdoust SAS, Alavian SM (2014) Hepatotoxicity of halogenated inhalation anesthetics. Iran Red Crescent Med J 16(9):e20153

44. Gaude GS, Chaudhury A, Hattiholi J (2015) Drug-induced hepatitis and the risk factors for liver injury in pulmonary tuberculosis patients. J Family Med Prim Care 4:238–243. https://doi.org/10.4103/2249-4863.154661

45. Lee SS, Lee CM, Kim TH, Kim JJ, Lee JM, Kim HJ, Ha CY, Kim HJ, Jung WT, Lee OJ, Kim DY (2016) Frequency and risk factors of drug-induced liver injury during treatment of multidrug-resistant tuberculosis. Int J Tuberc Lung Dis 20:800–805. https://doi.org/10.5588/ijtld.15.0668

46. Agarwal VK, McHutchison JG, Hoofnagle JH, Drug-Induced Liver Injury Network (DILIN) (2010) Important elements for the diagnosis of drug-induced liver injury. Clin Gastroenterol Hepatol 8:463–470

47. Davern TJ, Chalasani N, Fontana RJ, Hayashi PH, Protiva P, Kleiner DE, Engle RE, Nguyen H, Emerson SU, Purcell RH, Tillmann HL, Gu J, Serrano J, Hoofnagle JH, for the Drug-Induced Liver Injury Network (DILIN) (2011) Acute hepatitis E infection accounts for some cases of suspected drug-induced liver injury. Gastroenterology 141:1665–1672. https://doi.org/10.1053/j.gastro.2011.07.051

48. Hoofnagle JH, Nelson KE, Purcell RH (2012) Review article: hepatitis E. N Engl J Med 367:1237–1244

49. Teschke R, Schulze J, Eickhoff A, Wolff A, Frenzel C (2015) Review article: mysterious hawaii liver disease case—naproxen overdose as cause rather than OxyELITE Pro? J Liver Clin Res 2:1013. http://www.jscimedcentral.com/Liver/liver-2-1013.pdf. Last accessed 15 Dec 2016

50. Teschke R, Schwarzenboeck A, Frenzel C, Schulze J, Eickhoff A, Wolff A (2016) The mystery of the Hawaii liver disease cluster in summer 2013: a pragmatic and clinical approach to solve the problem. Ann Hepatol 15:91–119. http://www.annalsofhepatology.com.mx/revista/numeros/2016/HP161-12-Mystery%20(web)%20(FF_041215V)_PROTEGIDO%20(1).pdf. Last accessed 15 Dec 2016

51. Teschke R, Eickhoff A (2017) Suspected liver injury and the dilemma of causality. Dig Dis Sci 62:1095–1098. https://doi.org/10.1007/s10620-016-4442-5

52. Hennes EM, Zeniya M, Czaja AJ, Parés A, Dalekos GN, Krawitt EL, Bittencourt PL, Porta G, Boberg KM, Hofer H, Bianchi FB, Shibata M, Schramm C, Eisenmann de Torres B, Galle PR, McFarlane I, Dienes HP, Lohse AW, International Autoimmune Hepatitis Group (2008) Simplified criteria for the diagnosis of autoimmune hepatitis. Hepatology 48:169–176

53. National Institutes of Health (NIH) and LiverTox (2016) Agents included in LiverTox by drug class. Last updated 6 Sep 2016. http://livertox.nlm.nih.gov/index.html. Last accessed 15 Dec 2016

54. Teschke R, Frenzel C (2014) Drug induced liver injury: do we still need a routine liver biopsy for diagnosis today? Ann Hepatol 13:121–126

55. Teschke R, Eickhoff A, Schwarzenboeck A, Schmidt-Taenzer W, Genthner A, Frenzel C, Wolff A, Schulze J (2015) Clinical review: herbal hepatotoxicity and the call for systematic data documentation of individual cases. J Liver Clin Res 2(1):1008. http://www.jscimedcentral.com/Liver/liver-2-1008.pdf. Last accessed 15 December 2016

56. Teschke R, Danan G (2016) Diagnosis and management of drug-induced liver injury (DILI) in patients with pre-existing liver disease. Drug Saf 39:729–744. https://doi.org/10.1007/s40264-016-0423-z

57. Andrade RJ, Lucena MI, Fernández MC, Pelaez G, Pachkoria K, García-Ruiz E, García-Muñoz B, Gonzalez-Grande R, Pizarro A, Durán JA, Jiménez M, Rodrigo L, Romero-Gomez M, Navarro JM, Planas R, Costa J, Borras A, Soler A, Salmerón J, Martin-Vivaldi R, Spanish Group for the Study of Drug-induced Liver Disease (2005) Drug-induced liver injury: an analysis of 461 incidences submitted to the Spanish registry over a 10-year period. Gastroenterology 129:512–521

58. Wai CT (2016) Presentation of drug-induced liver injury in Singapore. Singapore Med J 47:116–120

59. Björnsson E, Olsson R (2007) Serious adverse liver reactions associated with herbal weight loss supplements. J Hepatol 47:295–297

60. EMA (European Medicine Agency) (2007) Assessment of case reports connected to herbal medicinal products containing cimicifugae racemosae rhizoma (black cohosh, root). Issued 8 May 2007. http://www.ema.europa.eu/docs/en_GB/document_library/Herbal_-_HMPC_assessment_report/2010/02/WC500074167.pdf. Last accessed 15 Dec 2016

61. García-Cortés M, Borraz Y, Lucena MI, Peláez G, Salmerón J, Diago M, Martínez-Sierra MC, Navarro JM, Planas R, Soria MJ, Bruguera M, Andrade RJ (2008) Liver injury induced by "natural remedies": an analysis of cases submitted to the Spanish Liver Toxicity Registry. Rev Esp Enferm Dig 100:688–695

62. García-Cortés M, Lucena MI, Pachkoria K, Borraz Y, Hidalgo R, Andrade RJ (2008) Evaluation of Naranjo Adverse Drug Reactions Probability Scale in causality assessment of drug-induced liver injury. Aliment Pharmacol Ther 27:780–789

63. Daly AK, Donaldson PT, Bhatnagar P, Shen Y, Pe'er I, Floratos A, Daly MJ, Goldstein DB, John S, Nelson MR, Graham J, Park BK, Dillon JF, Bernal W, Cordell HJ, Pirmohamed M, Aithal GP, Day CP, for the DILIGEN Study & International SAE Consortium (2009) *HLA-B*5701* genotype is a major determinant of drug-induced liver injury due to flucloxacillin. Nat Genet 41:816–819

64. Jung KA, Min HJ, Yoo SS, Kim HJ, Choi SN, Ha CY, Kim HJ, Kim TH, Jung WT, Lee OJ, Lee JS, Shim SG (2011) Drug-induced liver injury: twenty five cases of acute hepatitis following ingestion of *Polygonum multiflorum* Thun. Gut Liver 5:493–499

65. Chau TN, Cheung WI, Ngan T, Lin J, Lee KWS, Poon WT, Leung VKS, Mak T, Tse ML, the Hong Kong Herb-Induced Liver Injury Network (HK-HILIN) (2011) Causality assessment of herb-induced liver injury using multidisciplinary approach and the Roussel Uclaf Causality assessment Method (RUCAM). Clin Toxicol 49:34–39

66. Lucena MI, Molokhia M, Shen Y, Urban TJ, Aithal GP, Andrade RJ, Day CP, Ruiz-Cabello F, Donaldson PT, Stephens C, Pirmohamed M, Romero-Gomez M, Navarro JM, Fontana RJ, Miller M, Groome M, Bondon-Guitton E, Conforti A, Stricker BHC, Carvajal A, Ibanez L, Yue QY, Eichelbaum M, Floratos A, Pe'er I, Daly MJ, Goldstein DB, Dillon JF, Nelson MR, Watkins PB, Daly AK, Spanish DILI Registry, EUDRAGENE, DILIN, DILIGEN, and International SAEC (2011) Susceptibility to amoxicillin-clavulanate-induced liver injury is influenced by multiple HLA class I and II alleles. Gastroenterology 141:338–347

67. Stammschulte T, Treichel U, Pachl H, Gundert-Remy U (2016) Cases of liver failure in association with flupirtine in the German spontaneous reporting system. http://www.akdae.de/Kommission/Organisation/Aufgaben/Publikationen/PDF/Stammschulte2012.pdf. Last accessed 15 Dec 2016

68. Douros A, Bronder E, Andersohn F, Klimpel A, Thomae M, Orzechowski HD, Kreutz R, Garbe E (2014) Flupirtine-induced liver injury—seven cases from the Berlin Case–Control Surveillance Study and review of the German spontaneous adverse drug reaction reporting database. Eur J Clin Pharmacol 70:453–459

69. Robles-Diaz M, Gonzalez-Jimenez A, Medina-Caliz I, Stephens C, García-Cortes M, García-Muñoz B, Ortega-Alonso A, Blanco-Reina E, Gonzalez-Grande R, Jimenez-Perez M, Rendón P, Navarro JM, Gines P, Prieto M, Garcia-Eliz M, Bessone F, Brahm JR, Paraná R, Lucena MI, Andrade RJ, on behalf of the Spanish DILI Registry and the SLatinDILI Network (2015) Distinct phenotype of hepatotoxicity associated with illicit use of anabolic androgenic steroids. Aliment Pharmacol Ther 41:116–125

70. Douros A, Bronder E, Andersohn F, Klimpel A, Thomae M, Sarganas G, Kreutz R, Garbe E (2015) Drug-induced liver injury: results from the hospital-based Berlin Case–Control Surveillance Study. Br J Clin Pharmacol 79:988–999. https://doi.org/10.1111/bcp.12565

71. Flamenbaum M, Abergel A, Marcato N, Zénut KJL, Cassan P (1998) Regressive fulminant hepatitis, acute pancreatitis and renal

insufficiency after taking ketoprofen. Gastroenterol Clin Biol 22:975

72. Lucena MI, Carvajal A, Andrade RJ, Velasco A (2003) Antidepressant-induced hepatotoxicity. Expert Opinion Drug Saf 2:249–262

73. Stickel F, Baumüller HM, Seitz K, Vasilakis D, Seitz G, Seitz HK, Schuppan D (2003) Hepatitis induced by Kava (*Piper methysticum rhizoma*). J Hepatol 39:62–67

74. Masumoto T, Horiike N, Abe M, Kumaki T, Matsubara H, Fazle Akbar SM, Michitaka K, Hyodo I, Onji M (2003) Diagnosis of drug-induced liver injury in Japanese patients by criteria of the Consensus Meetings in Europe. Hepatol Res 25:1–7

75. Andrade RJ, Lucena MI, Alonso A, García-Cortés M, García-Ruiz E, Benitez R, Fernández MC, Pelaez G, Romero M, Corpas R, Durán JA, Jiménez M, Rodrigo L, Nogueras F, Martín-Vivaldi R, Navarro JM, Salmerón J, Sánchez de la Cuesta F, Hidalgo R (2004) HLA class II genotype influences the type of liver injury in drug-induced idiosyncratic liver disease. Hepatology 39:1603–1612

76. Arotcarena R, Bigué JP, Etcharry F, Pariente A (2004) Pioglitazone-induced acute severe hepatitis. Gastroenterol Clin Biol 28:609–618. Abstract in English, article in French

77. Lee WM, Larrey D, Olsson R, Lewis JH, Keisu M, Auclert L, Sheth S (2005) Hepatic findings in long-term clinical trials of ximelagatran. Drug Saf 28:351–370

78. Jorge OA, Jorge AD (2005) Hepatotoxicity associated with the ingestion of *Centella asiatica*. Rev Esp Enferm Dig 97:115–124

79. Gloro R, Hourmand-Ollivier I, Mosquet B, Mosquet L, Rousselot P, Salamé E, Piquet MA, Dao T (2005) Fulminant hepatitis during self-medication with hydroalcoholic extract of green tea. Eur J Gastroenterol Hepatol 17:1135–1137

80. Fontana RJ, Shakil O, Greenson JK, Boyd I, Lee WM (2005) Acute liver failure due to amoxicillin and amoxicillin/clavulanate. Dig Dis Sci 50(10):1785–1790

81. De Valle MB, Av Klinteberg V, Alem N, Olsson R, Björnsson E (2006) Drug-induced liver injury in a Swedish University hospital outpatient hepatology clinic. Aliment Pharmacol Ther 24:1187–1195

82. Yuen MF, Tam S, Fung J, Wong DKH, Wong BCY, Lai CL (2006) Traditional Chinese Medicine causing hepatotoxicity in patients with chronic hepatitis B infection: a 1-year prospective study. Aliment Pharmacol Ther 24:1179–1186

83. Jimenez-Saenz M, Martinez-Sanchez Mdel C (2006) Acute hepatitis associated with the use of green tea infusions. J Hepatol 44:616–617

84. Cárdenas A, Restrepo JC, Sierra F, Correa G (2006) Acute hepatitis due to shen-min: a herbal product derived from *Polygonum multiflorum*. J Clin Gastroenterol 40:629–632

85. Yan B, Leung Y, Urbanski SJ, Myers RP (2006) Rofecoxib-induced hepatotoxicity: a forgotten complication of the coxibs. Can J Gastroenterol 20:351–355

86. Hussaini SH, O'Brien CS, Despott EJ, Dalton HR (2007) Antibiotic therapy: a major cause of drug-induced jaundice in southwest England. Eur J Gastroenterol Hepatol 19:15–20

87. Stojanovski SD, Casavant MJ, Mousa HM, Baker P, Nahata MC (2007) Atomoxetine-induced hepatitis in a child. Clin Tox 45:51–55

88. Björnsson E, Kalaitzakis E, Klinteberg VAV, Alem E, Olsson R (2007) Long-term follow-up of patients with mild to moderate drug-induced liver injury. Aliment Pharmacol 26:79–85

89. Rigato I, Cravatari M, Avellini C, Ponte E, Crocè SL, Tiribelli C (2007) Drug-induced acute cholestatic liver damage in a patient with mutation of *UGT1A1*. Nat Clin Pract Gastroenterol Hepatol 4:403–408

90. Teschke R, Schwarzenboeck A, Hennermann KH (2008) Kava hepatotoxicity: a clinical survey and critical analysis of 26 suspected cases. Eur J Gastroenterol Hepatol 20:1182–1193

91. Kang SH, Kim JI, Jeong KH, Ko KH, Ko PG, Hwang SW, Kim EM, Kim SH, Lee HY, Lee BS (2008) Clinical characteristics of 159 cases of acute toxic hepatitis. Korean J Hepatol 14:483–492. Abstract in English, article in Korean

92. Sohn CH, Cha MI, Oh BJ, Yeo WH, Lee JH, Kim W, Lim KS (2008) Liver transplantation for acute toxic hepatitis due to herbal medicines and preparations. J Korean Soc Clin Toxicol 6:110–116. Abstract in English, article in Korean

93. Choi GY, Yang HW, Cho SH, Kang DW, Go H, Lee WC, Lee YJ, Jung SH, Kim AN, Cha SW (2008) Drug-induced hepatitis caused by albendazole. J Korean Med Sci 23:903–905

94. Teschke R, Bahre R (2009) Severe hepatotoxicity by Indian Ayurvedic herbal products: a structured causality assessment. Ann Hepatol 8:258–266

95. Mazzanti G, Menniti-Ippolito F, Moro PA, Cassetti F, Raschetti R, Santuccio C, Mastrangelo S (2009) Hepatotoxicity from green tea: a review of the literature and two unpublished cases. Eur J Clin Pharmacol 65:331–341

96. Stickel F, Droz S, Patsenker E, Bögli-Stuber K, Aebi B, Leib SL (2009) Severe hepatotoxicity following ingestion of Herbalife nutritionally

supplements contaminated with *Bacillus subtilis*. J Hepatol 50:111–117

97. Kang HS, Choi HS, Yun TJ, Lee KG, Seo YS, Yeon JE, Byun KS, Um SH, Kim CD, Ryu HS (2009) A case of acute cholestatic hepatitis induced by *Corydalis speciosa Max.* Korean J Hepatol 15:517–523. Abstract in English, article in Korean

98. Teschke R, Schwarzenboeck A (2009) Suspected hepatotoxicity by cimicifugae racemosae rhizoma (black cohosh, root): critical analysis and structured causality assessment. Phytomedicine 16:72–84

99. Teschke R, Bahre R, Fuchs J, Wolff A (2009) Black cohosh hepatotoxicity: quantitative causality evaluation in nine suspected cases. Menopause 16:956–965

100. Kim SY, Yim HJ, Ahn JH, Kim JH, Kim JN, Yoon I, Kim DI, Lee HS, Lee SW, Choi JH (2009) Two cases of toxic hepatitis caused by arrowroot juice. Korean J Hepatol 15:504–509. Abstract in English, article in Korean

101. Harugeri A, Parthasarathi G, Sharma J, D'Souza GA, Ramesh M (2009) Montelukast induced acute hepatocellular injury. J Postgrad Med 55:141–142

102. Licata A, Calvaruso V, Capello M, Craxi A, Almasio PL (2010) Clinical course and outcomes of drug-induced liver injury: nimesulide as the first implicated medication. Dig Liver Dis 42:143–148

103. Essaid A, Timraz A (2010) Cholestatic acute hepatitis induced by tadalafil (Cialis®). Gastroenterol Clin Biol 34:e1–e2. Abstract in English, article in French

104. Jóhannsson M, Ormarsdóttir S, Olafsson S (2010) Hepatotoxicity associated with the use of Herbalife. Laeknabladid 96:167–172

105. Bae SH, Kim DH, Bae YS, Lee KJ, Kim DW, Yoon JB, Hong JH, Kim SH (2010) Toxic hepatitis associated with *Polygoni multiflori*. Korean J Hepatol 16:182–186. Abstract in English, article in Korean

106. Treeprasertsuk S, Huntrakul J, Ridtitid W, Kullavanijaya P, Björnsson ES (2010) The predictors of complications in patients with drug-induced liver injury caused by antimicrobial agents. Aliment Pharmacol Ther 11: 1200–1207

107. Yang HN, Kim DJ, Kim YM, Kim BH, Sohn KM, Choi MJ, Choi YH (2010) Aloe-induced toxic hepatitis. J Korean Med Sci 25:492–495

108. Singla A, Hammad HT, Hammoud GM (2010) Uncommon cause of acute drug-induced liver injury following mammoplasty. Gastroenterol Res 3:171–172

109. Teschke R (2010) Kava hepatotoxicity: a clinical review. Ann Hepatol 9:251–265

110. Lin G, Wang JY, Li N, Li M, Gao H, Ji Y, Zhang F, Wang H, Zhou Y, Ye Y, Xu HX, Zheng J (2011) Hepatic sinusoidal obstruction syndrome associated with consumption of Gynura segetum. J Hepatol 54:666–673

111. Gluck N, Fried M, Porat R (2011) Acute amiodarone liver toxicity likely due to ischemic hepatitis. Isr Med Ass J 13:748–752

112. Sabaté M, Ibáñez L, Pérez E, Vidal X, Buti M, Xiol X, Mas A, Guarner C, Forné M, Solà R, Castellote J, Rigau J, Laporte JR (2011) Paracetamol in therapeutic dosages and acute liver injury: causality assessment in a prospective case series. BMC Gastroenterol 11:80. http://www.biomedcentral.com/1471-230X/11/80. Last accessed 15 December 2016

113. Teschke R, Glass X, Schulze J (2011) Herbal hepatotoxicity by Greater Celandine (*Chelidonium majus*): causality assessment of 22 spontaneous reports. Regul Toxicol Pharmacol 61:282–291

114. Teschke R, Schmidt-Taenzer W, Wolff A (2011) Spontaneous reports of assumed herbal hepatotoxicity by black cohosh: is the liver unspecific Naranjo scale precise enough to ascertain causality? Pharmacoepidemiol Drug Saf 20:567–582

115. Teschke R, Frenzel C, Schulze J, Eickhoff A (2012) Spontaneous reports of primarily suspected herbal hepatotoxicity by *Pelargonium sidoides*: was causality adequately ascertained? Regul Toxicol Pharmacol 63:1–9

116. Timcheh-Hariri A, Balali-Mood M, Aryan E, Sadeghi M, Riahi-Zanjani B (2012) Toxic hepatitis in a group of 20 male body-builders taking dietary supplements. Food Chem Toxicol 50:3826–3832

117. Teschke R, Frenzel C, Glass X, Schulze J, Eickhoff A (2012) Greater Celandine hepatotoxicity: a clinical review. Ann Hepatol 11:838–848

118. Moch C, Rocher F, Lainé P, Lacotte J, Biour M, Gouraud A, Bernard N, Descotes J, Vial T (2012) Etifoxine-induced acute hepatitis: a case review. Clin Res Gastroenterol Hepatol 36:e85–e88

119. Kim YJ, Ryu SL, Shim JW, Kim DS, Shim JY, Park MS, Jung HL (2012) A pediatric case of toxic hepatitis induced by Hovenia dulcis. Pediatr Gastroenterol Hepatol Nutr 15: 111–116

120. Gao H, Li N, Wang JY, Zhang SC, Lin G (2012) Definitive diagnosis of hepatic sinusoidal obstruction syndrome induced by pyrrolizidine alkaloids. J Dig Dis 13:33–39

121. Sprague D, Bamha K (2012) Drug-induced liver injury due to varenicline. BMC Gastroenterol 12:65

122. Suk KT, Kim DJ, Kim CH, Park SH, Yoon JH, Kim YS, Baik GH, Kim JB, Kweon YO, Kim BI, Kim SH, Kim IH, Kim JH, Nam SW, Paik YH, Suh JI, Sohn JH, Ahn BM, Um SH, Lee HJ, Cho M, Jang MK, Choi SK, Hwang SG, Sung HT, Choi JY, Han KH (2012) A prospective nationwide study of drug-induced liver injury in Korea. Am J Gastroenterol 107:1380–1387

123. Hou FQ, Zeng Z, Wang GQ (2012) Hospital admissions for drug-induced liver injury: clinical features, therapy, and outcomes. Cell Biochem Biophys 64:77–83

124. Nabha L, Balba GP, Tuanzon C, Kumar PN (2012) Etravirine induced severe hpersensitivity reaction and fulminant hepatitis: a case report and review of the literature. J AIDS Clin Res S2:005. https://doi.org/10.4172/2155-6113.S2-005

125. Teschke R, Frenzel C, Wolff A, Herzog J, Glass X, Schulze J, Eickhoff A (2012) Initially purported hepatotoxicity by *Pelargonium sidoides*: the dilemma of pharmacovigilance and proposals for improvements. Ann Hepatol 11:500–512

126. Ripault MP, Pinzani V, Fayolle V, Pageaux GP, Larrey D (2013) Crizotinib-induced acute hepatitis: first case with relapse after reintroduction with reduced dose. Clin Res Gastroenterol Hepatol 37:e21–e23

127. Carrier P, Godet B, Crepin S, Magy L, Debette-Gratien M, Pillegand B, Jacques J, Sautereau D, Vidal E, Labrousse F, Gondran G, Loustaud-Ratti V (2013) Acute liver toxicity due to methylprednisolone: consider this diagnosis in the context of autoimmunity. Clin Res Gastroenterol Hepatol 37:100–104

128. Ríos D, Restrepo JC (2013) Abendazole-induced liver injury: a case report. Colombia Méd 44:118–120

129. Teschke R, Frenzel C, Schulze J, Schwarzenboeck A, Eickhoff A (2013) Herbalife hepatotoxicity: evaluation of cases with positive reexposure tests. World J Hepatol 5:353–363

130. Goossens N, Spahr L, Rubbia-Brandt L (2013) Severe immune-mediated drug-induced liver injury linked to ibandronate: a case report. J Hepatol 59:1139–1142

131. Markova SM, De Marco T, Bendjilali N, Kobashigawa EA, Mefford J, Sodhi J, Le H, Zhang C, Halladay J, Rettie AE, Khojasteh C, McGlothlin D, AHB W, Hsueh WC, Witte JS, Schwartz JB, Kroetz DL (2013) Association of *CYP2C9*2* with bosentan-induced liver injury. Clin Pharmacol Ther 94:678–686

132. Abenavoli L, Milic N, Beaugrand M (2013) Severe hepatitis by cyproterone acetate: role of corticosteroids. A case report. Ann Hepatol 12:152–155

133. Marumoto A, Roytman MM, Tsai NCS (2013) Trial and error: investigational drug induced liver injury, a case series report. Hawaii J Med Publ Health 72(Suppl 4):30–33

134. Adnan MM, Khan M, Hashmi S, Hamza M, AbdulMujeeb S, Amer S (2014) Black cohosh and liver toxicity: is there a relationship? Case Rep Gastrointest Med 2014:860614. https://doi.org/10.1155/2014/860614

135. Lin J, Moore D, Hockey B, Di Lernia R, Gorelik A, Liew D, Nicoll A (2014) Drug-induced hepatotoxicity: incidence of abnormal liver function tests consistent with volatile anaesthetic hepatitis in traumatic patients. Liver Int 34:576–586

136. Cheetham TC, Lee J, Hunt CM, Niu F, Reisinger S, Murray R, Powell G, Papay J (2014) An automated causality assessment algorithm to detect drug-induced liver injury in electronic medical record data. Pharmacoepidemiol Drug Saf 23:601–608

137. Russmann S, Niedrig DF, Budmiger M, Schmidt C, Stieger B, Hürlimann S, Kullak-Ublick GA (2014) Rivaroxaban postmarketing risk of liver injury. J Hepatol 61:293–300

138. Bohm N, Bohm N, Makowski C, Machado M, Davie A, Seabrook N, Wheless L, Bevill B, Clark B, Kyle TR III (2014) Case report and cohort analysis of drug-induced liver injury associated with daptomycin. Antimicrob Agents Chemother 58:4902–4903

139. Saiful-Islam M, Wright G, Tanner P, Lucas R (2014) A case of anastrazole-related drug-induced autoimmune hepatitis. Clin J Gastroenterol 7:414–417

140. Im SG, Yoo SH, Jeon DO, Cho HJ, Choi JY, Paik S, Park YM (2014) *Chelidonium majus*-induced acute hepatitis. Ewha Med J 37:60–63

141. Lim R, Choundry H, Conner K, Karnsakul W (2014) A challenge for diagnosing acute liver injury with concomitant/sequential exposure to multiple drugs: can causality assessment scales be utilized to identify the offending drug? Case Rep Pediatr 2014:156389

142. Hao K, Yu Y, He C, Wang M, Wang S, Li X (2014) RUCAM scale-based diagnosis, clinical features and prognosis of 140 cases of drug-induced liver injury. Zhonghua gan zang bing za zhi 22: 938-941. Abstract in English, article in Chinese

143. Veluswamy RR, Ward SC, Yum K, Abramovitz RB, Isola LM, Jagannath S, Parekh S (2014) Adverse drug reaction: pomalidomide-induced liver injury. Lancet 383:2125–2126

144. Teschke R, Zhang L, Melzer L, Schulze J, Eickhoff A (2014) Green tea extract and the risk of drug-induced liver injury. Expert Opin Drug Metab Toxicol 10:1663–1676. https://doi.org/10.1517/17425255.2014.971011

145. Pillukat MH, Bester C, Hensel A, Lechtenberg M, Petereit F, Beckebaum S, Müller KM, Schmidt HHJ (2014) Concentrated green tea extract induces severe acute hepatitis in a 63-year-old woman—a case report with pharmaceutical analyis. J Ethnopharmacol 155:165–170. https://doi.org/10.1016/j.jep.2014.05.015

146. Lee WJ, Kim HW, Son CG (2015) Systematic review on herb induced liver injury in Korea. Food Chem Toxicol 84:47–54. https://doi.org/10.1016/j.fct.2015.06.004

147. Yilmaz B, Yilmaz B, Aktaş B, Unlu O, Roach EC (2015) Lesser celandine (pilewort) induced acute toxic liver injury: the first case report worldwide. World J Hepatol 7:285–288

148. Mazzanti G, Di Soto A, Vitalone A (2015) Hepatotoxicity of green tea: an update. Arch Toxicol 89:1175–1191

149. Tauqeer A, Pandey R, Shah R, Black J (2015) Resolution of ipilimumab induced severe hepatotoxicity with triple immunosuppressants therapy. BMJ Case Rep. https://doi.org/10.1136/bcr-2014-208102. Last accessed 15 Dec 2016

150. Son CG (2015) Drug-induced liver injury by Western medication. J Int Korean Med 36:69–75

151. Baig M, Wool KJ, Halalnych JH, Sarmad RA (2015) Acute liver failure after initiation of rivaroxaban: a case report and review of the literature. N Am J Med Sci 7:407–410

152. Tang DM, Koh C, Twaddell WS, von Rosenvinge EC, Han H (2015) Acute hepatocellular drug-induced liver injury from bupropion and doxycycline. ACG Case Rep J 3:66–68

153. Zambrone FAD, Corrêa CL, Sampaio do Amaral LM (2015) A critical analysis of the hepatotoxicity cases described in the literature related to Herbalife products. Braz J Pharm Sci 51. https://doi.org/10.1590/S1984-82502015000400004

154. Woo HJ, Kim HY, Choi ES, Cho Y, Kim Y, Lee JH, Jang E (2015) Drug-induced liver injury: a 2-year retrospective study of 1169 hospitalized patients in a single medical center. Phytomedicine 13:1201–1205. http://www.sciencedirect.com/science/article/pii/S0944711315003049

155. Wang J, Ma Z, Niu M, Zhu Y, Liang Q, Zhao Y, Song J, Bai Z, Zhang Y, Zhang P, Li N, Meng Y, Li Q, Qin L, Teng G, Cao J, Li B, Chen S, Li Y, Zou Z, Zhou H, Xiao X (2015) Evidence chain-based causality identification in herb-induced liver injury: exemplification of a well-known liver-restorative herb *Polygonum multiflorum*. Front Med 9:457–467. https://doi.org/10.1007/s11684-015-0417-8

156. Zhu Y, Li YG, Wang JB, Liu SH, Wang LF, Zhao YL, Bai YF, Wang ZX, Li JY, Xiao XH (2015) Causes, features, and outcomes of drug-induced liver injury in 69 children from China. Gut Liver 9:525–533. https://doi.org/10.5009/gnl14184

157. Zhu Y, Liu SH, Wang JB, Song HB, Li YG, He TT, Ma X, Wang ZX, Wang LP, Zhou K, Bai YF, Zou ZS, Xiao XH (2015) Clinical analysis of drug-induced liver injury caused by Polygonum multiflorum and its preparations. Zhongguo Zhong Xi Yi Jie He Za Zhi 35:1442–1447. (Abstract in English, article in Chinese)

158. Zhu Y, Niu M, Chen J, Zou ZS, Ma ZJ, Liu SH, Wang RL, He TT, Song HB, Wang ZX, SB P, Ma X, Wang LF, Bai ZF, Zhao YL, Li YG, Wang JB, Xiao XB (2016) Comparison between Chinese herbal medicine and Western medicine-induced liver injury of 1985 patients. J Gastroenterol Hepatol 31:1476–1482. https://doi.org/10.1111/jgh.13323.

159. Zhu Y, Li YG, Wang Y, Wang LP, Wang JB, Wang RL, Wang LF, Meng YK, Wang ZX. Xiao XH (2016) Analysis of clinical characteristics in 595 patients with herb-induced liver injury. Zhongguo Zhong Xi Yi Jie He Za Zhi, CJITWM 36: 43-47.

160. Papafragkakis C, Ona MA, Reddy A, Anand S (2016) Acute hepatitis after ingestion of a preparation of Chinese Skullcap and Black Catechu for joint pain. Case Rep Hepatol 2016:4356749. https://doi.org/10.1155/2016/4356749

161. Zhang P, Ye Y, Yang X, Jiao Y (2016) Systematic review on Chinese herbal medicine induced liver injury. Evid-Based Complement Alternat Med 2016, 3560812. DOI: https://doi.org/10.1155/2016/3560812

162. Ocak T, Duran A, Katırcı Y, Erkuran MK, Kurt BB (2016) Hepatorenal syndrome associated with the use of Reishi Fungus. J Emerg Medicine Case Rep. http://www.akatos.com/sayilar/231/buyuk/1-1477.pdf

163. Melchart D, Hager S, Dai J, Weidenhammer W (2016) Quality control and complication screening programme of Chinese medicinal drugs at the first German hospital of Traditional Chinese Medicine—a retrospective analysis. Forsch Komplementmed 23:21–28. https://doi.org/10.1159/000444983

164. Dyson JK, Hutchinson J, Harrison L, Rotimi O, Tiniakos D, Foster GR, Aldersley MA, McPherson S (2016) Liver toxicity associated with sofosbuvir, an NS5A inhibitor and ribavirin use. J Hepatol 64:234–238

165. Taneja S, Kumar P, Rathi S, Duseja A, Singh V, Dhiman RK, Chawla Y (2017) Acute liver failure due to Etodolac, a selective cycloxygenase-2 (COX-2) inhibitor non-steroidal anti-inflammatory drug established by RUCAM-based causality assessment. Ann Hepatol 16(5):818–821

166. Ferrajolo C, Verhamme KMC, Trifirò G, 't Jong GW, Picelli G, Giaquinto C, Mazzaglia G, Stricker BH, Rossi F, Capuano A, Sturkenboom MC (2017) Antibiotic-induced liver injury in pediatric outpatients: a case-control study in primary care databases. Drug Saf 40(4): 305–315

167. García-Cortés M, Stephens C, Lucena MI, Fernández-Castañer A, Andrade RJ, on behalf of the Spanish Group for the Study of Drug-Induced Liver Disease (2011) Causality assessment methods in drug induced liver injury: strengths and weaknesses. J Hepatol 55:683–669

168. Takikawa H (2010) Recent status of drug-induced liver injury and its problems in Japan. Jap Med Ass J 53:243–247

169. Teschke R, Eickhoff A, Schulze J (2013) Drug and herb induced liver injury in clinical and translational hepatology: causality assessment methods, quo vadis? J Clin Translat Hepatol 1:59–74

170. Fontana RJ, Watkins PB, Bonkovsky HL, Chalasani N, Davern T, Serrano J, Rochon J, for the DILIN Study Group (2009) Drug-induced liver injury Network (DILIN) prospective study. Rationale, design and conduct. Drug Saf 32:55–68

171. Tajiri K, Shimizu Y (2008) Practical guideline for diagnosis and early management of drug-induced liver injury. World J Gastroenterol 14:6774–6785

172. Teschke R, Wolff A (2011) Regulatory causality evaluation methods applied in kava hepatotoxicity: are they appropriate? Regul Toxicol Pharmacol 59:1–7

173. BfArM (Bundesinstitut für Arzneimittel und Medizinprodukte, Bonn. Federal Institute for Drugs and Medicinal Products in Germany) (2002) Rejection of Drug Risks, Step II. As related to: Kava-Kava (*Piper methysticum*)-containing, and kavain-containing drugs, including homeopathic preparations with a final concentration up to, and including D4. 14 June 2002. http://www.spc.int/cis/documents/02_0714_BfArM_Kava_Removal.pdf. Last accessed 15 Dec 2016

174. Liss G, Lewis JH (2009) Drug-induced liver injury: what was new in 2008? Expert Opin Drug Metab Toxicol 5:843–860. https://doi.org/10.1517/17425250903018904

175. Teschke R, Schulze J (2012) Suspected herbal hepatotoxicity: requirements for appropriate causality assessment by the US Pharmacopeia. Drug Saf 35:1091–1097

176. Teschke R, Schwarzenboeck A, Schmidt-Taenzer W, Wolff A, Hennermann KH (2011) Herb induced liver injury presumably caused by black cohosh: a survey of initially purported cases and herbal quality specifications. Ann Hepatol 11:249–259

177. Teschke R, Schmidt-Taenzer W, Wolff A (2012) USP suspected herbal hepatotoxicity: quality of causality assessment is more important than quantity of counted cases, not vice versa. Pharmacoepidemiol Drug Saf 21:336–338

178. Mahady GB, Low Dog T, Barrett ML, Chavez ML, Gardiner P, Ko R, Marles RJ, Pellicore LS, Giancaspro GI, Sarma DN (2008) United States Pharmacopeia review of the black cohosh case reports of hepatotoxicity. Menopause 15:628–638

179. Sarma DN, Barrett ML, Chavez ML, Gardiner P, Ko R, Mahady GB, Marles RJ, Pellicore LS, Giancaspro GI, Low Dog T (2008) Safety of green tea extract: a systematic review by the US Pharmacopeia. Drug Saf 31:469–484

180. WHO (World Health Organization) (2007) Assessments of the risk of hepatotoxicity with kava products. WHO Document Production Services, Geneva, Switzerland

181. Teschke R, Eickhoff A, Wolff A, Frenzel C, Schulze J (2013) Herbal hepatotoxicity and WHO global introspection method. Ann Hepatol 12:11–21

182. Teschke R, Andrade R (2015) Editorial. Drug-induced liver injury: expanding our knowledge by enlarging population analysis with prospective and scoring causality assessment. Gastroenterology 148:1271–1273. https://doi.org/10.1053/j.gastro.2015.04.027.

Part VI

New Emerging Technologies

Chapter 28

Circulating MicroRNAs as Novel Biomarkers of Drug-Induced Liver Injury in Humans

Julian Krauskopf, Jos C. Kleinjans, and Theo M. de Kok

Abstract

MicroRNAs have become a promising candidate for responding to the need for more specific and sensitive biomarkers for drug-induced liver injury (DILI). These small noncoding RNA molecules exert a regulatory function on biological processes by fine tuning gene expression levels. MicroRNAs are the most abundant and stable class of small RNAs in the cell and they are expressed in a cell type- and organ-specific manner. The expression of miRNAs changes with disease state and cells are actively and/or passively secreting miRNAs into the peripheral circulation. These extracellular, circulating miRNAs have been found to reflect the condition of distant organs. Numerous studies have shown elevated serum levels of miR-122, a liver-enriched miRNA, upon drug-induced hepatotoxicity and as a consequence of other liver injuries. These studies demonstrate the potential use of blood samples as minimally invasive, miRNA based "liquid biopsies," able to interrogate hepatotoxic mechanisms and liver pathology. The purpose of this review is to summarize the recent advances on miRNA-based biomarker research for drug-induced liver injury.

Key words Drug-induced liver injury, microRNAs, Acetaminophen, Biomarker

1 Introduction

Despite extensive safety testing at various stages during drug development, drug-induced liver injury (DILI) is one of the major reasons for failure of candidate drugs during clinical trials or withdrawal of pharmaceutical products from the market [1]. The current gold standard for liver damage is the measurement of proteins that are leaking from disrupted hepatocytes as a consequence of liver toxicity (e.g., alanine aminotransferase (ALT) and aspartate aminotransferase (AST)). However, the use of these marker proteins has its limitations in view of the lack of both sensitivity and organ specificity. For instance, ALT and AST are also leaking into the circulation from damaged muscle cells already upon moderate physical activity [2]. Additionally, about 12% of type-2 diabetes mellitus patients (T2DM) show increased serum ALT levels without suffering from liver damage [3]. These conventionally used biomarkers also show an inability

Minjun Chen and Yvonne Will (eds.), *Drug-Induced Liver Toxicity*, Methods in Pharmacology and Toxicology,
https://doi.org/10.1007/978-1-4939-7677-5_28, © Springer Science+Business Media, LLC, part of Springer Nature 2018

to differentiate between mild and severe liver damage as well as between the various types of liver impairments [4]. These limitations demonstrate the need to develop improved biomarkers that are capable of predicting hepatotoxicity and liver pathogenesis with improved sensitivity and a higher level of specificity.

Recently, the potential biomarker role of microRNAs (miR-NAs) has been brought to attention in view of their acclaimed superiority to reflect liver injury [5]. These small noncoding RNAs play a major role in complex gene regulatory networks and are therefore involved in many fundamental biological processes [6]. Numerous reports have shown that intracellular miRNAs are aberrantly expressed in various liver diseases such as viral hepatitis [7], DILI [8], and hepatocellular carcinoma [9]. Disease-specific miRNA expression patterns may also be reflected in the circulation as a consequence of tissue damage and/or active secretion [10]. Recent advances in the field of next-generation sequencing (NGS) enable high throughput quantification of the entire miRNome including all its isoforms (termed isomiRs) [11]. Screening the totality of the circulating miRNAs enables the identification of miRNA signatures which can be developed into blood-based diagnostic tests (referred to as "liquid biopsies" [12]) which may well represent liver pathology without the necessity to take highly invasive liver samples. These signatures are potentially capable to discriminate between the presences of different types of liver damage and to identify the mechanisms potentially involved in the induction of hepatotoxic responses. The purpose of this review is to summarize the recent progress made in development of miRNA-based biomarkers for DILI.

2   MicroRNA Biogenesis and Regulatory Function

Since the first miRNA was discovered in 1993 in *Caenorhabditis elegans* [13], 2588 human miRNAs have been identified [14]. These small noncoding RNAs of about 22 nucleotides play a major role in post transcriptional gene regulation and have been identified as more abundant than any other class of small RNAs in the cell [6]. MicroRNAs are transcribed from DNA by the *RNA polymerase II* into primary miRNAs, in which the mature miRNAs are embedded. The hairpin-structured primary miRNAs are processed by *DROSHA* into the shorter precursor miRNAs before they are exported into the cytoplasm. In the cytoplasm, the precursor miRNAs are cleaved by DICER and further processed into the mature, single stranded miRNAs [15].

Several NGS-based studies have shown that the mature miRNAs occur in several isoforms [16, 17]. These isoforms, also called isomiRs, originate from deviations in the cleavage position by

DROSHA or DICER during miRNA maturation and/or from post-transcriptional trimming or tailing of nucleotides by enzymatic reactions. It is assumed that these modifications of the miRNA sequence have an impact on miRNA half-life and miRNA target specificity [18].

To exert its function in gene regulation, the mature miRNA assembles together with *Argonaute2* and high-density lipoproteins to the RNA-induced silencing complex (RISC). The role of the miRNA in this complex is the detection and base pairing with the target mRNA sequence. Responsible for the base pairing is a 7 nucleotide long region, called the seed, that complementary binds to the 3'-untranslated region of the target mRNA. The specific binding enables the RISC to promote the decay and/or directly suppresses the translation of the respective target gene [6]. An overview of the microRNA biogenesis and functioning of miRNAs is presented in Fig. 1.

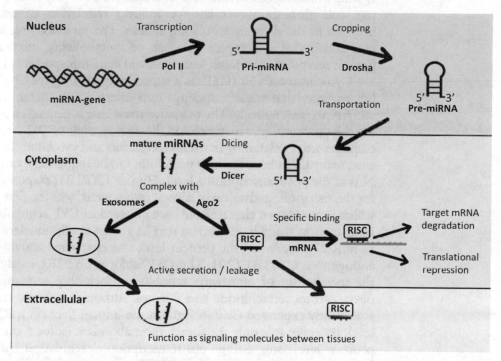

Fig. 1 MicroRNA biogenesis, regulatory function, and secretion/leakage to the circulation. In the nucleus miRNA genes are transcribed by the *RNA polymerase II* to double stranded pri-miRNAs, which are cropped by an enzyme called *Drosha* to the shorter pre-miRNAs. These pre-miRNAs are then transported into the cytoplasm where they are cleaved by the endoribonuclease *Dicer* to the single stranded mature miRNAs. At this point the miRNAs assemble with *Argonaute2* and lipoproteins to the RNA induced silencing complex (RISC) to exert their regulatory function in mRNA silencing. The protein bound miRNAs can enter the extracellular by active secretion through protein carriers or passive leakage from damaged cells. Alternatively, the mature miRNAs are also embedded into exosomes or microvesicles before they are actively secreted. In the extracellular the miRNAs, embedded to microvesicles or bound to proteins, can function as signaling molecules between tissues

In this manner, a miRNA can fine-tune the biological processes mediated by hundreds of genes whereas one gene can be regulated by several miRNAs. This creates substantial complexity in the ability to modulate gene regulatory networks. Hence, the influence of a miRNA is not always suppressive, as the inhibition of one transcription factor/gene can enhance the expression of another gene.

MicroRNAs are expressed in all cell types and exhibit crucial roles in liver (dys)functionalities such as apoptosis and necrosis, cell cycle and proliferation, and liver fibrosis [5]. Therefore, a connection between miRNAs and liver disease or drug metabolism is obvious and makes them promising candidates as biomarkers for DILI.

3   MicroRNAs in Drug Metabolism and the Development of DILI

During the metabolic breakdown of drugs, miRNAs play an important role through direct and/or indirect regulation of genes involved in the drug metabolizing system. The metabolizing system consists of a complex network of metabolizing enzymes, nuclear receptors, transferase enzymes, and drug transporters [19].

Cytochrome P450 (CYP) is a superfamily of drug metabolizing enzymes that transform drugs into intermediate metabolites and free oxygen radicals. The oxidative stress that is generated during this process plays a major role in the pathogenesis of DILI. CYP enzymes are regulated by transcription factors and cytokines, however, many CYPs have recently been found to be regulated by miRNAs at the posttranscriptional level. Human CYP1B1, responsible for the metabolic activation of several carcinogens, was the first for which it was shown that miRNAs are involved in CYP regulation. In an in vitro study it was shown that an antisense oligonucleotide of miR-27b increased the protein level and enzymatic activity of endogenous CYP1B1 [20]. The CYP isoform CYP2E1 catalyzes the metabolism of numerous xenobiotics, including acetaminophen, carbon tetrachloride and ethanol. Although it is the most abundantly expressed CYP isoform in the human liver on mRNA level, however, it is only the fourth most abundant isoform on the protein level suggesting posttranscriptional regulation [21]. Indeed, miR-378 transfected HEK293 cells showed significantly decreased CYP2E1 protein levels and activity [22]. Furthermore, in rat hepatocytes it was shown that administration of insulin increased miR-132 and miR-212 levels and the enhanced expression of these two miRNAs appeared to correlate significantly with decreased CYP2E1 mRNA expression [23].

The hepatocyte-nuclear 4α factor (HNF4A) is a nuclear receptor that plays an important role in the induction of many genes involved in drug metabolism (including CYPs). HNF4A activates the expression of CYP mRNAs by direct binding as well as through the regulation of other transcription factors such as pregnane x receptor (PXR). In HepG2 cells it was demonstrated that upon overexpression of miR-24 and miR-34a the protein levels of HNF4A were markedly decreased. Furthermore, a decrease of numerous HNF4A target genes such as CYP7A1 and CYP8B1, was observed [24].

PXR is also recognized as a major transcription factor that induces many drug metabolizing enzymes. Another study in HepG2 revealed that the PXR protein level was decreased by the overexpression of miR-148a, whereas it was increased by inhibition of miR-148a. Furthermore, in a panel of 25 human liver samples the expression levels of miR-148a inversely correlated with the translational efficiency of PXR (PXR protein–PXR mRNA ratio) [25].

In addition to these metabolizing enzymes and nuclear receptors, miRNAs were also identified as regulators of transferase enzymes and transporters. The UDP-glucuronosyltransferase (UGT) catalyzes the conjugation of a sugar molecule to its substrate (e.g., drugs, carcinogens) to enable the substrates excretion from the body, thus preventing DILI [26]. Enzyme activity and mRNA levels of hepatic UGT1A, a family of nine isoforms of UGT, showed inverse correlation with miR-491-3p in vitro and in vivo [27]. The same group additionally showed that also some isoforms of the UGT2B family are targeted and suppressed by miR-216b-5p [28]. Furthermore, the protein level of ABCG2, an important transporter responsible for cellular drug disposition, appeared to be affected by multiple miR-NAs, including miR-328, miR-519c, and miR-520h [29].

These examples of the complex interplay between drug metabolizing enzymes, transcription factors, transferase enzymes, drug transporters and posttranscriptional regulation by miRNAs shows the important role of these small RNAs as mediators of drug metabolism and DILI (Table 1).

Table 1
Examples of miRNA-mediated regulation of genes involved in the metabolizing system

Gene	Function	miRNAs	References
CYP1B1	Drug-metabolizing enzyme	miR-27b	[20]
CYP2E1	Drug-metabolizing enzyme	miR-378, miR-132, miR-212	[22, 23]
HNF4A	Nuclear receptor	miR-24, miR-34a	[24]
PXR	Nuclear receptor	miR-148a	[25]
UGT1A	Transferase enzymes	miR-491-3p	[27]
UGT2B	Transferase enzymes	miR-216b-5p	[28]
ABCG2	Drug transporter	miR-328, miR-519c, miR-520h	[29]

4   Circulating miRNAs

In 2008, the first evidence was published showing the presence of miRNAs in body fluids [30]. These circulating miRNAs were found to be stable even under conditions as harsh as boiling, extreme pH, long-time storage at room temperature, and multiple freeze-thaw cycles. Additionally, the study showed that synthetic miRNAs added to the sample were quickly degraded [31]. This suggests that, in contrast to the synthetic miRNAs, the endogenous miRNAs are stabilized by some protective mechanism. It has indeed been reported that circulating miRNAs are protected from RNase activity either by being bound to proteins such as *Agronaute2* or incorporated into microvesicles [32].

The fact that miRNAs in the circulatory system are to some extent also embedded into microvesicles and exosomes led to the hypothesis that they may also play a role in cell-to-cell communication (Fig. 1). It has been shown that human blood cells can secrete miRNAs and deliver them into recipient cells where the exogenous miRNAs can regulate target gene expression [33].

However, the majority of the miRNAs present in biofluids is not found inside microvesicles but is rather bound to RNA-binding proteins such as *Argonaute2* and high-density lipoproteins [34]. This suggests that a significant portion of miRNAs is leaked passively into the circulatory system by tissue disruption or possibly, by active secretion through protein carrier systems (Fig. 1).

The stability of miRNAs in the circulation, the accessibility through minimally invasive "liquid biopsies" and the advantage that miRNAs can be detected in a quantitative manner by relatively simple methods such as a real-time PCR, makes them a very promising new class of biomarkers for drug-induced liver injury.

5   Drug-Induced Liver Injury

With acetaminophen (APAP) toxicity being the most common cause of DILI, the first evidence of circulating miRNAs as novel biomarkers for DILI was identified in APAP-treated mice. The study showed that the liver-enriched miRNAs (miRNAs that are consistently highly expressed in the liver such as miR-122 and miR-192) exhibited dose- and duration-dependent elevations in plasma, and showed higher sensitivity than serum ALT [8]. The elevation of both miRNAs was later confirmed in human acetaminophen poisoning [35]. A clinical study also demonstrated that miR-122 is more sensitive than ALT and opposed to ALT, miR-122 remained stable in a cohort with muscle injury [36]. However, these two circulating miRNAs are not solely induced upon DILI. Numerous studies report increased levels of circulating miR-122 and miR-192 in other liver diseases such as hepatitis B and C infection [37, 38], hepatocellular carcinoma [39, 40] or nonalcoholic fatty liver disease [41, 42]. Therefore, the individual miRNAs seem to be promising biomarkers for general liver disease rather than specific for DILI and neither of these separately qualifies for differentiating between liver diseases.

Therefore, a panel of 221 miRNAs was screened in a total of 49 human subjects by qPCR and it was reported that the plasma levels of hundreds of miRNAs had increased more than eightfold change in patients suffering from APAP overdose [43]. The first NGS-based study in this context was conducted by our group, analyzing the complete circulating miRNome of six accidentally acetaminophen-overdosed subjects, including serial samples taken at various days during treatment with *N*-acetyl cysteine. The study reported serum elevations of 36 miRNAs (including the liver enriched miR-122, miR192, miR-194, miR-210, and miR-483, as well as 3 putative novel miRNAs) that returned to baseline after *N*-acetyl cysteine administration. Moreover, we identified varying isomiR proportions between healthy and APAP-overdosed subjects and this led to the hypothesis that isomiR fingerprints add to the complexity and capability of miRNA-based differentiation among liver pathologies [16] (see Sect. 6). Of the 20 most elevated miRNAs reported by Ward et al. (2014) only 3 (miR-122, miR-193, and miR-483) were overlapping with the 36 miRNAs identified in our study. Surprisingly, Ward et al. did not detect an elevation for miR-192, which was highly significant in our study, the study by Wang et al. (2009) and Starkey-Lewis et al. (2011). These differences are most likely due to various quantification methods, study designs, and variation in exposure to APAP.

The finding that several miRNAs were affected by APAP-overdose suggested that signatures of miRNAs are specific for various liver diseases. In a study on miRNA levels in APAP-overdose patients with and without organ injury, it was shown that the identified 16 miRNA signature accurately diagnosed APAP toxicity in a test cohort [44] (see Sect. 7). In a NGS study we screened the totality of circulating miRNAs in a group of subjects suffering from a broader range of liver pathologies, including acetaminophen-induced DILI, hepatitis B infection, liver cirrhosis and type-2 diabetes. The study revealed a total number of 179 miRNAs being altered by the liver pathologies and each disease could be differentiated by specific miRNA signatures with minimal overlap among the signatures. Bioinformatics analysis of the miRNA signatures and its potential mRNA targets showed that the altered miRNAs were in line with the mechanisms of disease [45]. Furthermore, the study suggests that varying proportions of isomiRs support the discrimination between the liver pathologies.

As liver injury changes the abundance and cargo of liver-born extracellular microvesicles [46], several recent studies have been exploring the potential of exosomal miRNAs as biomarkers of liver injury [47, 48]. Depending on the type of liver injury— alcoholic liver disease or DILI—serum miR-122 and miR-155 were predominantly present in either the exosome or the protein-rich fraction, respectively [49]. Two independent studies have shown that there is no strict correlation between miRNA elevations in serum and expression in the liver, supporting the hypothesis of active secretion of miRNAs by the liver [43, 50].

Besides miRNAs circulating in blood, also in other biofluids detectable levels of miRNAs have been described. A study revealed that in urine more than 200 different miRNA species are present. This is far less than miRNAs found in serum or plasma, suggesting that not all miRNAs are excreted into the urine. However, as urine can be collected even easier in a noninvasive manner, urinary miRNAs may have great prognostic value [51]. Indeed, a recent study investigating circulating miRNAs in APAP-overdosed children profiled next to serum also the urinary miRNAs. The study found significantly increased levels of four miRNAs (including miR-375) in the urine of children with an APAP overdose [52].

In addition to the studies on APAP, a limited number of studies have been investigating other hepatotoxic compounds. Several studies associated circulating miRNAs with exposure to hepatotoxic compounds such as herbal medicines (miR-122, miR-192, and miR193) [53], perfluorooctanoic acid (miR-122, miR-192, miR-26b, miR-28, and miR-32) [54] and Toll-like receptor (TLR) ligand-induced inflammatory cell-mediated liver damage (miR-122) [49]. Yet another study reported significant increases of 28 urinary miRNAs upon carbon tetrachloride-induced liver injury [55]. These findings demonstrate the potential of miRNAs to not only distinguish between various types of liver injury but also between hepatotoxic compounds that induced the liver damage. Table 2 lists important studies reporting on circulating miRNAs in drug-induced liver injury.

6   Study Case 1

The study by Krauskopf et al. (2015) investigated global circulating miRNA profiles in serum samples from six subjects with liver injury caused by accidental APAP-overdose as well as six healthy subjects. Blood samples were taken immediately after the patient's arrival at the hospital as well as during the treatment with N-acetyl cysteine (2–6 samples). A single blood sample from each healthy subject was used for analysis. After the serum was recovered from the total 24 blood samples, circulating miRNAs were isolated with the miRNeasy Mini Kit (QUIAGEN, Valencia, CA) and consequently sequenced using the Illumina HiSeq 2000 sequencing platform according to the manufacturer's protocol. After quality

Table 2
Studies on circulating miRNAs in drug-induced liver injury

Compound	Species	Sample	Quantification	Altered miRNA levels	References
APAP	Mouse	Plasma	qPCR	miR-122↑, miR-192↑, miR-193↑, miR-483↓ miR-710↓, miR-711↓, (total 44)	[8]
APAP	Human	Plasma	qPCR	miR-122↑, miR-192↑	[35]
APAP	Human	Plasma	qPCR	miR-122↑, miR-193↑, miR-3646↑, miR-412↑, miR-483↑, miR-885↑ (total >100)	[43]
APAP	Human	Serum	NGS	miR-122↑, miR192↑, miR-193↑, miR-320↑, miR-483↑ miR-885↑ (total 36)	[16]
APAP	Human	Plasma	qPCR	miR-122↑, miR-1468↓, miR-151a↑, miR-378i↓, miR-483↓, miR-885↑ (total >100)	[44]
APAP	Human	Serum	NGS	miR-122↑, miR-125b↑, miR-204↑, miR-30d↑, miR-375↑, miR-423↑ (total 8)	[52]
APAP	Human	Urine	qPCR	miR-375↑, miR-302↑, miR-9↑, miR-940↑	[52]
Herbal medicines	Rat	Serum	qPCR	miR122↑, miR101a↑, miR-101b↑, miR192↑, miR193↑, miR-200↑ (total 42)	[53]
Perfluorooctanoic acid	Mouse	Serum	qPCR	miR-122↑, miR-194↑, miR-28↑, miR-295↑, miR-339↑, miR-466j↑ (total 73)	[54]
TLR	Mouse	Plasma/serum	qPCR	miR-122↑	[49]
Carbon tetrachloride	Rat	Urine	qPCR	miR-291a↑, miR-296↑, miR-31↑, miR-330↑, miR-34c↑, let-7b↑ (total 28)	[55]

assessment and processing of the sequencing data a total of 355 miRNAs were detected across all serum samples. The statistical data analysis revealed that the serum levels of 36 miRNAs, including the liver enriched miR-122 and miR-192, were significantly elevated in the overdosed subjects and returned to baseline during the treatment with N-acetyl cysteine. The set of elevated miRNAs was functionally associated with liver-specific biological processes and mechanisms of toxicity. Despite the limited number of patients investigated, the study suggests that profiles of circulating miRNAs in human serum might provide additional biomarker candidates and possibly mechanistic information relevant to drug-induced liver injury [16].

7   Study Case 2

Ward et al. quantified 221 miRNAs by real-time PCR in a cohort of 49 patients suffering from APAP overdose or ischemic hepatitis. The study identified hundreds of miRNAs markedly elevated in the plasma or serum of APAP overdose patients. During treatment with N-acetyl cysteine most of these circulating miRNAs returned to normal levels. Furthermore, a set of 11 miRNAs was identified to clearly discriminate between APAP hepatotoxicity and ischemic hepatitis. The elevation of certain miRNAs could be detected before the rise of ALT, and some miRNAs also responded more rapidly than ALT to N-acetyl cysteine treatment. Ward et al. suggest that miRNAs can serve as sensitive diagnostic and prognostic clinical tools for severe liver injury and could be useful for monitoring drug-induced liver injury during drug discovery [43].

8   Conclusion and Future Perspectives

In summary these studies have shown that circulating miRNAs are potentially superior to the conventional biomarkers for diagnosing DILI. The liver-enriched miRNA miR-122 has been shown to outperform ALT in sensitivity and specificity. Signatures of miRNAs enable differentiating between liver pathologies, as well as monitoring mechanisms of liver disease. Taken the increasing body of evidence that miRNAs are also actively secreted in order to act as signaling molecules, miRNAs may hold a major advantage over the classical biomarkers as they may detect more sensitively early signs of liver diseases occurring before the actual onset of severe liver injury that is needed for proteins to leak out of the damaged tissue. Furthermore, the observation of specific isomiR proportions among different liver diseases adds a new level of complexity and opportunities to miRNA-based biomarkers.

Next to these promising findings, miRNAs hold several challenges that need to be addressed. Foremost is the lack of knowledge when it comes to the biological interpretation of induced circulating miRNAs. The function of most miRNAs, particularly in the liver and circulation, is still unknown. To fill this knowledge gap, more functional studies, including multi-omics studies investigating the relationship between miRNA, mRNA and proteins are needed to improve biological interpretations. Furthermore, several of the studies mentioned in this review found contradicting results when it comes down to the miRNA signatures. This inconsistency is mainly a result of a lack of standardization. Not only variation in preparation of the serum/plasma that possibly leads to contamination of blood cells is a source of bias. But also different study designs, various screening platforms and different data handling and analysis influence the outcome of such studies.

The main challenge, however, is to validate and integrate these findings within clinical studies where they may serve as early biomarkers for DILI as well as aid to the treatment of liver injuries by monitoring the progress of disease. The personalized effects of pharmacotherapy during the curative process could be screened and adjusted individually. Furthermore, as a consequence of the higher specificity of miRNA-based biomarkers diagnostic misclassifications would be reduced, allowing DILI patients to receive the appropriate treatment according to the severity of their liver injury.

In conclusion, the research on circulating miRNAs laid a foundation for a superior diagnostic test based on minimally invasive "liquid biopsies" capable of interrogating hepatotoxic mechanisms and liver pathology, and possibly, of differentiating between hepatotoxic compounds.

References

1. Regev A (2014) Drug-induced liver injury and drug development: industry perspective. Semin Liver Dis 34(2):227–239. https://doi.org/10.1055/s-0034-1375962

2. Pettersson J, Hindorf U, Persson P, Bengtsson T, Malmqvist U, Werkstrom V, Ekelund M (2008) Muscular exercise can cause highly pathological liver function tests in healthy men. Br J Clin Pharmacol 65(2):253–259. https://doi.org/10.1111/j.1365-2125.2007.03001.x

3. West J, Brousil J, Gazis A, Jackson L, Mansell P, Bennett A, Aithal GP (2006) Elevated serum alanine transaminase in patients with type 1 or type 2 diabetes mellitus. QJM 99(12):871–876. https://doi.org/10.1093/qjmed/hcl116

4. Amacher DE, Schomaker SJ, Aubrecht J (2013) Development of blood biomarkers for drug-induced liver injury: an evaluation of their potential for risk assessment and diagnostics. Mol Diagn Ther 17(6):343–354. https://doi.org/10.1007/s40291-013-0049-0

5. Szabo G, Bala S (2013) MicroRNAs in liver disease. Nat Rev Gastroenterol Hepatol 10(9):542–552. https://doi.org/10.1038/nrgastro.2013.87

6. Bartel DP (2009) MicroRNAs: target recognition and regulatory functions. Cell 136(2):215–233. https://doi.org/10.1016/j.cell.2009.01.002

7. Jopling CL, Yi M, Lancaster AM, Lemon SM, Sarnow P (2005) Modulation of hepatitis C virus RNA abundance by a liver-specific MicroRNA. Science 309(5740):1577–1581. https://doi.org/10.1126/science.1113329

8. Wang K, Zhang S, Marzolf B, Troisch P, Brightman A, Hu Z, Hood LE, Galas DJ (2009) Circulating microRNAs, potential biomarkers for drug-induced liver injury. Proc Natl Acad Sci U S A 106(11):4402–4407. https://doi.org/10.1073/pnas.0813371106

9. Hou J, Lin L, Zhou W, Wang Z, Ding G, Dong Q, Qin L, Wu X, Zheng Y, Yang Y, Tian W, Zhang Q, Wang C, Zhang Q, Zhuang SM, Zheng L, Liang A, Tao W, Cao X (2011) Identification of miRNomes in human liver and hepatocellular carcinoma reveals miR-199a/b-3p as therapeutic target for hepatocellular carcinoma. Cancer Cell 19(2):232–243. https://doi.org/10.1016/j.ccr.2011.01.001

10. Falcon-Perez JM, Royo F (2015) Circulating RNA: looking at the liver through a frosted glass. Biomarkers 20(6-7):339–354. https://doi.org/10.3109/1354750X.2015.1101785

11. Schwarzenbach H, Nishida N, Calin GA, Pantel K (2014) Clinical relevance of circulating cell-free microRNAs in cancer. Nat Rev Clin Oncol 11(3):145–156. https://doi.org/10.1038/nrclinonc.2014.5

12. Diaz LA Jr, Bardelli A (2014) Liquid biopsies: genotyping circulating tumor DNA. J Clin Oncol 32(6):579–586. https://doi.org/10.1200/JCO.2012.45.2011

13. Lee RC, Feinbaum RL, Ambros V (1993) The C. elegans heterochronic gene lin-4 encodes small RNAs with antisense complementarity to lin-14. Cell 75(5):843–854

14. Griffiths-Jones S (2006) miRBase: the microRNA sequence database. Methods Mol Biol 342:129–138. https://doi.org/10.1385/1-59745-123-1:129

15. Ha M, Kim VN (2014) Regulation of microRNA biogenesis. Nat Rev Mol Cell Biol 15(8):509–524. https://doi.org/10.1038/nrm3838

16. Krauskopf J, Caiment F, Claessen SM, Johnson KJ, Warner RL, Schomaker SJ, Burt DA, Aubrecht J, Kleinjans JC (2015) Application of high-throughput sequencing to circulating microRNAs reveals novel biomarkers for drug-induced liver injury. Toxicol Sci 143(2):268–276. https://doi.org/10.1093/toxsci/kfu232

17. Williams Z, Ben-Dov IZ, Elias R, Mihailovic A, Brown M, Rosenwaks Z, Tuschl T (2013) Comprehensive profiling of circulating microRNA via small RNA sequencing of cDNA libraries reveals biomarker potential and limitations. Proc Natl Acad Sci U S A 110(11): 4255–4260. https://doi.org/10.1073/pnas.1214046110

18. Ameres SL, Zamore PD (2013) Diversifying microRNA sequence and function. Nat Rev Mol Cell Biol 14(8):475–488. https://doi.org/10.1038/nrm3611

19. Yokoi T, Nakajima M (2013) microRNAs as mediators of drug toxicity. Annu Rev Pharmacol Toxicol 53:377–400. https://doi.org/10.1146/annurev-pharmtox-011112-140250

20. Tsuchiya Y, Nakajima M, Takagi S, Taniya T, Yokoi T (2006) MicroRNA regulates the expression of human cytochrome P450 1B1. Cancer Res 66(18):9090–9098. https://doi.org/10.1158/0008-5472.CAN-06-1403

21. Shimada T, Yamazaki H, Mimura M, Inui Y, Guengerich FP (1994) Interindividual variations in human liver cytochrome P-450 enzymes involved in the oxidation of drugs, carcinogens and toxic chemicals: studies with liver microsomes of 30 Japanese and 30 Caucasians. J Pharmacol Exp Ther 270(1):414–423

22. Mohri T, Nakajima M, Fukami T, Takamiya M, Aoki Y, Yokoi T (2010) Human CYP2E1 is regulated by miR-378. Biochem Pharmacol 79(7):1045–1052. https://doi.org/10.1016/j.bcp.2009.11.015

23. Shukla U, Tumma N, Gratsch T, Dombkowski A, Novak RF (2013) Insights into insulin-mediated regulation of CYP2E1: miR-132/-212 targeting of CYP2E1 and role of phosphatidylinositol 3-kinase, Akt (protein kinase B), mammalian target of rapamycin signaling in regulating miR-132/-212 and miR-122/-181a expression in primary cultured rat hepatocytes. Drug Metab Dispos 41(10):1769–1777. https://doi.org/10.1124/dmd.113.052860

24. Takagi S, Nakajima M, Kida K, Yamaura Y, Fukami T, Yokoi T (2010) MicroRNAs regulate human hepatocyte nuclear factor 4alpha, modulating the expression of metabolic enzymes and cell cycle. J Biol Chem 285(7):4415–4422. https://doi.org/10.1074/jbc.M109.085431

25. Takagi S, Nakajima M, Mohri T, Yokoi T (2008) Post-transcriptional regulation of human pregnane X receptor by micro-RNA affects the expression of cytochrome P450 3A4. J Biol Chem 283(15):9674–9680. https://doi.org/10.1074/jbc.M709382200

26. Court MH, Duan SX, Von Moltke LL, Greenblatt DJ, Patten CJ, Miners JO, Mackenzie PI (2001) Interindividual variability in acetaminophen glucuronidation by human liver microsomes: identification of relevant acetaminophen UDP-glucuronosyltransferase isoforms. J Pharmacol Exp Ther 299(3):998–1006

27. Dluzen DF, Sun DX, Salzberg AC, Jones N, Bushey RT, Robertson GP, Lazarus P (2014) Regulation of UDP-glucuronosyltransferase 1A1 expression and activity by microRNA 491-3p. J Pharmacol Exp Ther 348(3):465–477. https://doi.org/10.1124/jpet.113.210658

28. Dluzen DF, Sutliff AK, Chen G, Watson CJW, Ishmael FT, Lazarus P (2016) Regulation of UGT2B expression and activity by miR-216b-5p in liver cancer cell lines. J Pharmacol Exp Ther 359(1):182–193. https://doi.org/10.1124/jpet.116.235044

29. Li X, Pan YZ, Seigel GM, Hu ZH, Huang M, Yu AM (2011) Breast cancer resistance protein BCRP/ABCG2 regulatory microRNAs (hsa-miR-328, -519c and -520h) and their differential expression in stem-like ABCG2+ cancer cells. Biochem Pharmacol 81(6):783–792. https://doi.org/10.1016/j.bcp.2010.12.018

30. Mitchell PS, Parkin RK, Kroh EM, Fritz BR, Wyman SK, Pogosova-Agadjanyan EL, Peterson A, Noteboom J, O'Briant KC, Allen A, Lin DW, Urban N, Drescher CW, Knudsen BS, Stirewalt DL, Gentleman R, Vessella RL, Nelson PS, Martin DB, Tewari M (2008) Circulating microRNAs as stable blood-based markers for cancer detection. Proc Natl Acad Sci U S A 105(30):10513–10518. https://doi.org/10.1073/pnas.0804549105

31. Chen X, Ba Y, Ma L, Cai X, Yin Y, Wang K, Guo J, Zhang Y, Chen J, Guo X, Li Q, Li X, Wang W, Zhang Y, Wang J, Jiang X, Xiang Y, Xu C, Zheng P, Zhang J, Li R, Zhang H, Shang X, Gong T, Ning G, Wang J, Zen K, Zhang J, Zhang CY (2008) Characterization of microRNAs in serum: a novel class of biomarkers for diagnosis of cancer and other diseases. Cell Res 18(10):997–1006. https://doi.org/10.1038/cr.2008.282

32. Skog J, Wurdinger T, van Rijn S, Meijer DH, Gainche L, Sena-Esteves M, Curry WT Jr, Carter BS, Krichevsky AM, Breakefield XO (2008) Glioblastoma microvesicles transport RNA and proteins that promote tumour growth and provide diagnostic biomarkers. Nat Cell Biol 10(12):1470–1476. https://doi.org/10.1038/ncb1800

33. Zhang YJ, Liu DQ, Chen X, Li J, Li LM, Bian Z, Sun F, JW L, Yin YA, Cai X, Sun Q, Wang KH, Ba Y, Wang QA, Wang DJ, Yang JW, Liu PS, Xu T, Yan QA, Zhang JF, Zen K, Zhang CY (2010) Secreted monocytic miR-150 enhances targeted endothelial cell migration. Mol Cell 39(1):133–144. https://doi.org/10.1016/j.molcel.2010.06.010

34. Arroyo JD, Chevillet JR, Kroh EM, Ruf IK, Pritchard CC, Gibson DF, Mitchell PS, Bennett CF, Pogosova-Agadjanyan EL, Stirewalt DL, Tait JF, Tewari M (2011) Argonaute2 complexes carry a population of circulating microRNAs independent of vesicles in human plasma. Proc Natl Acad Sci U S A 108(12):5003–5008. https://doi.org/10.1073/pnas.1019055108

35. Starkey-Lewis PJ, Dear J, Platt V, Simpson KJ, Craig DG, Antoine DJ, French NS, Dhaun N, Webb DJ, Costello EM, Neoptolemos JP, Moggs J, Goldring CE, Park BK (2011) Circulating microRNAs as potential markers of human drug-induced liver injury. Hepatology 54(5):1767–1776. https://doi.org/10.1002/hep.24538

36. Thulin P, Nordahl G, Gry M, Yimer G, Aklillu E, Makonnen E, Aderaye G, Lindquist L, Mattsson CM, Ekblom B, Antoine DJ, Park BK, Linder S, Harrill AH, Watkins PB, Glinghammar B, Schuppe-Koistinen I (2014) Keratin-18 and microRNA-122 complement alanine aminotransferase as novel safety biomarkers for drug-induced liver injury in two human cohorts. Liver Int 34(3):367–378. https://doi.org/10.1111/liv.12322

37. Cermelli S, Ruggieri A, Marrero JA, Ioannou GN, Beretta L (2011) Circulating microRNAs in patients with chronic hepatitis C and non-alcoholic fatty liver disease. PLoS One 6(8):e23937. https://doi.org/10.1371/journal.pone.0023937

38. Ji F, Yang B, Peng X, Ding H, You H, Tien P (2011) Circulating microRNAs in hepatitis B virus-infected patients. J Viral Hepat 18(7):e242–e251. https://doi.org/10.1111/j.1365-2893.2011.01443.x

39. Qu KZ, Zhang K, Li H, Afdhal NH, Albitar M (2011) Circulating microRNAs as biomarkers for hepatocellular carcinoma. J Clin Gastroenterol 45(4):355–360. https://doi.org/10.1097/MCG.0b013e3181f18ac2

40. Bandiera S, Baumert TF, Zeisel MB (2016) Circulating microRNAs for early detection of hepatitis B-related hepatocellular carcinoma. Hepatobiliary Surg Nutr 5(3):198–200. 10.21037/hbsn.2016.03.08

41. Tryndyak VP, Latendresse JR, Montgomery B, Ross SA, Beland FA, Rusyn I, Pogribny IP (2012) Plasma microRNAs are sensitive indicators of inter-strain differences in the severity of liver injury induced in mice by a choline- and folate-deficient diet. Toxicol Appl Pharmacol 262(1):52–59. https://doi.org/10.1016/j.taap.2012.04.018

42. Pirola CJ, Fernandez Gianotti T, Castano GO, Mallardi P, San Martino J, Mora Gonzalez Lopez Ledesma M, Flichman D, Mirshahi F, Sanyal AJ, Sookoian S (2015) Circulating microRNA signature in non-alcoholic fatty liver disease: from serum non-coding RNAs to liver histology and disease pathogenesis. Gut 64(5):800–812. https://doi.org/10.1136/gutjnl-2014-306996

43. Ward J, Kanchagar C, Veksler-Lublinsky I, Lee RC, McGill MR, Jaeschke H, Curry SC, Ambros VR (2014) Circulating microRNA profiles in human patients with acetaminophen hepatotoxicity or ischemic hepatitis. Proc Natl Acad Sci U S A 111(33):12169–12174. https://doi.org/10.1073/pnas.1412608111

44. Vliegenthart AD, Shaffer JM, Clarke JI, Peeters LE, Caporali A, Bateman DN, Wood DM, Dargan PI, Craig DG, Moore JK, Thompson AI, Henderson NC, Webb DJ, Sharkey J, Antoine DJ, Park BK, Bailey MA, Lader E, Simpson KJ, Dear JW (2015) Comprehensive microRNA profiling in acetaminophen toxicity identifies novel circulating biomarkers for human liver and kidney injury. Sci Rep 5:15501. https://doi.org/10.1038/srep15501

45. Krauskopf J, Caiment F, De Kok TM, Johnson KJ, Warner RL, Schomaker SJ, Chandler P, Aubrecht J, Kleinjans JC (2016) High-throughput sequencing of circulating miRNAs in human reveals novel biomarkers for drug-induced liver injury, hepatitis B, liver cirrhosis and type 2 diabetes. Toxicol Lett 258 (Supplement):S79. https://doi.org/10.1016/j.toxlet.2016.06.1364

46. Royo F, Falcon-Perez JM (2012) Liver extracellular vesicles in health and disease. J Extracell Vesicles 1. https://doi.org/10.3402/jev.v1i0.18825

47. Yang X, Weng Z, Mendrick DL, Shi Q (2014) Circulating extracellular vesicles as a potential source of new biomarkers of drug-induced liver injury. Toxicol Lett 225(3):401–406. https://doi.org/10.1016/j.toxlet.2014.01.013

48. Momen-Heravi F, Saha B, Kodys K, Catalano D, Satishchandran A, Szabo G (2015) Increased number of circulating exosomes and their microRNA cargos are potential novel biomarkers in alcoholic hepatitis. J Transl Med 13:261. https://doi.org/10.1186/s12967-015-0623-9

49. Bala S, Petrasek J, Mundkur S, Catalano D, Levin I, Ward J, Alao H, Kodys K, Szabo G (2012) Circulating microRNAs in exosomes indicate hepatocyte injury and inflammation in alcoholic, drug-induced, and inflammatory liver diseases. Hepatology 56(5):1946–1957. https://doi.org/10.1002/hep.25873

50. Wang K, Yuan Y, Li H, Cho JH, Huang D, Gray L, Qin S, Galas DJ (2013) The spectrum of circulating RNA: a window into systems toxicology. Toxicol Sci 132(2):478–492. https://doi.org/10.1093/toxsci/kft014

51. Weber JA, Baxter DH, Zhang S, Huang DY, Huang KH, Lee MJ, Galas DJ, Wang K (2010) The microRNA spectrum in 12 body fluids. Clin Chem 56(11):1733–1741. https://doi.org/10.1373/clinchem.2010.147405

52. Yang X, Salminen WF, Shi Q, Greenhaw J, Gill PS, Bhattacharyya S, Beger RD, Mendrick DL, Mattes WB, James LP (2015) Potential of extracellular microRNAs as biomarkers of acetaminophen toxicity in children. Toxicol Appl Pharmacol 284(2):180–187. https://doi.org/10.1016/j.taap.2015.02.013

53. Su YW, Chen X, Jiang ZZ, Wang T, Wang C, Zhang Y, Wen J, Xue M, Zhu D, Zhang Y, Su YJ, Xing TY, Zhang CY, Zhang LY (2012) A panel of serum MicroRNAs as specific biomarkers for diagnosis of compound- and herb-induced liver injury in rats. PLos One 7(5):e37395. https://doi.org/10.1371/journal.pone.0037395

54. Yan S, Wang J, Zhang W, Dai J (2014) Circulating microRNA profiles altered in mice after 28 d exposure to perfluorooctanoic acid. Toxicol Lett 224(1):24–31

55. Yang X, Greenhaw J, Shi Q, ZQ S, Qian F, Davis K, Mendrick DL, Salminen WF (2012) Identification of urinary microRNA profiles in rats that may diagnose hepatotoxicity. Toxicol Sci 125(2):335–344. https://doi.org/10.1093/toxsci/kfr321

Chapter 29

Systems Microscopy Approaches in Unraveling and Predicting Drug-Induced Liver Injury (DILI)

Marije Niemeijer, Steven Hiemstra, Steven Wink, Wouter den Hollander, Bas ter Braak, and Bob van de Water

Abstract

The occurrence of drug-induced liver injury (DILI) after drug approval has often led to withdrawal from the market. Especially idiosyncratic DILI forms a major problem for pharmaceutical companies. Due to its independency of dose or duration of exposure, idiosyncratic DILI is considered as unpredictable. New in vitro test systems are now evoking to improve the prediction of DILI in the preclinical phase of drug development. Most conventional compound toxicity screening systems rely on single end-point assays most of which are based on relatively late-stage toxicity markers. When monitoring key events upstream in various adaptive stress signaling pathways combined in a single assay, the sensitivity to pick up hepatotoxic drugs will be increased while also mechanistic insight will be gained. Integrating with high-content imaging (HCI), time and high resolution single cell dynamics can be captured together with features for translocation between specific subcellular compartments. Efforts have been made to use specific dyes, antibodies or nanosensors in a multiplexed fashion using HCI, to assess multiple toxicity markers. However, these markers are still relatively downstream of toxicity signaling pathways which do not pinpoint to the molecular initiation event (MIE) of a drug. Here, we describe the application of a HepG2 BAC GFP reporter platform for the assessment of DILI liabilities by monitoring key components of adaptive stress pathways combining with HCI. Detailed insight in the regulation of these adaptive stress pathways during drug adversity can be reached by integrating these reporters with RNAi screening. Ultimately, this may lead to the recognition of novel biomarkers which can be used in the development of novel toxicity testing strategies.

Key words Systems microscopy, Drug-induced liver injury, Stress-response dynamics, BAC-GFP reporter platform, Mechanism-based toxicity screening

1 Introduction

Drug-induced liver injury (DILI) can present in various different pathologies: e.g., cholestasis (accumulation of bile), steatosis (accumulation of fatty acids) or phospholipidosis (accumulation of phospholipids). Mostly, these are mild perturbations, which will be counteracted by the target tissue ultimately establishing a new physiological homeostasis. However, DILI can also lead to severe

Minjun Chen and Yvonne Will (eds.), *Drug-Induced Liver Toxicity*, Methods in Pharmacology and Toxicology,
https://doi.org/10.1007/978-1-4939-7677-5_29, © Springer Science+Business Media, LLC, part of Springer Nature 2018

liver failure due to a necrotic liver or extensive inflammatory responses. Of all liver failures presented in the clinic, >50% are caused by drugs [1]. A large amount of these liver failures is caused by an overdose of acetaminophen. However, still 13% of all liver failures are caused by drugs taken on other prescribed dose regimens [1]. In most cases, these adverse reactions are called idiosyncratic reactions; idiosyncratic DILI (iDILI) occurs in rare cases and has a variable latency time. These features are the main reason these drugs are missed during preclinical safety testing and that liver injury is the leading cause for drug market withdrawal [2].

Cellular and biochemical perturbations that contribute to adverse outcomes underlie DILI, primarily in hepatocytes [3]. In the past decade, the field of predictive toxicology has initiated the integration of mechanistic insights in chemical adversity in toxicological screening approaches. Adaptive stress response pathways are central in toxicological responses [4, 5]. The amplitude of adaptive stress response pathway activation is the determining factor in the switch between adaptation and cell death, which makes them essential in toxicity. Quantitative assessment of adaptive stress responses and key event activation likely will contribute to a more accurate prediction of DILI based on mechanistic insight [6].

For quantitatively monitoring the adaptive stress response activation in drug safety assessment, systems microscopy will be essential. We define systems microscopy as the systematic high-throughput and high-content quantitative understanding of cell biology. Systems microscopy can be used to grasp detailed single cell protein dynamics, providing its own niche to cover the mechanistic insight spectrum in toxicological screening. Various imaging-based approaches have been established that enable the quantification of biological changes during chemical exposure [7–20]. These approaches have largely been based on the use of specific cell permeable dyes in a multiplexed fashion as indicators for the development of cellular injury in real time in combination with automated high-content screening (HCS). In these assays, cellular structures such as nuclei, mitochondria or the cellular membrane as well as specific functional characteristics like transporter activity, or mitochondrial function can be assessed and applied in the prediction of DILI [7–17]. While these approaches allow the quantification of various biochemical markers for toxicants, these are conventional late markers of cell injury and in close proximity to the tipping point toward cell death. These markers provide limited insight in adaptive stress response pathway activation, which typically occurs earlier and at lower concentrations and are likely more representative for the mode of action (MoA). More MoA-related markers that reflect the adaptive stress response pathways may increase the sensitivity to identify hepatotoxicity liabilities. Ideally, high resolution time dynamics of multiple key events in the early phase of stress signaling pathways would be monitored on single cell level to improve the prediction and understanding of DILI liabilities. In this chapter, we discuss the application of fluorescent protein reporter cell lines to monitor these adaptive stress signaling pathways using a systems microscopy approach to improve DILI liability assessments.

2 Adaptive Stress Response Pathway Activation and DILI

Cellular stress can lead to adaptation via activation of adaptive stress responses; however when the cell cannot cope with the severity of the stress, adaptive stress responses will switch to adversity and will induce cytotoxicity. The mechanism of how these stress responses exert their function in adaptation is reviewed extensively in previous reviews [4, 5, 21–25]. Therefore, here, we will briefly discuss four prominent main stress response pathways and their involvement in adaptation and relationship to cellular adverse outcomes.

Antioxidant response: Xenobiotic exposure can induce large amounts of reactive oxygen species (ROS). ROS accumulation may affect KEAP1 cysteine residues determining Nrf2 stabilization and subsequent nuclear translocation. In the nucleus, Nrf2 transcribes a large battery of antioxidant proteins which can detoxify the cell [21]. Yet, when the induced ROS is overwhelming, adaptation cannot rescue the overall overt cellular damage, thus leading to onset of cell death due to perturbation of both cellular bioenergetics and redox homeostasis [26]. The Nrf2-dependent oxidative stress response exemplifies the relevance of adaptive stress responses in the protection against liver injury: Nrf2 knock out mice are highly susceptible to various hepatotoxicants [27–29].

ER stress and unfolded protein response (UPR): When cells suffer from impaired protein folding, the load of unfolded proteins will accumulate in the endoplasmic reticulum (ER). To reduce the amount of unfolded proteins, three UPR signaling branches, involving PERK, IRE1α, and ATF6 activation, ensure production of chaperones including BiP, enlargement of the ER capacity and inhibition of the translational machinery. In addition, the UPR induces the expression of the transcription factor C/EBP homologous protein (Chop). Chop subsequently initiates transcription of target genes that trigger the onset of apoptotic signaling [30, 31]. Thus, Chop is a critical factor in the switch from adaptation to adversity in the unfolded protein response. This is illustrated by studies of Chop knock out mice which have reduced liver injury after acetaminophen treatment [32, 33].

DNA damage response: Upon accumulation of single or double stranded DNA breaks or covalent modification of nucleotides, various sensor and kinase signaling events result in the accumulation of p53. P53 is known as a tumor suppressor as it reduces the effects of massive DNA damage [24]. In the adaptive phase it activates cell cycle inhibitors, such as p21, and DNA repair mechanisms. However, upon severe DNA damage, p53 is able to transcribe apoptosis regulators as BAX, FAS, NOXA, and PUMA [34]. This results in a key role for p53 in the switch between adaptation and cell death by apoptosis.

Inflammatory TNFα signaling: Inflammatory signaling is initiated by the production of cytokines by immune cells such as resident liver Kupffer cells. Proinflammatory cytokine TNFα is able to bind the TNFα-receptor which results in NF-κB translocation and subsequent target gene expression [25]. Together these target genes induce an inflammation response to clear potential cellular damage and inhibit the onset of death receptor-mediated apoptosis. However, certain cytokine–drug combinations can induce synergistic cell death, whereby the antiapoptosis signaling by the TNFα-receptor is switched to a proapoptotic signaling route [35]. This exemplifies the subtle switch from adaptation to adversity by otherwise cytoprotective cytokine signaling.

These four adaptive stress responses demonstrate that cellular states can easily switch from reestablishment of cellular homeostasis after injury to necrosis and/or apoptosis. The amplitude and duration of stress response pathway activation are likely critical determinants for final cellular outcome. By quantitatively assessing the activation of these adaptive stress pathways by candidate drugs using a reporter system combined with systems microscopy, insight may be given in their DILI liabilities at the early phase of toxicity signaling.

3   A HepG2 BAC-GFP Reporter Platform as a Tool for Predicting and Unraveling DILI

To allow the assessment of adaptive stress response activation over time, we tagged different key components of the ER stress response, oxidative stress response, TNFα inflammation, and DNA damage response pathways with enhanced green fluorescent protein (eGFP) in hepatocellular carcinoma HepG2 cells. Confocal microscopy enables us to monitor live cell dynamics in a high-throughput fashion. GFP is integrated with bacterial artificial chromosome (BAC) recombineering technology: BACs are large plasmids (~150–200 kb) able to carry a whole eukaryotic locus including introns and promoter regions. In 2008, Poser et al. established a method to apply GFP-tagging of BACs in a high-throughput manner [36]. We used this BAC recombineering method to tag different components of adaptive stress responses with GFP [23, 37]. Transfection of BAC-GFP constructs allows the incorporation of very large pieces of DNA in the host genome, ultimately ensuring control of the engineered genes by the endogenous promotor region and other regulatory sequences. In relation to the earlier introduced adaptive stress response pathways, we have generated a broad range of BAC-GFP reporter lines aimed to capture the complexity of DILI [23, 37].

3.1 Development of the Reporter Platform

Below we describe the detailed approach to establish BAC-GFP reporters. We introduce these reporters in HepG2 cells, but any other cell line can be used.

3.1.1 Identification of a Stress Pathway Specific Biomarker

Both literature and transcriptomics mining allows the discovery of hepatotoxic drug responses (e.g., TG-GATES and Drug Matrix) and the identification of candidate biomarker genes that can be translated into reporter assays [38, 39]. In this way, key regulators of specific adaptive stress pathways have been identified. For our HepG2 BAC-GFP platform, both early sensors and downstream transcription factors along with their subsequent target genes were selected to resemble the activation of critical stress response pathways at different signaling levels.

3.1.2 Cloning of the BAC-GFP Plasmid

Using an online tool (http://www.mitocheck.org/cgi-bin/BACfinder), BAC constructs that contain the selected human gene of interest, containing all the regulatory elements, can be ordered; also the necessary GFP overhang primers can be found here. Using a multistep cloning strategy, the BAC-GFP fusion plasmid can be generated [36].

3.1.3 Transfection and Cell Reporter Cloning

HepG2 wild-type cells are seeded in a 6-well plate format and simultaneously transfected (Lipofectamine-based) to introduce the BAC-GFP construct to the cells. Geneticin (G418) selection is used to select BAC-GFP HepG2 positive clones. Monoclonal BAC-GFP HepG2 clones are picked (generally 10–24 clones) and expanded. PCR is used to confirm correct genomic integration of the BAC-GFP. Next, the expression of the target gene (quantitative PCR) and protein (Western blot) is determined to quantify the levels of GFP-tagged target gene or protein. The GFP-fusion protein size should correspond to the corresponding gene fusion product. Live cell imaging will then validate a correct localization of the GFP-protein fusion, the population variability, and the inducibility by xenobiotic treatment. At last, RNA interference experiments are performed to verify GFP-target gene specificity. See Fig. 1 for an overview of BAC-GFP reporter line generation.

4 Application of BAC-GFP HepG2 Reporters

The BAC-GFP reporter panel covers multiple adaptive stress responses (e.g., oxidative stress response, ER stress response, DNA damage response and NF-κB signaling) at different signaling levels and is able to reveal subcellular localization of the different components during stress induction when combined with confocal microscopy. Furthermore, intracellular translocation events and specific cellular accumulation can be captured with this system. The analysis of the GFP signal in each subcellular compartment needs a different image analysis strategy which is based on the usage of CellProfiler and ImageJ (Fig. 2). Retrieved data sets can

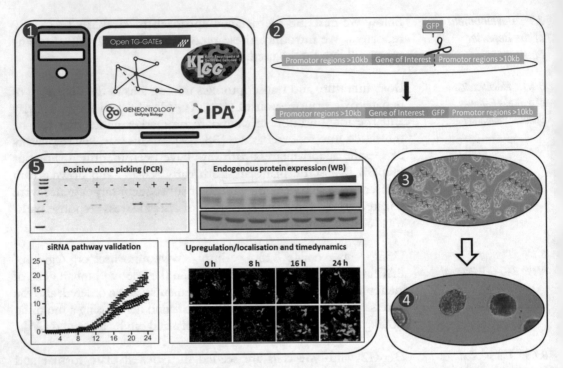

Fig. 1 Generation of the HepG2 BAC reporter platform. (1) Identifying the target proteins that can serve as biomarkers for certain stress responses. (2) Generating the BAC-GFP fusion plasmid. (3) Transfect HepG2 wt cells. (4) Selection and clonal expansion. (5) Validation of the HepG2 BAC reporters

contain cell population as well as single cell features making it possible to capture valuable single cell dynamics. Thus, the use of high-content high-throughput imaging of BAC-GFP reporter cell lines enables identification of spatial–temporal single cell dynamics of adaptive stress response cellular signaling underlying DILI.

We see two major application domains for BAC-GFP reporters in the context of DILI: prediction and mechanistic understanding. The application of the BAC-GFP reporter system in the DILI prediction domain allows to identify the activation levels of multiple adaptive stress responses giving a certain MoA toxicity fingerprint for each drug. These fingerprints can be linked to DILI liability classification and used for future hazard identification of potential new drugs. In this way, DILI liabilities can be predicted and simultaneously reveal the underlying MoA. The other domain, namely the application in mechanistic studies, focuses on the underlying cause of toxicity in contrast to DILI predictions and obtains a better understanding of why some patients are more prone to develop DILI. In addition, this may give more insight in the precise regulation of these adaptive stress responses and their balance between adaptation and adversity. Here, we will present examples of the application domains of these BAC-GFP reporters.

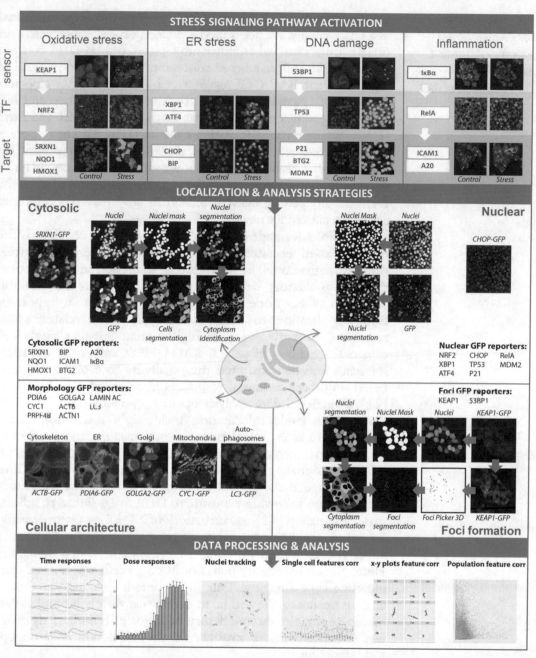

Fig. 2 Overview of HepG2 BAC-GFP reporter platform. Overview of different reporters for the oxidative stress, ER stress, DNA damage or inflammation response sensing at different levels with the signaling pathway. Depending on the specific reporter, GFP signal can be quantified either in the cytosol, nucleus, in foci or alterations in cellular structure can be examined. Each strategy has its own specific segmentation and analysis pipeline. In the end, high-content data can be further processed to obtain time or dose responses, single cell tracking, subpopulations identifications or specific translocation in between different subcellular compartments

4.1 Drug Testing for Cellular Stress Pathway Activation Supporting the Prediction of DILI

DILI prediction can make use of features specific to drugs attributed as a DILI liability. We performed an imaging-based screen with a set of 131 drugs classified as either most-, less-, or non-DILI concern by Chen et al. [40] in a broad concentration range using a panel of eight different BAC-GFP reporter cell lines. The BAC reporters used involved Srxn1 and Hmox1 (oxidative stress); Chop and BiP (ER stress pathway); Hspa1b (heat shock response); p21 and Btg2 (DNA damage); Icam1 (cytokine signaling) (Fig. 3). The responses of the different reporters together show clusters of drugs enriched for most-DILI classification which activates one or more adaptive stress responses. In this way, utilizing a classifier a prediction of the DILI liability can be made based on its adaptive stress responses activation pattern for newly developed drugs.

A major advantage of the BAC-GFP reporter cell lines is the imaging-based assessment of the dynamics of the cellular stress response activation. The definition of transcription factor activation and oscillatory behavior dynamics as well as the rate and induction of key-node signaling proteins will be an important future application to better understand DILI related stress responses. Recently, we used high-content imaging single cell temporal dynamics of several BAC-GFP reporters for statistical inference and demonstrated the possibility to capture imaging-based single cell temporal responses in so called base functions [41]. Functional data analysis opens up possibilities of detailed temporal dynamic information including transcription factor translocation rates, calculations of local maxima and oscillatory periods or dampening parameters; the latter finds applications for oscillatory signaling processes such as observed for NF-κB. Thus, we have applied the NF-κB reporter to quantify the oscillatory perturbations following exposure to DILI drugs linked to inflammatory signaling [42]. Perturbations of NF-kB oscillatory behavior will affect the downstream target gene activation and hence affect the biological outcome of cytokine-mediated signaling. Here, NF-κB oscillatory behavior in single cells was tracked during time-lapse imaging. Our high-content imaging and image analysis approach allowed us to define that diclofenac and carbamazepine inhibits the oscillatory behavior of NF-κB. This effect was associated with a sensitization to TNFα-induced proapoptotic signaling.

4.2 Identification of Novel Key Regulators of Stress Signaling Pathways

There is a need to gain insight in the underlying mechanisms of DILI. One aspect involves the unraveling how drugs perturb the cellular physiology and as a consequence switch on cellular stress responses that define cellular adaptation or adverse outcomes. Such improved mechanistic understanding will identify candidate biomarkers that can be integrated in safety testing strategies in either early drug development or as a part of the investigative toxicology tool box [43].

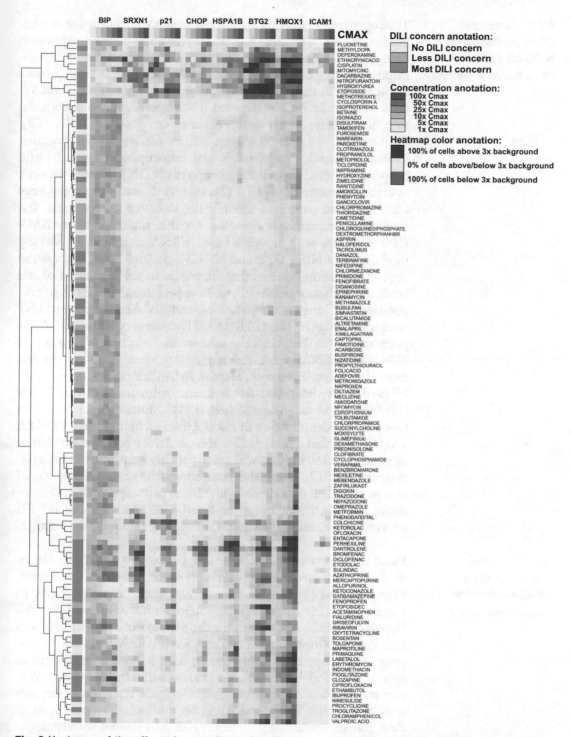

Fig. 3 Heat map of the effect of a set of 131 classified drugs on the activation of multiple adaptive stress BAC-GFP reporters. The drug set consists of drugs classified as either most-, less-, or non-DILI. HepG2 BAC-GFP reporters (BiP-, Srxn1-, p21-, Chop-, HSPA1B-, Btg2-, Hmox1-, and ICAM1-GFP) were exposed for 72 h to drugs in a broad concentration range (1–100× Cmax) and imaged using confocal microscopy. GFP activation levels are depicted as fraction of cells three times above the background levels

Toxicogenomics has been an efficient means to hypothesize mechanisms [38, 39, 44]. Yet, functional relevance of gene expression changes to mode-of-action of toxicity is hard to define. High-throughput functional siRNA-based screening provides direct functional insight in the role of individual genes in adverse outcome. We have successfully applied targeted RNAi approaches to discern the role of oxidative stress and ER stress in onset of DILI [43]. Furthermore, we applied a large siRNA survival screen targeting individual kinases, phosphatases, and transcription factors, to gain deeper understanding of the regulation of the DNA damage response in embryonic stem cells [45]. This success allowed us to apply large scale RNAi screening to identify the signaling components that modulate stress response signaling. For this, we integrate our BAC-GFP reporters with imaging-based siRNA screening to identify modulators of Nrf2, UPR and NF-κB signaling. As an example, to unravel novel components that are crucial in the regulation of this oscillatory behavior of NF-κB, we have performed an siRNA screen, consisting of kinases, ubiquitinases, and Toll-like Receptors/TNF receptors, using the HepG2 RelA-GFP reporter cell line. Diclofenac pretreatment of HepG2 cells inhibits the oscillatory behavior of NF-kB [35]; RNAi is an excellent means to identify modulators that cause this effect. Therefore, HepG2 RelA-GFP reporters were pre-exposed with diclofenac for 8 h and subsequently with TNFα (Fredriksson et al., unpublished data). Multiparametric analysis revealed the identification of novel genes, including A20, CDK12, and UFD1L, that could regulate this oscillatory behavior which may ultimately lead to insights why some patients are prone to the development of DILI. Using the same approach, key regulators could also be identified for other adaptive stress pathways, such as the oxidative stress pathway, using the Srxn1-GFP reporter, and the ER stress response, using the Chop-GFP reporter (unpublished data).

Based on improved mechanistic insight, better predictions can be made for the development of DILI, especially when this knowledge is placed in a structured adverse outcome pathway (AOP) framework. This opens up the opportunity to implement this knowledge into a test system for the assessment of DILI liabilities and, thereby, improving its accuracy for predictivity. Likewise, systems microscopy approaches can be used for the development of new AOPs. Work by Fredriksson et al. identified underlying molecular mechanisms of the synergistic apoptotic response of hepatotoxic drugs and TNFα and could be the basis for a novel AOP. First, transcriptomic analysis of HepG2 cells treated with synergistic hepatotoxic drugs (such as diclofenac and carbamazepine) with or without TNFα at different time points was performed and revealed after Ingenuity Pathway Analysis (IPA) the importance of EIF2/ER stress signaling, Nrf2-mediated oxidative stress response and death receptor signaling in this synergistic apoptotic response. Combining siRNA-mediated knockdowns of important genes in these pathways with high-content imaging of AnnexinV-Alexa633, a dye for apoptosis, and HepG2 oxidative stress GFP reporters, a model was proposed whereby compound-mediated activation of PERK and Chop together with oxidative stress sensitizes toward TNFα-induced apoptotic signaling [43]. This work highlights the strength of combining omics techniques and siRNA-based functional microscopy approaches to reveal new insight in the molecular mechanisms that define drug adversities.

4.3 3D Culture HepG2 BAC-GFP Reporter System with Improved Hepatic Phenotype Suitable for Long-Term Toxicity Assessment

HepG2 cells have reduced metabolic capacity and a lack in the resemblance with the liver phenotype [46]. Also the proliferative nature of HepG2 hinders chronic repeat testing. To overcome these issues, a method to culture HepG2 as spheroids in a 3D hydrogel was developed [47]. 3D HepG2 spheroids show enhanced metabolic capacity of phase I and phase II metabolizing enzymes, functional expression of liver phenotypical properties and enable culturing over several weeks due to lack of proliferation. We have established the application of our panel of BAC-GFP HepG2 reporters in 3D spheroids and defined their functionality using automated confocal live cell imaging applications. These models can be used for repeated dose toxicity evaluation for up to 2 weeks. This allowed us to quantify the activation of stress response pathways by DILI compounds in 3D spheroids [48]. Our findings indicate that 3D BAC-GFP HepG2 spheroids and integration with automated imaging, allows for high-throughput assessment of DILI liability.

5   Future Directions of DILI Testing Using Fluorescent Toxicity Pathway Reporter Technology

We have established the functionality of HepG2 BAC-GFP reporter cells to quantitatively assess stress response pathway activation using an automated confocal microscopy approach. Moreover, we demonstrated that these reporter cells are a valuable tool for DILI safety assessment [37, 49]. In addition, these reporters have further application in investigative toxicology as well as mechanistic molecular understanding of DILI. While the HepG2 cell line is a robust and cheap cell system which allows easy scaling for high-throughput screening [50], several issues may require further optimization.

Firstly, we need to address the limitation of the lack of drug metabolizing capacity in HepG2 cells and consequences for predicting DILI [51]. Various DILI drugs require metabolism for bioactivation and leading to toxicity [52–54]. By integrating drug metabolism in the reporter platform, thus increasing clearance as well as bioactivation capacity, we can address the question what the overall consequences will be for sensitivity and specificity of the reporter platform.

Secondly, the iPSC model in combination with CRISPR/Cas9 genome editing technology will allow the generation of iPSC-based fluorescent reporter systems. The CRISPR/cas9 tool makes it possible to make very specific genomic changes, including integration of fluorophores [55, 56]. These fluorescent hiPSC reporters can then be differentiated in hepatocyte-like cells (HLC), proposed as an improved model for toxicity screening [57, 58], using established differentiation protocols [59–61]. Further optimization of these differentiation protocols is still ongoing. These novel hiPSC derived HLC reporter lines can then be used for high-throughput screening. This work will require strong investments in generation of reporter systems and reassessing the sensitivity and specificity of these new reporters for DILI liability evaluation. Regardless of the outcome, these reporters can also be used for the generation of other cell lineages representing other target organs.

Thirdly, an advancement in generation of BAC-GFP HepG2 3D spheroids that contain additional nonparenchymal cell types that are critical for DILI, including Kupffer cells, stellate cells and endothelial cells, thus creating a microenvironment similar to the normal liver [62].

Finally, using either BAC-GFP approaches or CRISPR/Cas9-mediated GFP tagging technology will lead to expression of GFP-fusion products at the endogenous expression levels. We observed differences in the levels of GFP reporter expression, with in particular transcription factor GFP-fusion products being expressed at low levels. This requires in particular high-end image acquisition systems to allow sensitive and fast detection of reporters. Moreover, high resolution imaging at both the 2D and 3D level will facilitate the image segmentation and quantification of GFP-reporter levels as well as subcellular localization.

In conclusion, we have established an advanced cell stress reporter platform which finds its application in DILI liability evaluation in preclinical drug development. The above innovations will likely improve the quality and the applicability of these reporters in safety assessment.

Acknowledgments

This work was supported by the FP7 DETECTIVE project (grant agreement 266838), IMI MIP-DILI project (grant agreement 115336), and the H2020 EU-ToxRisk project (grant agreement 681002).

References

1. Ostapowicz G, Fontana RJ, Schiødt FV et al (2002) Results of a prospective study of acute liver failure at 17 tertiary care centers in the United States. Ann Intern Med 137:947–954

2. Wilke R, Lin D, Roden D (2007) Identifying genetic risk factors for serious adverse drug reactions: current progress and challenges. Nat Rev Drug Discov 6:904–916. https://doi.org/10.1038/nrd2423

3. Gu X, Manautou JE (2012) Molecular mechanisms underlying chemical liver injury. Expert Rev Mol Med 14:1–24. https://doi.org/10.1017/S1462399411002110

4. Simmons SO, Fan C-Y, Ramabhadran R (2009) Cellular stress response pathway system as a sentinel ensemble in toxicological screening. Toxicol Sci 111:202–225. https://doi.org/10.1093/toxsci/kfp140

5. Jennings P, Limonciel A, Felice L, Leonard MO (2013) An overview of transcriptional regulation in response to toxicological insult. Arch Toxicol 87:49–72. https://doi.org/10.1007/s00204-012-0919-y

6. Vinken M (2013) The adverse outcome pathway concept: a pragmatic tool in toxicology. Toxicology 312:158–165. https://doi.org/10.1016/j.tox.2013.08.011

7. O'Brien PJ, Irwin W, Diaz D et al (2006) High concordance of drug-induced human hepatotoxicity with in vitro cytotoxicity measured in a novel cell-based model using high content screening. Arch Toxicol 80:580–604. https://doi.org/10.1007/s00204-006-0091-3

8. Xu JJ, Henstock PV, Dunn MC et al (2008) Cellular imaging predictions of clinical drug-induced liver injury. Toxicol Sci 105:97–105. https://doi.org/10.1093/toxsci/kfn109

9. Persson M, Løye AF, Mow T, Hornberg JJ (2013) A high content screening assay to predict human drug-induced liver injury during drug discovery. J Pharmacol Toxicol Methods 68:302–313. https://doi.org/10.1016/j.vascn.2013.08.001

10. Tolosa L, Pinto S, Donato MT et al (2012) Development of a multiparametric cell-based protocol to screen and classify the hepatotoxicity potential of drugs. Toxicol Sci 127:187–198. https://doi.org/10.1093/toxsci/kfs083

11. Zhang J, Doshi U, Suzuki A et al (2016) Evaluation of multiple mechanism-based toxicity endpoints in primary cultured human hepatocytes for the identification of drugs with clinical hepatotoxicity: results from 152 marketed drugs with known liver injury profiles.

12. Tolosa L, Carmona A, Castell JV et al (2015) High-content screening of drug-induced mitochondrial impairment in hepatic cells: effects of statins. Arch Toxicol 89:1847–1860. https://doi.org/10.1007/s00204-014-1334-3

13. Bauch C, Bevan S, Woodhouse H et al (2015) Predicting in vivo phospholipidosis-inducing potential of drugs by a combined high content screening and in silico modelling approach. Toxicol In Vitro 29:621–630. https://doi.org/10.1016/j.tiv.2015.01.014

14. Germano D, Uteng M, Pognan F et al (2015) Determination of liver specific toxicities in rat hepatocytes by high content imaging during 2-week multiple treatment. Toxicol In Vitro 30:79–94. https://doi.org/10.1016/j.tiv.2014.05.009

15. van de Water FM, Havinga J, Ravesloot WT et al (2011) High content screening analysis of phospholipidosis: validation of a 96-well assay with CHO-K1 and HepG2 cells for the prediction of in vivo based phospholipidosis. Toxicol In Vitro 25:1870–1882. https://doi.org/10.1016/j.tiv.2011.05.026

16. Lechner C, Reichel V, Moenning U et al (2010) Development of a fluorescence-based assay for drug interactions with human multidrug resistance related protein (MRP2; ABCC2) in MDCKII-MRP2 membrane vesicles. Eur J Pharm Biopharm 75:284–290. https://doi.org/10.1016/j.ejpb.2010.03.008

17. De Bruyn T, Sempels W, Snoeys J et al (2014) Confocal imaging with a fluorescent bile acid analogue closely mimicking hepatic taurocholate disposition. J Pharm Sci 103:1872–1881. https://doi.org/10.1002/jps.23933

18. Perlman ZE, Slack MD, Feng Y et al (2004) Multidimensional drug profiling by automated microscopy. Science 306(5699):1194–1198. https://doi.org/10.1126/science.1100709

19. Shuhendler AJ, Pu K, Cui L et al (2014) Real-time imaging of oxidative and nitrosative stress in the liver of live animals for drug-toxicity testing. Nat Biotechnol 32:373–380. https://doi.org/10.1038/nbt.2838

20. Poon KL, Wang X, Lee SGP et al (2017) Transgenic Zebrafish reporter lines as alternative in vivo organ toxicity models. Toxicol Sci 156:133–148. https://doi.org/10.1093/toxsci/kfw250

21. Ray PD, Huang B-W, Tsuji Y (2012) Reactive oxygen species (ROS) homeostasis and redox

Chem Biol Interact 255:3–11. https://doi.org/10.1016/j.cbi.2015.11.008

regulation in cellular signaling. Cell Signal 24:981–990. https://doi.org/10.1016/j.cellsig.2012.01.008

22. Hetz C (2012) The unfolded protein response: controlling cell fate decisions under ER stress and beyond. Nat Rev Mol Cell Biol 13:89–102. https://doi.org/10.1038/nrm3270

23. Wink S, Hiemstra S, Huppelschoten S et al (2014) Quantitative high content imaging of cellular adaptive stress response pathways in toxicity for chemical safety assessment. Chem Res Toxicol 27:338–355. https://doi.org/10.1021/tx4004038

24. Banin S, Moyal L, Shieh S-Y et al (1998) Enhanced phosphorylation of p53 by ATM in response to DNA damage. Science 281:1674–1677. https://doi.org/10.1126/science.281.5383.1674

25. Varfolomeev E, Vucic D (2016) Intracellular regulation of TNF activity in health and disease. Cytokine. https://doi.org/10.1016/j.cyto.2016.08.035

26. Jaeschke H, McGill MR, Ramachandran A (2012) Oxidant stress, mitochondria, and cell death mechanisms in drug-induced liver injury: lessons learned from acetaminophen hepatotoxicity. Drug Metab Rev 44:88–106. https://doi.org/10.3109/03602532.2011.602688

27. Liu J, Wu KC, Lu YF et al (2013) NRF2 protection against liver injury produced by various hepatotoxicants. Oxidative Med Cell Longev 2013:305861. https://doi.org/10.1155/2013/305861

28. Enomoto A, Itoh K, Nagayoshi E et al (2001) High sensitivity of Nrf2 knockout mice to acetaminophen hepatotoxicity associated with decreased expression of ARE-regulated drug metabolizing enzymes and antioxidant genes. Toxicol Sci 59:169–177

29. Qu Q, Liu J, Zhou HH, Klaassen CD (2014) Nrf2 protects against furosemide-induced hepatotoxicity. Toxicology 324:35–42. https://doi.org/10.1016/j.tox.2014.02.008

30. Puthalakath H, O'Reilly LA, Gunn P et al (2007) ER stress triggers apoptosis by activating BH3-only protein Bim. Cell 129:1337–1349. https://doi.org/10.1016/j.cell.2007.04.027

31. Yamaguchi H, Wang HG (2004) CHOP is involved in endoplasmic reticulum stress-induced apoptosis by enhancing DR5 expression in human carcinoma cells. J Biol Chem 279:45495–45502. https://doi.org/10.1074/jbc.M406933200

32. Hur KY, So J-S, Ruda V et al (2012) IRE1α activation protects mice against acetaminophen-induced hepatotoxicity. J Exp Med 209:307–318. https://doi.org/10.1084/jem.20111298

33. Uzi D, Barda L, Scaiewicz V et al (2013) CHOP is a critical regulator of acetaminophen-induced hepatotoxicity. J Hepatol 59:495–503. https://doi.org/10.1016/j.jhep.2013.04.024

34. Yu J, Zhang L (2003) No PUMA, no death: implications for p53-dependent apoptosis. Cancer Cell 4:248–249. https://doi.org/10.1016/S1535-6108(03)00249-6

35. Fredriksson L, Herpers B, Benedetti G et al (2011) Diclofenac inhibits tumor necrosis factor-α-induced nuclear factor-κB activation causing synergistic hepatocyte apoptosis. Hepatology 53:2027–2041. https://doi.org/10.1002/hep.24314

36. Poser I, Sarov M, JR a H et al (2008) BAC TrangeneOmics: a high-throughput method for exploration of protein function in mammals. Nat Methods 5:409–415. https://doi.org/10.1038/nmeth.1199

37. Wink S, Hiemstra S, Herpers B, van de Water B (2017) High-content imaging-based BAC-GFP toxicity pathway reporters to assess chemical adversity liabilities. Arch Toxicol 91:1367–1383. https://doi.org/10.1007/s00204-016-1781-0

38. Igarashi Y, Nakatsu N, Yamashita T et al (2015) Open TG-GATEs: a large-scale toxicogenomics database. Nucleic Acids Res 43:D921–D927. https://doi.org/10.1093/nar/gku955

39. Suter L, Schroeder S, Meyer K et al (2011) EU framework 6 project: predictive toxicology (PredTox)-overview and outcome. Toxicol Appl Pharmacol 252:73–84. https://doi.org/10.1016/j.taap.2010.10.008

40. Chen M, Vijay V, Shi Q et al (2011) FDA-approved drug labeling for the study of drug-induced liver injury. Drug Discov Today 16:697–703. https://doi.org/10.1016/j.drudis.2011.05.007

41. Jiang X, Wink S, van de Water B, Koppschneider A (2016) Functional analysis of high-content high-throughput imaging data. J Appl Stat 44:1903–1919. https://doi.org/10.1080/02664763.2016.1238048

42. Herpers B, Wink S, Fredriksson L et al (2016) Activation of the Nrf2 response by intrinsic hepatotoxic drugs correlates with suppression of NF-κB activation and sensitizes toward TNFα-induced cytotoxicity. Arch Toxicol 90:1163–1179. https://doi.org/10.1007/s00204-015-1536-3

43. Fredriksson L, Wink S, Herpers B et al (2014) Drug-induced endoplasmic reticulum and oxidative stress responses independently sensitize toward TNFα-mediated hepatotoxicity. Toxicol Sci 140:144–159. https://doi.org/10.1093/toxsci/kfu072

44. Sutherland JJ, Jolly RA, Goldstein KM, Stevens JL (2016) Assessing concordance of drug-induced transcriptional response in rodent liver and cultured hepatocytes. PLoS Comput Biol 12:1–31. https://doi.org/10.1371/journal.pcbi.1004847

45. Carreras Puigvert J, von Stechow L, Siddappa R et al (2013) Systems biology approach identifies the kinase csnk1a1 as a regulator of the DNA damage response in embryonic stem cells. Sci Signal 6:ra5. https://doi.org/10.1126/scisignal.2003208

46. LeCluyse EL, Witek RP, Andersen ME, Powers MJ (2012) Organotypic liver culture models: meeting current challenges in toxicity testing. Crit Rev Toxicol 42:501–548. https://doi.org/10.3109/10408444.2012.682115

47. Ramaiahgari SC, den Braver MW, Herpers B et al (2014) A 3D in vitro model of differentiated HepG2 cell spheroids with improved liver-like properties for repeated dose high-throughput toxicity studies. Arch Toxicol 88:1083–1095. https://doi.org/10.1007/s00204-014-1215-9

48. Hiemstra S, Wink S, van den Nieuwendijk K, Ramaiaghari S, Dankers A, de Bont H and van de Water B. A 3D HepG2 GFP reporter platform to screen for drug-induced liver injury liabilities. Manuscript in preparation

49. Hiemstra S, Niemeijer M, Koedoot E et al (2016) Comprehensive landscape of Nrf2 and p53 pathway activation dynamics by oxidative stress and DNA damage. Chem Res Toxicol 30:923–933. https://doi.org/10.1021/acs.chemrestox.6b00322

50. Jennen DGJ, Magkoufopoulou C, Ketelslegers HB et al (2010) Comparison of HepG2 and HepaRG by whole-genome gene expression analysis for the purpose of chemical hazard identification. Toxicol Sci 115:66–79. https://doi.org/10.1093/toxsci/kfq026

51. Bader A (2003) Comparison of primary human hepatocytes and hepatoma cell line Hepg2 with regard to their biotransformation properties. Drug Metab Dispos 31:1035–1042

52. Gómez-Lechón MJ, Tolosa L, Donato MT (2016) Metabolic activation and drug-induced liver injury: in vitro approaches for the safety risk assessment of new drugs. J Appl Toxicol 36:752–768. https://doi.org/10.1002/jat.3277

53. Amacher DE (2012) The primary role of hepatic metabolism in idiosyncratic drug-induced liver injury. Expert Opin Drug Metab Toxicol 8:335–347. https://doi.org/10.1517/17425255.2012.658041

54. Leung L, Kalgutkar AS, Obach RS (2012) Metabolic activation in drug-induced liver injury. Drug Metab Rev 44:18–33. https://doi.org/10.3109/03602532.2011.605791

55. Jinek M, East A, Cheng A et al (2013) RNA-programmed genome editing in human cells. elife 2:e00471. https://doi.org/10.7554/eLife.00471

56. Cong L, Ran FA, Cox D et al (2013) Multiplex genome engineering using CRISPR/Cas systems. Science 339:819–823. https://doi.org/10.1126/science.1231143

57. Gómez-Lechón MJ, Tolosa L (2016) Human hepatocytes derived from pluripotent stem cells: a promising cell model for drug hepatotoxicity screening. Arch Toxicol 90:2049–2061. https://doi.org/10.1007/s00204-016-1756-1

58. Gao X, Liu Y (2017) A transcriptomic study suggesting human iPSC-derived hepatocytes potentially offer a better in vitro model of hepatotoxicity than most hepatoma cell lines. Cell Biol Toxicol 33:407–421. https://doi.org/10.1007/s10565-017-9383-z

59. Asplund A, Pradip A, van Giezen M et al (2016) One standardized differentiation procedure robustly generates homogenous hepatocyte cultures displaying metabolic diversity from a large panel of human pluripotent stem cells. Stem Cell Rev Rep 12:90–104. https://doi.org/10.1007/s12015-015-9621-9

60. Raju R, Chau D, Cho DS et al (2017) Cell expansion during directed differentiation of stem cells toward the hepatic lineage. Stem Cells Dev 26:274–284. https://doi.org/10.1089/scd.2016.0119

61. Chen Y-F, Tseng C Y, Wang H-W et al (2012) Rapid generation of mature hepatocyte-like cells from human induced pluripotent stem cells by an efficient three-step protocol. Hepatology 55:1193–1203. https://doi.org/10.1002/hep.24790

62. Ware BR, Berger DR, Khetani SR (2015) Prediction of drug-induced liver injury in micropatterned co-cultures containing iPSC-derived human hepatocytes. Toxicol Sci 145:252–262. https://doi.org/10.1093/toxsci/kfv048

Chapter 30

Noninvasive Preclinical and Clinical Imaging of Liver Transporter Function Relevant to Drug-Induced Liver Injury

J. Gerry Kenna, John C. Waterton, Andreas Baudy, Aleksandra Galetin, Catherine D.G. Hines, Paul Hockings, Manishkumar Patel, Daniel Scotcher, Steven Sourbron, Sabina Ziemian, and Gunnar Schuetz

Abstract

Imaging technologies can evaluate many different biological processes in vitro (in cell culture models) and in vivo (in animals and humans), and many are used routinely in investigation of human liver diseases. Some of these methods can help understand liver toxicity caused by drugs in vivo in animals, and drug-induced liver injury (DILI) which arises in susceptible humans. Imaging could aid assessment of the relevance to humans in vivo of toxicity caused by drugs in animals (animal/human translation), plus toxicities observed using in vitro model systems (in vitro/in vivo translation). Technologies and probe substrates for quantitative evaluation of hepatobiliary transporter activities are of particular importance. This is due to the key role played by sinusoidal transporter mediated hepatic uptake in DILI caused by many drugs, plus the strong evidence that inhibition of the hepatic bile salt export pump (BSEP) can initiate DILI. Imaging methods for investigation of these processes are reviewed in this chapter, together with their scientific rationale, and methods of quantitative data analysis. In addition to providing biomarkers for investigation of DILI, such approaches could aid the evaluation of clinically relevant drug–drug interactions mediated via hepatobiliary transporter perturbation.

Key words Drug-induced liver injury, Drug labelling, Causality assessment, Hepatotoxicity, Hepatobiliary transporters, Bile salt export pump, Gadoxetate, Drug-drug interactions

1 Introduction

Many hundreds of different drugs cause liver injury in humans which occurs only infrequently and in certain susceptible individuals, and cannot be anticipated from nonclinical safety studies undertaken in vivo in experimental animals [1, 2]. Hence their ability to cause human drug-induced liver injury (DILI) only starts to be appreciated in Phase 2 or Phase 3 clinical trials, or even post-licensing [2, 3]. The consequences in affected patients may be marked symptomatic liver damage, or even acute liver failure, and currently it is not possible to predict and identify "at risk" patients

Minjun Chen and Yvonne Will (eds.), *Drug-Induced Liver Toxicity*, Methods in Pharmacology and Toxicology,
https://doi.org/10.1007/978-1-4939-7677-5_30, © The Author(s) 2018

prior to their exposure to the relevant drugs [1, 2]. Because of this, unexpected "idiosyncratic" human DILI continues to be a leading cause of failed development of new drugs, of withdrawal from use of previously licensed drugs and of cautionary labeling that restricts prescribing [1–5].

The mechanisms by which drugs cause human idiosyncratic DILI are complex, and involve both drug-related adverse biochemical processes and susceptibility factors specific to susceptible patients [1, 2]. Important drug-related adverse processes which can initiate idiosyncratic DILI include formation of chemically reactive metabolites, injury to mitochondria, and inhibition of the activity of the bile salt export pump (BSEP), which mediates efflux of toxic bile salts from hepatocytes into bile [6–8]. The susceptibility factors that explain why only some patients develop DILI are less well defined, although it is clear that these can include activation of both innate and adaptive immune responses [9].

Several of the key drug-related events that initiate idiosyncratic DILI can be quantified using various in vitro assays. These assays can be used during drug discovery, to enable early identification and deselection of compounds with high propensity to cause DILI and other serious adverse reactions [6–8]. Many different methodologies have been described, and are used routinely in pharmaceutical companies. They are discussed in Chap. 17 of this volume, by Light et al., and can reduce the likelihood that compounds progressed into clinical trials will cause DILI in humans. However, in vitro toxicity assays have several important limitations. The most commonly used in vitro toxicity assays fail to reproduce many of the key molecular events that influence hepatic drug uptake, biotransformation and excretion in vivo. Furthermore, the assays do not reproduce all of the mechanisms by which DILI occurs in vivo. Consequently, the precise relationship between potencies of effects observed in in vitro safety assays and functional consequences that may arise within the liver in vivo, and may result in DILI in susceptible drug exposed humans, remains poorly understood.

One approach which can help to address this important translational gap is medical imaging. Several imaging modalities can measure the hepatic uptake and clearance of probe substrates. Many are well suited to in vivo studies in animals and humans, while others can be utilized in cellular systems in vitro. Mechanistically relevant processes include the transporters that mediate drug uptake into and excretion from the liver, plus BSEP and other hepatobiliary transporters that mediate bile flow. Suitable imaging modalities and probe substrates are reviewed in Sect. 2. Key issues that need to be considered when generating reproducible data and undertaking quantitative analyses of imaging data are discussed in Sect. 3. These include assessing interaction between investigational drugs and the probe substrates used in imaging studies. Some of these interactions provide insight into undesired drug–drug interactions and this aspect is addressed in Sect. 4. An imaging approach to investigate and characterize liver injury with potential to provide novel insight into DILI risk is dynamic contrast-enhanced magnetic resonance imaging (DCE-MRI) using the contrast agent gadoxetate. This is reviewed in Sect. 5, which discusses the value and limitations of the approach. Finally, challenges and opportunities in using imaging technologies to understand and risk-manage DILI are considered in Sect. 6.

2 Hepatobiliary Imaging Modalities and Tracers

Imaging techniques can measure the appearance of probe substrates in different compartments (blood, hepatocyte, and bile) and, if imaging is repeated with high temporal resolution (the so-called dynamic imaging), then transporter kinetics can be inferred. The added value of spatially resolving the liver signal (as opposed to simply monitoring tracer disappearance from blood) was recognized over 60 years ago [10], although it is only recently that the uptake and elimination rates or kinetics have been employed to derive absolute kinetic rate constants. Hepatic uptake of drugs is mediated primarily by solute carriers expressed on the sinusoidal plasma membrane domain of hepatocytes and is an essential first step before DILI can be initiated. Consequently, data provided by imaging technologies which provide quantitative insights into hepatic uptake transporter kinetics has the potential to improve interpretation of the in vivo DILI relevance of in vitro toxicity assay data, which currently poses a major challenge (e.g., see Chaps. 6, 8, and 17). In addition, inhibition of the activity of the biliary efflux transporter BSEP plays a direct role in the mechanism by which numerous drugs can initiate DILI, while upregulation of the activity of other biliary efflux transporters plays an important hepatoprotective role in response to BSEP inhibition by drugs [11] (see also Chap. 15). Furthermore, a recent genetic analysis undertaken in a Chinese patient cohort has revealed an association between genetic variants in the gene encoding BSEP (*ABCB11*) and cholestatic liver injury caused by treatment for between 6 and 9 months with antituberculous drugs (a combination of isoniazid, rifampicin, pyrazinamide, ethambutol, and/or streptomycin) [12]. Hence imaging methods that enable direct quantitative evaluation of drug-induced hepatic uptake and efflux transporter kinetics in vivo, and can be used to investigate perturbation of transporter function following administration of test drugs, have the potential to improve understanding of DILI mechanisms, and of DILI risk.

Several different imaging modalities can be used to assess hepatobiliary transporter kinetics (Table 1) [13]. A suitable imaging modality requires sufficient spatial resolution to resolve compartments, and adequate temporal resolution to enable characterization

Table 1
Imaging modalities used in liver transporter research in rats and humans [13]

	Typical region electromagnetic spectrum[a]	Ionizing radiation	Tissue depth	Typical spatial resolution/mm (human liver; rat liver)
Magnetic resonance imaging (MRI)	63–500 MHz	No	Full	$2 \times 2 \times 4$; $0.2 \times 0.2 \times 2$
Fluorescence or optoacoustic	500–1000 nm	No	20 mm	–; 1×1
Radiography and X-ray computed tomography (CT)	20–50 keV	Yes	Full	$1 \times 1 \times 1$; $0.1 \times 0.1 \times 0.1$
Scintigraphy and single-photon emission computed tomography (SPECT)	141–159 keV	Yes	Full	$5 \times 5 \times 5$; $0.5 \times 0.5 \times 0.5$
Positron emission tomography (PET)	511 keV	Yes	Full	$2 \times 2 \times 2$

[a]In the electromagnetic spectrum, a wavelength of 1 m corresponds to a frequency of 300 MHz and an energy of 1.24×10^{-6} eV

of kinetics. In addition, its signals must penetrate tissue to the depth of the liver in the species of interest (e.g., rat, human), and the modality must be able to detect exogenous substances which are transporter substrates. Ideally the imaging technology, and the substance detected, must also be widely available and of sufficiently low risk to allow studies to be performed in humans. Exogenous imaging substances used at high doses in imaging studies are called contrast media or contrast agents: these have the potential to saturate transporters. Conversely, exogenous imaging substances used in microdoses are called tracers. Many contrast agents and tracers will be discussed below, with priority given to those approved for human use as such approval demonstrates successful preclinical to clinical translatability for hepatobiliary function assessment.

Each modality exploits the different chemistry of the probe substances it detects [14]. Nuclear medicine modalities, i.e., positron emission tomography (PET) and single-photon emission computed tomography (SPECT)/scintigraphy, detect trace (subnanomolar) amounts of a substance radiolabeled with an isotope possessing a particular emission characteristic. SPECT studies detect gamma-emitting isotopes such as technetium-99m ($t_{1/2} = 6$ h) or iodine-123 ($t_{1/2} = 13$ h). PET studies detect positron-emitting isotopes such as carbon-11 ($t_{1/2} = 20$ min) or fluorine-18 ($t_{1/2} = 110$ min). CT and X-radiography can detect high micromolar or millimolar amounts of a heavy atom such as iodine in organoiodine contrast agents. MR can detect high micromolar or millimolar amounts of substances which accelerate the nuclear magnetic relaxation of water protons, such as gadolinium-chelate contrast agents. Fluorescence or optoacoustic imaging detects chromophores that emit visible or near-infrared light when excited by light of a specific wavelength. A final imaging modality, ultrasound, will not be discussed further as, although it is used clinically to evaluate hepatobiliary structures, there are no known chemistries that could generate hepatobiliary tracers suitable for ultrasound studies.

In principle, any adequately nontoxic substance with significant clearance through the liver can be used to measure liver transporter kinetics by imaging, provided that the substance is detectable using one of the imaging modalities in Table 1 and the mechanism of clearance is well understood. Since the 1920s, many tracers and contrast agents (Table 2, Fig. 1) have been developed specifically for medical imaging of the hepatobiliary system [15]. This allowed different medical imaging procedures to be devised, including radiographic visualization of the bile duct (cholangiography) and gall bladder (cholecystography), or visualization of the bile duct by SPECT and scintigraphy (cholescintigraphy) [16]. More recently, contrast agents have been developed for liver imaging via MRI, of which gadoxetate is most notable. Such agents are taken up by normal hepatocytes (but not neoplasms), and appear in the biliary tree. Quantitation of their uptake and biliary excretion provides an assessment of liver function [17, 18], and (through imaging) a functional liver volume. These tracers and contrast agents were optimized iteratively by medicinal chemists. For cholangiography, cholecystography, and cholescintigraphy, the ideal molecule reaches the biliary tree as a bolus requiring both very rapid uptake into the hepatocyte and very rapid elimination from the hepatocyte into the bile. However, for more modern applications such as detecting neoplasms and measuring functional liver volume) the ideal molecule is taken up rapidly into the hepatocyte but is eliminated rather slowly, to allow flexibility in the timing of imaging.

Few of the reported tracers and contrast agents are currently marketed. Others are or were investigational, or were formerly marketed then withdrawn (Table 2). From the perspective of an investigator planning a clinical imaging study on transporter function, a marketed agent is much more appealing than an investigational or withdrawn agent. The former (such as gadoxetate or mebrofenin) can be sourced readily from the pharmacy: ethical review would note off-label use of an approved medicinal product (with due consideration of radiation dose and other potential harms). On the other hand, use of a nonapproved agent (such as gadocoletic acid or arclofenin) would introduce many complications, requiring an IND (investigational new drug) application and establishing production according to Good Manufacturing Practice. It is for this reason that gadoxetate is of particular interest.

Table 2
Imaging tracers and contrast agents which are liver transporter substrates

Modality: Chemical class	Currently used in man	Investigational or formerly used
MRI: Gadolinium chelate	Gadoxetate (Primovist, Eovist) Gadobenate (Multihance)	Gadocoletate
Fluorescence	Indocyanine green Fluorescein	Bromosulfophthalein; tauro-nor-THCA-24-DBD; 5-chloromethylfluorescein diacetate; chloromethylfluorescein; dichlorofluorescein
CT: Triiodophenyl		Bunamiodyl; iobenzamic acid; iocetamic acid; iopanoic acid; ipodic acid; iophenoxic acid; iopronic acid; tyropanote; iosumetic acid; phenobutiodil; RCK-136
CT: Bistriiodophenyl	Iodipamide (Cholografin) Iotroxinate (Biliscopin)	Iodoxamate; ioglycamic acid; iosefamate; iosulamide
SPECT: [99mTc] iminodiacetic acid conjugates	[99mTc]disofenin (Hepatolite) [99mTc]mebrofenin (Choletec)	[99mTc]arclofenin; [99mTc]bultifenin; [99mTc]etifenin; [99mTc]galtifenin; [99mTc]iprofenin; [99mTc] lidofenin
SPECT: Radioiodophenyl		[131I]iodipamide; [123I]iodoxamate; [131I]ipodate; [131I]ioglycamate; [131I]rose bengal
SPECT: [99mTc] pyridoxal derivative	[99mTc]-N-pyridoxyl-5-methyltryptophan	
PET: [11C]-labeled therapeutic drug or metabolite		[11C]dehydropravastatin; [11C]erlotinib; [11C] metformin; [11C]rosuvastatin; [11C]SC-62807; [11C]telmisartan; [11C](15R)-16-m-tolyl-17,18,19,20-tetranorisocarbacyclin methyl ester
PET: [11C]-labeled bile acid derivative		N-[Methyl-11C]cholylsarcosine; N-[methyl-11C] taurocholic acid; N-[methyl-11C]taurolithocholic acid; N-[methyl-11C]tauroursodeoxycholic acid

References are cited in Sect. 2

2.1 Radiography and CT

Radiography and CT have been used clinically to evaluate the hepatobiliary system, employing contrast agents that assess hepatocyte function. The contrast agents for radiography and CT incorporate one or two triiodophenyl moieties, providing respectively three or six heavy atoms (i.e., nonradioactive [127I]) per molecule. Many such agents have been developed and marketed (see Table 2) in multiple jurisdictions, for cholangiography and cholecystography. These include iodipamide [19–21] and iotroxate [22]. These agents are cleared via the biliary system and, although there were early studies of transport of ipodate, iodipamide [23], and bunamiodyl [24],

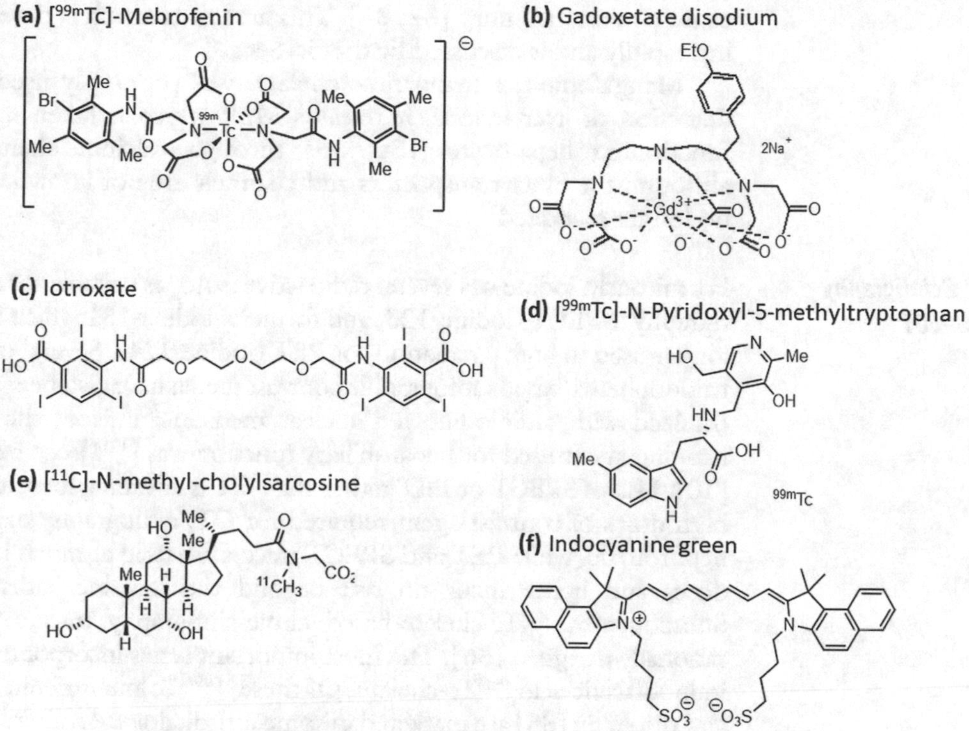

(a) [99mTc]-Mebrofenin

(b) Gadoxetate disodium

(c) Iotroxate

(d) [99mTc]-N-Pyridoxyl-5-methyltryptophan

(e) [11C]-N-methyl-cholylsarcosine

(f) Indocyanine green

Fig. 1 Tracers and contrast agents used for liver transporter assessment in vivo. (**a**) [99mTc]-Mebrofenin (scintigraphy/SPECT). (**b**) Gadoxetate disodium (MRI). (**c**) Iotroxate (radiography/CT). (**d**) [99mTc]-N-Pyridoxyl-5-methyltryptophan (scintigraphy/SPECT). (**e**) [11C]-N-Methyl-cholylsarcosine (PET). (**f**) Indocyanine green (optical)

the clearance of biliary CT agents remains poorly understood [19] and does not yet provide specific information on liver transporters; rather, these tracers are used primarily for gross assessment of the biliary tract. Most have now been withdrawn from the market because of nephrotoxicity or lack of demand. However, iodipamide [25] and iotroxate [26] are still marketed in some jurisdictions.

2.2   MRI

Several gadolinium chelates have been rationally designed for liver MRI. These agents are detected in MRI because they are effective at enhancing the nuclear magnetic relaxation of water protons, i.e., they have high relaxivity.

Gadoxetate [27] and gadobenate [28], which undergo partial hepatocyte-mediated elimination, are approved for use in multiple jurisdictions. Gadoxetate is FDA-approved for detection and characterization of focal liver lesions and exhibits high biliary clearance. Gadoxetate also has affinity for various liver transporters in multiple species (human OATP1B1, OATP1B3, MRP2, and NTCP; rat OATP1a1, Mrp2, Mrp3, and Oatp1A2) [29–32], and has been used preclinically and clinically to investigate liver transporter dysfunction or inhibition that may decrease hepatobiliary function or cause cholestatic injury [32, 33]. This area of research is developing rapidly and is discussed further in Sect. 4.

Mangafodipir, a manganese chelate, was previously used for detection of liver lesions: it releases Mn^{2+} which is taken up by functioning hepatocytes [34, 35] through calcium channels, although the exact transporters and channels are not known. It is no longer marketed.

2.3 Scintigraphy and SPECT

Fortuitously, iodine has several radioactive isotopes suitable for scintigraphy/SPECT (iodine-123, and formerly iodine-131 which is no longer used to high β radiation) or PET (iodine-124). Several of the triiodophenyl-based radiographic contrast media have also been synthesized with radioiodine for nuclear medicine: indeed, the first imaging agent used for hepatobiliary function was [^{131}I]rose bengal [10]. Use of SPECT or PET rather than CT is advantageous, as the high doses of contrast agent required for CT/radiography may be nephrotoxic, while PET and SPECT tracers are used at much lower doses and hence incur no risk beyond the ionizing radiation. Subsequently, [99mTc]-chelate-based cholescintigraphy tracers were rationally designed [36]. The most important series incorporates an iminodiacetic acid [99mTc]-chelate. Of these, [[99mTc]mebrofenin [37] and disofenin [38] are marketed in some jurisdictions. An alternative technetium chelate chemistry uses pyridoxal derivatives [39]: [[99mTc]N-pyridoxyl-5-methyltryptophan ([[99mTc]PMT) [40, 41] is used clinically in Japan. Human hepatic uptake of [[99mTc]PMT is mediated by OATP1B1 and OATP1B3, while its efflux into bile is via MDR1 and MRP2 [42]. [[99mTc]mebrofenin is used in assessment of liver function and functional liver volume before and after surgery and has also been used to investigate hepatobiliary transporter dysfunction in vitro and in vivo [43, 44]. [[99mTc]mebrofenin is almost exclusively taken up into the liver by OATP1B1 and OATP1B3 and is excreted into the bile primarily by MRP2 [44–46].

[[99mTc]sestamibi is marketed in several jurisdictions for assessment of myocardial function, and also has been used in vitro to study basolateral efflux [46]. [[99mTc]sestamibi likely enters hepatocytes passively and undergoes partial fecal clearance, as efflux is modulated by hepatocyte P-gp and the tracer undergoes preferential basolateral efflux into the bile. [[99mTc]galactosyl-human serum albumin is also used in Japan [17, 47] to assess liver function, but is not a known transporter substrate.

Gadolinium has a gamma-emitting isotope (gadolinium-153), so gadolinium-chelates can be detected using scintigraphy/SPECT, although the rather long half-life of this isotope ($t_{1/2} = 270$ d) restricts its use to animal studies [48].

2.4 PET

More recently, specific transporter-targeted positron-emitting tracers have been synthesized and used in animals or man, with particular emphasis on hepatobiliary transporters, although none has yet gained regulatory approval for use as a diagnostic product. Several of these (Table 2) are carbon-11 versions of small molecule drugs or drug metabolites which are known liver transporter substrates (e.g., erlotinib [49]; metformin [50], rosuvastatin [51], dehydropravastatin [52], telmisartan [53], and celecoxib metabolite [54]). ^{11}C-labeled bile acid derivatives have also been synthesised, such as [^{11}C]cholylsarcosine [55–57]; these have been used to investigate the kinetics of hepatobiliary tracer uptake and secretion in healthy pigs and humans in vivo, and to quantify perturbations that occur in patients with cholestasis.

2.5 Fluorescence

Fluorescent tracers offer the ability to image hepatobiliary processes at a cellular resolution and in real time, thereby granting opportunities to gain insights into detailed mechanistic perturbations of drugs on a high throughput level. Therefore they are well suited to in vitro studies of isolated cells or cell aggregates that can be imaged directly, although in general they are not appropriate for in vivo studies of cells within the liver or other internal organs. Methodologically, direct immunofluorescent antibody-based imaging of multiple transporters can answer whether the total amount of protein or localization (e.g., downregulation or receptor internalization) has occurred (e.g., [58, 59]), whereas studies undertaken with fluorescein analogues and fluorescently tagged bile acid derivative probes enable kinetic measures of uptake and efflux transport rates.

Each fluorescent probe has its own characteristic transporter substrate affinity, which may vary depending on the species and complexity of the transport system that is investigated. Cholyl-lysyl-fluorescein (CLF), a bile acid analogue, is a particularly widely used probe, with data that have spanned in vitro and in vivo studies involving both animals and humans. CLF is an OATP1B3, MRP2, and MRP3 substrate [60]. Measurement of drug inhibition of CLF transport has been used to discern cholestatic mechanisms [61, 62], and a positive association has been demonstrated between cholestatic DILI in humans and inhibition of apical CLF efflux from rat hepatocytes in sandwich culture [63]. Moreover, CLF has been shown to have 100% sensitivity when used to detect liver cirrhosis in patient cohorts [64, 65].

Additional fluorescent substrates have also been developed for examining specific uptake and efflux transporter routes. Sodium fluorescein is an OATP1B1, OATP1B3, and MRP2 substrate and has been used effectively in vivo to study impaired hepatic transport in animals [66]. Similarly, a fluorescent bile acid derivative (N-(24-[7-(4-N,N-dimethylaminosulfonyl-2,1,3-benzoxadiazole)]amino-3α,7α,12α-trihydroxy-27-nor-5β-cholestan-26-oyl)-2′-aminoethanesulfonate) may be used to investigate NTCP-mediated uptake in both primary rat and human hepatocyte suspensions, and apical efflux from hepatocytes cultures in sandwich configuration which is presumed to be mediated by BSEP [67]. 5-Chloromethyl-fluorescein diacetate, a fluorescein analog, is an example of a reagent that can freely diffuse into hepatocytes and is then metabolized to glutathione methylfluorescein, a cell-impermeant fluorescent product and Mrp2 substrate [68]. Finally, 5-(and 6)-carboxy-2′,7′-dichlorofluorescein has been used to quantify Mrp2 efflux from primary rat hepatocytes cultured in sandwich configuration, and inhibition of this process by drugs and their metabolites [69]. Interestingly, such reagents can also be used alone or in combination with bright field time course imaging to study the dilation and constriction dynamics of the bile canaliculi, which have recently been shown to be altered by cholestatic drugs [70].

Indocyanine Green (ICG) is transported by OATP1B3 and NTCP [45], and is established for estimating global liver function. Feng et al. [71] demonstrated improved accuracy of predicting 3-month mortality in acute liver failure patients, using a combination of ICG clearance measured with a pulse spectrometer and the model-for-end-stage liver disease (MELD) score, when compared to conventional scores. Subsequently, this result was extrapolated further to develop a human ex vivo model for acetaminophen-induced liver injury, in which ICG clearance was used as the outcome measure [72]. While probes that are more specific for liver transporter dysfunction have been reported, ICG is still used relatively routinely and has been approved for in vivo measurement of human hepatic function [73].

3   Quantitative Analyses of Hepatic Imaging Data

3.1   Absolute Quantification of Hepatocellular Transporter Expression with Dynamic Imaging

Imaging approaches to quantifying transporter expression follow the principles of standard pharmacokinetic measurements [74]. A suitable probe indicator (Sect. 2) is injected into the bloodstream and its concentration "c" in a tissue of interest is measured as a function of time "t" (min). The temporal structure of these concentration-time profiles is then interpreted using kinetic models of the motion of indicator molecules through tissue compartments (blood, interstitium, cells, bile, etc.).

Two different types of parameter can be derived from such dynamic imaging experiments [75, 76]. The distribution volumes "v" (ml/g) measure the space (ml) occupied by the indicator inside the compartments in a unit (g) of tissue (examples are plasma, interstitial, and intracellular distribution volumes). The transfer constants "k" (ml/min/g) measure the indicator flux (mmol/min/g) out of a compartment per unit concentration "c" (mM). For instance, if c_i is the indicator concentration in the interstitium, then the indicator flux from interstitium to intracellular space is $k_{hi}c_i$. Physiologically, k_{hi} is the volume of interstitial fluid (ml) in a unit of tissue (g) that is cleared of indicator in a minute. At the low concentrations that are used in imaging experiments it is assumed that the transfer constants are not concentration-dependent (linearity). Other parameters can be derived from the transfer constants, such as the hepatic extraction fraction (%), i.e., the percentage of indicator molecules that is extracted from the blood stream in one pass through the liver [77].

An accurate measurement requires at least two different concentration-time curves. One is the tissue concentration $c(t)$, which may be measured over the entire liver, an individual lobe, a liver segment, a smaller region within a segment or even a single imaging voxel (=3D pixel). The second curve, the input function, is measured in the arterial or portal venous inlet to the liver. Input functions are required as a reference to eliminate effects of systemic changes in the circulation, or differences in the way the tracer is injected. In measurements that also target perfusion, arterial and portal venous input functions are both required to separate out their individual contributions. In some cases outlet data are needed—in particular for indicators that are excreted from hepatocytes through biliary and interstitial routes.

The technical details of the image acquisition have a strong effect on parameter accuracy, but choosing the right approach involves trade-offs between accuracy, precision, practicality and cost. For instance, at higher sampling rates more rapid processes can be resolved, but this comes at a cost of image resolution and organ coverage. Equivalently, very long data collections (>45 min) are required to characterize slow processes such as biliary excretion, but this has significant implications on patient comfort and scan costs. Another important consideration in the liver is to minimize the effect of breathing motion, which is detrimental to image quality [78]. The best compromise depends critically on the exact purpose of the measurement and requires careful application-specific optimization.

3.2 Semiquantitative Imaging Analysis

Clinical evaluation of gadoxetate-enhanced MRI is based on evaluation of imaging features such as observation size, presence of arterial phase hyper- versus hypo- or iso-enhancement, washout appearance, capsule appearance, and threshold growth [79]. Quantitation of the disposition of the contrast agent can be undertaken by calculation of maximum relative enhancement (RE) when compared with pre-contrast images [29] and measurement of area under the curve (AUC) of the liver enhancement. In addition, curve fitting of the intensity profile in the liver after a bolus injection of contrast agent enables estimation of kinetic parameters which include rate of hepatic wash-in and wash-out, and hepatic extraction fraction [80]. These descriptive analysis techniques can exhibit good signal-to-noise ratio and low variance at individual sites in comparison to the compartmental modeling techniques described in the previous section. However, the results often display a greater dependence on experimental parameters, making comparisons between sites difficult and they lack direct relationship to transporter function that can provide additional and useful insights into pharmacologically and toxicologically relevant effects which otherwise may be difficult to obtain. For example, inhibition of hepatobiliary efflux transporters at the apical plasma membrane domain of hepatocytes membrane may lead to changes in drug exposure in the hepatocyte that have potential toxicological significance, but result only in minor changes in drug plasma exposure [81] (see also next section).

4 Hepatobiliary Transporter Mediated Drug–Drug Interactions

Hepatocytes express a range of transporter proteins mediating either active uptake of drugs/endogenous compounds from the blood (e.g., OATP1B1, which is expressed on the basolateral plasma membrane domain) or their active secretion into the bile (e.g., BCRP, expressed on the apical plasma membrane domain) [82, 83]. Characterization of drug transporters in the liver (also in the intestine, kidney and brain) and their effect on drug pharmacokinetics and drug–drug interaction (DDI) risk is now an integral part of drug development, and is required by regulatory agencies [84–86]. P-gp (MDR1/ABCB1), BCRP, OATP1B1, OATP1B3, OAT1, OAT3, and OCT2 are currently identified as key transporters for screening in drug development, with increased recognition of the clinical relevance of other transporters (e.g., MATE, BSEP, and OATP2B1) [87, 88]. Increasingly, clinical evidence raises concerns about transporter-mediated DDIs, where changes in drug exposure in blood or plasma (commonly used as metric) may not be reflective of the changes in the tissue/cellular drug exposure (local DDI) that may have consequences on drug safety and efficacy. For example, modulation of OCT/MATE transporters has resulted in minimal or no changes in metformin systemic exposure in a number of cases, yet modified glucose lowering effect was reported (which was attributed to modified liver exposure to metformin) [88].

In addition to the important role of transporters, hepatic drug exposure may be influenced by passive diffusion through biological membranes, intracellular binding, metabolism and organelle sequestration (Fig. 2) [82]. In recent years, a range of cellular systems have been used to characterize complex interplay of these processes in vitro. These range from transporter-transfected cell lines to three-dimensional microphysiological systems; although the utility of the latter as a tool for quantitative in vitro metabolism/transporter evaluation and in vitro/in vivo translation is yet to be established [89–91]. Characterization of transporter–metabolism interplay in these holistic in vitro systems is supported by mechanistic modeling of in vitro data, which allows estimation of

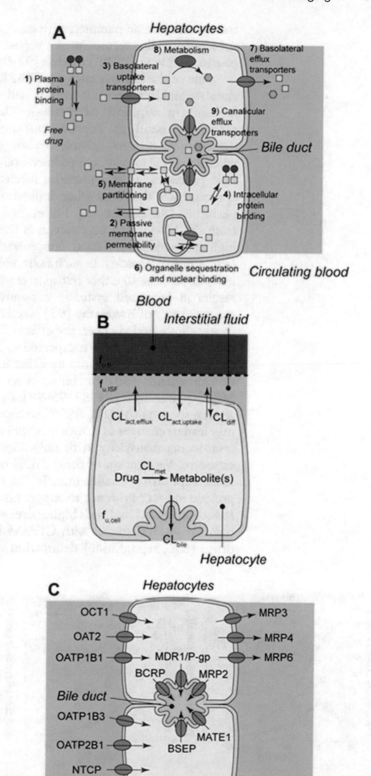

Fig. 2 Processes affecting intracellular drug concentration in the hepatocyte [82]

transporter kinetic parameters (e.g., K_m, V_{max}, and k_i) to be used subsequently for translational purposes in physiologically based pharmacokinetic (PBPK) models [92–94].

One of the key advantages of PBPK modeling is the ability to simulate and interpret concentration-time profiles in the tissues of interest (in addition to plasma). This modeling approach is extremely useful to improve our understanding of the rate-determining process driving hepatic exposure of a drug, i.e., whether this is uptake, efflux/metabolism or a composite of multiple processes. It also provides mechanistic insight into in vivo consequences that arise when individual disposition processes are perturbed [81, 82, 94–97]. For example, active uptake via OATPs from the blood into hepatocytes is the major process leading to high unbound liver–blood concentration ratio of many statins (e.g., simvastatin acid). In such cases, reduced activity in OATP1B1 transporter (due to either transporter inhibition or polymorphism) results in increased systemic exposure of simvastatin acid and increased risk of myopathy [95] (see Fig. 3). For drugs predominantly eliminated via liver, the effect of reduced OATP activity on liver exposure (AUC_{liver}) is expected to be marginal, as this parameter is determined primarily by either metabolic clearance (in case of simvastatin acid) or biliary excretion (BCRP-rosuvastatin, MRP2-pravastatin) [81, 82, 95–98]. In contrast, inhibition of biliary transporters (MRP2, BSEP) or metabolic enzymes (CYP3A4) may lead to changes in drug exposure in the liver and consequently even to hepatotoxicity, with only minor changes in drug plasma exposure. Verification of these PBPK model-predicted changes in tissue exposure is challenging. In the case of statins, clinical data provide indirect evidence to support this, as enhanced cholesterol reduction (associated with higher liver exposure of simvastatin) was reported in DDI studies with CYP3A4 inhibitors [95]. For certain drugs (e.g., repaglinide) delineation of the rate limiting step is

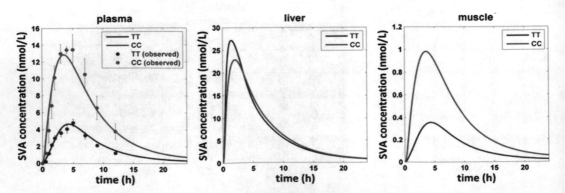

Fig. 3 Simulated concentration-time profiles for simvastatin acid (SVA) in plasma, liver tissue and muscle tissue for individuals with the homozygous wild-type TT (black line) and homozygous variant CC (red line) SLCO1B1 c.521T>C. Full symbols represent observed mean ± SE plasma SVA concentrations for individuals with the TT (black circles) and CC (red circles) genotype [95]

not as straightforward as in the case of simvastatin acid, as hepatic disposition is a composite of multiple contributing processes. Drugs like repaglinide highlight the utility of PBPK modeling to gain mechanistic insight into interplay of processes and prediction of DDI risk [97].

In all the cases above, quantification of drug exposure in the liver (and other tissues) is crucial to support modeling and simulation efforts. Emerging data on tissue concentrations obtained by advanced imaging methods [33, 99], in conjunction with mechanistic PBPK modeling, is envisaged as a powerful tool to improve predictability and understanding of implications of transporter-mediated tissue distribution and interactions.

5   Liver Imaging with Gadoxetate

5.1 Current Clinical Use of Gadoxetate in Liver Disease Diagnosis

The disodium salt of gadoxetic acid (gadoxetate, gadolinium-ethoxybenzyl-diethylenetriaminepentaacetic acid, SH L569 B, Gd-EOB-DTPA) is marketed by Bayer as Primovist® in Europe and Japan and as Eovist® in the USA and has been clinically approved as a liver-specific contrast agent for detection of focal liver lesions by magnetic resonance imaging. Gadoxetate exhibits a favorable safety profile [29, 100–104]. It has been demonstrated that gadoxetate does not trigger nephrogenic systemic fibrosis (NSF), even in the presence of moderate to severe renal impairment [105, 106], as a result of its dual excretion pathway. Recently, trace amounts of gadolinium have been detected in the brain of patients after several injections of the linear gadolinium-containing contrast agents gadodiamide, gadopentetate dimeglumine, gadobenate dimeglumine, and gadoversetamide. For gadoxetate, one report has indicated a correlation between the number of prior gadoxetate administrations and increase signal on nonenhanced T1-weighted images in the dentate nucleus [107], while a second report did not find such a correlation [108]. Currently it is not known whether persistence of gadolinium in the brain following therapeutic administration of contrast agents is associated with adverse health consequences.

Gadoxetate combines the well-established imaging characteristics of extracellular nonspecific gadolinium contrast agents during dynamic phases with further imaging information during the hepatobiliary disposition phase. This enables enhanced detection, classification and characterization of focal liver lesions, as well as improved assessment of liver function in diffuse liver diseases. Gadoxetate-enhanced liver MRI is most commonly used for clinical diagnosis of hepatocellular carcinoma, classification of focal liver lesions and cirrhotic nodules [109], but also is used in a large number of further conditions [110]. The possibility to distinguish between benign and malignant liver tumors, due to differences in accumulation of gadoxetate in hepatocytes, allows imaging based formulation of the therapeutic strategy [110, 111]. For instance, hemangiomas and focal nodular hyperplasia do not require any therapeutic intervention, whereas adenomas possess a risk for malignant transformation, and therefore require treatment [112]. Dynamic hepatocyte contrast enhanced MRI is a valuable tool for the assessment of liver volume and liver functional capacity in patients with primary sclerosing cholangitis [113]. Gadoxetate uptake and enhancement in patients with diffuse chronic liver disease is generally lower than in healthy individuals, due to differences in transporter number or activity. Therefore it allows differentiation between two subgroups of nonalcoholic fatty liver disease, plus between simple steatosis and nonalcoholic steatohepatitis [114]; and also can be used for assessment and staging of fibrosis [76] and cirrhosis [115], as well as in predicting liver transplant graft survival [116]. In addition, gadoxetate enhanced MR imaging together with T2-weighted MR cholangiography may be a useful tool in providing information about the biliary system, like biliary injury, bile duct obstruction, diagnosis of cholecystitis, and differentiation of biliary from extrabiliary lesions [117, 118].

Hepatocellular uptake of gadoxetate from blood is mediated in humans by the sinusoidal solute carriers OATP1B1, OATP1B3, and NTCP [119]. Its active secretion into bile in rats is via the apical transporter Mrp2 [120] and it is presumed that the human ortholog (MRP2) mediates its biliary excretion in humans. The extensive biliary clearance of gadoxetate (healthy human: 50% of administered dose [101]) facilitates its use for evaluation of hepatobiliary transporter inhibition by drugs as a DILI risk factor [32, 33]. This aspect is discussed further in the next section. In addition, gadoxetate-enhanced MRI was successful in prediction of hyperbilirubinemia which occurred during treatment of hepatitis C patients with a triple therapy of simeprevir, pegylated interferon plus ribavirin [121]. Simeprevir is a substrate of the same transporters for hepatic uptake and excretion as gadoxetate [121]. In rats, a transient impairment of bile flow induced with a single dose of estradiol-17β D-glucuronide was associated with a sixfold decrease in gadoxetate elimination rate [122]. Prednisolone, doxorubicin hydrochloride, cisplatin, and propranolol hydrochloride can lead to a slight but significant increase in the hepatic MRI enhancement observed following administration of gadoxetate to rats, most likely due to the longer retention of the contrast agent in hepatocytes because of its competition with these drugs for biliary excretion into the bile duct [123].

5.2 Effects on Gadoxetate Hepatic Clearance of an Investigational Drug Which Cause DILI in Rats

The investigational drug used in these studies [33] is a chemokine receptor antagonist (CKA) whose intended clinical use was in the treatment of systemic inflammatory diseases. Livers from rats dosed orally with the compound for 7 days exhibited dose dependent centrilobular degeneration and necrosis, which was accompanied by neutrophil infiltration and associate sinusoidal congestion. These abnormalities in liver histopathology were accompanied by marked elevations in plasma levels of alanine aminotransferase activity, bilirubin and bile acids, which also exhibited clear dose dependency. In vitro studies revealed that the CKA was a potent inhibitor of human OATP1B1 (IC_{50} <3 μM), plus a less potent inhibitor of both rat Mrp2 (IC_{50} 69 μM) and rat BSEP (IC_{50} 130 μM).

To investigate whether these in vitro findings might have in vivo functional relevance, anaesthetized rats were given either a single dose of gadoxetate alone, or CKA plus gadoxetate, then were evaluated by DCE-MRI [33]. Imaging data are shown in Fig. 4. The data were quantified following development of a nonlinear two-compartment model. This provided a good description of gadoxetate disposition in animals dosed with the contrast agent alone, and yielded a rate constant for its hepatic uptake and Michaelis–Menten constants (K_m and V_{max}) for biliary secretion. Coadministration of the CKA with gadoxetate resulted in marked inhibition of the rate of hepatic uptake of gadoxetate, plus resulted in a reduced V_{max} and increased K_m for biliary gadoxetate excretion. These effects were dose dependent and correlated well with the abnormalities in plasma bilirubin and bile acids observed in rats dosed for multiple days with the CKA.

These findings suggest that gadoxetate DCE-MRI can characterize functional consequences in vivo of compounds that perturb hepatobiliary transporters. Furthermore, since gadoxetate is

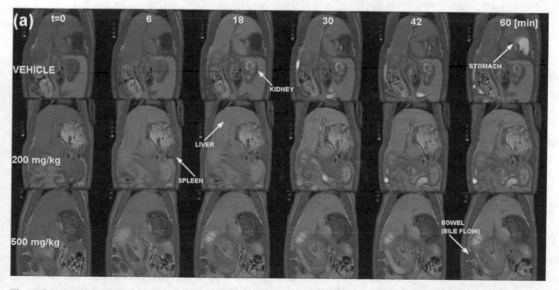

Fig. 4 Examples of dynamic images for animals treated with vehicle (top), 200 mg/kg (middle) or 500 mg/kg (bottom) CKA at t = 0, 6, 18, 30, 42, and 60 min after contrast injection. Note the enhancement of the small bowel lumen at about 30 min after contrast injection and also the reflux of gadoxetate into the stomach at the end of the acquisition in the vehicle treated animal. No enhancement was observed in the bowel of the animal treated with 500 mg/kg CKA. From [33]. Reproduced by permission of John Wiley & Sons

already used clinically to aid the assessment and management of liver disease in patients, this may be a translatable biomarker that can aid human risk assessment of new investigational drugs during clinical trials [33].

6 Future Opportunities and Challenges

Many different imaging methodologies and probe substrates have been used to explore processes in the liver that may be relevant to DILI. These methods could provide important additional tools to detect and investigate DILI, and to gain new insight into underlying mechanisms and susceptibility factors.

An especially promising method is gadoxetate DCE-MRI. This is due to the current widespread use of MRI in human liver disease diagnosis and management, plus the very promising data already obtained in rats dosed with an investigational drug that inhibited several hepatobiliary transporters and caused liver injury [33] (see Sect. 5). Nonetheless, substantial further work is required to develop and validate the use of gadoxetate DCE-MRI for DILI risk assessment in animals, and also as a translational biomarker technology that can be used during clinical trials. It is intended that the necessary additional work will be undertaken as part of the TRISTAN project, which is a large collaborative public-private partnership that is cofunded jointly by the European Union and industry via the Innovative Medicines Initiative [124]. The TRISTAN project will also investigate the potential value of gadoxetate DCE-MRI for the assessment of undesired and clinically important drug–drug interactions that occur via hepatobiliary transporter perturbations (see Sect. 4).

A limitation of gadoxetate DCE-MRI is that, since gadoxetate is not transported by BSEP, it does not enable direct investigation of drug-induced inhibition of BSEP activity, which is considered to play an important role in DILI caused by many drugs [11]. Other probe substrates that are transported by BSEP, and ideally are BSEP-specific, are needed. The chemistries described in Sect. 2 might provide compounds suitable for this purpose. Imaging studies undertaken using a BSEP probe substrate could improve our understanding the in vivo significance of in vitro BSEP inhibition data, and in particular the relationship between BSEP inhibition and DILI.

The present chapter covers hepatobiliary transporter interactions, and their role in DILI and drug–drug interactions. Imaging probes and technologies that evaluate other processes relevant to DILI would be complementary. Processes meriting particular attention include oxidative stress and inflammation, in view of their known role in DILI pathogenesis [1, 9].

Acknowledgment

Preparation of this chapter was funded by the Innovative Medicines Initiative 2 Joint Undertaking, Grant Agreement number 116106-IB4SD-TRISTAN.

References

1. Leise MD, Poterucha JJ, Talwalkar JA (2014) Drug-induced liver injury. Mayo Clinic Proc 89:95–106

2. Regev A (2014) Drug-induced liver injury and drug development: industry perspective. Semin Liver Dis 34:227–239

3. Waring MJ, Arrowsmith J, Leach AR, Leeson PD, Mandrell S, Owen RM, Pairaudeau G, Pennie WD, Pickett SD, Wang J, Wallace O, Weir A (2015) An analysis of the attrition of drug candidates from four major pharmaceutical companies. Nat Rev Drug Discov 14:475–486

4. Chen M, Vijay V, Shi Q, Liu Z, Fang H, Tong W (2011) FDA-approved drug labeling for the study of drug-induced liver injury. Drug Discov Today 16:697–703

5. Onakpoya IJ, Heneghan CJ, Aronson JK (2016) Post-marketing withdrawal of 462 medicinal products because of adverse drug reactions: a systematic review of the world literature. BMC Med 14:10. https://doi.org/10.1186/s12916-016-0553-2

6. Thompson RA, Isin EM, Li Y, Weaver R, Weidolf L, Wilson I, Claesson A, Page K, Dolgos H, Kenna JG (2011) Risk assessment and mitigation strategies for reactive metabolites in drug discovery and development. Chem Biol Interact 192:65–71

7. Thompson RA, Isin EM, Li Y, Weidolf L, Page K, Wilson I, Swallow S, Middleton B, Stahl S, Foster AJ, Dolgos H, Weaver R, Kenna JG (2012) In vitro approach to assess the potential for risk of idiosyncratic adverse reactions caused by candidate drugs. Chem Res Toxicol 25:1616–1632

8. Aleo MD, Luo Y, Swiss R, Bonin PD, Potter DM, Will Y (2014) Human drug-induced liver injury severity is highly associated with dual inhibition of liver mitochondrial function and bile salt export pump. Hepatology 60:1015–1022

9. Ju C, Reilly T (2012) Role of immune reactions in drug-induced liver injury (DILI). Drug Metab Rev 44:107–115

10. Taplin GV, Meredith OM Jr, Kade H (1955) The radioactive (I^{131} tagged) rose bengal uptake-excretion test for liver function using external gamma-ray scintillation counting techniques. J Lab Clin Med 45:665–678

11. Kenna JG (2014) Current concepts in drug-induced bile salt export pump (BSEP) interference. Curr Protoc Toxicol 61:23.7.1–23.715

12. Chen R, Wang J, Tang S, Zhang Y, Lv X, Wu S, Yang Z, Xia Y, Chen D, Zhan S (2016) Role of polymorphic bile salt export pump (BSEP, ABCB11) transporters in anti-tuberculosis drug-induced liver injury in a Chinese cohort. Sci Rep 6:27750. https://doi.org/10.1038/srep27750

13. Flower MA (2012) Webb's physics of medical imaging, 2nd edn. CRC, UK. ISBN: 9780750305730

14. Waterton JC (2011) Medical imaging: overview and the importance of contrast. In: Braddock M (ed) biomedical imaging: the chemistry of labels, probes and contrast agents. RSC Press, Cambridge, UK. ISBN: 978-1-84973-014-3, pp 1–20. https://doi.org/10.1039/9781849732918-00001

15. Freeman LM, Lan JA (1990) Radiopharmaceutical evaluation of the hepatobiliary pathway. Int J Rad Appl Instrum B 17:129–139

16. Ziessman HA (2014) Hepatobiliary scintigraphy in 2014. J Nucl Med 55:967–975

17. Geisel D, Lüdemann L, Hamm B, Denecke T (2015) Imaging-based liver function tests—past, present and future. Fortschr Röntgenstr 187:863–871

18. Hoekstra LT, de Graaf W, Nibourg GA, Heger M, Bennink RJ, Stieger B, van Gulik TM (2014) Physiological and biochemical basis of clinical liver function tests: a review. Ann Surg 257(1):27–36

19. Yeh BM, Liu PS, Soto JA, Corvera CA, Hussain HK (2009) MR imaging and CT of the biliary tract. Radiographics 29:1669–1688

20. Miller GA, Yeh BM, Breiman RS, Roberts JP, Qayyum A, Coakley FV (2004) Use of CT cholangiography to evaluate the biliary tract after liver transplantation: initial experience. Liver Transpl 10:1065–1070

21. Stockberger SM, Sherman S, Kopecky KK (1996) Helical CT cholangiography. Abdom Imaging 21:98–104

22. Cabada Giadás T, Sarría Octavio de Toledo L, Martínez-Berganza Asensio MT, Cozcolluela Cabrejas R, Alberdi Ibáñez I, Alvarez López A, García-Asensio S (2002) Helical CT cholangiography in the evaluation of the biliary tract: application to the diagnosis of choledocholithiasis. Abdom Imaging 27:61–70

23. Frimmer M, Giessen FRG (1988) The transport of bile acids in liver cells. Biochim Biophys Acta 947:75–99

24. Hargreaves T, Lathe GH (1963) Inhibitory aspects of bile secretion. Nature 200:1172–1176

25. FDA (2015) NDA 09-321; Cholografin® Meglumine (Iodipamide Meglumine Injection USP 52%). http://www.accessdata.fda.gov/drugsatfda_docs/label/2015/009321s028lbl.pdf. Accessed 4 April 2017

26. Bayer (2007) Product information Biliscopin® for infusion. http://www.bayerresources.com.au/resources/uploads/PI/file9317.pdf. Accessed 4 April 2017

27. MHRA (2016) Summary of product characteristics: Primovist 0.25 mmol/ml, solution for injection, prefilled syringe https://www.medicines.org.uk/emc/medicine/15927. Accessed 4 April 2017

28. FDA (2013) Highlights of prescribing information MultiHance (gadobenate dimeglumine) injection. https://www.accessdata.fda.gov/drugsatfda_docs/label/2013/02135 7s013,021358s012lbl.pdf. Accessed 4 April 2017

29. Hamm B, Staks T, Muhler A, Bollow M, Taupitz M, Frenzel T, Wolf KJ, Weinmann HJ, Lange L (1995) Phase I clinical evaluation of Gd-EOB-DTPA as a hepatobiliary MR contrast agent: safety, pharmacokinetics, and MR imaging. Radiology 195:785–792

30. Nassif A, Jia J, Keiser M, Oswald S, Modess C, Nagel S, Weitschies W, Hosten N, Siegmund W, Kühn JP (2012) Visualization of hepatic uptake transporter function in healthy subjects by using gadoxetic acid-enhanced MR imaging. Radiology 264:741–750

31. Jia J, Puls D, Oswald S, Jedlitschky G, Kühn JP, Weitschies W, Hosten N, Siegmund W, Keiser M (2014) Characterization of the intestinal and hepatic uptake/efflux transport of the magnetic resonance imaging contrast agent gadolinium-ethoxylbenzyl-diethylenetriamine-pentaacetic acid. Investig Radiol 49(2):78–86

32. Georgiou L, Penny J, Nicholls G, Woodhouse N, Blé F-X, Hubbard Cristinacce PL, Naish JH (2017) Quantitative assessment of liver function using Gadoxetate-enhanced magnetic resonance imaging: monitoring transporter-mediated processes in healthy volunteers. Investig Radiol 52:111–119

33. Ulloa JL, Stahl S, Yates J, Woodhouse N, Kenna JG, Jones HB, Waterton JC, Hockings PD (2013) Assessment of gadoxetate DCE-MRI as a biomarker of hepatobiliary transporter inhibition. NMR Biomed 26:1258–1270

34. Gallez B, Bacic G, Swartz HM (1996) Evidence for the dissociation of the hepatobiliary MRI contrast agent Mn-DPDP. Magn Reson Med 35:14–19

35. Gallez B, Baudelet C, Adline J et al (1996) The uptake of Mn-DPDP by hepatocytes is not mediated by the facilitated transport of pyridoxine. Magn Reson Imaging 14:1191–1195

36. Nunn AD, Loberg MD (1981) Hepatobiliary agents. In: Spencer RD (ed) Radiopharmaceuticals: structure activity relationships. Grune & Stratton, New York

37. Bracco (2014) Choletec® kit for the preparation of technetium Tc 99m mebrofenin. http://imaging.bracco.com/sites/braccoimaging.com/files/technica_sheet_pdf/Choletec Prescribing Information.pdf. Accessed 4 April 2017

38. Pharmalucence (2008) Hepatolite® kit for the preparation of technetium Tc99m disofenin for injection. http://www.pharmalucence.com/images/HepatoliteInsert.pdf. Accessed 4 April 2017

39. Baker RJ, Bellen JC, Ronai PM (1975) Technetium 99m-pyridoxylideneglutamate: a new hepatobiliary radiopharmaceutical. I. Experimental aspects. J Nucl Med 16:720–727

40. Kato-Azuma M (1982) Tc-99m(Sn)-N-Pyridoxylaminates: a new series of hepatobiliary imaging agents. J Nucl Med 23:517–552

41. Fritzberg AR, Bloedow DC, Estima D, Johnson DL (1984) Comparison of 99mTc-N-pyridoxyl-5-methyltryptophan and 99mTc-N-3(-bromo-2,4,6-trimethylacetanilide)-iminodiacetate as hepatobiliary radiopharmaceuticals. J Pharm Sci 73:1861–1863

42. Kobayashi M, Nakanishi T, Nishi K, Higaki Y, Okudaira H, Ono M, Tsujiuchi T, Mizutani A, Nishii R, Tamai I, Arano Y, Kawai K (2014) Transport mechanisms of hepatic uptake and bile excretion in clinical hepatobiliary scintigraphy with 99mTc-N-pyridoxyl-5-methyltryptophan. Nucl Med Biol 41:338–342. https://doi.org/10.1016/j.nucmedbio.2014.01.004

43. Ghibellini G, Leslie EM, Pollack GM, Brouwer KL (2008) Use of tc-99m mebrofenin as a clinical probe to assess altered hepatobiliary transport: integration of in vitro, pharmacokinetic modeling, and simulation studies. Pharm Res 25:1851–1860

44. Neyt S, Huisman MT, Vanhove C, De Man H, Vliegen M, Moerman L, Dumolyn C, Mannens G, De Vos F (2013) In vivo visualization and quantification of (disturbed) Oatp-mediated hepatic uptake and Mrp2-mediated biliary excretion of 99mTc-mebrofenin in mice. J Nucl Med 54:624–630

45. de Graaf W, Häusler S, Heger M, van Ginhoven TM, van Cappellen G, Bennink RJ, Kullak-Ublick GA, Hesselmann R, van Gulik TM, Stieger B (2011) Transporters involved in the hepatic uptake of (99m)Tc-mebrofenin and indocyanine green. J Hepatol 54:738–745

46. Swift B, Yue W, Brouwer KL (2010) Evaluation of (99m)technetium-mebrofenin and (99m)technetium-sestamibi as specific probes for hepatic transport protein function in rat and human hepatocytes. Pharm Res 27:1987–1998

47. Satoh K, Yamamoto Y, Nishiyama Y, Wakabayashi H, Ohkawa M (2003) 99mTc-GSA liver dynamic SPECT for the preoperative assessment of hepatectomy. Ann Nucl Med 17:61–67

48. Wadas TJ, Sherman CD, Miner JH, Duncan JR, Anderson CJ (2010) The biodistribution of [153Gd]Gd-labeled magnetic resonance contrast agents in a transgenic mouse model of renal failure differs greatly from control mice. Magn Reson Med 64(5):1274–1280

49. Traxl A, Wanck T, Mairinger S, Stanek J, Filip T, Sauberer M, Müller M, Kuntner C, Langer O (2015) Breast cancer resistance protein and P-glycoprotein influence in vivo disposition of 11C-Erlotinib. J Nucl Med 56:1930–1936. https://doi.org/10.2967/jnumed.115.161273

50. Hume WE, Shingaki T, Takashima T, Hashizume Y, Okauchi T, Katayama Y, Hayashinaka E, Wada Y, Kusuhara H, Sugiyama Y, Watanabe Y (2013) The synthesis and biodistribution of [11C]metformin as a PET probe to study hepatobiliary transport mediated by the multi-drug and toxin extrusion transporter 1 (MATE1) in vivo. Bioorg Med Chem 21:7584–7590

51. He J, Yu Y, Prasad B, Link J, Miyaoka RS, Chen X, Unadkat JD (2014) PET imaging of Oatp-mediated hepatobiliary transport of [11C]rosuvastatin in the rat. Mol Pharmacol 11:2745–2754. https://doi.org/10.1021/mp500027c.

52. Shingaki T, Takashima T, Ijuin R, Zhang X, Onoue T, Katayama Y, Okauchi T, Hayashinaka E, Cui Y, Wada Y, Suzuki M, Maeda K, Kusuhara H, Sugiyama Y, Watanabe Y (2013) Evaluation of Oatp and Mrp2 activities in Hepatobiliary excretion using newly developed positron emission tomography tracer [11C]dehydropravastatin in rats. J Pharmacol Exp Ther 347:193–202

53. Takashima T, Hashizume Y, Katayama Y, Murai M, Wada Y, Maeda K, Sugiyama Y, Watanabe Y (2011) The involvement of organic anion transporting polypeptide in the hepatic uptake of telmisartan in rats: PET studies with [11C]telmisartan. Mol Pharmacol 8:1789–1798

54. Takashima-Hirano M, Takashima T, Katayama Y, Wada Y, Sugiyama Y, Watanabe Y, Doi H, Suzuki M (2011) Efficient sequential synthesis of PET probes of the COX-2 inhibitor [11C]celecoxib and its major metabolite [11C]SC-62807 and in vivo PET evaluation. Bioorg Med Chem 19:2997–3004

55. Takashima T, Wu C, Takashima-Hirano M, Katayama Y, Wada Y, Suzuki M, Kusuhara H, Sugiyama Y, Watanabe Y (2013) Evaluation of breast cancer resistance protein function in hepatobiliary and renal excretion using PET with 11C-SC-62807. J Nucl Med 54:267

56. Sørensen M, Munk OL, Ørntoft NW, Frisch K, Andersen KJ, Mortensen FV, Alstrup AK, Ott P, Hofmann AF, Keiding S (2016) Hepatobiliary secretion kinetics of conjugated bile acids measured in pigs by 11C-cholylsarcosine PET. J Nucl Med 57:961–966

57. Ørntoft NW, Munk OL, Frisch K, Ott P, Keiding S, Sørensen M (2017) Hepatobiliary transport kinetics of the conjugated bile acid tracer 11C-CSar quantified in healthy humans and patients by positron emission tomography (PET). J Hepatol S0168-8278(17):30120–30124

58. Zinchunk V, Zinchuk O, Okada T (2005) Experimental LPS-induced cholestasis alters subcellular distribution and affects colocalization of Mrp2 and Bsep proteins: a quantitative colocalization study. Microsc Res Tech 67:65–70

59. Hammad S, Hoehme S, Friebel A, von Recklinghausen I, Othman A, Begher-Tibbe B, Reif R, Godoy P, Johann T, Vartak A, Golka K, Bucur PO, Vibert E, Marchan R, Christ B, Dooley S, Meyer C, Ilkavets I, Dahmen U, Dirsch O, Böttger J, Gebhardt R, Drasdo D, Hengstler JG (2014) Protocols for staining of bile canalicular and sinusoidal networks of human, mouse and pig livers, three-dimensional reconstruction and

quantification of tissue microarchitecture by image processing and analysis. Arch Toxicol 88:1161–1183

60. de Waart DR, Häusler S, Vlaming ML, Kunne C, Hänggi E, Gruss HJ, Oude Elferink RP, Stieger B (2010) Hepatic transport mechanisms of cholyl-L-lysyl-fluorescein. J Pharmacol Exp Ther 334:78–86

61. Milkiewicz P, Mils CO, Huscher SG, Cardenas R, Cardenas T, Williams A, Elias E (2001) Visualization of the transport of primary and secondary bile acids across liver tissue in rats: in vivo study with fluorescent bile acids. J Hepatol 34:4–10

62. Milkiewicz P, Roma MG, Elias E, Coleman R (2002) Hepatoprotection with tauroursodeoxycholate and beta muricholate against taurolithocholate induced cholestasis: involvement of signal transduction pathways. Gut 51:113–119

63. Barber JA, Stahl SH, Summers C, Barrett G, Park BK, Foster JR, Kenna JG (2015) Quantification of drug-induced inhibition of canalicular cholyl-l-lysyl-fluorescein excretion from hepatocytes by high content cell imaging. Toxicol Sci 148(1):48–59

64. Milkiewicz P, Saksena S, Cardenas T, Mills CO, Elias E (2000) Plasma elimination of cholyl-lysyl-fluorescein (CLF): a pilot study in patients with liver cirrhosis. Liver 20:330–334

65. Ryan JC, Dunn KW, Decker BS (2014) Effects of chronic kidney disease on liver transport: quantitative intravital microscopy of fluorescein transport in the rat liver. Am J Physiol Regul Integr Comp Physiol 307:R1488–R1492

66. De Bruyn T, Fattah S, Stieger B, Augustijns P, Annaert P (2011) Sodium fluorescein is a probe substrate for hepatic drug transport mediated by OATP1B1 and OATP1B3. J Pharm Sci 100:5018–5032

67. De Bruyn T, Sempels W, Snoeys J, Holmstock N, Chatterjee S, Stieger B, Augustijns P, Hofkens J, Mizuno H, Annaert P (2014) Confocal imaging with a fluorescent bile acid analogue closely mimicking hepatic taurocholate disposition. J Pharm Sci 103:1872–1881

68. Reif R, Karlsson J, Günther G, Beattie L, Wrangborg D, Hammad S, Begher-Tibbe B, Vartak A, Melega S, Kaye PM, Hengstler JG, Jirstrand M (2015) Bile canalicular dynamics in hepatocyte sandwich cultures. Arch Toxicol 89:1861–1870

69. Nakanishi T, Ikenaga M, Fukuda H, Matsunaga N, Tamai I (2012) Application of quantitative time-lapse imaging (QTLI) for evaluation of Mrp2-based drug-drug inter-

action induced by liver metabolites. Toxicol Appl Pharmacol 263:244–250

70. Burbank MG, Burban A, Sharanek A, Weaver RJ, Guguen-Guillouzo C, Guillouzo A (2016) Early alterations of bile canaliculi dynamics and the rho kinase/myosin light chain kinase pathway are characteristics of drug-induced intrahepatic cholestasis. Drug Metabol Dispos 44:1780–1793

71. Feng HL, Li Q, Wang L, Yuan GY, Cao WK (2014) Indocyanine green clearance test combined with MELD score in predicting the short-term prognosis of patients with acute liver failure. Hepatobiliary Pancreat Dis Int 13:271–275

72. Schreiter T, Sowa JP, Schlattjan M, Treckmann J, Andreas P, Strucksberg KH, Baba HA, Odenthal M, Gieseler RK, Gerken G, Arteel GE, Canbay A (2016) Human ex-vivo liver model for acetaminophen-induced liver damage. Sci Rep 23(6):1–10

73. https://www.accessdata.fda.gov/drug-satfda_docs/label/2006/011525s017lbl.pdf

74. Ingrisch M, Sourbron S (2013) Tracer-kinetic modeling of dynamic contrast-enhanced MRI and CT: a primer. J Pharmacokinet Pharmacodyn 40:281–300

75. Giraudeau C, Leporq B, Doblas S, Lagadec M, Pastor CM, Daire J-L, Van Beers BE (2017) Gadoxetate-enhanced MR imaging and compartmental modelling to assess hepatocyte bidirectional transport function in rats with advanced liver fibrosis. Eur Radiol 27:1804–1811

76. Juluru K, Talal AH, Yantiss RK, Spincemaille P, Weidman EK, Giambrone AE, Jalili S, Sourbron SP, Dyke JP (2017) Diagnostic accuracy of intracellular uptake rates calculated using dynamic Gd-EOB-DTPA-enhanced MRI for hepatic fibrosis stage. J Magn Reson Imaging 45:1177–1185

77. Lagadec M, Doblas S, Giraudeau C, Ronot M, Lambert SA, Fasseu M, Paradis V, Moreau R, Pastor CM, Vilgrain V, Daire JL, Van Beers BE (2015) Advanced fibrosis: correlation between pharmacokinetic parameters at dynamic gadoxetate-enhanced MR imaging and hepatocyte organic anion transporter expression in rat liver. Radiology 274:379–386

78. Sourbron S, Sommer WH, Reiser MF, Zech CJ (2012) Combined quantification of liver perfusion and function with dynamic Gadoxetic acid-enhanced MR imaging. Radiology 263:874–883

79. Liver Imaging Reporting and Data System (LI-RADS). American College of Radiology website. www.acr.org/Quality-Safety/

Resources/LIRADS. Accessed 1 April 2013. http://www.ajronline.org/doi/full/10.2214/AJR.12.9491

80. Tamada T, Ito K, Higaki A, Yoshida K, Kanki A, Sato T, Higashi H, Sone T (2011) Gd-EOB-DTPA-enhanced MR imaging: evaluation of hepatic enhancement effects in normal and cirrhotic livers. Eur J Radiol 80(3):e311–e316

81. Watanabe T, Kusuhara H, Maeda K, Shitara Y, Sugiyama Y (2009) Physiologically based pharmacokinetic modeling to predict transporter-mediated clearance and distribution of pravastatin in humans. J Pharmacol Exp Ther 328:652–662

82. Chu X, Korzekwa K, Elsby R, Fenner K, Galetin A, Lai Y, Matsson P, Moss A, Nagar S, Rosania GR, Bai JP, Polli JW, Sugiyama Y, Brouwer KL, International Transporter Consortium (2013) Intracellular drug concentrations and transporters: measurement, modeling and implications in the liver. Clin Pharmacol Ther 94:126–141

83. International Transporter Consortium, Giacomini KM, Huang SM, Tweedie DJ, Benet LZ, Brouwer KL, Chu X, Dahlin A, Evers R, Fischer V, Hillgren KM, Hoffmaster KA, Ishikawa T, Keppler D, Kim RB, Lee CA, Niemi M, Polli JW, Sugiyama Y, Swaan PW, Ware JA, Wright SH, Yee SW, Zamek-Gliszczynski MJ, Zhang L (2010) Membrane transporters in drug development. Nat Rev Drug Discov 9:215–236

84. FDA (2012) FDA Guidance for industry 2012, drug interaction studies—study design, data analysis, implications for dosing, and labeling recommendations. https://www.fda.gov/downloads/Drugs/Guidances/ucm292362.pdf

85. Zamek-Gliszczynski MJ, Chu X, Polli JW, Paine MF, Galetin A (2014) Understanding the transport properties of metabolites: case studies and considerations for drug development. Drug Metab Dispos 42:650–664

86. European Medicines Agency (2012) Guideline on the investigation of drug interactions. EMA website [online]: http://www.ema.europa.eu

87. Zamek-Gliszczynski MJ, Hoffmaster KA, Tweedie DJ, Giacomini KM, Hillgren KM (2012) Highlights from the international transporter consortium second workshop. Clin Pharmacol Ther 92:553–556

88. Hibma JE, Zur AA, Castro RA, Wittwer MB, Keizer RJ, Yee SW, Goswami S, Stocker SL, Zhang X, Huang Y, Brett CM, Savic RM, Giacomini KM (2016) The effect of famotidine, a MATE1-selective inhibitor, on the pharmacokinetics and pharmacodynamics of metformin. Clin Pharmacokinet 55:711–721

89. Brouwer KL, Keppler D, Hoffmaster KA, Bow DA, Cheng Y, Lai Y, Palm JE, Stieger B, Evers R, International Transporter Consortium (2013) In vitro methods to support transporter evaluation in drug discovery and development. Clin Pharmacol Ther 94:95–112

90. Vivares A, Salle-Lefort S, Arabeyre-Fabre C, Ngo R, Penarier G, Bremond M, Moliner P, Gallas JF, Fabre G, Klieber S (2015) Morphological behaviour and metabolic capacity of cryopreserved human primary hepatocytes cultivated in a perfused multiwell device. Xenobiotica 45:29–44

91. Galetin A (2014) Rationalizing underprediction of drug clearance from enzyme and transporter kinetic data: from in vitro tools to mechanistic modeling. Methods Mol Biol 1113:255–288

92. Ménochet K, Kenworthy KE, Houston JB, Galetin A (2012) Use of mechanistic modelling to assess inter-individual variability and inter-species differences in active uptake in human and rat hepatocytes. Drug Metab Dispos 40:1744–1756

93. Zamek-Gliszczynski MJ, Lee CA, Poirier A, Bentz J, Chu X, Ellens H, Ishikawa T, Jamei M, Kalvass JC, Nagar S, Pang KS, Korzekwa K, Swaan PW, Taub ME, Zhao P, Galetin A, International Transporter Consortium (2013) ITC recommendations on transporter kinetic parameter estimation and translational Modeling of transport-mediated PK and DDIs in humans. Clin Pharmacol Ther 94:64–79

94. Jones HM, Barton HA, Lai Y, Bi YA, Kimoto E, Kempshall S, Tate SC, El-Kattan A, Houston JB, Galetin A, Fenner KS (2012) Mechanistic pharmacokinetic modeling for the prediction of transporter-mediated disposition in humans from sandwich culture human hepatocyte data. Drug Metab Dispos 40:1007–1017

95. Tsamandouras N, Dickinson G, Guo Y, Hall S, Rostami-Hodjegan A, Galetin A, Aarons L (2015) Development and application of a mechanistic pharmacokinetic model for simvastatin and its active metabolite simvastatin acid using an integrated population PBPK approach. Pharm Res 32:1864–1883

96. Gertz M, Cartwright CM, Hobbs MJ, Kenworthy KE, Rowland M, Houston JB, Galetin A (2013) Cyclosporine inhibition of hepatic and intestinal CYP3A4, uptake and efflux transporters: application of PBPK modeling in the assessment of

drug-drug interaction potential. Pharm Res 30:761–780

97. Gertz M, Tsamandouras N, Säll C, Houston JB, Galetin A (2014) Reduced physiologically-based pharmacokinetic model of repaglinide: impact of OATP1B1 and CYP2C8 genotype and source of in vitro data on the prediction of drug-drug interaction risk. Pharm Res 31:2367–2382

98. Jones HM, Chen Y, Gibson C, Heimbach T, Parrott N, Peters SA, Snoeys J, Upreti VV, Zheng M, Hall SD (2015) Physiologically based pharmacokinetic modeling in drug discovery and development: a pharmaceutical industry perspective. Clin Pharmacol Ther 97:247–262

99. Takashima T, Kitamura S, Wada Y, Tanaka M, Shigihara Y, Ishii H, Ijuin R, Shiomi S, Nakae T, Watanabe Y, Cui Y, Doi H, Suzuki M, Maeda K, Kusuhara H, Sugiyama Y, Watanabe Y (2012) PET imaging-based evaluation of hepatobiliary transport in humans with (15R)-11C-TIC-Me. J Nucl Med 53:741–748

100. Döhr O, Hofmeister R, Treher M, Schweinfurth H (2007) Preclinical safety evaluation of Gd-EOB-DTPA (Primovist). Investig Radiol 42:830–841

101. Reimer P, Rummeny EJ, Shamsi K, Balzer T, Daldrup HE, Tombach B, Hesse T, Berns T, Peters PE (1996) Phase II clinical evaluation of Gd-EOB-DTPA: dose, safety aspects, and pulse sequence. Radiology 199:177–183

102. Breuer J, Balzer T, Shamsi K, Carter R (2003) Clinical safety experience from phase II and III studies of Gd-EOB-DTPA: a new liver-specific MR contrast agent. Europ Radiol 13(Suppl 2):S109. Abstract No 7.05

103. Bluemke DA, Sahani D, Amendola M, Balzer T, Breuer J, Brown JJ, Casalino DD, Davis PL, Francis IR, Krinsky G, Lee FT Jr, Lu D, Paulson EK, Schwartz LH, Siegelman ES, Small WC, Weber TM, Welber A, Shamsi K (2005) Efficacy and safety of MR imaging with liver-specific contrast agent: U.S. multicenter phase III study. Radiology 237:89–98

104. Endrikat J, Kim SY, Sakaguchi T, Dohanish S, Breuer J (2016) Safety of gadoxetate disodium: results from six clinical phase IV studies in 8194 patients. Acta Radiol 57:1326–1333

105. Hope TA, Doherty A, Fu Y, Aslam R, Qayyum A, Brasch RC (2012) Gadolinium accumulation and fibrosis in the liver after administration of gadoxetate disodium in a rat model of active hepatic fibrosis. Radiology 264:423–427

106. Lauenstein T, Ramirez-Garrido F, Kim YH, Rha SE, Ricke J, Phongkitkarun S, Boettcher J, Gupta RT, Korpraphong P, Tanomkiat W, Furtner J, Liu PS, Henry M, Endrikat J (2015) Nephrogenic systemic fibrosis risk after liver magnetic resonance imaging with gadoxetate disodium in patients with moderate to severe renal impairment: results of a prospective, open-label, multicenter study. Investig Radiol 50:416–422

107. Kahn J, Posch H, Steffen IG, Geisel D, Bauknecht C, Liebig T, Denecke T (2017) Is there long-term signal intensity increase in the central nervous system on T1-weighted images after MR imaging with the hepatospecific contrast agent Gadoxetic acid? A cross-sectional study in 91 patients. Radiology 282:708–716

108. Ichikawa S, Motosugi U, Omiya Y, Onishi H (2017) Contrast agent-induced high signal intensity in dentate nucleus on unenhanced T1-weighted images: comparison of gadodiamide and gadoxetic acid. Invest Radiol 52(7):389–395. https://doi.org/10.1097/RLI.0000000000000360. [Epub ahead of print]

109. Neri E, Bali MA, Ba-Ssalamah A, Boraschi P, Brancatelli G, Caseiro Alves F, Grazioli L, Helmberger T, Lee JM, Manfredi R, Martì-Bonmatì L, Matos C, Merkle EL, Op De Beeck B, Schima W, Skehan S, Vilgrain V, Zech C, Bartolozzi C (2016) ESGAR consensus statement on liver MR imaging and clinical use of liver-specific contrast agents. Eur Radiol 26:921–931

110. Channual S, Pahwa A, DS L, Raman SS (2016) Enhancements in hepatobiliary imaging: the spectrum of gadolinium-ethoxybenzyl diethylenetriaminepentaacetic acid usages in hepatobiliary magnetic resonance imaging. Abdom Radiol 41:1825–1841

111. Suh CH, Kim KW, Kim GY, Shin YM, Kim PN, Park SH (2015) The diagnostic value of Gd-EOB-DTPA-MRI for the diagnosis of focal nodular hyperplasia: a systematic review and meta-analysis. Eur Radiol 25:950–960

112. Doyle M, Bagia JS, Yeo J, Teixeira-Pinto A, Tran S (2016) Differentiation of hepatic adenoma from focal nodular hyperplasia with primovist MRI: validation of diagnostic criteria. HPB 18:e730. https://doi.org/10.1016/j.hpb.2016.01.183

113. Nilsson H, Blomqvist L, Douglas L, Nordell A, Jacobsson H, Hagen K, Bergquist A, Jonas E (2014) Dynamic gadoxetate-enhanced MRI for the assessment of total and segmental liver function and volume in primary sclerosing cholangitis. J Magn Reson Imaging 39:879–886

114. Ba-Ssalamah A, Bastati N, Wibmer A, Fragner R, Hodge JC, Trauner M, Herold CJ, Bashir MR, Van Beers BE (2017) Hepatic gadoxetic

acid uptake as a measure of diffuse liver disease: where are we? J Magn Reson Imaging 45:646–659

115. Takeyama Y, Tsuchiya N, Kunimoto H, Fukunaga A, Sakurai K, Hirano G, Yokoyama K, Morihara D, Anan A, Irie M, Shakado S, Sohda T, Sakisaka S (2015) Gadolinium-ethoxybenzyl-diethylenetriamine pentaacetic acid-enhanced magnetic resonance imaging as a useful detection method for advanced primary biliary cirrhosis. Hepatol Res 45:E108–E114

116. Bastati N, Wibmer A, Tamandl D, Einspieler H, Hodge JC, Poetter-Lang S, Rockenschaub S, Berlakovich GA, Trauner M, Herold C, Ba-Ssalamah A (2016) Assessment of orthotopic liver transplant graft survival on gadoxetic acid-enhanced magnetic resonance imaging using qualitative and quantitative parameters. Investig Radiol 51:728–734

117. Lee NK, Kim S, Lee JW, Lee SH, Kang DH, Kim GH, Seo HI (2009) Biliary MR imaging with Gd-EOB-DTPA and its clinical applications. Radiographics 29:1707–1724

118. Blair P, Low G (2014) Biliary anastomotic leakage following orthotopic liver transplant: the use of primovist (gadoxetate disodium) as an intravenous MR cholangiography contrast agent for biliary leakage. J Clin Imaging Sci 4:75

119. Leonhardt M, Keiser M, Oswald S, Kühn J, Jia J, Grube M, Kroemer HK, Siegmund W, Weitschies W (2010) Hepatic uptake of the magnetic resonance imaging contrast agent Gd-EOB-DTPA: role of human organic anion transporters. Drug Metab Dispos 38:1024–1028

120. Saito S, Obata A, Kashiwagi Y, Abe K, Murase K (2013) Dynamic contrast-enhanced MRI of the liver in Mrp2-deficient rats using the hepatobiliary contrast agent Gd-EOB-DTPA. Investig Radiol 48:548–553

121. Okubo H, Kitamura T, Ando H, Fukada H, Igusa Y, Kokubu S, Miyazaki A, Fujimura A, Shiina S, Watanabe S (2017) Gadoxetic acid-enhanced MR imaging predicts Simeprevir-induced hyperbilirubinemia during hepatitis C virus treatment: a pilot study. J Clin Pharmacol 57:369–375

122. Ulloa J, Stahl S, Liess C, Bright J, McDermott A, Woodhouse N, Halliday J, Parmar A, Healing G, Kenna JG, Holmes AP, Barjat H, Waterton JC, Hockings PD (2010) Effects of a single intravenous dose of Estradiol-17? D-Glucuronide on biliary excretion: assessment with Gadoxetate DCEMRI. Procedings of the international society of magnetic resonance in medicine eighteenth scientific meeting and exhibition, Stockholm, Sweden, 2593

123. Kato N, Yokawa T, Tamura A, Heshiki A, Ebert W, Weinmann HJ (2002) Gadolinium-ethoxybenzyl-diethylenetriamine-pentaacetic acid interaction with clinical drugs in rats. Investig Radiol 37:680–684

124. http://www.eortc.org/news/new-tristan-project-leverages-potential-of-imaging-techniques-in-drug-safety-assessment/

Erratum to: Regulatory Toxicological Studies: Identifying Drug-Induced Liver Injury Using Nonclinical Studies

Elizabeth Hausner and Imran Khan

Erratum to:
Chapter 19 in: Minjun Chen and Yvonne Will (eds.), *Drug-Induced*
Liver Toxicity, **Methods in Pharmacology and Toxicology,**
https://doi.org/10.1007/978-1-4939-7677-5_19

The original version of Chapter 19 was inadvertently published with incorrect author name sequence as "Imran Khan and Elizabeth Hausner" instead of "Elizabeth Hausner and Imran Khan". The chapter has been updated.

The updated online version of this chapter can be found at
https://doi.org/10.1007/978-1-4939-7677-5_19

Minjun Chen and Yvonne Will (eds.), *Drug-Induced Liver Toxicity*, Methods in Pharmacology and Toxicology,
https://doi.org/10.1007/978-1-4939-7677-5_31, © Springer Science+Business Media, LLC, part of Springer Nature 2018

INDEX

Minjun Chen and Yvonne Will (eds.), *Drug-Induced Liver Toxicity*, Methods in Pharmacology and Toxicology,
https://doi.org/10.1007/978-1-4939-7677-5, © Springer Science+Business Media, LLC, part of Springer Nature 2018

Printed in the United States
By Bookmasters